Veterinary Parasitology

Veterinary Parasitology

Editor:

Patricia Marques, Ph.D.

Delve Publishing

www.delvepublishing.com

Veterinary Parasitology

Editor: Patricia Marques, Ph.D.

708 3rd Avenue, 6th Floor
New York, NY 10017
United States of America
www.delvepublishing.com

ISBN: 978-1-68095-872-0

Library of Congress Control Number: 2016951623

Delve Publishing LLC publishes wide variety of books and eBooks. For more information about Delve Publishing and its products, visit our website at **www.delvepublishing.com**

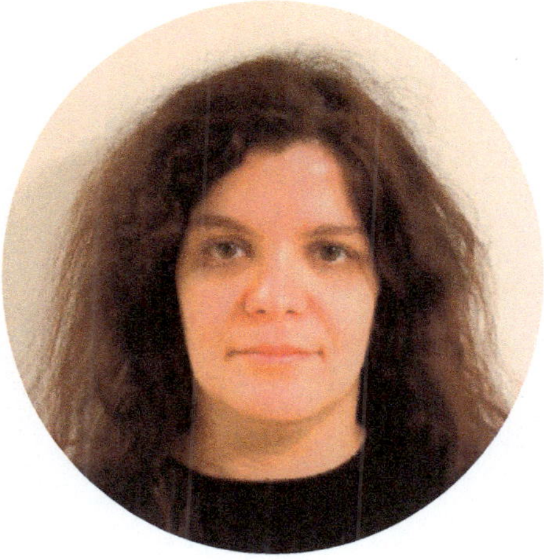

About the Editor

Patricia Marques, Ph.D.

Patricia obtained her PhD form University College Dublin in 2010. Her interests are on Microbiology and Parasitology. She is currently working as a Postdoc at University of Maryland Baltimore, USA on Chlamydia infections

Contents

Section IV: Parasites of Horses and Donkeys

Section V: Parasites of Pigs

List of Contributors

B. Y. Kaltungo
Veterinary Teaching Hospital, Ahmadu Bello University, Zaria, Nigeria

I. W. Musa
Department of Veterinary Medicine, Ahmadu Bello University, Zaria, Nigeria

Musa O Ng'ayo
Department of Biochemistry and Biotechnology, Kenyatta University, 00100 – Nairobi, Kenya
Molecular Biology and Biochemistry Department, International Centre of Insect Physiology and Ecolcgy, Duduville, Kasarani, 00100 – Nairobi, Kenya

Zablon K Njiru
Trypanosomiasis Research Centre, Kenya Agricultural Research Institute, Kikuyu, Kenya an
Western Australia Biomedical Research Institute, Division of Health Sciences, School of Veterinary and Biomedical Sciences, Murdoch University, Murdoch, WA 6150, Australia

Eucharia U Kenya
Department of Biochemistry and Biotechnology, Kenyatta University, 00100 – Nairobi, Kenya

Geoffrey M Muluvi
Department of Biochemistry and Biotechnology, Kenyatta University, 00100 – Nairobi, Kenya

Ellie O Osir
Molecular Biology and Biochemistry Department, International Centre of Insect Physiology and Ecology, Duduville, Kasarani, 00100 – Nairobi, Kenya

Daniel K Masiga
Department of Biochemistry and Biotechnology, Kenyatta University, 00100 – Nairobi, Kenya
Molecular Biology and Biochemistry Department, International Centre of Insect Physiology and Ecology, Duduville, Kasarani, 00100 – Nairobi, Kenya

Olubukola Deborah Adedipe
Department of Veterinary Public Health and Preventive Medicine, Faculty of Veterinary Medicine, University of Ibadan, Ibadan 200005, Nigeria

Emmanuel Chibuike Uwalaka
Department of Veterinary Microbiology and Parasitology, Faculty of Veterinary Medicine, University of Ibadan, Ibadan 200005, Nigeria

Victor Oluwatoyin Akinseye
Department of Veterinary Public Health and Preventive Medicine, Faculty of Veterinary Medicine, University of Ibadan, Ibadan 200005, Nigeria

Oyeduntan Adejoju Adediran
Department of Veterinary Microbiology and Parasitology, Faculty of Veterinary Medicine, University of Ibadan, Ibadan 200005, Nigeria

Simeon Idowu Babalola Cadmus
Department of Veterinary Public Health and Preventive Medicine, Faculty of Veterinary Medicine, University of Ibadan, Ibadan 200005, Nigeria

Lin Ai
State Key Laboratory of Veterinary Etiological Biology, Key Laboratory of Veterinary Parasitology of Gansu Province, Lanzhou Veterinary Research Institute, CAAS, Lanzhou, Gansu Province 730046, P R China
National Institute of Parasitic Diseases, Chinese Center for Disease Control and Prevention, Shanghai 200025, P R China
College of Veterinary Medicine, South China Agricultural University, Guangzhou, Guangdong Province 510642, P R China

Mu-Xin Chen
State Key Laboratory of Veterinary Etiological Biology, Key Laboratory of Veterinary Parasitology of Gansu Province, Lanzhou Veterinary Research Institute, CAAS, Lanzhou, Gansu Province 730046, P R China
National Institute of Parasitic Diseases, Chinese Center for Disease Control and Prevention, Shanghai 200025, P R China

Samer Alasaad
Estación Biológica de Doñana, Consejo Superior de Investigaciones Científicas (CSIC), Avda. Américo Vespucio s/n 41092 Sevilla, Spain

Hany M Elsheikha
School of Veterinary Medicine and Science, University of Nottingham, Sutton Bonington Campus, Loughborough, LE12 5RD, UK

Juan Li
College of Veterinary Medicine, South China Agricultural University, Guangzhou, Guangdong Province 510642, P R China

Hai-Long Li
College of Veterinary Medicine, South China Agricultural University, Guangzhou, Guangdong Province 510642, P R China

Rui-Qing Lin
College of Veterinary Medicine, South China Agricultural University, Guangzhou, Guangdong Province 510642, P R China

Xing-Quan Zhu
State Key Laboratory of Veterinary Etiological Biology, Key Laboratory of Veterinary Parasitology of Gansu Province, Lanzhou Veterinary Research Institute, CAAS, Lanzhou, Gansu Province 730046, P R China
College of Animal Science and Technology, Yunnan Agricultural University, Kunming, Yunnan Province 650201, P R China
College of Animal Science and Veterinary Medicine, Heilongjiang Bayi Agricultural University, Daqing, Heilongjiang Province 163319, P R China.

Jia-Xu Chen
National Institute of Parasitic Diseases, Chinese Center for Disease Control and Prevention, Shanghai 200025, P R China

Edouard Vannier
Division of Geographic Medicine and Infectious Diseases, Tufts Medical Center, 800 Washington Street, Boston, MA 02111, USA

Peter J. Krause
Department of Epidemiology and Public Health, Yale School of Medicine, 60 College Street, Room 600, New Haven, CT 06520, USA

Nikolaos Tzanidakis
Veterinary Research Institute – Hellenic Agricultural Organization Demeter, 57001 Thermi, Thessaloniki, Greece

Smaragda Sotiraki
Veterinary Research Institute – Hellenic Agricultural Organization Demeter, 57001 Thermi, Thessaloniki, Greece

Edwin Claerebout
Laboratory for Parasitology, Faculty of Veterinary Medicine, Ghent University, Salisburylaan 133, 9820 Merelbeke, Belgium

Amimul Ehsan
Laboratory for Parasitology, Faculty of Veterinary Medicine, Ghent University, Salisburylaan 133, 9820 Merelbeke, Belgium

Nikolaos Voutzourakis
Veterinary Research Institute – Hellenic Agricultural Organization Demeter, 57001 Thermi, Thessaloniki, Greece

Despoina Kostopoulou
Veterinary Research Institute – Hellenic Agricultural Organization Demeter, 57001 Thermi, Thessaloniki, Greece

Casaert Stijn
Laboratory for Parasitology, Faculty of Veterinary Medicine, Ghent University, Salisburylaan 133, 9820 Merelbeke, Belgium

Jozef Vercruysse
Laboratory for Parasitology, Faculty of Veterinary Medicine, Ghent University, Salisburylaan 133, 9820 Merelbeke, Belgium

Thomas Geurden
Laboratory for Parasitology, Faculty of Veterinary Medicine, Ghent University, Salisburylaan 133, 9820 Merelbeke, Belgium

Ovutor Owhoeli
Department of Animal and Environmental Biology, University of Port Harcourt, P.M.B 5323, Choba, Port Harcourt, Rivers State 500001, Nigeria

Kingsley Elele
Department of Biology, Ignatius Ajuru University of Education, P.M.B 5047, Port Harcourt, Rivers State 500001, Nigeria

Lebari Barine Gboeloh
Department of Biology, Ignatius Ajuru University of Education, P.M.B 5047, Port Harcourt, Rivers State 500001, Nigeria

Eric R. Morgan
School of Veterinary Sciences, University of Bristol, Langford House, Langford, North Somerset BS40 5DU, UK

Johannes Charlier
Laboratory of Parasitology, Faculty of Veterinary Medicine, Ghent University, Merelbeke B-9820, Belgium

Guy Hendrickx
Avia-GIS, Zoersel 2980, Belgium

Annibale Biggeri
Cooperativa Epidemiologia e Prevenzione "Giulio Alfredo Maccacaro", Milan 20148, Italy;

Dolores Catalan
Cooperativa Epidemiologia e Prevenzione "Giulio Alfredo Maccacaro", Milan 20148, Italy;

Georg von Samson-Himmelstjerna
Institute for Parasitology and Tropical Veterinary Medicine, Freie Universität Berlin, Berlin 14195, Germany

Janina Demeler
Institute for Parasitology and Tropical Veterinary Medicine, Freie Universität Berlin, Berlin 14195, Germany

Elizabeth Müller
Laboklin, Bad Kissingen D-97668, Germany

Jan van Dijk
Institute of Infection and Global Health, University of Liverpool, Liverpool L69 3BX, UK

Fiona Kenyon
Moredun Research Institute, Edinburgh EH26 0PZ, Scotland, UK

Philip Skuce
Moredun Research Institute, Edinburgh EH26 0PZ, Scotland, UK

Johan Höglund
Department of Biomedicine and Vet Public Health, Swedish University of Agricultural Sciences, Uppsala 753 12, Sweden
Department of Parasitology (SWEPAR), Swedish University of Agricultural Sciences and National Veterinary Institute, SE-751 89 Uppsala, Sweden

Padraig O'Kiely
Animal & Grassland Research and Innovation Centre, Teagasc, Grange, Dunsany, Co. Meath, Ireland

Bonny van Ranst
UNIFORM-AGRI BV, Assen 9401, The Netherlands

Theo de Waal
School of Veterinary Medicine, University College Dublin, Dublin 4, Ireland

Laura Rinaldi
Department of Pathology and Animal Health, Faculty of Veterinary Medicine, University of Naples "Federico II", Naples 80137, Italy

Giuseppe Cringoli
Department of Pathology and Animal Health, Faculty of Veterinary Medicine, University of Naples "Federico II", Naples 80137, Italy

Hubertus Hertzberg
Institute of Parasitology, Vetsuisse Faculty, University of Zürich, Zürich 8057, Switzerland

Paul Torgerson
Section of Epidemiology, Vetsuisse Faculty, University of Zürich, Zürich 8057, Switzerland

Adrian Wolstenholme
Department of Infectious Diseases, University of Georgia College of Veterinary Medicine, Athens, GA 30602, USA

Beniamino T Cenci-Goga
Dipartimento di Medicina Veterinaria, Università degli Studi di Perugia, Via San Costanzo, 06121, Perugia, Italy

Antonio Ciampelli
Veterinary practitioner, Tuscany, Italy

Paola Sechi
Dipartimento di Medicina Veterinaria, Università degli Studi di Perugia, Via San Costanzo, 06121, Perugia, Italy

Fabrizia Veronesi
Dipartimento di Medicina Veterinaria, Università degli Studi di Perugia, Via San Costanzo, 06121, Perugia, Italy

Iolanda Moretta
Dipartimento di Medicina Veterinaria, Università degli Studi di Perugia, Via San Costanzo, 06121, Perugia, Italy

Valentina Cambiotti
Dipartimento di Medicina Veterinaria, Università degli Studi di Perugia, Via San Costanzo, 06121, Perugia, Italy

Peter N Thompson
Epidemiology Section, Department of Production Animal Studies, Faculty of Veterinary Science, University of Pretoria, Private Bag X04, Onderstepoort 0110, South Africa

Weizhe Zhang
Department of Parasitology, Harbin Medical University, Harbin, People's Republic of China

Xiaoli Zhang
Department of Parasitology, Harbin Medical University, Harbin, People's Republic of China

Rongjun Wang
College of Animal Science and Veterinary Medicine, Henan Agricultural University, Zhengzhou, People's Republic of China

Aiqin Liu
Department of Parasitology, Harbin Medical University, Harbin, People's Republic of China

Yujuan Shen
National Institute of Parasitic Diseases, Chinese Center for Disease Control and Prevention, Key Laboratory of Parasite and Vector Biology, Ministry of Health, WHO Collaborating Centre for Malaria, Schistosomiasis and Filariasis, Shanghai, People's Republic of China

Hong Ling
Department of Parasitology, Harbin Medical University, Harbin, People's Republic of China

Jianping Cao
National Institute of Parasitic Diseases, Chinese Center for Disease Control and Prevention, Key Laboratory of Parasite and Vector Biology, Ministry of Health, WHO Collaborating Centre for Malaria, Schistosomiasis and Filariasis, Shanghai, People's Republic of China

Fengkun Yang
Department of Parasitology, Harbin Medical University, Harbin, People's Republic of China

Xiaoyun Zhang
Department of Parasitology, Harbin Medical University, Harbin, People's Republic of China

Longxian Zhang
College of Animal Science and Veterinary Medicine, Henan Agricultural University, Zhengzhou, People's Republic of China

Atle VM Domke
Norwegian School of Veterinary Science, Sandnes, Norway

Christophe Chartier
National College of Veterinary Medicine, Food Science and Engineering-ONIRIS, Nantes, France

Bjørn Gjerde
Norwegian School of Veterinary Science, Oslo, Norway

Nils Leine
Norwegian Goat Health Service, Oslo, Norway

Synnøve Vatn
Norwegian Sheep Health Service, Animalia, Oslo, Norway.

Olav Østerås
Norwegian School of Veterinary Science, Oslo, Norway

Snorre Stuen
Norwegian School of Veterinary Science, Sandnes, Norway

F. Iqbal
Institute of Pure and Applied Biology, Zoology Division, Bahauddin Zakariya University Multan, Pakistan

M. Fatima
Institute of Pure and Applied Biology, Zoology Division, Bahauddin Zakariya University Multan, Pakistan

S. Shahnawaz
Institute of Pure and Applied Biology, Zoology Division, Bahauddin Zakariya University Multan, Pakistan

M. Naeem
Institute of Pure and Applied Biology, Zoology Division, Bahauddin Zakariya University Multan, Pakistan

R.S. Shaikh
Institute of Biotechnology, Bahauddin Zakariya University Multan, Pakistan

M. Ali
Institute of Biotechnology, Bahauddin Zakariya University Multan, Pakistan

A.S. Shaikh
Institute of Pure and Applied Biology, Zoology Division, Bahauddin Zakariya University Multan, Pakistan

M. Aktas
Department of Parasitology, Faculty of Veterinary Medicine, University of Firat 23119, Elazig, Turkey

Saleh Mohammed Jajere
Department of Veterinary Public Health and Preventive Medicine, Faculty of Veterinary Medicine, University of Maiduguri, PMB 1069, Maiduguri, Borno State, Nigeria

Jallailudeen Rabana Lawal
Department of Veterinary Medicine, Faculty of Veterinary Medicine, University of Maiduguri, PMB 1069, Maiduguri, Borno State, Nigeria

Amina Mohammed Bello
Department of Veterinary Medicine, Faculty of Veterinary Medicine, University of Maiduguri, PMB 1069, Maiduguri, Borno State, Nigeria

Yakaka Wakil
Department of Veterinary Medicine, Faculty of Veterinary Medicine, University of Maiduguri, PMB 1069, Maiduguri, Borno State, Nigeria

Usman Aliyu Turaki
Department of Animal Science, Faculty of Agriculture, Federal University Kashere, PMB 0182, Kashere, Gombe State, Nigeria

Ibrahim Waziri
Ministry of Animal Husbandry and Nomadic Affairs, GSADP Block, Off Bauchi Road, PMB 0010, Gombe, Gombe State, Nigeria

Maristela Peckle
Animal Parasitology Department, Veterinary Institute, Universidade Federal Rural do Rio de Janeiro, BR 465, Km 7, Seropédica, Rio de Janeiro 23897-000, Brazil

Marcus S. Pires
Animal Parasitology Department, Veterinary Institute, Universidade Federal Rural do Rio de Janeiro, BR 465, Km 7, Seropédica, Rio de Janeiro 23897-000, Brazil

Tiago M. dos Santos
Zootechny Department, Agricultural Science and Technology Institute, Universidade Federal de Mato Grosso, Rondonópolis, Brazil

Erica C. R. Roier
Animal Parasitology Department, Veterinary Institute, Universidade Federal Rural do Rio de Janeiro, BR 465, Km 7, Seropédica, Rio de Janeiro 23897-000, Brazil

Claudia B. da Silva
Animal Parasitology Department, Veterinary Institute, Universidade Federal Rural do Rio de Janeiro, BR 465, Km 7, Seropédica, Rio de Janeiro 23897-000, Brazil

Joice A. R. Vilela
Animal Parasitology Department, Veterinary Institute, Universidade Federal Rural do Rio de Janeiro, BR 465, Km 7, Seropédica, Rio de Janeiro 23897-000, Brazil

Huarrisson A. Santos
Epidemiology and Public Health Department, Veterinary Institute, Universidade Federal Rural do Rio de Janeiro, Seropédica, Brazil

Carlos L. Massard
Animal Parasitology Department, Veterinary Institute, Universidade Federal Rural do Rio de Janeiro, BR 465, Km 7, Seropédica, Rio de Janeiro 23897-000, Brazil

Ana Patrícia Lopes
Department of Veterinary Sciences, School of Agrarian and Veterinary Sciences, University of Trás-os-Montes e Alto Douro (UTAD), Vila Real, Portugal
Animal and Veterinary Research Centre, UTAD, Vila Real, Portugal.

Susana Sousa
Parasite Disease Group, Instituto de Biologia Molecular e Celular (IBMC), Universidade do Porto , Porto, Portugal

JP Dubey
Animal Parasitic Diseases Laboratory, Beltsville Agricultural Research Center, Agricultural Research Service, United States Department of Agriculture, Beltsville, MD, USA

Ana J Ribeiro
Veterinary Hospital, UTAD, Vila Real, Portugal

Ricardo Silvestre
Parasite Disease Group, Instituto de Biologia Molecular e Celular (IBMC), Universidade do Porto , Porto, Portugal

Mário Cotovio
Department of Veterinary Sciences, School of Agrarian and Veterinary Sciences, University of Trás-os-Montes e Alto Douro (UTAD), Vila Real, Portugal
Animal and Veterinary Research Centre, UTAD, Vila Real, Portugal.

Henk DFH Schallig
Department of Parasitology, Koninklijk Instituut voor de Tropen (KIT), Royal Tropical Institute, Amsterdam, The Netherlands

Luís Cardoso
Department of Veterinary Sciences, School of Agrarian and Veterinary Sciences, University of Trás-os-Montes e Alto Douro (UTAD), Vila Real, Portugal
Parasite Disease Group, Instituto de Biologia Molecular e Celular (IBMC), Universidade do Porto , Porto, Portugal

Anabela Cordeiro-da-Silva
Parasite Disease Group, Instituto de Biologia Molecular e Celular (IBMC), Universidade do Porto , Porto, Portugal
Departamento de Ciências Biológicas, Faculdade de Farmácia, UP, Porto, Portugal

Qiang Miao
College of Animal Science and Technology, Yunnan Agricultural University, Yunnan Province 650201, Kunming, PR China

Xi Wang
College of Animal Science and Technology, Yunnan Agricultural University, Yunnan Province 650201, Kunming, PR China

Li-Na She
Yunnan Academy of Scientific and Technical Information, Yunnan Province 650091, Kunming, PR China

Ya-Ting Fan
College of Animal Science and Technology, Yunnan Agricultural University, Yunnan Province 650201, Kunming, PR China

Fei-Zhou Yuan
College of Animal Science and Technology, Yunnan Agricultural University, Yunnan Province 650201, Kunming, PR China

Jian-Fa Yang
College of Animal Science and Technology, Yunnan Agricultural University, Yunnan Province 650201, Kunming, PR China

Feng-Cai Zou
College of Animal Science and Technology, Yunnan Agricultural University, Yunnan Province 650201, Kunming, PR China
School of Life Sciences, Yunnan University, Yunnan Province 650091, Kunming, PR China.

I. Francisco
Animal Pathology Department, Epidemiology, Zoonoses and Parasitic Diseases, Veterinary Faculty, University of Santiago de Compostela, 27002-Lugo, Spain

M. Arias
Animal Pathology Department, Epidemiology, Zoonoses and Parasitic Diseases, Veterinary Faculty, University of Santiago de Compostela, 27002-Lugo, Spain

F. J. Cortiñas
Animal Pathology Department, Epidemiology, Zoonoses and Parasitic Diseases, Veterinary Faculty, University of Santiago de Compostela, 27002-Lugo, Spain

R. Francisco
Animal Pathology Department, Epidemiology, Zoonoses and Parasitic Diseases, Veterinary Faculty, University of Santiago de Compostela, 27002-Lugo, Spain

E. Mochales
Animal Pathology Department, Epidemiology, Zoonoses and Parasitic Diseases, Veterinary Faculty, University of Santiago de Compostela, 27002-Lugo, Spain

V. Dacal
Animal Pathology Department, Epidemiology, Zoonoses and Parasitic Diseases, Veterinary Faculty, University of Santiago de Compostela, 27002-Lugo, Spain

J. L. Suárez
Animal Pathology Department, Epidemiology, Zoonoses and Parasitic Diseases, Veterinary Faculty, University of Santiago de Compostela, 27002-Lugo, Spain

J. Uriarte
Centro de Investigación y Tecnología Agroalimentaria de Aragón (CITA), Animal Health Division, Avda. Montaña, 930 50059 Zaragoza, Spain

P. Morrondo
Animal Pathology Department, Epidemiology, Zoonoses and Parasitic Diseases, Veterinary Faculty, University of Santiago de Compostela, 27002-Lugo, Spain

R. Sánchez-Andrade
Animal Pathology Department, Epidemiology, Zoonoses and Parasitic Diseases, Veterinary Faculty, University of Santiago de Compostela, 27002-Lugo, Spain

P. Díez-Baños
Animal Pathology Department, Epidemiology, Zoonoses and Parasitic Diseases, Veterinary Faculty, University of Santiago de Compostela, 27002-Lugo, Spain

A. Paz-Silva
Animal Pathology Department, Epidemiology, Zoonoses and Parasitic Diseases, Veterinary Faculty, University of Santiago de Compostela, 27002-Lugo, Spain

Eva Osterman Lind
Department of Parasitology (SWEPAR), Swedish University of Agricultural Sciences and National Veterinary Institute, SE-751 89 Uppsala, Sweden

Erik Rautalinko
Department of Psychology, Uppsala University, SE-751 42 Uppsala, Sweden

Arvid Uggla
Department of Parasitology (SWEPAR), Swedish University of Agricultural Sciences and National Veterinary Institute, SE-751 89 Uppsala, Sweden

Peter J Waller
Department of Parasitology (SWEPAR), Swedish University of Agricultural Sciences and National Veterinary Institute, SE-751 89 Uppsala, Sweden

David A Morrison
Department of Parasitology (SWEPAR), Swedish University of Agricultural Sciences and National Veterinary Institute, SE-751 89 Uppsala, Sweden

Jing Yang
Department of Parasitology, School of Basic Medical Sciences, Capital Medical University, Beijing, China

Wei Pan
Department of Parasitology, School of Basic Medical Sciences, Capital Medical University, Beijing, China

Ximeng Sun
Department of Parasitology, School of Basic Medical Sciences, Capital Medical University, Beijing, China

Xi Zhao
Department of Parasitology, School of Basic Medical Sciences, Capital Medical University, Beijing, China

Gu Yuan
Department of Parasitology, School of Basic Medical Sciences, Capital Medical University, Beijing, China

Qing Sun
Department of Parasitology, School of Basic Medical Sciences, Capital Medical University, Beijing, China

Jingjing Huang
Department of Parasitology, School of Basic Medical Sciences, Capital Medical University, Beijing, China

Xinping Zhu
Department of Parasitology, School of Basic Medical Sciences, Capital Medical University, Beijing, China

Martha Betson
Department of Production and Population Health, Royal Veterinary College, Hatfield, Hertfordshire, United Kingdom
Department of Parasitology, Pembroke Place, Liverpool School of Tropical Medicine, United Kingdom

Peter Nejsum
Department of Veterinary Disease Biology, Faculty of Health and Medical Sciences, University of Copenhagen, Denmark

Richard P. Bendall
Department of Clinical Microbiology, Royal Cornwall Hospital, Truro

Rinki M. Deb
Department of Parasitology, Pembroke Place, Liverpool School of Tropical Medicine, United Kingdom

J. Russell Stothard
Department of Parasitology, Pembroke Place, Liverpool School of Tropical Medicine, United Kingdom

Ernatus Martin Mkupasi
Department of Veterinary Disease Biology, Faculty of Health and Medical Sciences, University of Copenhagen, Frederiksberg, Denmark

Chummy Sikalizyo Sikasunge
Department of Para-clinical Studies, School of Veterinary Medicine, University of Zambia, Lusaka, Zambia

Helena Aminiel Ngowi
Department of Veterinary Medicine and Public Health, Sokoine University of Agriculture, Morogoro, Tanzania

Maria Vang Johansen
Department of Veterinary Disease Biology, Faculty of Health and Medical Sciences, University of Copenhagen, Frederiksberg, Denmark

Zewdneh Tomass
Department of Biology, College of Natural and Computational Sciences, Mekelle University, Ethiopia (Africa)

Ekwal Imam
Department of Biology, College of Natural and Computational Sciences, Mekelle University, Ethiopia (Africa)

Tsegabirhan Kifleyohannes
College of Veterinary Medicine, Mekelle University, Ethiopia (Africa); #Association with Department of Wildlife Sciences, AMU, Aligarh, India.

Yohannes Tekle
College of Veterinary Medicine, Mekelle University, Ethiopia (Africa); #Association with Department of Wildlife Sciences, AMU, Aligarh, India.

Kidane Weldu
College of Veterinary Medicine, Mekelle University, Ethiopia (Africa); #Association with Department of Wildlife Sciences, AMU, Aligarh, India.

Papa Kofi Amissah-Reynolds
Department of Science Education, University of Education, Winneba, Mampong, Ashanti, Ghana

Isaac Monney
Department of Environmental Health and Sanitation Education, University of Education, Winneba, Mampong, Ashanti, Ghana

Lucy Mawusi Adowah
Department of Science Education, University of Education, Winneba, Mampong, Ashanti, Ghana

Samuel Opoku Agyemang
Department of Science Education, University of Education, Winneba, Mampong, Ashanti, Ghana

Joshua Kamani
Parasitology Division, National Veterinary Research Institute, Vom, Nigeria

Gad Baneth
Koret School of Veterinary Medicine, The Hebrew University of Jerusalem, Rehovot, Israel

Kosta Y. Mumcuoglu
Department of Microbiology and Molecular Genetics, The Kuvin Center for the Study of Infectious and Tropical Diseases, Hebrew University–Hadassah Medical School, Jerusalem, Israel

Ndadilnasiya E. Waziri
Central Diagnostic Division, National Veterinary Research Institute, Vom, Nigeria

Osnat Eyal
Koret School of Veterinary Medicine, The Hebrew University of Jerusalem, Rehovot, Israel

Yifat Guthmann
Koret School of Veterinary Medicine, The Hebrew University of Jerusalem, Rehovot, Israel

Shimon Harrus
Koret School of Veterinary Medicine, The Hebrew University of Jerusalem, Rehovot, Israel

Guadalupe Miró
Department of Animal Health, Veterinary Faculty, Universidad Complutense de Madrid, Madrid, Spain

Ana Montoya
Department of Animal Health, Veterinary Faculty, Universidad Complutense de Madrid, Madrid, Spain

Xavier Roura
Hospital Clínic Veterinari, Universitat Autònoma de Barcelona, Barcelona, Spain

Rosa Gálvez
Department of Animal Health, Veterinary Faculty, Universidad Complutense de Madrid, Madrid, Spain

Angel Sainz
Department of Animal Medicine and Surgery, Veterinary Faculty, Universidad Complutense de Madrid, Madrid, Spain.

Michele Podaliri Vulpiani
Settore Sanità Pubblica Veterinaria, Istituto "G. Caporale", Via Campo Boario, 64100 Teramo, Italy

Luigi Iannetti
Settore Sanità Pubblica Veterinaria, Istituto "G. Caporale", Via Campo Boario, 64100 Teramo, Italy

Daniela Paganico
Settore Sanità Pubblica Veterinaria, Istituto "G. Caporale", Via Campo Boario, 64100 Teramo, Italy

Filomena Iannino
Settore Sanità Pubblica Veterinaria, Istituto "G. Caporale", Via Campo Boario, 64100 Teramo, Italy

Nicola Ferri
Settore Sanità Pubblica Veterinaria, Istituto "G. Caporale", Via Campo Boario, 64100 Teramo, Italy

Domenico Otranto
Dipartimento di Sanità Pubblica e Zootecnia, Facoltà di Medicina Veterinaria, Università degli Studi di Bari, 70010 Valenzano, Bari, Italy

Filipe Dantas-Torres
Dipartimento di Sanità Pubblica e Zootecnia, Facoltà di Medicina Veterinaria, Università degli Studi di Bari, 70010 Valenzano, Bari, Italy

Peter J Irwin
Australasian Centre for Companion Animal Research, School of Veterinary and Biomedical Sciences, Murdoch University, Murdoch 6150, WA, Australia

Barakat Shehata Abd-Elmaleck
Zoology Department, Faculty of Science, Assiut University, Assiut, 71516, Egypt

Gamal Hassan Abed
Zoology Department, Faculty of Science, Assiut University, Assiut, 71516, Egypt

Ahmed Mohammad Mandour
Parasitology Department, Faculty of Medicine, Assiut University, Assiut, 71516, Egypt

Satya Kalluri
Raytheon Company, Upper Marlboro, Maryland, United States of America

Peter Gilruth
Raytheon Company, Upper Marlboro, Maryland, United States of America

David Rogers
TALA Research Group, Professor of Ecology, Department of Zoology, Oxford University, United Kingdom

Martha Szczur
Deputy Associate Director, National Library of Medicine, Specialized Information Services, Bethesda, Maryland, United States of America.

Hatem A Shalaby
Department of Parasitology and Animal Diseases, National Research Center, Giza, Egypt

Tarek K Farag
Department of Parasitology and Animal Diseases, National Research Center, Giza, Egypt

Amy B. Pedersen
Department of Biology, University of Virginia, Charlottesville, VA 22904, USA
Centre for Immunity, Infection and Evolution, School of Biological Sciences, University of Edinburgh, Edinburgh EH9 3JT, UK

Janis Antonovics
Department of Biology, University of Virginia, Charlottesville, VA 22904, USA

Luis Quihui-Cota
Departamento de Nutrición Pública y Salud, Coordinación de Nutrición, Centro de Investigación en Alimentación y Desarrollo, A.C. Carretera a La Victoria Km 0.6, 83304 Hermosillo, SON, Mexico

Rocio León-Trujillo
Departamento de Nutrición Pública y Salud, Coordinación de Nutrición, Centro de Investigación en Alimentación y Desarrollo, A.C. Carretera a La Victoria Km 0.6, 83304 Hermosillo, SON, Mexico

Humberto Astiazarán-García
Departamento de Nutrición y Metabolismo, Coordinación de Nutrición, Centro de Investigación en Alimentación y Desarrollo, A.C. Carretera a La Victoria Km 0.6, 83304 Hermosillo, SON, Mexico

Julián Esparza-Romero
Departamento de Nutrición Pública y Salud, Coordinación de Nutrición, Centro de Investigación en Alimentación y Desarrollo, A.C. Carretera a La Victoria Km 0.6, 83304 Hermosillo, SON, Mexico

María del Refugio Robles
Departamento de Ciencias de los Alimentos, Centro de Investigación en Alimentación y Desarrollo, A.C. Carretera a La Victoria Km 0.6, 83304 Hermosillo, SON, Mexico

Ramón E. Robles-Zepeda
Departamento de Ciencias Químico Biológicas, Universidad de Sonora, Bulevar Luis Encinas y Rosales s/n, 83000 Hermosillo, SON, Mexico

Rafael Canett
Departamento de Investigación y Posgrado en Alimentos, Universidad de Sonora, Bulevar Luis Encinas y Rosales s/n, 83000 Hermosillo, SON, Mexico

Jesús Sánchez-Escalante
Herbario USON, Departamento de Investigaciones Científicas y Tecnológica, Universidad de Sonora, Niños Héroes entre Rosales y José María Pino Suárez, Edificio 1A (Museo), Colonia Centro, 83000 Hermosillo, SON, Mexico

Prachi Bhargava
Amity Institute of Biotechnology, Amity University Uttar Pradesh, Sector 125, Noida 201303, India

Rajni Singh
Amity Institute of Microbial Biotechnology, Amity University Uttar Pradesh, Sector 125, Noida 201303, India

Marie Varloud
Ceva Santé Animale S. A, 10 Avenue de la Ballastière, 33500 Libourne, France

Elizabeth Hodgkins
Ceva Animal Health LLC, 8735 Rosehill Road, Suite 300, Lenexa, KS 66215, USA

Luís Cardoso
Department of Veterinary Sciences, School of Agrarian and Veterinary Sciences, University of Trás-os-Montes e Alto Douro (UTAD)

Concepta McManus
Vice-Coordinator INCT-Pecuaria, Universidade Federal do Rio Grande do Sul, Departamento de Zootecnia, Av. Bento Gonçalves, CEP 91540-000 Porto Alegre, Rio Grande do Sul, Brazil
Universidade de Brasília, Campus Darcy Ribeiro, 70910-900 Asa Norte, Brasilia, Distrito Federal, Brazil

Tiago do Prado Paim
INCT – Pecuaria, Universidade Federal de Minas Gerais, 30161-970 Belo Horizonte, Brazil
Instituto Federal de Educação, Ciência e Tecnologia Goiano – Campus Iporá, Avenida Oeste s/n, saída para Piranhas, CEP 76.200-000 Iporá, Goiás, Brazil

Cristiano Barros de Melo
Universidade de Brasília, Campus Darcy Ribeiro, 70910-900 Asa Norte, Brasilia, Distrito Federal, Brazil
INCT – Pecuaria, Universidade Federal de Minas Gerais, 30161-970 Belo Horizonte, Brazil

Bruno S. A. F. Brasil
EMBRAPA Agroenergia, Final W3 Norte, 70770-901 Brasília, Brazil

Samuel R. Paiva
Secretaria de Relações Internacionais, Embrapa, Final W5 Norte, 70770-901 Brasília, Brazil
EMBRAPA Recursos Genéticos e Biotecnologia, Final W5 Norte, 70770-901 Brasília, Brazil

Hany Elsheikha
School of Veterinary Medicine and Science, University of Nottingham, Sutton Bonington Campus, Loughborough, LE12 5RD, UK

Cyril Rauch
School of Veterinary Medicine and Science, University of Nottingham, Sutton Bonington Campus, Loughborough, LE12 5RD, UK

Radovan Václav
Institute of Zoology, Slovak Academy of Sciences, Dúbravská Cesta 9, 845 06 Bratislava, Slovakia

Jana Blažeková
Institute of Zoology, Slovak Academy of Sciences, Dúbravská Cesta 9, 845 06 Bratislava, Slovakia

Natasha M. Girgis
Department of Microbiology, New York University, New York, New York, United States of America

Uma Mahesh Gundra
Department of Microbiology, New York University, New York, New York, United States of America

P'ng Loke
Department of Microbiology, New York University, New York, New York, United States of America

Emmanuelle Moreau
UMR ENVN/INRA 1300 Bioagression, Épidémiologie et Analyse de Risques, Atlanpole-La Chantrerie, Route de Gachet, BP40706, 44307 Nantes, France

Alain Chauvin
UMR ENVN/INRA 1300 Bioagression, Épidémiologie et Analyse de Risques, Atlanpole-La Chantrerie, Route de Gachet, BP40706, 44307 Nantes, France

Edecio Cunha-Neto
Heart Institute (Incor), University of São Paulo School of Medicine, 05403-000 São Paulo, SP, Brazil

Christophe Chevillard
INSERM and Université Aix-Marseille, Marseille, France

Mauricio Martins Rodrigues
Escola Paulista de Medicina, Universidade Federal de São Paulo, 04044-010 São Paulo, SP, Brazil

Marcelo T. Bozza
Departamento de Imunologia, Instituto de Microbiologia, Universidade Federal do Rio de Janeiro, 21941-902 Rio de Janeiro, RJ, Brazil

Marcela F. Lopes
Instituto de Biofísica Carlos Chagas Filho, Universidade Federal do Rio de Janeiro, 21941-902 Rio de Janeiro, RJ, Brazil

Dario S. Zamboni
Departamento de Biologia Celular Molecular e Bioagentes Patogenicos, Faculdade de Medicina de Ribeirão Preto, Universidade de São Paulo, 14049-900 Ribeirão Preto, SP, Brazil

Hugo D. Lujan
Laboratorio de Bioquímica y Biología Molecular, Facultad de Medicina, Universidad Católica de Córdoba, X5004ASK Cordoba, Argentina

Mauricio M. Rodrigues
CINTERGEN, Escola Paulista de Medicina, UNIFESP, 04044-010 São Paulo, SP, Brazil

Ali Ouaissi
INSERM, IRD UR008 "Pathogénie des Trypanosomatidés", Centre IRD de Montpellier, 911 Avenue Agropolis, BP 64501, Montpellier 34394, France

Henryka Dlugonska
Department of Immunoparasitology, Institute of Microbiology and Immunology, University of Lodz, 90-237 Lodz, Poland

Eric Dumonteil
Laboratorio de Parasitología, Centro de Investigaciones Regionales "Dr. Hideyo Noguchi", Universidad Autónoma de Yucatán, Mérida, Yucatán 97000, Mexico

Preface

Veterinary parasitology is the study of animal parasites, especially relationships between parasites and animal hosts. Parasites of domestic animals, (livestock and pet animals), as well as wildlife animals are considered. Veterinary parasitologists study the genesis and development of parasites in animal hosts, as well as the taxonomy and systematics of parasites, including the morphology, life cycles, and living needs of parasites in the environment and in animal hosts. Using a variety of research methods, they diagnose, treat, and prevent animal parasites. Data obtained from parasitological research in animals helps in veterinary practice and improves animal breeding. The major goal of veterinary parasitology is to protect animals and improve their health, but because a number of animal parasites are transmitted to humans, veterinary parasitology is also important for public health. Veterinary parasitology comprises three big areas of study which are helminthology, protozoology and entomology. Helminthology is the study of parasitic worms which includes nematodes, cestodes and trematodes. Protozoology is the study of protozoan parasites. Entomology is the study of arthropods that can be ectoparasites and/or vectors of infection.

This book provides some examples of veterinary parasites in farm animals (Section 1), parasites of cattle (Section 2), parasites of sheep and goats (Section 3), parasites of horses and donkeys (Section 4) and parasites of pigs (Section 5). Section 6 provides examples of dogs and cats parasites and Section 7 of ungulates. The next Sections cover different aspects of parasitology, like entomology (Section 8), Antiparasitics, Antiprotozoals and Ectoparasiticides (Section 9), host resistance to parasitic infections (Section 10), Immunity to parasitic infections (Section 11), Protozoal infections (Section 12) and Vaccines (Section 13). These are only a few examples of the immense world of veterinary parasitology. It is concerned with those aspects of helminthology, protozoology and entomology which are of interest to animal health investigators, veterinary practitioners and others with a special interest in parasitology. Articles of the highest quality dealing with all aspects of disease prevention, pathology, treatment, epidemiology, and control of parasites in all domesticated animals.

Editor
Patricia Marques, Ph.D.

INTRODUCTION

Parasitology is the scientific study of parasites. Some parasitology studies evaluate the relationship between parasitic organisms and their hosts. Other studies look for and describe different types of parasites. Parasitology has applications in human and veterinary medicine. The study of parasites draws on other scientific disciplines, such as microbiology, organic chemistry, and cytology.

Though the name parasite has negative connotations, not all parasites adversely affect their hosts. In some cases, parasitology demonstrates how the relationship of a parasite to its host is mutually beneficial, called mutualism. The parasite and the host may gain protection from each other's presence or provide each other with food. When parasite and host cannot exist apart, their relationship is called symbiotic. The two organisms are equally and mutually dependent upon each other.

Parasitology, when used in applications in human and veterinary medicines, tends to examine the relationship between parasites that invade and cause damage to the animal or human body. For example, insects that are vectors for disease are studied to see to what degree they pass those diseases on to humans or animals. The mosquito is a parasite that affects not only human populations, but also birds and horses. Some mosquitoes carry West Nile Virus, which in severe cases can result in encephalitis and sometimes death. In order to improve medicine's understanding of West Nile Virus, parasitologists must understand the mosquito.

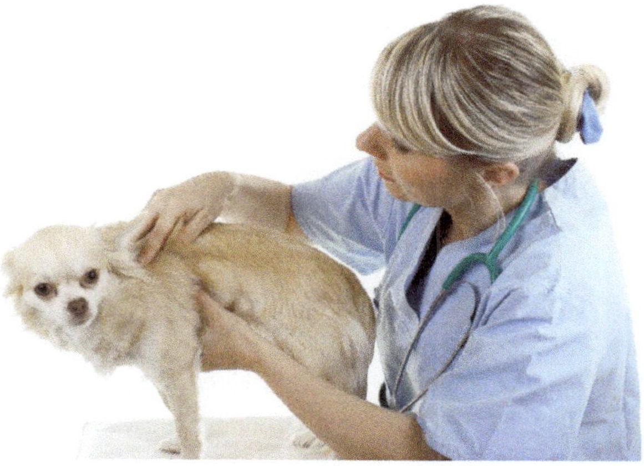

From past studies, parasitologists determined that not all mosquitoes are equally dangerous, and not all carry West Nile Virus. Only female mosquitoes bite, while male mosquitoes drink nectar. More recent parasitology studies have identified that mosquitoes that carry West Nile Virus have a tendency to survive and be present through winter in moderate climates. So from this, we know that the presence of a mosquito in December in the US means more risk to us of contracting West Nile Virus.

In veterinary medicine, parasitologists work specifically to eliminate flea infestation on cats and dogs. Recent technology has evolved to allow dogs or cats to either take a pill a month, or have a spot treatment on their back that either retards fleas from maturing, thus preventing bites, or directly kills fleas that bite. Some fleas can be vectors for diseases. Fleas on rats caused the Black Plague of the Middle Ages. Improved flea protection can minimize health risks and reduce flea infestation, providing relief to both pets and their owners.

Parasitology also studies the one-celled organisms that can make us ill, which can be either bacteria or fungi. Such studies depend on the ability to identify and describe cells, cytology, or microbiology at the microscopic level. Description of these cells and their presence has lead to better detection of certain bacterial and parasitic infections.

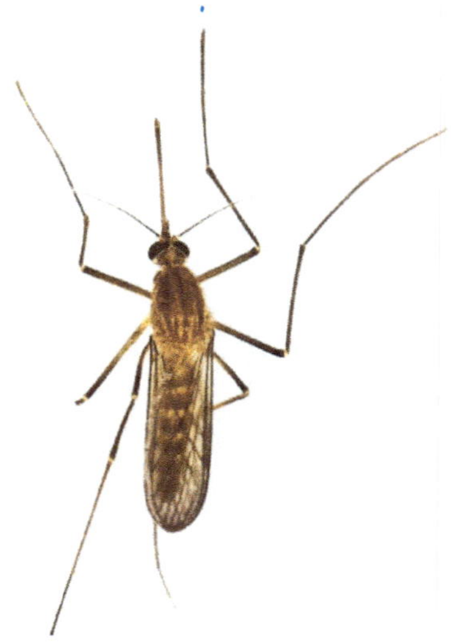

Parasitology must concentrate not only on identifying and describing harmful cells, but also on evolving methods for destroying them. From this information, medications are developed to treat specific infections. Understanding parasites led to the understanding of the role of antibiotics in treating bacterial infections, arguably one of the most significant medical developments in history.

What does a Parasitologist do?

A parasitologist is a scientist that studies parasites, and the relationship between the parasites and their hosts. While parasites can be found in any form of animal or plant life, parasitology is usually confined to the study of protozoan and metazoan parasites. A parasitologist also examines the way in which parasites move from host to host, and the effects that the parasites have upon on these hosts. He or she also looks for ways to fight parasites and prevent them from spreading disease. Because of the nature of living organisms, there is some overlap between the field of parasitology and other scientific disciplines, such as immunology, cell biology, microbiology, and molecular biology.

Given the complex nature of the field, parasitologists work in many different capacities. For example, a medical parasitologist studies parasites that are found in humans. These include common parasites such as lice, fleas, and ticks, as well as more invasive organisms, such as pinworms, which are usually found in the colon, and tapeworms, which result from eating undercooked beef. Medical parasitologists are also concerned with more serious parasitic infections. Ticks may infect humans with Lyme disease, and mosquitoes are not only responsible for the spread of malaria, but viral diseases such as yellow fever and encephalitis, as well.

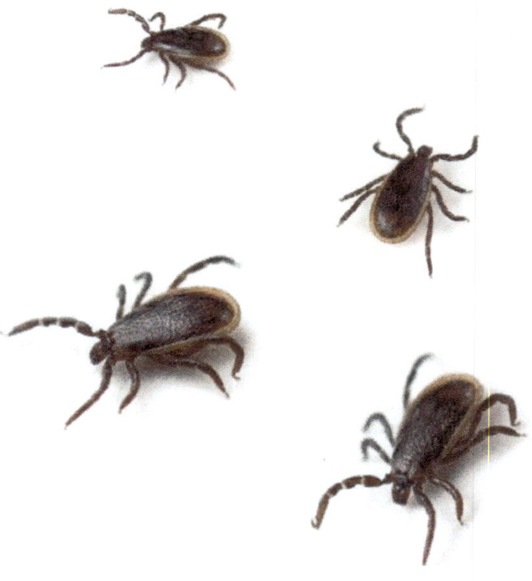

A medical parasitology's attempts to treat numerous conditions by performing research in several fields. Epidemiology, immunology, chemotherapy, and pathology are all areas of interest to the medical parasitology's. Through research, vaccines against certain types of parasites have been developed, and the spread of many parasitic diseases has been considerably slowed.

Parasitologists may also work in the veterinary field, studying parasites that attack animals. These include farm animals that are raised for food or work, as well as domesticated animals that are kept as pets. In addition, a veterinary parasitology's may also study the parasites that are found in wildlife.

Common veterinary parasites include fleas, ticks, mites, mange, and various worms. Heartworms are probably the best known parasites among pet owners, as heartworms can infect both dogs and cats. Veterinary parasitologists are often employed by pharmaceutical companies where they research therapies and vaccines that may eradicate parasites in animals. Since some parasites may be passed from animal to human, veterinary parasitologists can also play a role in public health issues.

Some parasitologists also work in the field of agriculture. They help farmers protect crops and plants from destructive parasites. An agricultural parasitolgoist may also research the possible use of parasites as a means of fighting insects that would also attack crops.

For a career as a parasitology's, an undergraduate degree in biology or chemistry is usually required, though many parasitologists have a Bachelor of Science in microbiology. A master's degree or PhD, however, typically is necessary for senior research positions in parasitology. If a career in medical parasitology is desired, a medical degree may also be required.

What are the Best Tips for Parasite Control?

A person can practice parasite control by preventing the ingestion and the spread of microbes. This is accomplished through simple measures such as washing hands frequently, particularly before eating; cooking meat until it is fully done; and using bleach water to clean surfaces in the kitchen and bathroom. Parasite control also involves never using toilet paper to serve as a facial tissue, covering one's mouth when sneezing or coughing, adding herbs that are natural antimicrobials to the diet and following an herbal parasite management program on a regular basis. People who have a compromised immune system are also urged to sterilize dairy products, including those that have already been pasteurized.

When hand-washing is not possible for any reason, a hand sanitizer can temporarily substitute for soap and water. This does not mean, however, that hand sanitizers should completely take the place of washing the hands. All meats, especially pork, should be thoroughly cooked, because rare and medium rare meats can and often do carry parasites that can cause serious health problems that can even be fatal. Wiping down kitchen counter surfaces while cooking, especially when cooking meats, is very valuable for parasite control. The same can be said about using a little bleach if dishes are washed by hand and about using bleach water to clean bathroom fixtures.

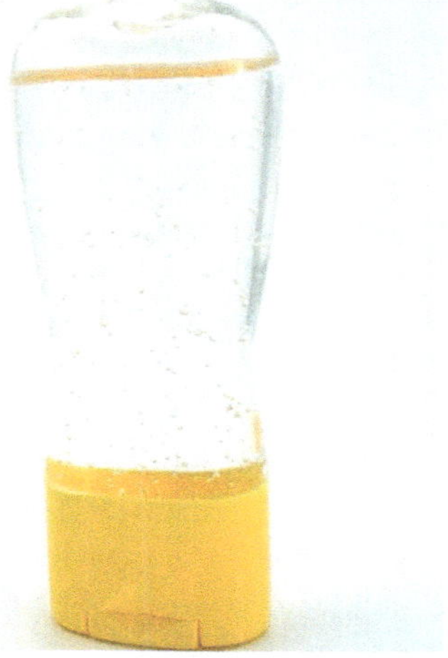

Dairy products, particularly those that are purchased in chain grocery stores, can put a person at risk for contracting parasites. Cancer patients, people who have the human immunodeficiency virus (HIV) and others who have weakened immunity might want to consider boiling or cooking dairy products. Milk could be boiled, all cheeses could be cooked, and yogurt could be homemade from boiled or sterilized milk. Cheese such as cottage cheese, which cannot be thoroughly sterilized even when cooked, because of the curds, would be avoided altogether.

Raw garlic is one of many natural antimicrobials used in parasite control. Cooked garlic, however, does not help to control parasites like the raw herb does. Garlic can be consumed with foods such as spaghetti, eaten in dip for chips or chewed alone once or twice per week as a kind of a maintenance program. A parasite cleanse and management program also can be achieved by taking other herbs known to be invaluable in parasite control. Freshly ground cloves and black walnut tincture are among the natural substances that, unlike chemical antibiotics, can be taken on a regular basis for parasite control.

What is Parasite Cleaning?

Parasite cleaning is the process of eliminating parasites from the body. It can be done with conventional medicines as well as with natural remedies. Treatments and parasite cleanses are designed to kill off and eliminate the parasites at the adult and developing stages. An effective treatment, or parasite cleanse will also focus on destroying the parasitic eggs to hasten the cleaning process.

During the parasite cleaning process, the parasites are either poisoned or forced to leave the body via natural cleansing methods. In general, they leave the body through the stool, but they can also leave through skin outbreaks. Crawling sensations, fatigue, and digestive problems are common signs that the parasites are leaving the body.

In alternative medicine, parasite cleaning is done with natural remedies and parasite cleanses. These cleanses are designed to purge all parasites and unhealthy bacteria and toxins from the body in order to prevent a future infestation. A colon cleanse is recommended prior to a parasite cleanse, as that opens the doorway for the parasites to leave the body more efficiently. It is also recommended to begin the parasite cleanse around the full moon. This is the time of the month when the parasites tend to be most active, and thus the efforts of the cleanse may be more effective.

The three main herbs that are used in alternative therapy include black walnut hulls, wormwood, and cloves. The black walnut hulls and wormwood are effective for killing off the parasites at all stages, and the cloves help to kill the parasitic eggs before they hatch. These herbs are available separately as well as in parasite cleansing kits for convenience. This type of parasite cleaning can take anywhere from one to eight weeks until all the parasites have left the body. In some cases, depending on the type of parasite, it can take even longer.

Conventional medicine offers specific drugs for different types of parasites. Some of the parasitic drugs are quite strong, and therefore, they should only be taken under the care of a physician. Depending on what type of parasites are present in the body, the treatment can be administered in a single dose, or it can be taken for several weeks until the parasites are gone. These treatments are effective when taken as prescribed and taken in conjunction with a healthy diet.

A healthy diet to assist parasite cleaning consists of plenty of antiparasitic foods, which include spicy foods such as hot peppers, garlic, and cayenne pepper. Plenty of fluids are also essential in helping to flush the parasites from the body. In addition, there are certain foods that should be avoided during parasite cleaning as they can potentially feed the parasites. Any type of sugar, including refined sugar and sugar substitutes, should be avoided. Breads and pastas, along with processed foods and unhealthy saturated fats, can also hinder the parasite cleaning process.

Best Parasite Diet?

There are several parasite diet options that can be easily added to the diet to get rid of parasites and well as prevent infestations. Most medical and holistic doctors recommend eating a well-balanced diet of lean proteins, though some suggest vegetarian diets, whole grains, and fresh fruits and vegetables. Some foods, such as refined sugar, should be avoided or consumed only rarely to ensure the body is inhospitable to most parasite species. Many medical professionals also advise specific types of cooking techniques that allow the whole foods to retain as much of their original nutrients as possible. A natural, healthy diet, along with regular exercise, is considered to be the most effective parasite program available.

A parasite diet often features meat cooked according to specific instructions. In an anti-parasite diet, lean meats such as chicken, pork, and some cuts of beef should be cooked thoroughly to avoid any potential contamination from uncooked meat. People who are concerned about or prone to parasite infestation should avoid eating red meat cooked either medium or rare. Fish and shellfish should also be completely cooked to avoid any possible parasite from entering the body. For the person who is already infected, choosing to eat meat and fish prepared in this manner helps create a less friendly environment for the parasites, and encourages the body to expel them naturally.

Another element of an effective parasite treatment diet is consuming whole grains, such as oats, bran, and barley. Many whole foods advocates also suggest adding some of the ancient grains to the person's diet, including kamet, quinoa, and whole wheat berries. These grains usually require a longer cooking time than rice and other common grains to be palatable. Kamet and quinoa can be prepared in about 45 minutes, and whole wheat berries are often cooked overnight in a slow cooker appliance. These foods are effective for eliminating parasites by ensuring the digestive system is in good health and able to flush toxins and other contaminants out of the body.

Like most other healthy diet, the parasite diet prominently features fresh vegetables and fruits. In particular, carrots, squash, and sweet potatoes are recommended for getting rid of parasites, as well as green, leafy vegetables. Fruits including papayas and pineapple are suggested as well. When possible, fruits and vegetables should be consumed raw to enhance their natural parasite fighting properties. With proper washing and preparation, these foods are ideal for naturally eliminating the parasitic threat.

What are the Different Types of Skin Parasites?

Skin parasites are tiny, often microscopic invertebrates that live on the skin of humans and animals. They burrow or bite in order to feed off the blood directly beneath the skin. Lice are considered one of the most common types of these parasites. Other common skin parasites include scabies, ticks, and fleas.

Most lice, though very tiny, are visible without the use of a microscope. The three different types of lice that live on human skin are head lice, body lice, and pubic lice. All three varieties of these skin parasites are blood feeders and very easy to spread from one person to another. In most cases, the presence of lice on the body causes itching and redness.

Scabies is a type of skin mite that causes extreme itching. People who have scabies often mistake the infestation for an allergic type reaction, because infested areas usually appear as bumpy red patches on the skin. These tiny bumps are actually the result of egg sacks that the mites lay when they burrow into the skin.

Treatment for both scabies and lice usually involves soaps and shampoos that kill the pests. Most of the time, these shampoos and washes must be repeated over a period of several days to be sure all of the parasites have been eliminated. It also usually necessary to thoroughly clean and wash home furnishings, carpets, and bed linens, because lice and scabies can be transferred to these items.

Fleas are often spread to humans from the pets inside their homes. Unlike other skin parasites whose bites often go unnoticed, flea bites can sometimes be painful. Most of the time, the bitten area becomes immediately red and irritated. Though it is considered rare, in some instances fleas have been known to transfer dangerous diseases, such as typhus and even plague.

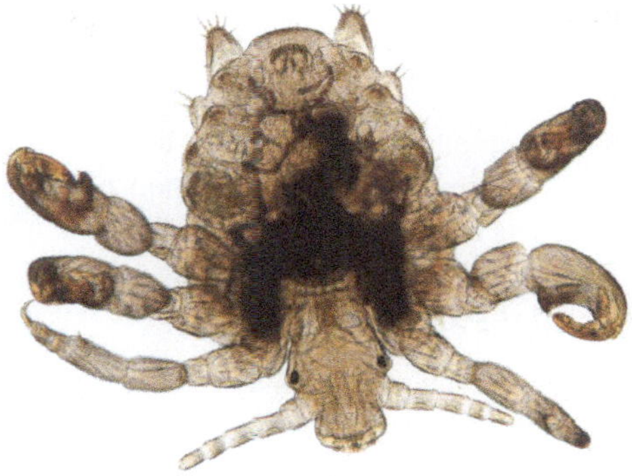

Ridding a home of fleas can be quite difficult, but usually must begin with flea treatment for pets. Unless the pets are free of fleas, there is little hope of keeping the home flea free. Most veterinarians can prescribe monthly flea applications that often do the trick. Flea sprays for the home can be purchased at most hardware stores, but in cases of severe infestation, it may be necessary to hire a professional exterminator.

Ticks are another type of skin parasite that is often spread from pets within the home. Ticks usually live in wooded habitats, so people who spend a lot of time outdoors are at greater risk of being bitten by a tick. When ticks bite, they attach themselves to the skin where they begin to feed on blood. In many cases, tick bites lead to infection, so the bites should be immediately cleaned and treated with disinfectant.

What are the Different Parasite Symptoms?

Contrary to popular belief, parasitic infection is not confined to undeveloped or Third World countries. Those who live in developed countries can be stricken with parasites. Many different parasites exist and, thus, parasite symptoms can be specific to the type of infestation experienced. However, the following is a list of general symptoms that may point to intestinal parasites.

Constipation is often seen among parasite symptoms. Intestinal parasites that live in the human body's gastrointestinal tract can obstruct the intestinal tract and bile duct, which can then lead to constipation. While multiple parasites can achieve this, constipation can also be the fault of one worm that is shaped and sized sufficiently enough to block the tract.

Diarrhea or loose and watery stools can also belong to the list of potential parasite symptoms. If an infection is present, protozoa infections are usually to blame for this symptom. Diarrhea can occur because the protozoa effect sodium and chloride levels in the body.

Irritable bowel syndrome can be a direct result of parasites negatively effecting the intestines. When parasites latch on or otherwise come into contact with the intestine, disruption of the bowel system can occur. As a result, a person can have some trouble absorbing nutrients entering his body and stool may be difficult to pass.

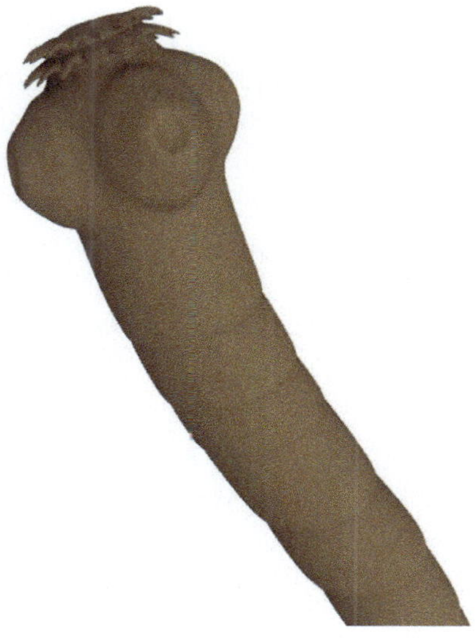

Bloating and excess gas may be attributed to parasitic infection. Parasite infections can irritate the upper part of the small intestine, causing both of these symptoms to arise. These symptoms may increase in severity when the infected person eats foods known for digestion difficulty, such as beans or certain raw vegetables.

Anemia can also be linked to parasite symptoms. It can develop after a parasite latches onto the intestine's mucosa and begins to drain the host of nutrients. An infection of this sort can result in pernicious anemia or severe iron deficiency.

Other potential parasite symptoms include those that may not be so obvious. Skin problems like rashes, hives, and eczema can potentially be the result of parasites. Teeth grinding or bruxism, especially in children, may be symptom of a foreign infection. Chronic fatigue, changes in memory and concentration abilities, flu-like symptoms, immune deficiency and the sudden onslaught of bacterial and viral illnesses may also be caused by a parasite infection. Weight loss, increased appetite, hemorrhoids, numb hands, bed wetting, depression, floaters in the eyes, arthritis-like symptoms and pain in the navel, back, thighs and shoulders may also find their root in parasites.

Simply having one or two of the above symptoms does not point to parasitic infection. However, those who experience any symptoms should consult with a doctor to determine the origin of their medical problem. If parasites exist in the body, the infection should be treated promptly, as symptoms can continue and infections can be contagious.

What are the Different Types of Intestinal Parasites?

There are two main groups of intestinal parasites: helminths and protozoa. Collectively, these organisms cause millions of infections around the world every year, in regions which vary from the urban United States to the remote areas of Africa. Left untreated, intestinal parasites can cause long term health problems or even death in the patient, and the patient can also act as a carrier to spread the parasites to other members of the community.

Intestinal parasites can be ingested in a variety of ways, with one of the leading modes of transmission being fecal to oral contact due to poor hygiene. Infections can also occur when parasites colonize water or soil, or in the case of zoonotic parasites which infect animals consumed by humans. In all cases, the parasites feed off the body to the detriment of the patient, interfering with nutrient absorption and causing a variety of symptoms.

People may develop symptoms right away, or they may be infected for years without being aware of it. When symptoms do appear, abdominal pain, nausea, vomiting, diarrhea, and cramping are all very common. The presence of intestinal parasites can be diagnosed with the use of a fecal sample which is examined for traces of organisms which could be causing infection. Patients should be aware that sometimes a sample may yield false negative or inconclusive results, necessitating another sample.

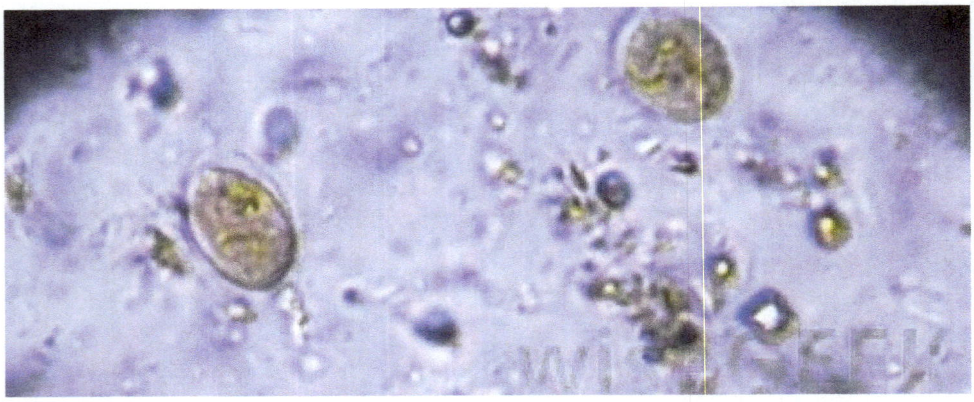

Helminths or worms are multi-celled organisms which are typically found in undercooked food, although it is also possible to be infected via contaminated water or soil. Tapeworms, roundworms, and pinworms are among the most famous and widespread. One of the classic signs of infection with worms is the presence of worms or segments in the feces.

Protozoa such as amoebas, giardia, and cryptosporidium are one celled organisms which can multiply freely in the intestinal tract. It can sometimes be difficult to identify protozoa because they are so small and difficult to identify in the feces. People who have traveled recently should alert their doctors to this fact when they request medical attention for symptoms which suggest infection with intestinal parasites, as travel is a major risk factor for infection.

Several medications can be used to eliminate intestinal parasites from the body. These drugs are generally available by prescription only to encourage patients to go to the doctor for a diagnosis so that the correct medication can be selected to eliminate the particular species causing the infection. Some patients also have success with herbal and other alternative therapies.

What is a Parasitic Infection?

Parasitic infection is contamination of one organism with another living organism that then begins to feed off or reside in the initial organism. In humans this generally means infections with very large parasites that can be seen, such as tapeworms or with tiny ones like amoeba that take intensive laboratory study to find. When most humans have a parasite infection they become ill, because their bodies are not supposed to play host to other large or small organisms of certain types, and these other organisms can cause destruction to the body including death if they are not somehow removed.

The greatest chance of getting parasitic infections tends to occur in underdeveloped countries, where methods of keeping the water supply free from amoeba or large parasites may not be as advanced. Certain parts of the world run much greater risk for people getting parasitic infections than do others, and these include parts of Asia, Africa and South America. In other parts of Asia, much of Western Europe and most of North America, the likelihood of getting a parasite infection is much lower, though it still exists.

It's fairly easy to get a parasitic infection from drinking untreated water for instance, and there are plenty of people who might do so on a camping trip and end up with conditions like giardia. Other ways in which parasites can be passed to a host are through the consumption of undercooked meats or through raw fruit or veggies contaminated by them, bites from certain insects, directly from another person with a parasite infection, or by direct contact with parasites, such as by playing in the dirt where there might be animal droppings.

Often, a parasite infection affects the gastrointestinal tract, and people's response especially to amoebic infection may be what seems like never-ending stomach flu. People have diarrhea and vomiting for long periods of time. Other large parasites like tapeworm may not cause stomach flu symptoms, but survive instead by taking away and consuming part of the food humans consume, and this can lead to severe malnutrition. Complications from a tapeworm may also arise as new worms are born and move into others areas of the body.

In order to appropriately treat a parasitic infection it must be diagnosed first, and best treatment must be considered for the specific parasite. Diagnosis may be made through a number of means. Many times, doctors evaluate stool samples to look for evidence of parasites, but they may also find parasites through x-ray or other scanning methods, and through skin swabs of certain areas of the body. Next, most people will go on a course of anti-parasitic medicine, which can last for several months. People are usually retested at this time to make sure the medicine has worked effectively, and they may be tested again some months later to make certain that another infection hasn't occurred.

As with many types of infections, a parasite infection tends to be most dangerous to people who are vulnerable medically. This can include people with autoimmune diseases like HIV, and those who are very young and very old. However, anyone can get parasitic infections, and when diagnosis is missed, this can result in extreme illness.

SECTION I: PARASITES IN FARM ANIMALS

CHAPTER 1

A REVIEW OF SOME PROTOZOAN PARASITES CAUSING INFERTILITY IN FARM ANIMALS

B. Y. Kaltungo and I. W. Musa

INTRODUCTION

Infertility is a major cause of economic losses and a major limitation to achievement of optimum efficiency in the livestock production system largely as a result of loss of milk production in the dairy sector and increase in culling rates. The causes of infertility can be numerous and complex [1]. They may relate to impairment in Graafian follicle development and maturation, onset of estrus, ovulation, successful coitus, fertilization, implantation, and the development and delivery of the foetus and its membranes. Any temporary state interfering with these routines, such as disease conditions, malnutrition, inadequate herd management, hereditary and congenital factors, hormonal disturbances, or environmental changes, makes the animal infertile [2].

Parasitic infections are typically associated with poor and often marginalized communities in low-income countries [3]. Protozoan parasites are a significant cause of abortion and infertility in domestic ruminants.Toxoplasma gondii and Sarcocystis species are a common cause of extensive abortion in livestock and they both have a two-host life cycle. Carnivorous definitive hosts spread the infection through their feces and domestic ruminants are intermediate hosts. A similar, recently recognized protozoon, Neospora spp., has emerged as an important cause of reproductive disease, especially as an abortifacient in cattle. Neospora is presumed to also have a two-host life cycle, although the definitive host(s) has not been identified. The venereally transmittedTritrichomonas foetus has also been reported to be an important cause of pregnancy loss in naturally bred cattle throughout the world [4].

Citation: B. Y. Kaltungo and I. W. Musa, "A Review of Some Protozoan Parasites Causing Infertility in Farm Animals," ISRN Tropical Medicine, vol. 2013, Article ID 782609, 6 pages, 2013. doi:10.1155/2013/782609.

NEOSPOROSIS

Neospora caninum is an obligate protozoan (Coccidian) parasite related to Toxoplasma gondii and was first associated with neuromuscular disease in dogs in the mid-1980s [5]. It is globally distributed and has been identified as a major cause of infertility in cattle resulting in considerable economic losses [6, 7]. The parasite has been reported to have a wide host range and infects all the major livestock species, as well as companion animals, and certain wildlife species [8, 9]. Clinical infections have also been reported in horses, goats, sheep, and deer. Direct production losses and treatment costs of N. caninum infection have been reported in the Maritime Provinces of Canada to be €1,921 annually [6]. Also, it has been estimated to result in an average annual cost of €249 with a maximum of €5,604 for a herd with 50 lactating cows [7]. Furthermore, the total annual losses due to N. caninum infections/abortions were estimated to range from a median US $1.1 million in the New Zealand beef industry to an estimated median total of US $546.3 million impact per annum in the US dairy population [10].

Infection in cattle was first recognized in 1988 as causing abortion and infertility in cattle, and it is now recognized as an important cause of reproductive problems and abortion in cattle worldwide [11]. Economic implication of this infection in livestock is as a result of reduction in productivity of affected animal in terms of reproduction losses, decrease in milk production, premature weaning of calves, and weight losses [12].

Transmission and Pathogenesis

Dog is both the definitive host and intermediate host for the parasite [13]. Whilst dogs act as definitive hosts to N. caninum and can spread the infection in their faeces, their role in the horizontal transmission of the disease is not usually considered as important as vertical, congenital transmission from dam to calf during terminal stages of gestation or postnatally via milk [11, 14, 15]. Horizontal transmission from cow to cow does not take place [16]. Dogs can shed infectious oocysts for a variable period of time after infection and because the oocysts are very resistant to harsh environmental conditions, it is unclear how long they survive in the environment [17]. Intermediate hosts (cattle) ingest oocysts that are found in contaminated food and water [18,19]. Infection spreads (as tachyzoites) to other tissues in the cow, for example, neural cells, macrophages, fibroblasts, vascular endothelial cells, hepatocytes, and, if pregnant, to the placenta, where damage to the placenta or transmission vertically through the placenta to the foetus can occur. Abortion may be a result of both the primary damage and the immune-mediated inflammatory response of the cow [20]. As a result of the immune response generated, the tachyzoites can transform into bradyzoites (a slowly dividing "dormant" stage or tissue cyst). They remain latent until the immune system of the cow is suppressed, when infection then can recrudesce [11]. Bradyzoites in tissue cysts can be consumed by dogs and then complete the life cycle of the parasite.

Clinical Signs

Infection due to N. caninum is common but seldom results in clinical disease [15]. However, it can result in abortion which can occur at any stage of pregnancy but mostly occurs between 3 and 9 months of pregnancy (particularly 5 to 6 months), with moderate rotting (autolysis) of the foetus. Immunologically competent foetus may be born alive but is congenitally infected, although still-birth may occur. Thus, foetuses may be resorbed, mummified, autolysed, still-born, born alive with clinical signs, or born clinically normal but chronically infected and may manifest nervous symptoms [21]. Such animals may remain malnourished leading to increased mortality, hydrocephalus, exophthalmos, underweight, and difficulty in growth [22]. Congenitally infected heifers may run the risk of abortion, especially in the first gestation and continue to pass the infection to their offspring, while horizontally infected heifers may or may not pass the infection on to their offsprings [4].

Diagnosis

Clinical signs are of little help in the diagnosis of neosporosis. Diagnosis can be made by combination of serology, for example, immunofluorescent antibody tests (IFAT) and enzyme linked immunosorbent assay (ELISA), with immune histochemistry and histopathology of aborted foetus [23]. The most promising specimens for the diagnosis of neosporosis are heart, liver, placenta, and body fluids or blood serum; examination of several tissues gives a higher diagnostic rate; the fetal brain is the most consistently affected organ and has the most characteristic lesion. Polymerase chain reaction (PCR) is also an important tool in the diagnosis of neosporosis, efficiency of which is dependent on the laboratory, stage of the autolysis of the foetus, and the sampling procedures [22, 23].

Prevention/Control

In herds free of N. caninum, prevention of the introduction of the infection through standard biosecurity measures is the primary goal [11], whereas, in N. caninum-infected herds, control programs are based on decreasing the vertical transmission in a herd by reduction of the number of seropositive cattle and/or decreasing the risk of horizontal transmission of N. caninum principally by controlling the definitive host population as a source of oocyst contamination [24, 25].

Treatment

There is no safe and effective treatment for bovine neosporosis. Drug therapy is not usually advocated because it is usually prophylactic involving long-term administration which can result in unacceptable milk and meat residues and withdrawal problems [15, 26].

SARCOCYSTOSIS

Sarcocystosis is a disease of birds and mammals caused by several species of single-celled coccidian protozoa in the group called Sarcocystis. The Greek word sarco refers to flesh or muscle, with sarcocyst referring literally to a cyst in muscle. Sarcocystis is a genus of Coccidian protozoan parasites that is associated with the presence of muscle cysts which are usually grossly evident, in striated muscle of an intermediate host species [27]. The muscle cyst stage in the intermediate host is relatively benign. However, the early developmental stages in other tissues of the intermediate host can prove that fatal. Sarcocystis species occasionally cause abortion in cattle [28]. Three species have been reported in bovine muscle; they are Sarcocystis cruzi with canids as definitive hosts, Sarcocystis hirsuta with felids as definitive hosts, and Sarcocystis hominis with primates as definitive hosts [29, 30]. Abortions are usually sporadic, but they may occur as "storms." Sarcocystis is spread by carnivores (wild and domestic) and cattle become infected by ingesting feed or forages contaminated by carnivore faeces. Abortions occur at any stage of gestation. Infection due to Sarcocystis results in economic losses as a result of weight loss, anorexia, decreased milk production, anemia, and prostration often culminating in death [31].

Transmission and Pathogenesis

Sarcocystis spp. normally develop in 2-host cycles consisting of an intermediate host (prey) and the final host (predator).

Species-specific prey-predator cycles have been demonstrated, for example, cattle-dog (S. cruzi), cattle-cat (S. hirsuta), and opossum-psittacine (S. falcatula) [26]. Definitive hosts which are carnivores become infected by feeding on preys whose tissues contain encysted Sarcocystis protozoa and subsequently shed the infectious sporocysts in their faeces. The intermediate host ingests the sporocysts, which develop into sarcocysts in the muscle of the host [32].

Clinical Signs

Most animals infected with Sarcocystis spp. are asymptomatic, and the parasites are seen mainly as an incidental finding at necropsy. However, clinical cases are occasionally reported, particularly in the intermediate host, but often depend on the number of sporocysts ingested and the species of infecting Sarcocystis. Clinical signs reported in heavily infected cattle include fever, anorexia, wasting, decreased milk production, diarrhoea, muscle spasms, weakness, hyperexcitability, pneumonia, haemorrhages, anaemia, icterus, prostration, and death. These signs may last several days to several weeks. When pregnant mammals ingest sporocysts, they may abort or give birth to a still-born foetus. Definitive hosts typically do not show any clinical signs of sarcocystosis [33].

Diagnosis

The diagnosis is usually done postmortem by examination of the skeletal muscles. The cysts are tan to white resembling parallel grains of rice, which may be observed throughout the breast muscle tissue and other muscles, including the heart. The affected tissue often produces a gritty sound when cut with a knife. In some species, the cysts may be visible to the naked eye (ducks, mice, rabbits, and sheep), but, in most species, microscopic examination is required, which includes peptic digestion, muscle squash, squeezing methods, and indirect fluorescent antibody test Antemortem diagnosis may be made with the use of dermal sensitivity test or complement fixation tests [34].

Prevention/Control

Dogs and other carnivores should not be allowed access to raw meat, offal, or dead animals as these may harbor cysts of sarcocystosis. Dogs and cats should not be allowed access to buildings where livestock feed or animals are kept [26, 33]. It has been reported that good sanitation is important in the control of this disease in domestic and captive animals. Freezing meat prior to cooking can also help to kill the organisms. Condemned carcasses as a result of sarcocystosis should be disposed of by deep burial to avoid consumption by scavenging animals.

Treatment

There is no effective treatment for cattle infected with Sarcocystis spp. However, anticoccidial drugs like amprolium and salinomycine have been used to prevent severe illness and death in experimentally infected calves [35, 36]. In addition, anti-inflammatory medications or vitamin E may be given, and supportive care may be necessary [37].

TOXOPLASMOSIS

Toxoplasma gondii is a systemic coccidian, a universal parasite, a protozoan, and a member of the suborderEimeriina [30]. It is a tissue protozoan infecting humans and warm blooded animals. It has three life stages, namely, tachyzoites, bradyzoites, and oocyst containing sporozoites, and is of zoonotic importance of worldwide distribution [38, 39]. A primary infection in pregnant animals is capable of establishing a placental and foetal infection, which may result in foetal death and resorption, abortion, or stillbirth [38]. The definitive host for this parasite is the cat and has, therefore, not developed resistance to the parasite [40]. In the definitive host for T. gondii, the organism undergoes both sexual and asexual life cycles. Other mammals and birds are intermediate hosts in which T. gondii undergoes only the asexual life cycle [41]. Infection with this parasite has been associated with a variety of mental health and brain problems in humans, including schizophrenia, neurosis, and brain cancer [42].

Transmission and Pathogenesis

The sexual cycle is initiated when a susceptible cat ingests oocysts or tissue cysts. In the latter case, bradyzoites excyst from the tissue, penetrate the epithelial cells of the small intestine, and disseminate to other tissues, such as striated muscle and the brain, where they encyst and are resistant to attacks by the host's immune system [41,42]. Bradyzoites in animal tissues are a source of toxoplasmosis in humans. In the enteroepithelial cells of the cat, the oocysts undergo gametogony, and the gametocytes are released into the lumen of the intestine and pass out in the faeces. Sporulation occurs in the environment within 1 to 5 days, with each oocyst containing 8 infectious sporozoites. Four days after ingesting tissue cysts, the cat is capable of shedding millions of oocysts in the faeces which can survive for 12–18 months in the environment, depending on climactic conditions, and they serve as an important source of infection for grazing animals [43, 44]. Oocysts may be shed in smaller numbers for a few days or not at all, 20 days after a cat ingests oocysts or tachyzoites [41].

Clinical Signs

Clinical signs develop as a result of inflammation in infected tissues. The course of the disease varies a great deal between animal species and between age groups being more of a problem of the young. If organism replication is attenuated by immune response, tissue cysts may develop containing the more slowly dividing bradyzoites. Bradyzoites can later be reactivated under conditions of immunosuppression to divide rapidly as tachyzoites, potentially resulting in clinical disease. Bradyzoites can persist in affected tissues for the lifetime of the host. Infection of ewes during early pregnancy may result in embryonic death and resorption due to the immature nature of the foetal immune system. Infection during mid-pregnancy may result in either foetal death followed by mummification or foetal retardation due to compromised placental nutrition and foetal infection. Characteristic lesions on the infected placenta are white spots visible to the naked eye due to areas of necrosis, resulting in the impaired function of the placenta [45]. Late pregnancy infection may result in abortion of freshly dead lambs or birth of weak lambs with high neonatal mortality rates [43].

Prevention/Control

Measures should be taken to limit breeding of cats and their prevention from gaining access to livestock feed and pasture. The coccidiostat drug, decoquinate, can be fed to pregnant ewes as an aid to prevention of abortions due to toxoplasmosis. Despite the current knowledge of immunology, pathology, and genetics related to the parasite, a safe vaccine for prevention of the infection in both humans and animals does not exist [46]. However, a live, attenuated vaccine, containing the S48 strains (Toxovax), has been used to vaccinate sheep. The vaccine should be given at least three weeks before mating. One dose of the vaccine is enough to protect sheep for a period of 18 months [47]. T-263 strain of T. gondii, ME-49 strain, and 60Co irradiated tachyzoites of the Beverley strain of T. gondii have been used to control oocyst shedding in cats [48–50].

Treatment

In the face of a late abortion storm, injectable or oral sulphonamide antibiotics can be used to reduce losses, a combination of sulfamethazine and pyrimethamine has also been reported to give good results.

TRICHOMONIASIS

Trichomoniasis is a venereal disease of cattle, characterized primarily by early pregnancy loss and, occasionally, by abortion and pyometra leading to significant infertility. It is worldwide in distribution and has been reported to possibly be the third most common cause of abortion in cattle (after Brucellosis and Leptospirosis) [51]. The causative agent, Tritrichomonas foetus, is a flagellated protozoan parasite transmitted from infected, asymptomatic bulls to heifers or cows at the time of coitus [52]. The infection has been reported in dogs [53] and in cats as a cause of large-bowel diarrhea [54, 55]. Furthermore, Tritrichomonas suis has been reported to be a gastrointestinal commensal of pig [53].

Aetiology and Pathogenesis

The parasite has characteristic three anterior flagellae about the same length as the body of the parasite and an undulating membrane [4]. Younger bulls are less liable to become persistent carriers than older bulls because the crypts of the penile integument and prepucial mucosa are less developed in young than older animals [26]. The parasite colonises the uterus, cervix, and vagina but survives less in the vulva; it does not prevent fertilisation but causes early embryonic death, resulting in irregular extended return to oestrus [4].

Clinical Signs

Neither the cow nor the bull appears ill at any time, when they are infected with this organism [56]. However, there is marked subfertility, extended return to oestrus, and long calving intervals. There is presence of pyometra and early gestation abortions (1–6 weeks). In some cases, despite infection, pregnancy is not terminated by abortion and a normal, full-term calf is born [55]. Infected cows or heifers may have a uterine discharge for several months [26]. The aborted foetus is usually fresh and parasites disappear quickly from vaginal discharges after abortion (usually within 7 days) [4].

Diagnosis

Diagnosis is confirmed by demonstrating T. foetus organisms from specimens obtained from genital tract of female cattle, prepucial material of bulls or aborted foetal, and placental tissues [57]. Other diagnostic procedures include culture of the organism, polymerase chain reaction (PCR), and immunological tests [58–60].

Prevention/Control

Trichomoniasis is a "self-limiting" disease in the nonpregnant cow with an involuted uterus. After being sexually rested for 3 or 5 cycles, many cows develop some immunity and their fertility improves. Once infected, however, males become permanent carriers of the pathogen; therefore, only clean bulls or semen should be used for breeding and cows with abnormal genital tracts should be culled [52]. "Carrier" bulls can reinfect treated, recovered, and susceptible females and should, therefore, be culled.

Treatment

There is no approved chemotherapeutic agent for treatment of trichomoniasis in cattle [60].

CONCLUDING REMARK

The most serious deterrent to efficient animal production and herd profitability is pregnancy loss, of which parasitic infections can be a possible cause. These infections are, however, often poorly considered during investigations for a diagnosis. This may lead to inaccurate diagnosis of the cause of infertility. Maximizing reproductive efficiency, however, is a major production management goal and cannot be compromised, for the success and financial profitability of enterprises. Therefore, parasitic infections should be borne in mind during such investigations.

REFERENCES

1. G. H. Arthur, Veterinary Reproduction and Obstetrics, Bailliere Tindall, London, UK, 5th edition, 1982.
2. S. T. Osmanu, "Studies on bovine infertility at the agricultural research Station (Legon) over half a decade (1972–77)," Ghana University, Department of Animal Science Studies, Legon, Ghana, pp. 82, 2009.
3. CDC, "Neglected parasitic infections in the United States," 2012, http://www.cdc.gov/parasites/npi.html.
4. T. Parkinson, "Subfertility and infertility," in Veterinary Reproduction and Obstetrics, G. H. Arthur, D. E. Noakes, and H. Pearson, Eds., pp. 476–516, ELBS Bailliere Tindall, London, UK, 9th edition, 2009.
5. I. Bjerkas, S. F. Mohn, and J. Presthus, "Unidentified cyst-forming sporozoon causing encephalomyelitis and myositis in dogs," Zeitschrift für Parasitenkunde, vol. 70, no. 2, pp. 271–274, 1984. ·
6. J. Chi, J. A. VanLeeuwen, A. Weersink, and G. P. Keefe, "Direct production losses and treatment costs from bovine viral diarrhoea virus, bovine leukosis virus, Mycobacterium aviumsubspeciesparatuberculosis, and

Neospora caninum," Preventive Veterinary Medicine, vol. 55, no. 2, pp. 137–153, 2002.

7. H. Hogeveen and S. Van der Heijden, "Economic consequences of Neospora caninumon dairy farms," inProceedings of the 10th International Society for Veterinary Epidemiology and Economics, Vina del Mar, Chile, November 2003.

8. J. P. Dubey and D. S. Lindsay, "A review of Neospora caninum and neosporosis," Veterinary Parasitology, vol. 67, no. 1–2, pp. 1–59, 1996.

9. J. Gharekhani, G. Tavoosidana, and G. Naderisefat, "Seroprevalence of Neospora infection in horses and donkeys in Hamedan province, Western Iran," Veterinary World, vol. 6, no. 9, pp. 620–622, 2013.

10. M. P. Reichel, M. A. Ayanegui-Alcérreca, L. F. P. Gondim, and J. T. Ellis, "What is the global economic impact of Neospora caninum in cattle—the billion dollar question," International Journal for Parasitology, vol. 43, no. 2, pp. 133–142, 2013.

11. J. P. A. Haddad, I. R. Dohoo, and J. A. VanLeewen, "A review of Neospora caninum in dairy and beef cattle—a Canadian perspective," Canadian Veterinary Journal, vol. 46, no. 3, pp. 230–243, 2005.

12. K. Reiterová, S. Špilovská, D. Antolová, and P. Dubinský, "Neospora caninum, potential cause of abortions in dairy cows: the current serological follow-up in Slovakia," Veterinary Parasitology, vol. 159, no. 1, pp. 1–6, 2009.

13. M. M. McAllister, J. P. Dubey, D. S. Lindsay, W. R. Jolley, R. A. Wills, and A. M. McGuire, "Dogs are definitive hosts of Neospora caninum," International Journal for Parasitology, vol. 28, no. 9, pp. 1473–1478, 1998.

14. L. F. P. Gondim, M. M. McAllister, N. E. Mateus-Pinilla, W. C. Pitt, L. D. Mech, and M. E. Nelson, "Transmission of Neospora caninum between wild and domestic animals," Journal of Parasitology, vol. 90, no. 6, pp. 1361–1365, 2004.

15. J. P. Dubey and G. Schares, "Neosporosis in animals—the last five years," Veterinary Parasitology, vol. 180, no. 1–2, pp. 90–108, 2011.

16. M. L. Anderson, P. C. Blanchard, B. C. Barr, J. P. Dubey, R. L. Hoffman, and P. A. Conrad, "Neospora-like protozoan infection as a major cause of abortion in California dairy cattle," Journal of the American Veterinary Medical Association, vol. 198, no. 2, pp. 241–244, 1991.

17. A. F. A. Neto, L. A. Bandini, S. M. Nishi et al., "Viability of sporulated oocysts of Neospora caninum after exposure to different physical and chemical treatments," Journal of Parasitology, vol. 97, no. 1, pp. 135–139, 2011.

18. A. J. Trees and H. C. Davison, "Current understanding of the epidemiology of bovine neosporosis and its control," Cattle Practice, vol. 7, no. 3, pp. 271–272, 1999.

19. H. C. Davison, C. S. Guy, J. W. McGarry et al., "Experimental studies on the transmission of Neospora caninum between cattle," Research in Veterinary Science, vol. 70, no. 2, pp. 163–168, 2001.

20. S. W. Maley, D. Buxton, A. G. Rae et al., "The pathogenesis of neosporosis in pregnant cattle: inoculation at mid-gestation," Journal of Comparative Pathology, vol. 129, no. 2–3, pp. 186–195, 2003.

21. J. P. Dubey, "Recent advances in Neospora and neosporosis," Veterinary Parasitology, vol. 84, no. 3–4, pp. 349–367, 1999.

22. J. P. Dubey, "Review of Neospora caninum and neosporosis in animals," Korean Journal of Parasitology, vol. 41, no. 1, pp. 1–16, 2003.

23. D. P. Moore, J. Regidor-Cerrillo, E. Morrell et al., "The role of Neospora caninum and Toxoplasma gondiiin spontaneous bovine abortion in Argentina," Veterinary Parasitology, vol. 156, no. 3–4, pp. 163–167, 2008.

24. J. P. Dubey, "Review of Neospora caninum and neosporosis in animals," The Korean Journal of Parasitology, vol. 41, no. 1, 2003.

25. C. A. Hall, M. P. Reichel, and J. T. Ellis, "Neospora abortions in dairy cattle: diagnosis, mode of transmission and control," Veterinary Parasitology, vol. 128, no. 3–4, pp. 231–241, 2005.

26. M. K. Cynthia, "Trichomoniasis," in Merck Veterinary Manual, pp. 1142–1143, Merck & Co., Whitehouse Station, NJ, USA, 9th edition, 2005.

27. S. L. Clubb, "Sarcocystosis in psittacine birds," 2010, http://www.avianweb.com/sarcocystosis.html.

28. B. Abbitt and D. O. Rae, "Infertility in horses," in Current Therapy in Large Animal Thereogenology, R. S. Yoyngquist and W. R. Threlfall, Eds., pp. 409–413, Saunders Elsevier, St. Louis, Mo, USA, 2nd edition, 2007.

29. A.-O. Heydorn, R. Gestrich, H. Mehlhorn, and M. Rommel, "Proposal for a new nomenclature of theSarcosporidia," Zeitschrift für Parasitenkunde, vol. 48, no. 2, pp. 73–82, 1975.

30. O. M. Radostits, C. C. Gay, D. C. Blood, and K. W. Hinchcliff, "Diseases associated with protozoa," inVeterinary Medicine: A Textbook of the Diseases of Cattle, Sheep, Pigs, Goats and Horses, pp. 1483–1530, W.B. Saunders, St. Louis, Mo, USA, 10th edition, 2005.

31. A. M. Dafedar, P. E. D'Souza, K. J. Ananda, and G. C. Puttalakshmamma, "Prevalence of Sarcocystosis in goats slaughtered at an abattoir in Bangalore, Karnataka state," Veterinary World, vol. 1, no. 11, pp. 335–337, 2008.

32. M. B. Markus, J. J. Van der Lugt, and J. P. Dubey, Infectious Diseases of Livestock, Oxford University Press, Oxford, UK, 2004.

33. R. Fayer, "Sarcocystis spp. in human infections," Clinical Microbiology Reviews, vol. 17, no. 4, pp. 894–902, 2004.

34. B. M. A. Latif, J. K. Al-Delemi, B. S. Mohammed, S. M. Al-Bayati, and A. M. Al-Amiry, "Prevalence ofSarcocystis spp. in meat-producing animals in Iraq," Veterinary Parasitology, vol. 84, no. 1–2, pp. 85–90, 1999.

35. R. Fayer and A. J. Johnson, "Effect of amprolium on acute sarcocystosis in experimentally infected calves,"Journal of Parasitology, vol. 61, no. 5, pp. 932–936, 1975.

36. R. G. Leek and R. Fayer, "Experimental Sarcocystis ovicanis infection in lambs: salinomycin chemoprophylaxis and protective immunity," Journal of Parasitology, vol. 69, no. 2, pp. 271–276, 1983. ·

37. M. Sutherland-Smith and P. Morris, "Combination therapy using trimethoprim-sulfamethoxazole, pyrimethamine, and diclazuril to treat Sarcocystosis in a pied imperial pigeon (Ducula bicolor bicolor),"Journal of Avian Medicine and Surgery, vol. 18, no. 3, pp. 151–154, 2004.

38. D. Buxton and D. Henderson, "Infectious abortion in sheep," In Practice, vol. 21, no. 7, pp. 360–368, 1999.

39. S. Bayarri, M. J. Gracia, R. Lá Zaro, C. Pérez-Arquillué, M. Barberán, and A. Herrera, "Determination of the viability of Toxoplasma gondii in cured ham using bioassay: influence of technological processing and food safety implications," Journal of Food Protection, vol. 73, no. 12, pp. 2239–2243, 2010.

40. J. P. Dubey and C. P. Beattie, Toxoplasmosis of Animals and Man, CRC Press, Boca Raton, Fla, USA, 1988.

41. J. Weissmann, "Presumptive Toxoplasma gondii abortion in a sheep," Canadian Veterinary Journal, vol. 44, no. 4, pp. 322–324, 2003.

42. S. Pappas, "Cat parasite linked to suicide attempts in humans," 2012, http://www.livescience.com/21345-t-gondii-parasite-suicide-attempts.html.

43. D. Buxton, "Protozoan infections (Toxoplasma gondii , Neospora caninum and Sarcocystis spp.) in sheep and goats: recent advances," Veterinary Research, vol. 29, no. 3–4, pp. 289–310, 1998.

44. A. M. Tenter, A. R. Heckeroth, and L. M. Weiss, "Toxoplasma gondii: from animals to humans,"International Journal for Parasitology, vol. 30, no. 12–13, pp. 1217–1258, 2000.

45. D. Buxton and S. M. Rodger, "Toxoplasmosis and neosporosis," in Diseases of Sheep, I. D. Aitken, Ed., pp. 112–118, Wiley-Blackwell, Hoboken, NJ, USA, 4th edition, 2008.

46. J. L. Garcia, "Vaccination concepts against toxoplasma gondii," Expert Review of Vaccines, vol. 8, no. 2, pp. 215–225, 2009.

47. D. Buxton and E. Innes, "A commercial vaccine for ovine toxoplasmosis," Parasitology, vol. 110, pp. 11–16, 1995.

48. A. Freyre, L. Choromanski, J. L. Fishback, and I. Popiel, "Immunization of cats with tissue cysts, bradyzoites, and tachyzoites of the T-263 strain of toxoplasma gondii," Journal of Parasitology, vol. 79, no. 5, pp. 716–719, 1993.

49. Y. Omata, Y. Aihara, M. Kanda, A. Saito, I. Igarashi, and N. Suzuki, "Toxoplasma gondii: experimental infection in cats vaccinated with 60 Co-irradiated tachyzoites," Veterinary Parasitology, vol. 65, no. 3–4, pp. 173–183, 1996.

50. A. Freyre, J. Falcón, J. Méndez, T. Gastell, and J. M. Venzal, "Toxoplasma gondii: cross-immunity against the enteric cycle," Experimental Parasitology, vol. 115, no. 1, pp. 48–52, 2007.

51. N. S. Silva, S. M. Machado, F. C. S. Filho, and C. P. Soares, "Basic biological aspects of Tritrichomonas foetus of relevance to the treatment of bovines suffering of trichomoniasis," Open Journal of Animal Sciences, vol. 1, no. 3, pp. 112–120, 2011.

52. L. B. Corbeil, C. M. Campero, K. Van Hoosear, and R. H. BonDurant, "Detection of trichomonad species in the reproductive tracts of breeding and virgin bulls," Veterinary Parasitology, vol. 154, no. 3–4, pp. 226–232, 2008.

53. M. K. Tolbert, C. M. Leutenegger, R. Lobetti, J. Birrell, and J. L. Gookin, "Species identification of trichomonads and associated coinfections in dogs with diarrhea and suspected trichomonosis,"Veterinary Parasitology, vol. 187, no. 1–2, pp. 319–322, 2012. ·

54. M. K. Tolbert and J. L. Gookin, "Tritrichomonas fetus: a new agent of feline diarrhea," Compendium on Continuing Education for the Practicing Veterinarian, vol. 31, no. 8, pp. 374–381, 2009.

55. C. Profizi, A. Cian, D. Meloni et al., "Prevalence of Tritrichomonas foetus infections in french catteries,"Veterinary Parasitology, vol. 196, no. 1-2, pp. 50–55, 2013.

56. R. BonDurant, "Trichomoniasis," 1997, http://www.vetmed.ucdavis.edu/vetext/INF-BE_cca/INF-BE_cca97/INF-BE_cca9706.htm.

57. N. Mukhufhi, P. C. Irons, A. Michel, and F. Peta, "Evaluation of a PCR test for the diagnosis ofTritrichomonas foetus infection in bulls: effects of sample collection method, storage and transport medium on the test," Theriogenology, vol. 60, no. 7, pp. 1269–1278, 2003.

58. L. A. Bryan, J. R. Campbell, and A. A. Gajadhar, "Effects of temperature on the survival ofTritrichomonas foetus in transport, Diamond›s and InPouch TF media," Veterinary Record, vol. 144, no. 9, pp. 227–232, 1999.

59. J. C. Rhyan, K. L. Wilson, B. Wagner et al., "Demonstration of Tritrichomonas foetus in the external genitalia and of specific antibodies in preputial secretions of naturally infected bulls," Veterinary Pathology, vol. 36, no. 5, pp. 406–411, 1999.

60. C. M. Campero, C. Rodriguez Dubra, A. Bolondi et al., "Two-step (culture and PCR) diagnostic approach for differentiation of non-T. foetus trichomonads from genitalia of virgin beef bulls in Argentina," Veterinary Parasitology, vol. 112, no. 3, pp. 167–175, 2003.

CHAPTER 2

DETECTION OF TRYPANOSOMES IN SMALL RUMINANTS AND PIGS IN WESTERN KENYA: IMPORTANT RESERVOIRS IN THE EPIDEMIOLOGY OF SLEEPING SICKNESS?

Musa O Ng'ayo, Zablon K Njiru, Eucharia U Kenya, Geoffrey M Muluvi, Ellie O Osir and Daniel K Masiga

Keywords: *Trypanosoma brucei rhodesiense* - Human African Trypanosomosis, sleeping sickness, epidemiology - Serum Resistance Associated (SRA) gene - small ruminants - pigs - reservoirs.

BACKGROUND

African trypanosomosis has profoundly affected settlement and economic development in much of the African continent, especially south of the Sahara desert where it is transmitted mainly by tsetse flies. Overlaying a map of the distribution of livestock and that of tsetse infestation highlights the extent to which tsetse and trypanosomosis impede livestock development [1]. Additionally, sleeping sickness or Human African Trypanosomosis (HAT) is responsible for considerable morbidity and mortality in many countries of sub-Saharan Africa. Sleeping sickness is caused by two protozoan parasites of genus *Trypanosoma*:*Trypanosoma brucei rhodesiense* and *T. b. gambiense*. The latter is characterized by a chronic disease in man, often lasting several years, and is distributed mainly in western and central Africa. *T. b. rhodesiense* is more acute, with clinical signs apparent within weeks of infection and is confined to eastern and southern Africa. For a long time, wildlife were considered the most important, perhaps the only reservoir for both sleeping sickness and trypanosomosis in livestock. However, this changed when it was demonstrated that cattle were reservoirs of *T. b. rhodesiense* in Kenya [2]. With respect to *T. b. gambiense* on the other hand, it has been shown that pigs are reservoirs [3], although a direct man-fly-man transmission cycle is considered the more important [4]. The acute nature of sleeping sickness due to *T. b. rhodesiense* appears to preclude this, making the presence of a non-human reservoir obligatory in maintaining an endemic focus. Recent cases from areas where wildlife are protected, such as Serengeti National Park in Tanzania, indicate that wildlife continue to play a role in transmission of sleeping sickness [5].

Unlike cattle, sheep and goats are kept in a very broad range of agro-ecological zones [1], where they contribute considerably to the rural economies as a source of meat, milk, manure and readily disposable income [6]. Early reports suggested that trypanosomosis was not an important disease in small ruminants [7]. However, more recent studies have clearly demonstrated that sheep and goats acquire natural infections [8, 9,10, 11, 12], and suffer economic loss [13, 14]. Trypanosomes have also been shown to infect pigs, with reports of natural infections in different regions of Africa [9, 11, 15, 16].

Citation: Musa O Ng'ayo, Zablon K Njiru, Eucharia U Kenya, Geoffrey M Muluvi, Ellie O Osir and Daniel K Masiga, "Detection of trypanosomes in small ruminants and pigs in western Kenya: important reservoirs in the epidemiology of sleeping sickness?," Kinetoplastid Biology and Disease20054:5. DOI: 10.1186/1475-9292-4-5.

This study was undertaken in western Kenya, an area that is endemic for Human African Trypanosomosis (HAT) or sleeping sickness, and several species of trypanosomes of veterinary importance. We sought to investigate the role of small ruminants and pigs in the transmission dynamics of trypanosomosis. In this area, pigs are increasingly kept as free-range livestock, presumably thriving as a result of the varied nature of their diet. Our efforts to identify *T. b. rhodesiense* have benefited from evidence that the Serum Resistance Associated gene (SRA) is ubiquitous among all *T. b. rhodesiense* isolates tested so far that have also been characterized by other biochemical criteria [17, 18, 19].

RESULTS

Detection of Trypanosomes

The buffy coat and haematocrit centrifuge technique (HCT) [20] examination of blood from the 402 animals detected 5 trypanosome infections as shown in Table 1. The infections detected by microscopy were one *T. congolense*, one *T. vivax* and three *T. brucei*; no mixed infections were detected using microscopy alone. All 402 animals sampled were subjected to PCR analysis for detection of trypanosomes, based on primers specific for different species and subspecies (Table 2). Eighty-six (18.9%) animals out of the 402 were found infected by PCR. Thirty-one (27.7%) out of 112 animals sampled from Obuchun were infected by various species of trypanosomes. The infection rate was 28.05% (23/82) in Amoni, 22.1% (15/68) in Ongariama, 19.2% (10/52) in Amase and 7.9% (7/88) in Rukada. Twenty-four of the 95 sheep sampled (25.3%) were infected, while 52/255 goats (20.0%) and 10/52 pigs (19.2%) were infected. There was no significant difference in infection between animals ($p > 0.05$).

Table 1: Identification of trypanosome species using PCR

Amoni								
Goats	42	2	3	1	0	2	8	**19.04**
Sheep	37	0	6	5	0	4	15	**40.54**
Pigs	3	0	0	0	0	0	0	**0**
Amase								
Goats	35	0	0	0	4	1	5	**14.29**
Sheep	8	0	0	0	0	1	1	**12.5**
Pigs	9	1	0	0	1	2	4	**44.44**
Ongariama								
Goats	55	0	0	7	5	1	13	**23.64**
Sheep	7	0	0	0	0	0	0	**0**
Pigs	6	0	0	1	1	0	2	**33.33**
Obuchun								
Goats	86	4	0	8	8	3	23	**26.74**
Sheep	13	0	1	0	1	2	4	**30.77**
Pigs	13	0	0	0	3	1	4	**30.77**
Rukada								
Goats	37	1	1	0	0	1	3	**8.11**
Sheep	30	1	1	0	0	2	4	**13.33**
Pigs	21	0	0	0	0	0	0	**0**
TOTAL	**402**	**9**	**12**	**22**	**23**	**20**	**86**	**21.39%**

Table 2: Sequences of primers used for PCR and expected product size

Trypanosome species	Primer sequence 5'-3'	Size (bp)	Reference
T. Congolense savannah	For: CGAGAACGGGCACTTTGCGA	316	[28]
	Rev: GGACAAACAAATCCCGCACA		
T. congolense Kilifi	For: GTGACCAAATTTGAAGTGAT	294	[28]
	Rev: ACTCAAAATCGTGCACCTCG		
T. vivax	For: CCCGGCAGGTTGGCCGCCATC	399	[29]

	Rev: TCGCTACCACAGTCGCAATCGCAATCGTCGTCT-CAAGG		
T. simiae	For: CCGGTCAAAAACGCATT	437	[28]
	Rev: AGTCGCCCGGAGTCGAT		
T. brucei	For: GAATATTAAACAATGCGCAG	164	[28]
	Rev: CCATTTATTAGCTTTGTTGC		
SRA – T. b. rhod-esiense	SRA-A: 5'GACAACAAGTACCTTGGCGC	460	[18]
	SRA-E: 5'TACTGTTGTTGTACCGCCGC)		

Prevalence of Trypanosome Species

The prevalence of *Trypanosoma vivax* as detected by PCR was 23 (5.7%), *T. simiae* 22 (5.5%), *T. congolense* savannah 9 (2.2%), *T. congolense* Kilifi 12 (3.0%) and *T. brucei* ssp 20 (5.0%). A number of mixed infections were reported in this study; *T. congolense* Savannah and *T. brucei* were encountered twice, and there was one mixed infection of *T. congolense* savannah and *T. simiae*. Sheep carried significantly more infections of *T. congolense* Kilifi than goats ($\chi^2 = 9.8$, df = 1, $p < 0.05$) and similarly with *T. brucei* ssp ($\chi^2 = 6.6$, df = 1, $p < 0.05$). There were more *T. vivax* infections in goats and pigs than in sheep respectively, and this difference was significant ($p < 0.05$).

Presence of Serum Resistance Associated (SRA) Gene

Twenty samples in which T. brucei spp. was detected by PCR were further analyzed for the presence of the SRA. This analysis resulted in 3 positive samples for the SRA gene (from a goat, pig and sheep) (Figure 1), demonstrating the presence of this gene associated with human infectivity in trypanosomes infecting livestock other than cattle.

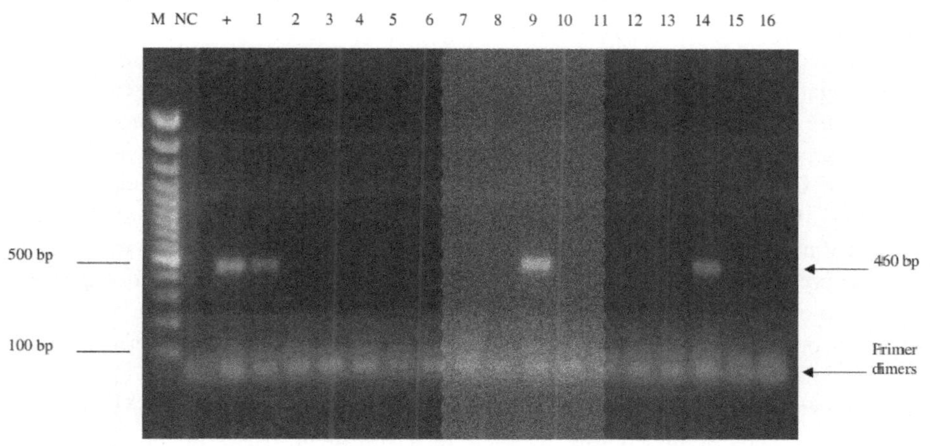

Figure 1: Map of study area showing sampling locations. Sampling was undertaken in 5 villages (4 in Teso and 1 in Busia Districts), whose GPS locations are shown in this map.

DISCUSSION

Trypanosomes in Small Ruminants

Few records exist on the effect of trypanosomosis in small ruminants in East Africa. However, the work of Griffin and Allonby [8, 13], who used microscopic examination of blood smears to demonstrate that the disease was an important natural infection, is a notable exception. These authors also reported that small ruminants survived better than cattle under medium tsetse challenge. More recent studies undertaken in an area of high tsetse fly challenge have shown that small ruminants succumb to trypanosomosis and that heavy economic loss is occasioned [12, 14]. Although the microscopic techniques used in these studies have limitations of sensitivity [20], they provided an important basis for investigations into the importance of trypanosomosis in small ruminants. In the present study, using PCR raised the number of infections detected from 5 to 86, considerably improving our understanding of the prevalence of trypanosomosis in small ruminants and pigs.

A greater percentage of sheep were infected compared to goats and pigs, findings that are consistent with other studies that have shown sheep to be more frequently infected than goats under natural conditions [9,11, 12], [21, 22, 23, 24]. All these findings, drawn from experiments on different breeds suggest that goats are more refractory to trypanosome infections than sheep. The presence of many small ruminants with *T. simiae*(5 sheep and 16 goats) shows that this trypanosome has the potential to impact negatively on the growing importance of pig farming in the study area. Our data also show that sheep were more frequently infected with *T. congolense* Kilifi and

T. brucei, while pigs and goats were more frequently infected with *T. vivax*.

All the 5 villages, except Ongariama, had infections of *T. congolense*, arguably the most important pathogens of cattle in Africa. Also, with the exception of Rukada and Amoni, *T. vivax* infections were identified. These two species constitute the most important trypanosomes of livestock in Africa. Considering the greater trypanotolerance of small ruminants, they may be acting as reservoirs of these pathogens, therefore limiting the economic impact of the cattle industry.

Trypanosome Infections in Pigs

The presence of trypanosomes in pigs has been documented from different parts of Africa [9, 11, 15, 16]. In the present study, out of the 10 pigs infected, 3 carried *T. brucei* ssp., 5 had *T. vivax*, and there was one infection each of *T. congolense* savannah and *T. simiae*. Of important relevance to sleeping sickness epidemiology, the SRA gene was detected in one pig carrying *T. brucei*. These data show that pigs play a role in the epidemiology of both human and animal trypanosomosis.

Reservoirs of Sleeping Sickness

Small ruminants and pigs constitute a key component of livestock kept in the study area. It is now well recognized that these livestock naturally acquire trypanosome infections. On the basis of DNA amplification of the SRA gene, this study shows that sheep, goats and pigs may harbour *T. b. rhodesiense*. It is in this context that investigations were undertaken in these livestock as potential reservoirs of *T. b. rhodesiense*. Reports implicating cattle date back to the infection of human subjects with pathogens isolated from cattle [2]. In the intervening period, descriptions of human infective trypanosomes in cattle have been made on the basis of multilocus DNA fingerprinting [15], and more recently the presence of the SRA gene as a marker [17, 18]. The epidemiology of HAT in western Kenya is very complex, and key factors can vary within very short geographical distances. The existence of two species of tsetse flies, *G. pallidipes* and *G. fuscipes fuscipes*, which have different habitats, and feeding preferences, adds to this complexity. *G. fuscipes fuscipes* feeds primarily on the Nile monitor lizard, *Varanus niloticus* [25]. This probably prompted experiments that led to the isolation of *T. brucei* from one monitor lizard [26], but the ability of these cold-blooded reptiles to support trypanosomes, other than Stercorarian forms such as *T. grayi* remains unconfirmed.

The ability to identify *T. b. rhodesiense* in reservoirs and tsetse provides a means for estimating disease risk, even in the absence of current human infections. Our study also identified one pig that was infected with trypanosomes bearing the SRA gene. It is estimated that there are more than 10,000 pigs reared in a free-range management system in the area (Dr. Samuel Maina, personal communication). Their large number, and the evidence that they can act as reservoirs underscores the importance of this study on the health and economic development of rural Africa, even on a small geographical scale.

CONCLUSION

To date, no significant efforts are made, either by the relevant government agents, or farmers to control trypanosomosis in small ruminants and pigs. This study contributes to the understanding of the epidemiology of sleeping sickness and livestock trypanosomosis in this area, with implications for the entire lake Victoria basin. Our conclusion is that small ruminants and pigs may constitute an enduring reservoir of trypanosomes that infect both humans and their livestock. Concerted efforts to control trypanosomes in these livestock can contribute significantly to a multi-disciplinary approach to trypanosomosis control in western Kenya, and other areas where the disease is endemic, and have an impact on the well being of the inhabitants of this region.

METHODS

Study Area

The study area included two districts in western Kenya, Busia and Teso. Sampling was carried out in five villages: Rukada in Busia district; Amoni, Amase, Obuchun and Ongariama in Teso district (Figure 2). These villages were selected on the basis of having reported cases of sleeping sickness within a period of about 10 years prior to the study. Samples were collected in August 2001 over a period of two weeks. The two districts lie between latitude 0° 1'South and 0° 46' North; and longitude 33° 54' West and 34° 26' East (Figure 2). The altitude varies from 1130 m to 1375 m. The mean annual rainfall is 1500 mm divided between two seasons, while annual maximum temperature ranges from 26°C to 30°C and minimum temperatures vary from 14°C to 18°C. Busia District borders Lake Victoria and the entire study area is traversed by two tributaries (rivers Sio and Malaba) and several streams that feed into them. It is a mixed farming area, with a variety of livestock species, mainly cattle, sheep and goats. Over the past two decades, free-range pig rearing has increased steadily. Two species of tsetse flies (Diptera: *Glossinidae*) infest the area. *G. fuscipes fuscipes*, which is a riverine species, associated with rivers/streams and the shores of Lake Victoria, while *G. pallidipes* is more widely distributed and associated with shrubs, thickets and open grassland. The distribution of *G. pallidipes* is discontinuous and occurs in several small foci of infestation (Kenya Trypanosomiasis Research Institute, unpublished). In areas infested with *G. pallidipes*, bushes of *Lantana camara*, a suitable habitat for resting and larviposition are widespread.

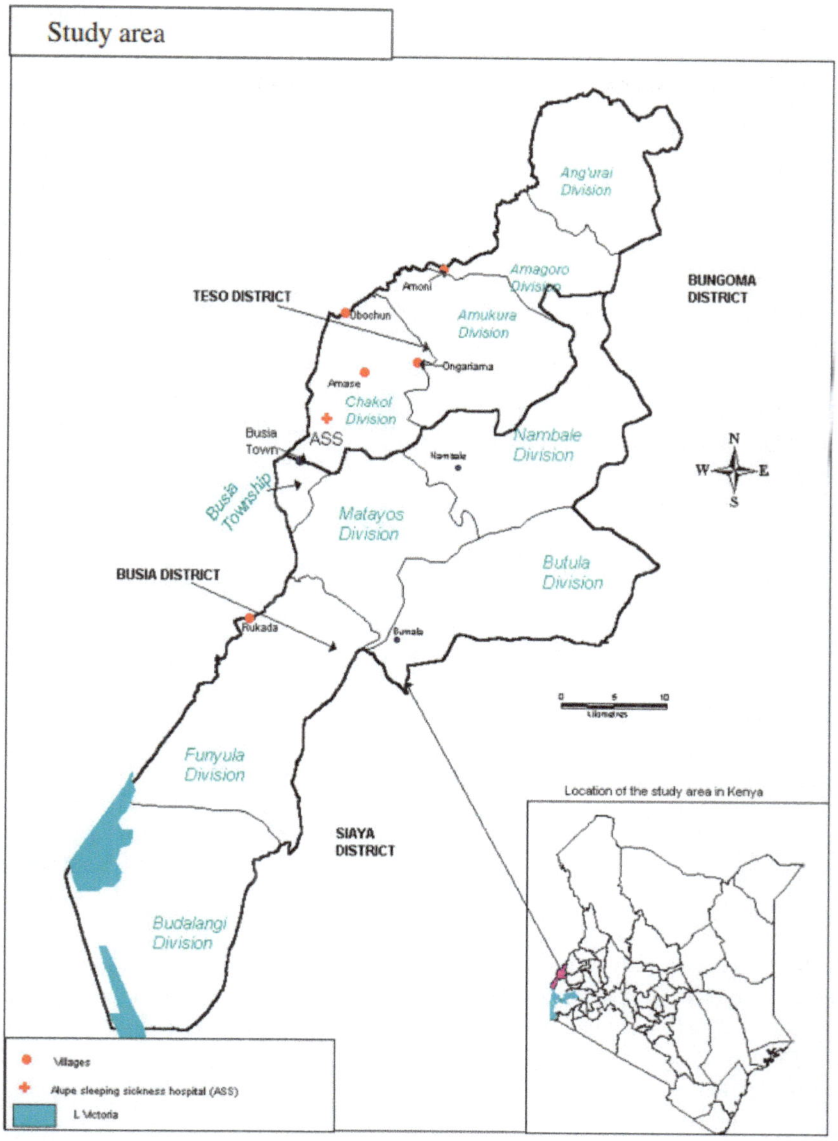

Figure 2: Detection of SRA gene. Ethidium Bromide stained 1.5% agarose gel showing PCR identification of samples containing putative *T. b. rhodesiense* using SRA A and E primers. M, 100 bp DNA marker; NC, Negative Control, +, positive control. Lanes 1 (pig), 9 (sheep) and 14 (goat) show the expected fragment of 460 bp, which indicates the detection of the SRA gene in these samples.

Animal Sampling

Blood samples were collected from 402 animals (255 goats, 95 sheep and 52 pigs) that were brought to the sampling site by local farmers. The animals were bled from the ear vein into two capillary tubes. One capillary tube was used to estimate the percentage Packed Cell Volume (%PCV) and microscopic examination for trypanosomes, and also to make an initial diagnosis on the basis of morphology and movement [20, 27]. Animals were also bled from the jugular vein into 2 ml vials containing EDTA, and stored in liquid nitrogen for further analysis.

Template Preparation and PCR Cycling

For each sample, 500 µl of cryopreserved blood was thawed into a single 1.5 ml microcentrifuge containing 500 µl of Saponin lysis buffer (0.15% w/v Saponin, 0.2% w/v NaCl and 1 mM EDTA) and mixed by vortexing. The mixture was then centrifuged at 11,000 g for 10 min in a microcentrifuge, followed by four washes in the same buffer. The resulting pellet was then resuspended in 100 µl of PCR buffer (50 mM KCl, 1.5 mM $MgCl_2$ 10 mM Tris-Cl, pH 8.3) and incubated at 95°C for 20 minutes, cooled and stored at -20°C for.

Standard PCR cycling was carried out in 25 µl reaction mixtures containing; 75 mM Tris-HCl, pH 8.8, 20 mM $(NH_4)_2SO_4$, 0.1 % Tween 20), 200 µM of each of the four deoxynucleoside triphosphates (dNTPs), primers at 1 µM, 1 µl DNA template (except for screening the presence of SRA gene, where 4 µl of template was used), and 1 unit of *Taq* DNA polymerase (Fermentas MBI, Lithuania). The PCR cycling involved an initial denaturation step at 94°C for 3 minutes, followed by 30 cycles of denaturing at 94°C for 30 s, annealing at 60°C for 45 s and extension at 72°C for 30 s, with a final elongation step at 72°C for 5 minutes. Five microlitres of each PCR product was mixed with standard loading dye (Fermentas MBI, Lithuania) and electrophoresed in 1.5% agarose, with ethidium staining (5 µg/ml) and photographed under ultraviolet illumination. A positive control (with reference DNA) and a negative control (without DNA) were included with each set of reactions. PCR primers and their source references are given in Table 2.

Statistical Analysis

Statistical analysis was performed using SPSS v11. The prevalence of trypanosome species and infection between animals were determined using chi-square test and odds ratios and their 95% confidence intervals. The level of significant difference was set at 0.05.

ACKNOWLEDGEMENTS

The authors gratefully acknowledge funding from the International Foundation for Science, IFS and the International Centre for Scientific Culture (ICSC) – World Laboratory. This study was carried out at KETRI and ICIPE, and we gratefully acknowledge the support from the Directors of the two institutions. This study benefited from the excellent fieldwork with support from staff at the KETRI Alupe station, which we hereby acknowledge. We are grateful to Dr. George Matete, head of Alupe station at the time of the study for coordinating the sampling.

AUTHORS' CONTRIBUTIONS

MNO undertook this study as part of his training for the Master of Science degree at Kenyatta University, where he was supervised by EUK and GMM. Field and laboratory activities were jointly supervised by ZKN (at KETRI), DKM and EOO (at ICIPE). All authors read and approved the final manuscript.

REFERENCES

1. Okech G, Masinde A, Stevenson P, Ndung'u JM: The role of isometamidium chloride in chemoprophylaxis against trypanosomosis of small ruminants in Kenya. Proceedings of the 24th meeting of the International Scientific Council for Trypanosomiasis Research and Control (ISCTRC), Maputo, Mozambique). Edited by: Njogu AR. 1999, Nairobi, OAU/STRC, 390-397.
2. Onyango RJ, Van Hoeve K, De Raadt P: The epidemiology of *Trypanosoma rhodesiense* sleeping sickness in Alego location central Nyanza, Kenya. I. Evidence that cattle may act as a reservoir host of trypanosomes infectious to man. Trans R Soc Trop Med Hyg. 1966, 60: 175-182. 10.1016/0035-9203(66)90024-1.
3. Mehlitz D, Zillmann U, Scott CM, Godfrey DG: Epidemiological studies on the animal reservoir of Gambian sleeping sickness. Trypanozoon. 1982, 33: 113-118.
4. Gibson WC: Will the real *Trypanosoma brucei gambiense* please stand up?. Parasitol Today. 1986, 2: 255-257. 10.1016/0169-4758(86)90011-6.
5. Jelinek T, Bisoffi Z, Bonazzi L, van Thiel P, Bronner U, de Frey A, Gundersen SG, McWhinney P, Ripamonti D: Cluster of African trypanosomiasis in travellers to Tanzanian national parks. Emerging Infect Dis. 2002, 8: 643-635.
6. Luckins AG: Trypanosomiasis in small ruminants – a major constraint to livestock production. Brit Vet J. 1992, 148: 471-472.
7. Stephen LE: Clinical manifestations of the trypanosomiasis in livestock and other domestic animals. The African trypanosomiases (George Allen and UNWIM/Ministry of overseas Development, London). 1970, 774-794.
8. Griffin L, Allonby EW: Disease syndromes in sheep and goats at a range research station in Kenya. J Comp Path. 1979, 89: 457-464. 10.1016/0021-9975(79)90037-9.
9. Katunguka-Rwakishaya E: The prevalence of trypanosomosis in small ruminants and pigs in a sleeping sickness endemic area of Buikwe country Mukono district, Uganda. Rev Elev Med Vet Trop. 1996, 49: 56-58.
10. Snow WF, Wacher TJ, Rawlings P: Observations on the prevalence of trypanosomiasis in small ruminants, equines and cattle, in relation to tsetse challenge, in The Gambia. Vet Parasitol. 1996, 66: 1-11. 10.1016/S0304-4017(96)01003-5.
11. Makumyaviri A, Mehlitz D, Kageruka P, Kazyumba GL, Molisho D: Animal reservoir hosts of *T. b. gambiense* in Zaire: trypanosome infections in two foci in Bas-Zaire. Trop Med Parasitol. 1989, 40: 258-62.
12. Masiga DK., Okech G., Irungu P, Ouma J, Wekesa S, Ouma B, Guya SO, Ndung'u JM: Growth and mortality in sheep and goats under high tsetse challenge in Kenya. Trop Anim Health Pro. 2002, 34: 489-501. 10.1023/A:1021241220575.
13. Griffin L, Allonby EW: The economic effects of trypanosomiasis in sheep and goats of a range research station in Kenya. Trop Anim Health Pro. 1979, 11: 127-132.
14. Irungu P, Nyamwaro SO, Masiga DK: Financial implication of rearing sheep and goats under natural trypanosomosis challenge at Galana ranch Kenya. Trop Anim Health Pro. 2002, 34: 503-513. 10.1023/A:1021293204645.
15. Hide G, Welburn SC, Tait A, Maudlin I: Epidemiological relationship of *Trypanosoma brucei* stock from Southeast Uganda: Evidence for different population structure in human-infective and non-human infective. Parasitol. 1994, 109: 95-111.
16. Asoganyi T, Suh S, Tetuh MD: Prevalence of domestic animal trypanosomiasis in the Fontem sleeping sickness focus, Cameroon. Rev Elev Med Vet Trop. 1990, 43: 69-74.
17. Welburn SC, Picozzi K, Fevre EM, Coleman PG, Odiit M, Carrington M, Maudlin I: Identification of human-infective trypanosomes in animal reservoir of sleeping sickness in Uganda by means of serum-resistance-associated (SRA) gene. Lancet. 2001, 358: 2017-2019. 10.1016/S0140-6736(01)07096-9.
18. Gibson W, Backhous T, Griffiths A: The human serum resistance associated gene is ubiquitous and conserved in *T. b. rhodesiense* throughout East Africa. Infect Genet Evol. 2002, 1: 207-214. 10.1016/S1567-1348(02)00028-X.
19. Radwanska M, Chamekh M, Vanhamme L, Claes F, Magez S, Magnus E, De Baetselier P, Buscher P, Pays E: The serum resistance-associated gene as a diagnostic tool for the detection of Trypanosoma brucei rhodesiense. Am J Trop Med Hyg. 2002, 67: 684-690.

20. Murray M, Murray PK, Mclntyre WM: An improved parasitological technique for the diagnosis of African trypanosomiasis. Trans R Soc Trop Med Hyg. 1977, 71: 325-326. 10.1016/0035-9203(77)90110-9.

21. Bealby KA, Connor RJ, Rowlands GJ: Trypanosomosis in Goats in Zambia. ILRI (International Livestock Research Institute), Nairobi, Kenya. 1996, 88-

22. Kalu AU, Uzoukwu M, Ikeme M: Prevalence of tsetse fly and ruminant trypanosomosis in Katsina-Ala Local Government Area, Nigeria. Roum Arch Microbiol Immunol. 1996, 55: 341-52.

23. Osear S, Goossens B, Kora S, Gaye M, Darboe L: Health and productivity of traditionally managed Djallonke sheep and West African dwarf goats under high and moderate trypanosomosis risk. Vet Parasitol. 1999, 82: 101-109. 10.1016/S0304-4017(99)00011-4.

24. Kayang BB, Bosompem KM, Assoku RK, Awumbla B: Detection of *T. brucei*, *T. congolense* and *T. vivax* infections in cattle, sheep and goats using latex agglutination. Int J Parasiot. 1997, 27: 83-7. 10.1016/S0020-7519(96)00160-9.

25. Mohamed-Ahmad MM, Odulaja A: Diet activity patterns and host preferences of *Glossina fuscipes fuscipes* (Diptera: Glossinidae) along the shores of Lake Victoria, Kenya. Bull Ent Res. 1997, 89: 179-186.

26. Njagu Z, Mihok S, Kokwaro E, Verloo D: Isolation of *Trypanosoma brucei* from the monitor lizard (*Varanus niloticus*) in an endemic focus of Rhodesian sleeping sickness in Kenya. Acta Trop. 1999, 72: 137-148. 10.1016/S0001-706X(98)00092-8.

27. Hoare CA: 1972, trypanosomes of mammals. Blackwell scientific publications. Oxford and Edinburgh, 483-484.

28. Masiga DK, Smyth AJ, Bromidge TJ, Hayes P, Gibson WC: Sensitive detection of trypanosomes in tsetse flies by DNA amplification. Int J Parasitol. 1992, 22: 909-918. 10.1016/0020-7519(92)90047-O.

29. Morlais I, Ravel S, Grebaut P, Dumas V, Cuny G: New molecular marker for *Trypanosoma* (*Duttonella*) *vivax*identification. Acta Trop. 2001, 80: 207-213. 10.1016/S0001-706X(01)00160-7.

SECTION II: PARASITES OF CATTLE

CHAPTER 3

GASTROINTESTINAL HELMINTHS IN SLAUGHTERED CATTLE IN IBADAN, SOUTH-WESTERN NIGERIA

Olubukola Deborah Adedipe, Emmanuel Chibuike Uwalaka, Victor Oluwatoyin Akinseye, Oyeduntan Adejoju Adediran, and Simeon Idowu Babalola Cadmus

INTRODUCTION

Cattle, the most prominent domesticated livestock in Nigeria, represent a valuable asset in both traditional and modern agriculture; in addition, they also provide meat, milk, skin, and draught power for farming [1]. In some traditional settings, they also play an essential role in the socioeconomic system, representing family wealth or they can be regarded as a survival kit by nomadic people [2]. In Nigeria, the livestock sector contributes 5.2% of the gross domestic products (GDP) while cattle production solely contributes 50% of the total meat [3]. Meat is one of the most important livestock products, although there could be losses due to various diseases including helminth infections. The quantity of meat and revenue obtained from domestic livestock is far below the national demand due to factors such as death and ill health with associated reduced productivity and increased cost of treatment [4–6].

Helminths are known to be a major constraint to ruminants' well-being and productive performance [7–9]. Gastrointestinal helminths are ubiquitous parasitic agents of livestock especially ruminants and are known to limit cattle production in many areas and countries [7, 9]. Mortality of animals due to parasitic diseases may not be alarming at times but their indirect effects on livestock productivity and their zoonotic impact on human health are considerably greater [10–12]. Indirect losses associated with helminth infections include the reduction in productive potential such as decreased growth rate, weight loss, diarrhea, anorexia, and sometimes anaemia [13–15].

The most important predisposing factors of helminth infections are grazing habits, climate, nutritional deficiency, pasture management, immunological status, vector, presence of intermediate host, and the number of infective larvae and eggs in the environment [16]. The effect of helminth infections is determined by a combination of factors, of which the varying susceptibility of the host species, the pathogenicity of the parasite species, the host/parasite interaction, and the infective dose are the most important [17].

A literature review of the last decade reveals paucity of information on the prevalence of gastrointestinal helminths of slaughtered cattle in south-western Nigeria. This current study therefore aims at determining the prevalence of gastrointestinal helminths of slaughtered cattle in south-western Nigeria. This is with a view of providing a baseline epidemiological data on this group of parasites and other livestock diseases of economic and zoonotic importance in an ongoing study in Nigeria.

Citation: Olubukola Deborah Adedipe, Emmanuel Chibuike Uwalaka, Victor Oluwatoyin Akinseye, Oyeduntan Adejoju Adediran, and Simeon Idowu Babalola Cadmus, "Gastrointestinal Helminths in Slaughtered Cattle in Ibadan, South-Western Nigeria," Journal of Veterinary Medicine, vol. 2014, Article ID 923561, 6 pages, 2014. doi:10.1155/2014/923561.

MATERIALS AND METHODS

Study Area

This study was carried out at the Bodija Municipal Abattoir, a major abattoir located in Ibadan, south-western Nigeria. Cattle slaughtered in this abattoir are mostly sourced from different cattle rearing regions of Nigeria (mainly northern Nigeria) and some neighboring African countries including Burkina Faso, Cameroon, Chad, Mali, and Niger. Hence, this abattoir serves as a good source of sentinel survey for diseases (including helminthic infections) from different regions of Nigeria and beyond. Again, because of its location and large number of animals slaughtered, this abattoir serves as a major source of meat consumed in Ibadan, a cosmopolitan city with a population of about 4 million people.

Sample Collection and Identification

Systematic random sampling method was employed in selecting cattle that were screened at antemortem. For each animal screened, parameters such as the sex, breed, and body condition score were recorded. Faecal samples were collected per rectum into well-labeled sterile polythene bags and transported in ice packs to the Parasitology Laboratory, Department of Veterinary Microbiology and Parasitology, Faculty of Veterinary Medicine, University of Ibadan, where they were examined for helminth egg according to the protocols earlier described by Thienpoint [18] and Khin-Khin [19]. Eggs were identified on the basis of their morphological features as described by Soulsby [20].

Data Analysis

Data were subjected to descriptive statistical analysis using percentages in determining the prevalence rates in the different breeds, sex, and body condition score groups. Prevalence of helminthosis in relation to sex, breed, and body condition score was analyzed using Chi-square statistical test.

RESULTS

In all, 397 cattle were screened and 163 (41.6%) were positive for gastrointestinal helminth eggs. We found several helminths from eight genera, including four nematodes (strongyle-type eggs, Strongyloides spp.,Toxocara vitulorum, and Nematodirus spp.) (Figure 1); three trematodes (Paramphistomum spp., Fasciola gigantica, and Dicrocoelium dendriticum) (Figure 2); and one cestode (Moniezia benedeni) (Figure 3). The prevalence of all identified parasitic helminth eggs (Table 1) showed that strongyle-type eggs had the highest prevalence, and Nematodirus spp. present the least occurrence.

Table 1: Prevalence of gastrointestinal helminths obtained from slaughtered cattle in south-western Nigeria

Species of helminth	Number of examined samples	Number of positive samples (n)	Prevalence (%)
Strongyle-type eggs	397	260	65.50
Strongyloides species	397	19	4.86
Toxocara vitulorum	397	4	1.01
Nematodirus sp.	397	1	0.3
Paramphistomum cervi	397	61	15.37
Fasciola gigantica	397	34	8.56
Dicrocoelium dendriticum	397	10	2.52
Moniezia benedeni	397	8	2.01

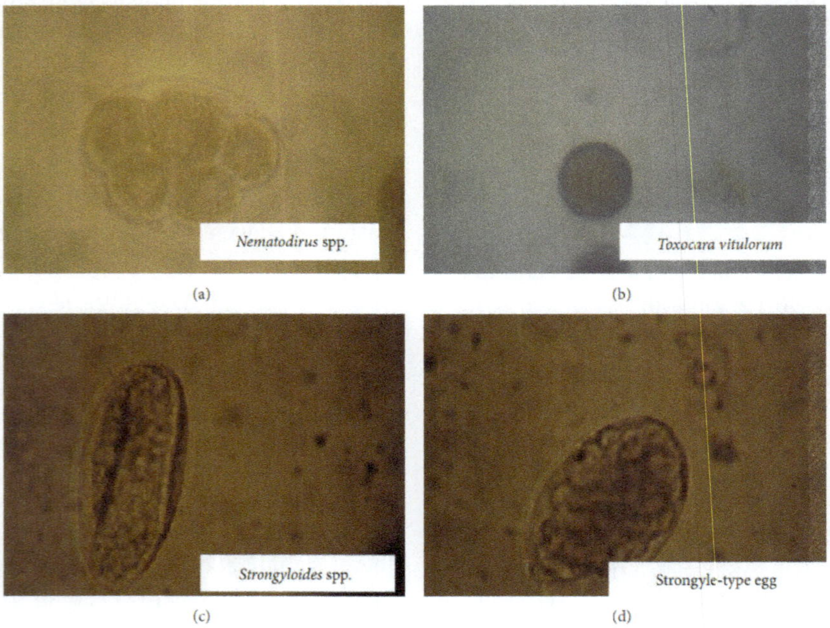

Figure 1: Micrograph of gastrointestinal nematode eggs (magnification ×40) obtained from slaughtered cattle in south-western Nigeria.

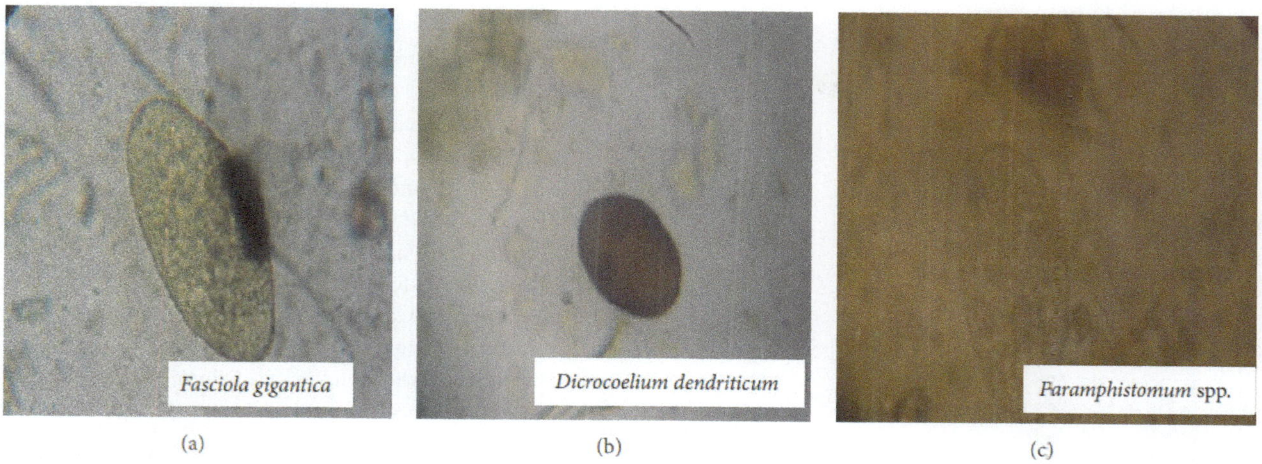

Figure 2: Micrograph of gastrointestinal trematode eggs (magnification ×40) obtained from slaughtered cattle in south-western Nigeria.

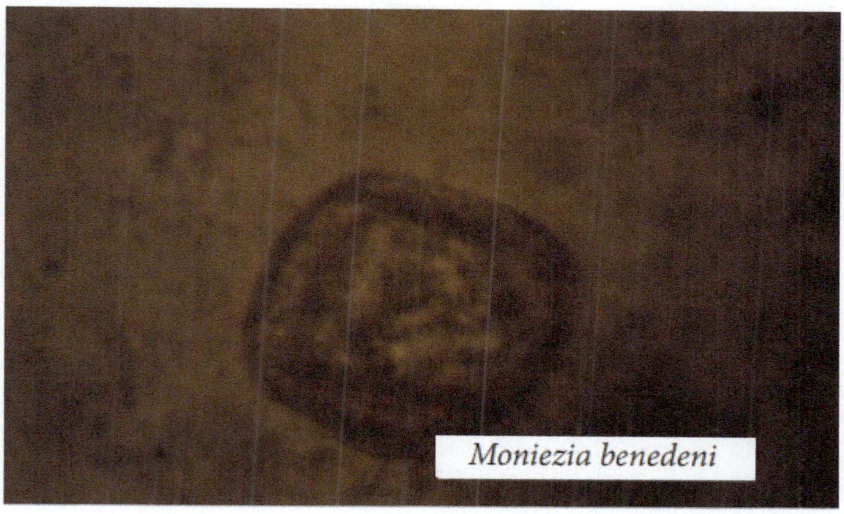

Figure 3: Micrograph of gastrointestinal cestode egg (magnification ×40) obtained from slaughtered cattle in south-western Nigeria.

The prevalence of helminths in relation to sex reveals that 40.0% (24/60) of the male and 41.25% (139/337) of the female were infected, respectively (Table 2). The percentage of the male infected was similar to that of the female, with the female (OR = 1.1; 95% CI: 0.60–1.84) showing slightly higher likelihood of being infected with gastrointestinal helminth when compared to the male. The Bunaji breed of cattle had the highest infection rate of 46% (69/150) followed by Sokoto Gudali (39.13%; 39/92) and the Rahaji (37.42%; 58/155), respectively. The Rahaji (OR = 0.7; 95% CI: 0.44–1.11) and Sokoto Gudali (OR = 0.8; 95% CI: 0.45–1.32) breeds showed lower likelihood of being infected with gastrointestinal helminth when compared to the Bunaji breed (Table 2). A higher percentage of gastrointestinal helminth infection of 48.1% (93/397) was however observed in cattle with moderate body score; and this group of cattle showed higher likelihood of being infected with gastrointestinal helminth when compared to those that were emaciated (OR = 1.2; 95% CI: 0.80–1.79; Table 2).

Table 2: Prevalence of gastrointestinal helminths obtained from slaughtered cattle in south-western Nigeria in relation to sex, breed, and body condition score

Variable	Category	RBT		OR	95% CI	value
		Positive n (%)	Negative n (%)			
Breed	Bunaji	69 (46.00)	81 (54.00)	1		
	Rahaji	58 (37.42)	97 (62.58)	0.7	0.44–1.11	0.16
	Sokoto Gudali	36 (39.13)	56 (60.87)	0.8	0.45–1.32	0.36
Sex	Male	24 (40.00)	36 (60.00)	1		
	Female	139 (41.25)	198 (58.75)	1.1	0.60–1.84	0.97
Body condition score	Emaciated	70 (38.67)	111 (61.33)			
	Moderate	93 (43.06)	123 (56.94)	1.2	0.80–1.79	0.43

In all, the nature of parasitism among the cattle was observed to range from single to varying mixed infections (Figure 4).

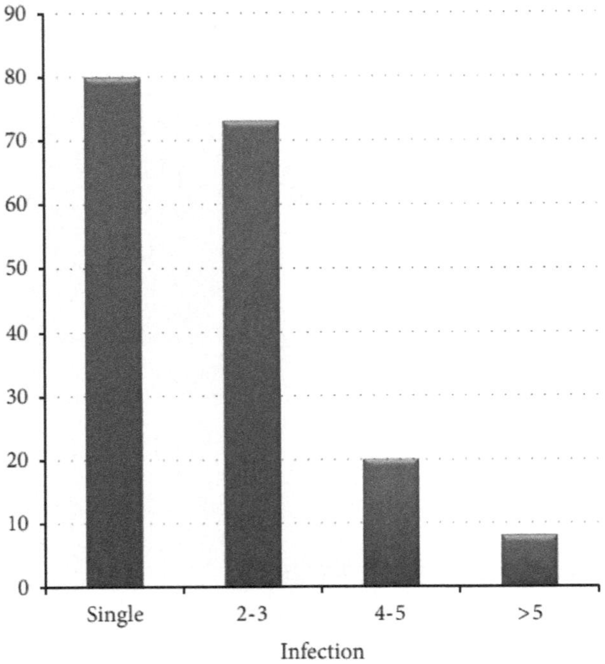

Figure 4: Distribution of gastrointestinal helminth infection among slaughtered cattle in south-western Nigeria.

DISCUSSION

The findings of this study show that 41.6% (163/397) of the cattle screened had helminth infection, thus providing valuable information on the burden of helminths among cattle in Nigeria since animals slaughtered in this abattoir are representative of cattle in the country. Precisely, nematode infections were particularly high, as they accounted for 71.7% of the total helminth burden. High nematode infection has huge impact on livestock production since they result in reduced milk, meat, wool, hide products, and stamina of working animals [10–12], hence resulting in the diminution of production potentials such as decreased growth rate, weight loss in young growing calves, and late maturity of the animals [15]. Trematode (26.5%) and cestode (2.01%) infections were lower; however, they are of significant public health importance. Fasciola gigantica andDicrocoelium dendriticum are both liver trematodes known to be zoonotic and have caused considerable economic losses and health problems [21, 22].

The overall prevalence of 41.6% of helminth infection obtained in this study is similar to that of Edosomwan and Shoyemi [23] who reported a prevalence of 47.4% in south-south region of Nigeria but lower than the 50.8% and 62.1% earlier reported in south-eastern and south-southern Nigeria, respectively [24, 25]. The differences observed could be due to the periods or seasons in which the studies were conducted as well as the sources of cattle sampled in the various regions. Furthermore, our findings revealed that strongyle-type eggs were the most prevalent among the helminths; however, this is at variance with previous reports by Hailu et al. [26], Mir et al. [27], and Nwigwe et al. [24] who reported trematodes as the most prevalent helminths in studies carried out in India, Ethiopia, and eastern Nigeria, respectively. This difference could however be associated with the differences in geographical and/or climatic conditions and ecology since the presence of trematode infections is dependent on availability of the intermediate hosts.

Again, the helminths identified in this study were similar to those identified by Edosomwan and Shoyemi [23] and Elele et al. [25] in earlier studies carried out in Benin and Port Harcourt, south-south Nigeria. Findings from these studies showed that 12 and 16 different helminths were obtained from Benin and Port Harcourt, respectively, and some of the helminths are similar to those found in our study. It can therefore be suggested that the similarity in the helminth profile indicates exposure of these animals to common conditions (e.g., ecology, pasture, and humidity) which are prevalent in northern Nigeria where majority of these animals are sourced from before being transported to different abattoirs in Nigeria.

Furthermore, this study reveals that both the male and female animals have equal likelihood of being infected with gastrointestinal helminths. One major factor that would have accounted for this is the fact that both the male and female cattle under the local setting in Nigeria are exposed to poor feeding and veterinary care, factors accountable for equal susceptibility to helminth infections. Though earlier findings by Raza et al. [28] indicated that the male cattle were more likely to be infected with helminth than the female, reason given was that male animals were more aggressive when feeding and thus likely to pick up more ova of helminths on the pasture. Furthermore, male domestic ungulates are said to be more susceptible to infections with gastrointestinal tract parasites than females due to hormones debilitating immune functions, which favor the growth and spread of parasites in male guts [29, 30]. Despite these, the phenomenon of parasitism during pregnancy due to stress and decreased immune competence [31] in female animals may have neutralized the possibility of more male infection in our study. Although we do not have the exact number of pregnant female animals during this study, some were found pregnant at slaughter. This factor, we believe, would also have contributed to the similarity in the prevalence of helminth infection in both the male and female animals.

The breed prevalences of 46.00%, 37.42%, and 39.13% obtained for Bunaji, Rahaji, and Sokoto Gudali breeds of cattle, respectively, were lower compared to the 62% (Bunaji) and 62.2% (Sokoto Gudali) as earlier reported by Elele et al. [25]. The difference in the prevalence obtained could be attributed to the existence of favorable environmental factors necessary for the prolonged survival and development of infective larval stage of most helminths [32]. Furthermore, management system of animals could also be accountable for the difference in prevalence [33]. Cattle with moderate body condition score had higher prevalence of gastrointestinal helminths when compared to those that were emaciated. Possible reason for this could be that those with moderate body condition for a number of reasons, including good nutrition, tolerated helminth infections better or that both host and parasites had reached a state of equilibrium and were asymptomatic at the point of faecal collection [34]. In addition, we also found that more mixed infections were prevalent in comparison to single infections in our study. Mixed infection was characterized by the presence of two or more helminths. The phenomenon of mixed infection has been suggested to be an important cause of morbidity and reduced production in livestock [35]. Furthermore, the immunosuppression of the host immune system by mixed infections increases host susceptibility to other diseases or parasites [36].

Coincidentally, farmers and meat consumers (including abattoir workers) are known to be susceptible to zoonotic helminthic infections resulting from some strongyle-type eggs (i.e., Trichostrongylus sp. andOesophagostomum radiatum), Dicrocoelium dendriticum, and Fasciola gigantica [12, 37, 38]. Again, earlier reports have also indicated very high human infections among farmers in the developing world, where close contact exists between humans and animals and where minimal hygiene and sanitation occurs [39]. Furthermore, the bovine species due to their susceptibility to various zoonotic diseases are known to be a source of higher health risk to humans given their close interactions and cohabitation with humans [12, 40].

CONCLUSION

The result of this study shows a moderately high prevalence of gastrointestinal helminth infection of both economic and zoonotic importance among trade cattle slaughtered in south-western Nigeria. This has negative impact on both animal production and public health. Therefore, to mitigate these problems, appropriate anthelminthic regimen and control measures (i.e., comprehensive parasite control program, pasture management, and environmental sanitation) in cattle and public health awareness should be encouraged. Finally, there is a need to monitor gastrointestinal parasites of cattle to promote animal production and public health in Nigeria.

ACKNOWLEDGMENTS

The authors sincerely thank the abattoir workers at the Bodija Municipal Abattoir, Ibadan, Oyo State, Nigeria, for their cooperation while carrying out this project. They also thank the laboratory technologists of the Department of Veterinary Microbiology and Parasitology, University of Ibadan, for their laboratory support. The funding support received by Dr. Cadmus from the John D. and Catherine T. MacArthur Foundation, USA, under the Higher Education Initiative in Africa (Grant no. 97944-0-800/406/99) is appreciated.

REFERENCES

1. O. O. Tewe, Sustainability and Development: Paradigms from Nigeria's Livestock Industry, Inaugural Lecture series, University of Ibadan Press, Ibadan, Nigeria, 1997.
2. J. P. Fabiyi, "Seasonal fluctuations of nematode infestations in goats in the savanna belt of Nigeria,"Bulletin of Epizootic Diseases of Africa, vol. 21, pp. 227–286, 1973.
3. N. O. Adedipe, J. S. Bakshi, O. A. Odegbaro, and A. Aliyu, Evolving the Nigeria Agricultural Research Strategy Plan: Agro-Ecological Inputs, National Agricultural Research Project (NARP), 1996.
4. M. M. Hossain, S. Paul, M. M. Rahman, F. M. A. Hossain, M. T. Hossain, and M. R. Islam, "Prevalence and economic significance of caprine fascioliasis at sylhet district of Bangladesh," Pakistan Veterinary Journal, vol. 31, no. 2, pp. 113–116, 2011. ·
5. M. B. Bolajoko, G. D. Moses, K. O. Gambari-Bolajoko, V. I. Ifende, P. Emenna, and A. Bala, "Participatory rural appraisal of livestock diseases among the Fulani community of the Barkin Ladi local government area," Journal of Veterinary Medicine and Animal Health, vol. 3, no. 1, pp. 11–13, 2011.
6. P. O. Ozung, P. U. Owai, and K. O. Oni, "An assessment of the prevalence of fascioliasis of ruminants in Ikom Abattoir of Cross River State Nigeria," Continental Journal of Veterinary Sciences, vol. 5, no. 1, pp. 1–5, 2011.
7. J. D. Keyyu, J. Monrad, N. C. Kyvsgaard, and A. A. Kassuku, "Epidemiology of Fasciola gigantica and amphistomes in cattle on traditional, small-scale dairy and large-scale dairy farms in the southern highlands of Tanzania," Tropical Animal Health and Production, vol. 37, no. 4, pp. 303–314, 2005.
8. Z. I. Rajput, S.-H. Hu, W.-J. Chen, A. G. Arijo, and C.-W. Xiao, "Importance of ticks and their chemical and immunological control in livestock," Journal of Zhejiang University Science B, vol. 7, no. 11, pp. 912–921, 2006.
9. U. W. Hesterberg, R. Bagnall, K. Perrett, R. Horner, and B. Gummow, "A questionnaire survey of perceptions and preventive measures related to animal health amongst cattle owners of rural communities in KwaZulu-Natal, South Africa," Journal of the South African Veterinary Association, vol. 78, no. 4, pp. 205–208, 2007. ·
10. L. R. Ballweber, "Diagnostic methods for parasitic infections," Veterinary Clinics of North America, vol. 22, no. 3, pp. 695–705, 2006.
11. C. O. Nwosu, P. P. Madu, and W. S. Richards, "Prevalence and seasonal changes in the population of gastrointestinal nematodes of small ruminants in the semi-arid zone of north-eastern Nigeria,"Veterinary Parasitology, vol. 144, no. 1-2, pp. 118–124, 2007. · ·
12. P. S. Ekong, R. Juryit, N. M. Dika, P. Nguku, and M. Musenero, "Prevalence and risk factors for zoonotic helminth infection among humans and animals—Jos, Nigeria, 2005–2009," The Pan African Medical Journal, vol. 12, article 6, 2012. ·
13. J. Nahed-Toral, Q. López-Tirado, G. Mendoza-Martínez, A. Aluja-Schunemann, and F. J. Trigo-Tavera, "Epidemiology of parasitosis in the Tzotzil sheep production system," Small Ruminant Research, vol. 49, no. 2, pp. 199–206, 2003.
14. R. Gonzalez and A. C. Gonzalez, "Alternatives for the control of gastrointestinal nematodes in sheep," inProceedings of the European Population Forum (EEPF ‹04), Matanzas, Cuba, 2004.
15. E. S. Swai, P. F. Mtui, A. N. Mbise, E. Kaaya, P. Sanka, and P. M. Loomu, "Prevalence of gastro intestinal parasite infections in Maasai cattle in Ngorongoro District, Tanzania," Livestock Research for Rural Development, vol. 18, no. 8, 2006. ·
16. O. M. Radostits, D. C. Blood, and C. C. Gay, "Diseases caused by helminth parasites," in Veterinary Medicine: A Textbook of Diseases of Cattle, Sheep, Pigs, Goats and Horses, pp. 1223–1230, Bailliere Tindall, London, UK, 8th edition, 1994.
17. Food and Agricultural Organisation, "Distribution and impact of helminth diseases of livestock in developing countries," in FAO Corporate Document Repository—Agriculture and Consumer Protection, 2000.

18. D. Thienpoint, Diagnosing Helminthiasis through Coprological Examination, Janssen Research Foundation, Beerse, Belgium, 1979.
19. L. Khin-Khin, Prevalence of Cryptosporidium, Giardia and other gastrointestinal parasites in dairy calves in Mandalay, Myanmar, Chuang Mai University and Freie Universität Berlin, 2007.
20. E. J. L. Soulsby, Helminths, Arthropods and Protozoa of Domesticated Animals, Bailliere Tindall, London, UK, 7th edition, 1982.
21. M. H. M. Ghazani, M. R. Valilou, F. B. Kharati, and K. Zirak, "Prevalence of sheep liver hydatid cyst in the Northwest region of Iran," Asian Journal of Animal and Veterinary Advances, vol. 3, no. 1, pp. 30–35, 2008.
22. A. Zuko and A. Hodžić, "A slaughterhouse study on prevalence of sheep liver helminths in region of Sarajevo," MESO, vol. 13, pp. 102–104, 2011.
23. E. U. Edosomwan and O. O. Shoyemi, "Prevalence of gastrointestinal helminth parasites of cattle and goats slaughtered at abattoirs in Benin City, Nigeria," African Scientist, vol. 13, no. 2, pp. 109–114, 2012.
24. J. O. Nwigwe, O. O. Njoku, O. O. Odikamnoro, and C. A. Uhuo, "Comparative study of intestinal helminths and protozoa of cattle and goats in Abakaliki metropolis of Ebonyi State, Nigeria," Advances in Applied Science Research, vol. 4, no. 2, pp. 223–227, 2013.
25. K. Elele, O. Owhoeli, and L. B. Gboeloh, "Prevalence of species of helminths parasites in cattle slaughtered in selected abattoirs in Port Harcourt, south-south, Nigeria," International Research on Medical Sciences, vol. 1, no. 2, pp. 10–17, 2013.
26. D. Hailu, A. Cherenet, Y. Moti, and T. Tadele, "Study on gastrointestinal helminth infections in small-scale dairy cattle farms of Jimma town, Ethiopia," Ethiopian Journal of Applied Sciences and Technology, vol. 2, no. 1, pp. 31–37, 2011.
27. M. R. Mir, M. Z. Chishti, M. Rashid et al., "Point prevalence of gastrointestinal helminthiasis in large ruminants of Jammu, India," International Journal of Scientific and Research Publications, vol. 3, no. 3, pp. 5–8, 2013.
28. M. A. Raza, M. M. Ayaz, S. Murtaza et al., "Prevalence of GIT helminths in cattle at the vicinities of Tehsil Jatoi, Punjab," Science International (Lahore), vol. 25, no. 2, pp. 305–309, 2013.
29. N. Hillgarth and J. C. Wingfield, "Parasite-mediated sexual selection: endocrine aspects," in Host-Parasite Evolution: General Principals and Avian Models, D. H. Clayton and J. Moore, Eds., pp. 78–104, Oxford University Press, New York, NY, USA, 1997.
30. A. Apio, M. Plath, and T. Wronski, "Patterns of gastrointestinal parasitic infections in the bushbuckTragelaphus scriptus from the Queen Elizabeth National Park, Uganda," Journal of Helminthology, vol. 80, no. 3, pp. 213–218, 2006.
31. G. M. Urquhart, J. Armour, J. L. Duncan, A. M. Dunn, and F. W. Jennings, Veterinary Parasitology, vol. 28, Blackwell Science, 2nd edition, 1996.
32. C. E. Rossanigo and L. Gruner, "Moisture and temperature requirements in faeces for the development of free-living stages of gastrointestinal nematodes of sheep, cattle and deer," Journal of Helminthology, vol. 69, no. 4, pp. 357–362, 1995.
33. F. Regassa, T. Sori, R. Dhuguma, and Y. Kiros, "Epidemiology of gastrointestinal parasites of ruminants in Western Oromia, Ethiopia," International Journal of Applied Research of Veterinary Medicine, vol. 4, no. 1, pp. 51–57, 2006.
34. E. Moreau and A. Chauvin, "Immunity against helminths: interactions with the host and the intercurrent infections," Journal of Biomedicine and Biotechnology, vol. 2010, Article ID 428593, 9 pages, 2010.
35. B. Kumsa, T. Tadesse, T. Sari, R. Duguma, and B. Hussen, "Helminths of sheep and goats in Central Oromia (Ethiopia) during the dry season," Journal of Animal and Veterinary Advances, vol. 10, no. 14, pp. 1845–1849, 2011.
36. C. R. Wang, J. H. Qiu, J. P. Zhao, L. M. Xu, W. C. Yu, and X. Q. Zhu, "Prevalence of helminthes in adult dogs in Heilongjiang Province, the People›s Republic of China," Parasitology Research, vol. 99, no. 5, pp. 627–630, 2006.
37. J. McCarthy and T. A. Moore, "Emerging helminth zoonoses," International Journal for Parasitology, vol. 30, no. 12-13, pp. 1351–1359, 2000.
38. J. M. Goldsmid, R. Speare, and S. Bettiol, "The parasitology of foods," in Foodborne Microorganisms of Public Health Significance, A. D. Hocking, Ed., pp. 705–722, AIFST, Waterloo, Canada, 6th edition, 2003.
39. V. J. Adams, M. B. Markus, J. F. Adams et al., "Paradoxical helminthiasis and giardiasis in Cape Town, South Africa: epidemiology and control," African Health Science, vol. 5, pp. 276–280, 2005.
40. S. I. B. Cadmus, "The transmission chain of Mycobacterium bovis from cattle to humans and within the human setting in Nigeria: facts, reality and way forward," Tropical Veterinarian, vol. 28, no. 1, pp. 1–12, 2010.

CHAPTER 4

GENETIC CHARACTERIZATION, SPECIES DIFFERENTIATION AND DETECTION OF FASCIOLA SPP. BY MOLECULAR APPROACHES

Lin Ai, Mu-Xin Chen, Samer Alasaad, Hany M Elsheikha, Juan Li, Hai-Long Li, Rui-Qing Lin, Feng-Cai Zou, Xing-Quan Zhu and Jia-Xu Chen

BACKGROUND

Fascioliasis is an important food-and water-borne parasitic zoonosis caused by liver flukes of the genus *Fasciola* (Platyhelminthes: Digenea: Fasciolidae) [1, 2]. *Fasciola* spp. have a cosmopolitan distribution, with high frequency in tropical areas [1, 3, 4]. Human fascioliasis has been reported in numerous countries [1, 3, 5]. It is estimated that millions of people are infected worldwide and the number of people at risk exceeds 180 million [6]. Also, fascioliasis is one of the most important parasitic diseases in grazing animals with over 700 million production animals being at risk of infection and economic losses were estimated at > US$ 2 billion per year worldwide [6].

A few species have been described within the genus *Fasciola*, but only three species, *Fasciola hepatica, Fasciola gigantica* and *Fasciola jacksoni* are commonly recognized as taxonomically valid, with *F. hepatica*mainly occurring in temperate areas, *F. gigantica* in tropical zones, and both taxa overlapping in subtropical areas [6, 7, 8, 9, 10, 11]. *F. jacksoni* is known as the fasciolid of Asian elephants and its phylogenetic position is still uncertain [12]. Given the adverse impact of *Fasciola* infection on human health and its economic significance, rapid and accurate identification of *Fasciola* species is necessary for successful clinical management of infection, and for epidemiological surveys.

For a long time, the identification of *Fasciola* spp. has been based solely on traditional morphological approaches. However, due to the limitations of morphological methods, various molecular approaches have been developed and used for the identification and differentiation of *Fasciola* species. Importantly, these molecular methods have raised questions and spurred debate on the recognition of the "intermediate*Fasciola*" as a hybrid/introgressed form between *F. hepatica* and *F. gigantica* [8, 13, 14, 15, 16, 17, 18, 19, 20]. This hybrid *Fasciola* represents the emergence of a natural diversity previously undetected using conventional approaches, probably because of the inadequacy of their discriminatory power.

This article reviews molecular techniques used to identify and detect genetic variation among *Fasciola* spp.

The Identification and Recognition of the "Intermediate *Fasciola*"

A number of genetic and phylogenetic studies (Table 1) using different molecular targets have shown the existence of novel "intermediate *Fasciola*" [13, 14, 15, 16, 17, 18, 19, 21, 22, 23]. Ribosomal DNA (rDNA) is one of the most useful markers in genetic studies because it is available in high copy number and contains variable regions flanked by more conserved regions [24]. Previous studies have demonstrated that the first and second internal transcribed spacers (ITS-1 and ITS-2) of rDNA located between the nuclear small and large subunit rRNA genes can provide genetic markers for species-level identification of *Fasciola* [14, 18, 21, 22, 25] (Table 1). The ITS-2 sequence motifs were considered the DNA barcodes for *Fasciola* spp. [26]. Comparing ITS-2 sequences, six sites at which *F. gigantica* and *F. hepatica* differ were found, and one of these is a deletion in *F. gigantica* relative to *F. hepatica* [18, 22, 25, 27]. Whereas, the "intermediate *Fasciola*" has nucleotides shared between the two *Fasciola* species. In agreement with results obtained by using ITS-2 sequences, *F. gigantica*was found to be different from *F. hepatica* at five nucleotide positions in the ITS-1 sequences, whereas the "intermediate *Fasciola*" has the ITS-1 sequence of both *F. gigantica* and *F.*

Citation: Ai et al.: Genetic characterization, species differentiation and detection of Fasciola spp. by molecular approaches. Parasites & Vectors 2011 4:101. doi:10.1186/1756-3305-4-101.

hepatica [15, 16, 17, 21]. In addition to the ITS sequences, the D2 region of 28S rDNA provided genetic evidence for the existence of natural hybridization between *F. gigantica* and *F. hepatica* in Korea [18].

Table 1: Summary of molecular approaches used for the detection and/or genetic differentiation of *Fasciola* spp..

Molecular approach	**Species investigated**			**Developmental stage**			**DNA target regions**	**References**
	F. hepatica	***F. gigantica***	**Intermediate form**	**Adult**	**Cercaria**	**Eggs**		
Conventional PCR	√			√			ITS2	38
	√	√	√	√			ITS2	14, 27
	√	√		√			ITS1, ITS2	25
	√			√			*nad* 1, *cox* 1	28
	√	√	√	√			*nad* 1, *cox* 1	13, 17
	√	√	√	√			ITS2, *cox* 1	9
	√	√	√	√			ITS1, *nad* 1	16
	√	√	√	√			*cox* 1, ITS1, ITS2	15
	√	√	√	√			*nad* 1, *cox* 1, ITS2, 28S	18
	√			√			Complete mitochondrial genome	30
		√			√		124 bp repetitive DNA sequence	49
	√				√		124 bp repetitive DNA sequence	50
	√			√			28S	39
Multiplex PCR	√				√		*cox* 1, ITS1, ITS2	52
Specific PCR	√	√	√	√	√	√	ITS2	47
PCR-RFLP	√	√	√	√			ITS2	22
		√		√			*cox* 1, ITS2	23
	√	√	√	√			ITS1	8, 21
PCR-SSCP	√	√		√			Repetitive DNA sequences	46
RAPD-PCR		√		√			Random nucleotide sequence	43
	√	√	√	√			Random nucleotide sequence	53
SRAP	√			√			Random nucleotide sequence	42
	√	√	√	√			Random nucleotide sequence	10

DNA probe		√			√		Repetitive DNA fragments	48
TaqMan real-time PCR	√	√	√	√			ITS2	54
LAMP	√	√	√	√	√	√	IGS	58
PCR	√			√			Microsatellites	59

Other molecular markers being used frequently are mitochondrial DNA (mtDNA) sequences. Almost all of eukaryotes contain a mitochondrial genome which evolves at a faster rate than the nuclear genome and, is thus suitable for discriminating closely related organisms [28, 29, 30], especially at the species and sub-species levels [31, 32, 33]. mtDNA sequence analysis also provided evidence for the existence of the "intermediate*Fasciola*" [15, 16, 19].

Genetic Variation among and within *Fasciola* spp

Revealing genetic variation has been the focus of many studies because accurate analysis of genetic variability has important implications for studying population biology, epidemiology, and genetic structure of these parasites, and thus the efficient control of the diseases they cause.

Examination of *Fasciola* specimens from geographical areas where *F. hepatica* and *F. gigantica* co-exist, such as Egypt and Iran, demonstrated the existence of phenotypic variations in adult flukes [20, 34]. Molecular approaches utilizing a number of genetic makers are useful for genetic characterization and studies of genetic variability among parasite populations [35, 36, 37]. A recent study investigated the extent of genetic variation among *Fasciola* collected from different host species and geographical localities in Spain using ITS rDNA as genetic markers, and concluded that only a single species *F. hepatica* exists in Spain, although a slight sequence variation in the ITS-2 was detected among *F. hepatica* samples from different host species and geographical areas [38]. Spanish *F. hepatica* examined in that study differed from *F. hepatica* from elsewhere by two nucleotides in the ITS-2 [38]. Another study detected some genetic variations in *F. hepatica* from northwest of Spain using the 28S rDNA as genetic marker, and there were nucleotide differences in a number of sequence positions [39].

Sequence related amplified polymorphism (SRAP) is a molecular technique for detecting genetic variation in the open reading frames (ORFs) of genomes of related organisms [40, 41]. A recent study showed that the SRAP technique was useful for revealing genetic variability within and between *F. hepatica, F. gigantica* and the "intermediate *Fasciola*", which substantiated the evidence for the existence of the "intermediate *Fasciola*" [10]. Using the same technique, genetic variability among a number of *F. hepatica* samples collected from six host species and 16 geographical locations in Spain was investigated [42], and a low genetic variation in the coding regions of the genomes was found, indicating the lack of genetic association between *F. hepatica* and their hosts and/or geographical locations in Spain [42].

Randomly amplified polymorphic DNA (RAPD) is a useful genetic marker for the identification and genetic characterization of parasite populations [37]. RAPD is a useful technique for the identification and differentiation of *F. hepatica* and *F. gigantica*. Using the RAPD technique, some degree of genetic variation was detected among *F. gigantica* isolates from cattle, buffalo, and goat. Cattle and buffalo isolates of *F. gigantica* showed 100% homogeneity, whereas goat and cattle/buffalo isolates displayed 92.68% similarity [43].

mtDNA sequences provided useful markers for studies of genetic variability and population structures [28,44]. Walker et al. (2007) examined DNA polymorphism in the entire mitochondrial genome and showed that genetic diversity exist among and within *F. hepatica* populations from cattle and sheep and provided evidence for the existence of multiple mitochondrial lineages within infra-populations of *F. hepatica* [44]. Another study examined genetic variation in eastern European and western Asian populations of *F. hepatica* using partial mitochondrial NADH dehydrogenase subunits 1 (*nad* 1) and cytochrome *c* oxidase subunit 1 gene (*cox* 1) as genetic markers, and revealed the existence of two well-defined lineages with two main haplotypes and a number of shared divergent haplotypes among the examined *F. hepatica* populations [28].

Molecular Detection and Identification of *Fasciola* spp

In order to overcome the limitation of the phenotypic methods, genotypic approaches have been used for the identification and differentiation of *Fasciola* spp. [9, 10, 21, 22, 45, 46, 47]. Before the availability of PCR-based approaches, DNA probes were the alternative choice for the genotypic detection of *Fasciola* spp. [48]. However, DNA probe-based assays usually require the use of radioactive isotopes and can have bio-safety concerns.

Over the last two decades, several PCR-based approaches (Table 1), including PCR-linked restriction fragment length polymorphism (PCR-RFLP), PCR-linked single-strand conformation polymorphism (PCR-SSCP) and specific PCR assays, have been developed for the accurate identification of *Fasciola* spp. [8, 21, 22, 45, 46]. For example, a simple and rapid PCR-RFLP assay targeting a 618-bp sequence of the 28S rDNA was developed for the differentiation between *F. hepatica* and *F. gigantica* [45]. A similar PCR-RFLP assay using restriction endonucleases *Hsp* 92 II and *Rca* I was developed to differentiate between *F. hepatica, F. gigantica* and the "intermediate *Fasciola*" in China utilizing the ITS-2 rDNA as genetic marker [22]. Using the ITS-1 rDNA as genetic marker, Lin et al. (2007) established a PCR-SSCP assay for the accurate identification and differentiation between *F. hepatica,*

F. gigantica and the "intermediate *Fasciola*" [21]. A very recent study established a fluorescence-based SSCP (F-PCR-SSCP) for the identification of *Fasciola* spp. [46].

Recently, several specific PCR assays have been developed to differentiate *F. hepatica* from *F. gigantica* and detect *Fasciola* infections in the intermediate host snail and definitive hosts (such as buffalo), utilizing various genetic markers, such as *cox* 1, ITS, non-coding repetitive DNA fragment as well as RAPD-derived sequences [47, 49, 50, 51, 52, 53]. For example, Ai et al. (2010) established a specific PCR method based on the ITS-2 sequences to identify *F. hepatica, F. gigantica* and the "intermediate *Fasciola*". The method was sensitive as it was able to amplify target DNA fragment from a single *Fasciola* egg [47]. Specific PCR assays, using two primer sets derived from RAPD-derived sequences from English *F. hepatica* and Ghanaian *F. gigantica*, were able to distinguish *F. hepatica* from *F. gigantica* from cattle and sheep hosts from different countries [53]. Alasaad et al. (2011) developed a highly specific, sensitive, and simple TaqMan-based real-time PCR assay for the identification of *F. hepatica* and *F. gigantica*, as well as the "intermediate *Fasciola*" based on sequences of the ITS-2 rDNA [54].

A PCR assay was used to detect *F. gigantica* infection in the snail vector host, *Lymnaea auricularia* [49]. The specific primers amplified a *F. gigantica* specific 124-bp non-coding repetitive DNA fragment from infected *L. auricularia* snails. Kaplan et al. (1995) also identified a 124-bp repetitive DNA sequence which was used as a specific probe for detection of *F. hepatica* infections in intermediate host snails (*Fossaria cubensis* and*Pseudosuccinea columella*) [51]. A multiplex PCR assay was able to detect *F. hepatica* DNA in *L. viatrix* snails, which were even formalin-fixed and paraffin-embedded [52]. TaqMan chemistry was adopted by Schweizer et al. (2007) to establish a real-time PCR assay. The combined use of primers and probe targeting an 86-bp target of a repetitive 449-bp genomic DNA fragment facilitated the detection of *L. truncatula* naturally infected with *F. hepatica*. These PCR assays are highly specific and sensitive, providing useful and practical tools for the epidemiological investigation of *Fasciola* in the snail hosts [55].

Loop-mediated isothermal amplification (LAMP) allows amplification of target nucleic acids under isothermal conditions with high sensitivity, specificity, rapidity and precision, which has found broad applications for the detection of pathogens [56, 57]. Ai et al. (2010) developed a LAMP assay for the sensitive and rapid detection and discrimination of *F. hepatica* and *F. gigantica*. The assay can be done in 45 min under isothermal conditions at 61°C or 62°C by employing a set of 4 species-specific primer mixtures and the results can be checked visually. This LAMP assay was approximately 10^5 times more sensitive than the conventional specific PCR assays, and may find applicability in the field settings or in poorly-equipped laboratories in endemic countries [58].

CONCLUSIONS AND FUTURE PERSPECTIVES

Much of the current knowledge of *Fasciola* spp. taxonomy and epidemiology has stemmed from numerous observational and morphological studies. However, conventional methods of detection and differentiation of*Fasciola* do not accurately reflect the full diversity of *Fasciola* spp. Nevertheless, molecular genetics studies over the past two decades have added significantly to our understanding of *Fasciola* taxonomy, genetics, and contributed to the development of advanced approaches for the accurate identification and differentiation of*Fasciola* spp. Importantly, these molecular methods have facilitated the identification of the hybrid "intermediate *Fasciola*". However, presently there is no molecular diagnostic method (e.g. a Copro-PCR) developed and validated for use with human stools.

We are still far from a complete understanding of the molecular evolution of the hybrid *Fasciola*, and many questions remain unanswered. For example, what is the outcome of experimental crosses between *F. hepatica* and *F. gigantica*? What are the differences between the "intermediate *Fasciola*" and other *Fasciola* species at the genomic and transcriptomic levels? Comprehensive genetic characterization using more variable markers such as microsatellites (eg. [59]) along with transcriptional analysis of *Fasciola* species can be used to refine the taxonomic status of the "intermediate *Fasciola*" and to assess its potential as a zoonotic agent.

On the analytical methods front, there is a clear need for the application of high-throughput molecular techniques such as next-generation sequencing, transcriptomics, proteomics and large-scale analysis of single nucleotide polymorphisms. The successful application of these and other techniques should bring more insights into the population genetic structure and the evolutionary process in *Fasciola*.

Recently, there have been increasing interests in the studies of transcriptome and proteome of *F. hepatica* [60,61, 62]. More studies in these promising areas of research will expand our understanding of the complex biology of different *Fasciola* species, which, in turn, will facilitate the development of novel means of therapeutic and immunological intervention.

ACKNOWLEDGEMENTS

This work was supported, in part, by the National S & T Major Program (Grant No. 2008ZX10004-011, 2009ZX10004-302, 2009ZX10004-201), the National Key Technology R & D Program (Grant No. 2008BAI56B03), the State Key Laboratory of Veterinary Etiological Biology, Lanzhou Veterinary Research Institute, Chinese Academy of Agricultural Sciences, the Yunnan Provincial Program for Introducing High-level Scientists (Grant No. 2009CI125) and the Program for Changjiang Scholars and Innovative Research Team in University (Grant No. IRT0723).

AUTHORS' CONTRIBUTIONS

XQZ, JXC, SA and HME conceived and designed the review, and critically revised the manuscript. LA and MXC drafted the manuscript. JL, HLL, RQL and FCZ contributed to drafting the manuscript. All authors read and approved the final manuscript.

REFERENCES

1. Mas-Coma S, Bargues MD, Valero MA: Fascioliasis and other plant-borne trematode zoonoses. Int J Parasitol. 2005, 35: 1255-1278. 10.1016/j.ijpara.2005.07.010.
2. Zhou P, Chen N, Zhang RL, Lin RQ, Zhu XQ: Food-borne parasitic zoonoses in China: perspective for control. Trends Parasitol. 2008, 24: 190-196. 10.1016/j.

pt.2008.01.001.

3. Mas-Coma MS, Esteban JG, Bargues MD: Epidemiology of human fascioliasis: a review and proposed new classification. Bull World Health Organ. 1999, 77: 340-346.

4. Spithill TW, Dalton JP: Progress in development of liver fluke vaccines. Parasitol Today. 1998, 14: 224-228. 10.1016/S0169-4758(98)01245-9.

5. Le TH, De NV, Agatsuma T, Blair D, Vercruysse J, Dorny P, Nguyen TG, McManus DP: Molecular confirmation that *Fasciola gigantica* can undertake aberrant migrations in human hosts. J Clin Microbiol. 2007, 45: 648-650. 10.1128/JCM.01151-06.

6. Mas-Coma S, Valero MA, Bargues MD: *Fasciola*, lymnaeids and human fascioliasis, with a global overview on disease transmission, epidemiology, evolutionarygenetics, molecular epidemiology and control. Adv Parasitol. 2009, 69: 41-146.

7. Caple IW, Jainudeen MR, Buick TD, Song CY: Some clinico-pathologic findings in elephants (Elephas maximus) infected with *Fasciola Jacksoni*. J Wildl Dis. 1978, 14: 110-115.

8. Ichikawa M, Itagaki T: Discrimination of the ITS1 types of *Fasciola* spp. based on a PCR-RFLP method. Parasitol Res. 2010, 106: 757-761. 10.1007/s00436-010-1724-2.

9. Nguyen TG, Van De N, Vercruysse J, Dorny P, Le TH: Genotypic characterization and species identification of *Fasciola* spp. with implications regarding the isolates infecting goats in Vietnam. Exp Parasitol. 2009, 123: 354-361. 10.1016/j.exppara.2009.09.001.

10. Li QY, Dong SJ, Zhang WY, Lin RQ, Wang CR, Qian DX, Lun ZR, Song HQ, Zhu XQ: Sequence-related amplified polymorphism, an effective molecular approach for studying genetic variation in *Fasciola* spp. of human and animal health significance. Electrophoresis. 2009, 30: 403-409. 10.1002/elps.200800411.

11. Kramer F, Schnieder T: Sequence heterogeneity in a repetitive DNA element of *Fasciola*. Int J Parasitol. 1998, 28: 1923-1929. 10.1016/S0020-7519(98)00162-3.

12. Lotfy WM, Brant SV, DeJong RJ, Le TH, Demiaszkiewicz A, Rajapakse RP, Perera VB, Laursen JR, Loker ES: Evolutionary origins, diversification, and biogeography of liver flukes (Digenea, Fasciolidae). Am J Trop Med Hyg. 2008, 79: 248-255.

13. Itagaki T, Tsutsumi KI, Ito K, Tsutsumi Y: Taxonomic status of the Japanese triploid forms of *Fasciola*: comparison of mitochondrial ND1 and COI sequences with *F. hepatica* and *F. gigantica*. J Parasitol. 1998, 84: 445-448. 10.2307/3284510.

14. Itagaki T, Tsutsumi K: Triploid form of *Fasciola* in Japan: genetic relationships between *Fasciola hepatica* and *Fasciola gigantica* determined by ITS-2 sequence of nuclear rDNA. Int J Parasitol. 1998, 28: 777-781. 10.1016/S0020-7519(98)00037-X.

15. Itagaki T, Kikawa M, Sakaguchi K, Shimo J, Terasaki K, Shibahara T, Fukuda K: Genetic characterization of parthenogenic*Fasciola* sp. in Japan on the basis of the sequences of ribosomal and mitochondrial DNA. Parasitology. 2005, 131: 679-685. 10.1017/S0031182005008292.

16. Itagaki T, Kikawa M, Terasaki K, Shibahara T, Fukuda K: Molecular characterization of parthenogenic *Fasciola* sp. in Korea on the basis of DNA sequences of ribosomal ITS1 and mitochondrial NDI gene. J Vet Med Sci. 2005, 67: 1115-1118. 10.1292/jvms.67.1115.

17. Itagaki T, Sakaguchi K, Terasaki K, Sasaki O, Yoshihara S, Van Dung T: Occurrence of spermic diploid and aspermic triploid forms of *Fasciola* in Vietnam and their molecular characterization based on nuclear and mitochondrial DNA. Parasitol Int. 2009, 58: 81-85. 10.1016/j.parint.2008.11.003.

18. Agatsuma T, Arakawa Y, Iwagami M, Honzako Y, Cahyaningsih U, Kang SY, Hong SJ: Molecular evidence of natural hybridization between *Fasciola hepatica* and *F. gigantica*. Parasitol Int. 2000, 49: 231-238. 10.1016/S1383-5769(00)00051-9.

19. Le TH, De NV, Agatsuma T, Thi NT, Nguyen QD, McManus DP, Blair D: Human fascioliasis and the presence of hybrid/introgressed forms of *Fasciola hepatica* and *Fasciola gigantica* in Vietnam. Int J Parasitol. 2008, 38: 725-730. 10.1016/j.ijpara.2007.10.003.

20. Ashrafi K, Valero MA, Panova M, Periago MV, Massoud J, Mas-Coma S: Phenotypic analysis of adults of *Fasciola hepatica, Fasciola gigantica* and intermediate forms from the endemic region of Gilan, Iran. Parasitol Int. 2006, 55: 249-260. 10.1016/j.parint.2006.06.003.

21. Lin RQ, Dong SJ, Nie K, Wang CR, Song HQ, Li AX, Huang WY, Zhu XQ: Sequence analysis of the first internal transcribed spacer of rDNA supports the existence of the intermediate *Fasciola* between *F. hepatica* and *F. gigantica* in mainland China. Parasitol Res. 2007, 101: 813-817. 10.1007/s00436-007-0512-0.

22. Huang WY, He B, Wang CR, Zhu XQ: Characterisation of *Fasciola* species from mainland China by ITS-2 ribosomal DNA sequence. Vet Parasitol. 2004, 120: 75-83. 10.1016/j.vetpar.2003.12.006.

23. Hashimoto K, Watanobe T, Liu CX, Init I, Blair D, Ohnishi S, Agatsuma T: Mitochondrial DNA and nuclear DNA indicate that the Japanese *Fasciola* species is *F. gigantica*. Parasitol Res. 1997, 83: 220-225.

24. Chilton NB: The use of nuclear ribosomal DNA markers for the identification of bursate nematodes (order Strongylida) and for the diagnosis of infections. Anim Health Res Rev. 2004, 5: 173-187. 10.1079/AHR200497.

25. Ali H, Ai L, Song HQ, Ali S, Lin RQ, Seyni B, Issa G, Zhu XQ: Genetic characterisation of *Fasciola* samples from different host species and geographical localities revealed the existence of *F. hepatica* and *F. gigantica* in Niger. Parasitol Res. 2008, 102: 1021-1024. 10.1007/s00436-007-0870-7.

26. Prasad PK, Tandon V, Biswal DK, Goswami LM, Chatterjee A: Use of sequence motifs as barcodes and secondary structures of internal transcribed spacer 2 (ITS2, rDNA) for identification of the Indian liver fluke, *Fasciola* (Trematoda: Fasciolidae). Bioinformation. 2009, 3: 314-320.

27. Adlard RD, Barker SC, Blair D, Cribb TH: Comparison of the second internal transcribed spacer (ribosomal DNA) from populations and species of Fasciolidae (Digenea). Int J Parasitol. 1993, 23: 423-425. 10.1016/0020-7519(93)90022-Q.

28. Semyenova SK, Morozova EV, Chrisanfova GG, Gorokhov VV, Arkhipov IA, Moskvin AS, Movsessyan SO, Ryskov AP: Genetic differentiation in Eastern European and Western Asian populations of the liver fluke, *Fasciola hepatica*, as revealed by mitochondrial *nad* 1 and *cox* 1 genes. J Parasitol. 2006, 92: 525-530. 10.1645/GE-673R.1.

29. Boore JL: Animal mitochondrial genomes. Nucleic Acids Res. 1999, 27: 1767-1780. 10.1093/nar/27.8.1767.

30. Le TH, Blair D, McManus DP: Complete DNA sequence and gene organization of the mitochondrial genome of the liverfluke, *Fasciola hepatica* L. (Platyhelminthes; Trematoda). Parasitology. 2001, 123: 609-621.

31. Galtier N, Nabholz B, Glémin S, Hurst GD: Mitochondrial DNA as a marker of molecular diversity: a reappraisal. Mol Ecol. 2009, 18: 4541-4550. 10.1111/j.1365-294X.2009.04380.x.

32. Santamaria M, Lanave C, Vicario S, Saccone C: Variability of the mitochondrial genome in mammals at the inter-species/intra-species boundary. Biol Chem. 2007, 388: 943-946. 10.1515/BC.2007.121.

33. Li MW, Lin RQ, Song HQ, Sani RA, Wu XY, Zhu XQ: Electrophoretic analysis of sequence variability in three mitochondrial DNA regions for Ascaridoid parasites of human and animal health significance. Electrophoresis. 2008, 29: 2912-2917.

34. Periago MV, Valero MA, El SM, Ashrafi K, El WA, Mohamed MY, Desquesnes M, Curtale F, Mas-Coma S: First phenotypic description of *Fasciola hepatica/Fasciola gigantica* intermediate forms from the human endemic area of the Nile Delta, Egypt. Infect Genet Evol. 2008, 8: 51-58. 10.1016/j.meegid.2007.10.001.

35. Zhu XQ, Podolska M, Liu JS, Yu HQ, Chen HH, Lin ZX, Luo CB, Song HQ, Lin RQ: Identification of Anisakid nematodes with zoonotic potential from Europe and China by single-strand conformation polymorphism analysis of nuclear ribosomal DNA. Parasitol Res. 2007, 101: 1703-1707. 10.1007/s00436-007-0699-0.

36. Zhu XQ, Gasser RB, Chilton NB, Jacobs DE: Molecular approaches for studying Ascaridoid nematodes with zoonotic potential, with an emphasis on *Toxocara* species. J Helminthol. 2001, 75: 101-108.

37. Gasser RB: Molecular tools-advances, opportunities and prospects. Vet Parasitol. 2006, 136: 69-89. 10.1016/j.vetpar.2005.12.002.

38. Alasaad S, Huang CQ, Li QY, Granados JE, Garcia-Romero C, Perez JM, Zhu XQ: Characterization of *Fasciola* samples from different host species and geographical localities in Spain by sequences of internal transcribed spacers of rDNA. Parasitol Res. 2007, 101: 1245-1250. 10.1007/s00436-007-0628-2.

39. Vara-Del RM, Villa H, Martinez-Valladares M, Rojo-Vazquez FA: Genetic heterogeneity of *Fasciola hepatica* isolates in the northwest of Spain. Parasitol Res. 2007, 101: 1003-1006. 10.1007/s00436-007-0574-z.

40. Dinler G, Budak H: Analysis of expressed sequence tags (ESTs) from *Agrostis* species obtained using sequence related amplified polymorphism. Biochem Genet. 2008, 46: 663-676. 10.1007/s10528-008-9181-7.

41. Han XY, Wang LS, Shu QY, Liu ZA, Xu SX, Tetsumura T: Molecular characterization of tree peony *Germplasm* using sequence-related amplified polymorphism markers. Biochem Genet. 2008, 46: 162-179. 10.1007/s10528-007-9140-8.

42. Alasaad S, Li QY, Lin RQ, Martin-Atance P, Granados JE, Diez-Banos P, Perez JM, Zhu XQ: Genetic variability among*Fasciola hepatica* samples from different host species and geographical localities in Spain revealed by the novel SRAP marker. Parasitol Res. 2008, 103: 181-186. 10.1007/s00436-008-0952-1.

43. Gunasekar KR, Tewari AK, Sreekumar C, Gupta SC, Rao JR: Elucidation of genetic variability among different isolates of*Fasciola gigantica* (giant liver fluke) using random-amplified polymorphic DNA polymerase chain reaction. Parasitol Res. 2008, 103: 1075-1081. 10.1007/s00436-008-1095-0.

44. Walker SM, Prodohl PA, Fletcher HL, Hanna RE, Kantzoura V, Hoey EM, Trudgett A: Evidence for multiple mitochondrial lineages of *Fasciola hepatica* (liver fluke) within infrapopulations from cattle and sheep. Parasitol Res. 2007, 101: 117-125. 10.1007/s00436-006-0440-4.

45. Marcilla A, Bargues MD, Mas-Coma S: A PCR-RFLP assay for the distinction between *Fasciola hepatica* and *Fasciola gigantica*. Mol Cell Probes. 2002, 16: 327-333. 10.1006/mcpr.2002.0429.

46. Alasaad S, Soriguer RC, Abu-Madi M, El Behairy A, Baños PD, Píriz A, Fickel J, Zhu XQ: A fluorescence-based polymerase chain reaction-linked single-strand conformation polymorphism (F-PCR-SSCP) assay for the identification of *Fasciola* spp. Parasitol Res. 2011, 108: 1513-1517. 10.1007/s00436-010-2209-z.

47. Ai L, Dong SJ, Zhang WY, Elsheikha HM, Mahmmod YS, Lin RQ, Yuan ZG, Shi YL, Huang WY, Zhu XQ: Specific PCR-based assays for the identification of *Fasciola* species: their development, evaluation and potential usefulness in prevalence surveys. Ann Trop Med Parasitol. 2010, 104: 65-72. 10.1179/136485910X12607012373713.

48. Heussler V, Kaufmann H, Strahm D, Liz J, Dobbelaere D: DNA probes for the detection of *Fasciola hepatica* in snails. Mol Cell Probes. 1993, 7: 261-267. 10.1006/mcpr.1993.1039.

49. Velusamy R, Singh BP, Raina OK: Detection of *Fasciola gigantica* infection in snails by polymerase chain reaction. Vet Parasitol. 2004, 120: 85-90. 10.1016/j.vetpar.2003.11.009.

50. Cucher MA, Carnevale S, Prepelitchi L, Labbe JH, Wisnivesky-Colli C: PCR diagnosis of *Fasciola hepatica* in field-collected*Lymnaea columella* and *Lymnaea viatrix* snails. Vet Parasitol. 2006, 137: 74-82. 10.1016/j.vetpar.2005.12.013.

51. Kaplan RM, Dame JB, Reddy GR, Courtney CH: A

repetitive DNA probe for the sensitive detection of *Fasciola hepatica*infected snails. Int J Parasitol. 1995, 25: 601-610. 10.1016/0020-7519(94)00159-L.

52. Magalhaes KG, Jannotti-Passos LK, Caldeira RL, Berne ME, Muller G, Carvalho OS, Lenzi HL: Isolation and detection of*Fasciola hepatica* DNA in *Lymnaea viatrix* from formalin-fixed and paraffin-embedded tissues through multiplex-PCR. Vet Parasitol. 2008, 152: 333-338. 10.1016/j.vetpar.2007.12.019.

53. McGarry JW, Ortiz PL, Hodgkinson JE, Goreish I, Williams DJ: PCR-based differentiation of *Fasciola* species (Trematoda: Fasciolidae), using primers based on RAPD-derived sequences. Ann Trop Med Parasitol. 2007, 101: 415-421. 10.1179/136485907X176508.

54. Alasaad S, Soriguer RC, Abu-Madi M, El BA, Banos PD, Piriz A, Fickel J, Zhu XQ: A TaqMan real-time PCR-based assay for the identification of *Fasciola* spp. Vet Parasitol. 2011, 179: 266-271. 10.1016/j.vetpar.2011.01.059.

55. Schweizer G, Meli ML, Torgerson PR, Lutz H, Deplazes P, Braun U: Prevalence of *Fasciola hepatica* in the intermediate host *Lymnaea truncatula* detected by real time TaqMan PCR in populations from 70 Swiss farms with cattle husbandry. Vet Parasitol. 2007, 150: 164-169. 10.1016/j.vetpar.2007.08.006.

56. Notomi T, Okayama H, Masubuchi H, Yonekawa T, Watanabe K, Amino N, Hase T: Loop-mediated isothermal amplification of DNA. Nucleic Acids Res. 2000, 28: E63. 10.1093/nar/28.12.e63.

57. Nagamine K, Hase T, Notomi T: Accelerated reaction by loop-mediated isothermal amplification using loop primers. Mol Cell Probes. 2002, 16: 223-229. 10.1006/mcpr.2002.0415.

58. Ai L, Li C, Elsheikha HM, Hong SJ, Chen JX, Chen SH, Li X, Cai XQ, Chen MX, Zhu XQ: Rapid identification and differentiation of *Fasciola hepatica* and *Fasciola gigantica* by a loop-mediated isothermal amplification (LAMP) assay. Vet Parasitol. 2010, 174: 228-233. 10.1016/j.vetpar.2010.09.005.

59. Hurtrez-Boussés S, Durand P, Jabbour-Zahabr R, Guegan JF, Meunier C, Bargues MD, Mas-Coma S, Renaud F: Isolation and characterization of microsatellite markers in the liver fluke (*Fasciola hepatica*). Mol Ecol Notes. 2004, 4: 689-690. 10.1111/j.1471-8286.2004.00786.x.

60. Young ND, Jex AR, Cantacessi C, Hall RS, Campbell BE, Spithill TW, Tangkawattana S, Tangkawattana P, Laha T, Gasser RB: A portrait of the transcriptome of the neglected trematode, *Fasciola gigantica*-biological and biotechnological implications. PLoS Negl Trop Dis. 2011, 5: e1004. 10.1371/journal.pntd.0001004.

61. Robinson MW, Menon R, Donnelly SM, Dalton JP, Ranganathan S: An integrated transcriptomics and proteomics analysis of the secretome of the helminth pathogen *Fasciola hepatica*: proteins associated with invasion and infection of the mammalian host. Mol Cell Proteomics. 2009, 8: 1891-1907. 10.1074/mcp.M900045-MCP200.

62. Moxon JV, LaCourse EJ, Wright HA, Perally S, Prescott MC, Gillard JL, Barrett J, Hamilton JV, Brophy PM: Proteomic analysis of embryonic *Fasciola hepatica*: characterization and antigenic potential of a developmentally regulated heat shock protein. Vet Parasitol. 2010, 169: 62-75. 10.1016/j.vetpar.2009.12.031.

CHAPTER 5 UPDATE ON BABESIOSIS

Edouard Vannier and Peter J. Krause

INTRODUCTION

Human babesiosis is an emerging tick-borne infectious disease caused by an intraerythrocytic protozoan and has many clinical features similar to those of malaria. The parasite was first described in cattle by Babes in 1888 [1]. The first human case was described in 1957 [2]. Over the past 50 years, the epidemiology of the disease has changed from a few isolated cases to the establishment of endemic areas in southern New England, New York, New Jersey, and the northern Midwest [3–8]. Isolated cases are reported over a wide geographic range in Europe, Asia, Africa, and South America [9–17]. We will review the epidemiology, clinical characteristics, diagnosis, and treatment of infections caused by the four Babesia species that most commonly infect people: B. microti, B. duncani, B. divergens, and B. venatorum.

EPIDEMIOLOGY

United States

B. microti Infection

The most common cause of human babesiosis is Babesia microti, a Babesia of mice and other small rodents that is endemic in the United States [5–8]. Most cases occur along the northeastern seaboard. The first confirmed case was a normosplenic individual on Nantucket Island off the coast of Massachusetts [18]. Additional cases were soon identified and the disease became known as Nantucket fever. Other islands off the coast of southern New England subsequently became recognized as endemic areas, including Martha's Vineyard, the Elizabeth Islands, Block Island, Shelter Island, the eastern part of Long Island, and Fire Island [19]. Endemic areas on the mainland include Cape Cod, the southwestern counties of Rhode Island, and southeastern Connecticut [6, 19,20]. Babesiosis has been diagnosed in individuals from the Lower Hudson Valley (Westchester, Putnam, Dutchess, and Columbia counties) in New York State, and is endemic in New Jersey [21–23]. B. microti is also the etiologic agent of babesiosis in the northern midwestern region of the United States, particularly in Wisconsin and Minnesota [24–26]. A few isolated cases have been noted in Indiana [27, 28]. Human babesiosis due to B. microti recently has been reported from Europe while B. microti-like species have been described as the cause of infection in people living in Asia [13, 17, 29].

The distribution of B. microti overlaps with that of Borrelia burgdorferi, the agent of Lyme disease, as both organisms are transmitted by Ixodes scapularis in the United States [19, 30]. Although the geographic distribution of babesiosis appears to be restricted to certain foci within the areas of endemicity for B. burgdorferi, the endemic range is expanding. For this reason and because the number of reported cases has dramatically increased over the last two decades, babesiosis is recognized as an emerging infectious disease [8,31, 32]. The increase in incidence has often been attributed to the expansion of the deer population because these vertebrates are the primary host for adult ticks, although they are not competent reservoirs for B. microti. Other factors include better awareness of the disease by local physicians, an encroachment of humans on wildlife habitat, and increasing travel of immunosuppressed individuals to endemic areas.

Although most B. microti infections are acquired by tick bites from May through October, at least 70 patients in the United States have acquired babesiosis by transfusion of contaminated blood products from asymptomatic donors [33–36]. Blood products typically are fresh or frozen packed red blood cells, although one case has been attributed to platelet transfusion. Several cases of neonatal babesiosis have been

Citation: Edouard Vannier and Peter J. Krause, "Update on Babesiosis," Interdisciplinary Perspectives on Infectious Diseases, vol. 2009, Article ID 984568, 9 pages, 2009. doi:10.1155/2009/984568.

reported, and these were acquired by tick bite, transfusion, or transplacental transmission [37, 38].

B. duncani Infection

B. duncani is the name given to the previously designated WA1 Babesia [3]. All nine documented cases of B. duncani infection have occurred on the west coast of the United States. Two people acquired the babesial infection by transfusion of blood products while the remaining cases were attributed to tick bites [39, 40]. One blood donor was asymptomatic at time of donation whereas the other reported a 10-day episode of nausea. Both recipients were immunologically at risk; one was an elderly man and the other was a premature infant. Among the five other symptomatic cases, one was a young normosplenic adult living in Washington State (index case) whereas four were splenectomized and lived in California [41, 42]. One of these four men died. Sequence analysis of the entire 18S rRNA gene indicated that the organisms causing babesial illness in the index case from Washington State and in the two cases acquired by blood transfusion were phylogenetically indistinguishable whereas the organisms acquired by three of the four splenectomized cases in California formed a separate but closely related phylogenetic group [3, 43]. The seroprevalence of B. duncani infection has been found to vary from 4% to 17% [41].

B. divergens-Like Infection

B. divergens-like organisms have been identified in three cases, two from the Midwest (Missouri and Kentucky) and one from Washington State [4, 44, 45]. All three patients had risk factors for severe babesial disease, namely, age greater than 50 years and splenectomy. Sequence analysis of the entire 18S rRNA gene indicated that the Missouri isolate (MO1) and the Kentucky isolate (KY) were identical to each other and to piroplasms found in eastern cottontail rabbits on Nantucket Island [46]. These isolates differed by a few bp in their 18S rRNA gene from the isolate of the Washington State patient and from the B. divergens organisms of European cattle. Because the piroplasms isolated from eastern cottontail rabbits are not infectious to cattle, the isolates obtained from the three US patients are now referred to as B. divergens-like organisms.

EUROPE

B. divergens Infection

About 40 cases of B. divergens infection have been documented in Europe, mostly from countries with extensive cattle industry such as France, Ireland, and Great Britain [47–49]. Cases have sporadically been reported from Sweden, Switzerland, Spain, Portugal, and Croatia (index case). Nearly all patients were splenectomized prior to the onset of Babesia infection. Because cattle are the reservoir for B. divergens, persons at risk of contracting babesiosis are farmers or people vacationing in rural areas. Limited data suggest that infection with B. divergens can be asymptomatic in normosplenic individuals [47]. There are no reports of B. divergens infection acquired by blood transfusion [49].

B. venatorum (EU1) Infection

Because the advent of PCR allows for molecular characterization of babesial organisms, a new Babesia species has been identified in Europe. Originally referred to as EU1, the name "B. venatorum" was later proposed [12].B. venatorum, together with B. odocoilei that infects white-tail deer in the United States, form a sister group to that of B. divergens. Three cases of infection with B. venatorum have been documented [12, 50]. All three were men beyond 50 years of age who had been splenectomized. Unlike B. divergens infections that are fulminant and often fatal, B. venatorum infections have varied from mild to severe but have not been fatal.

CLINICAL CHARACTERISTICS

B. microti Infection

The severity of B. microti infection is variable, depending primarily on the immune status of the host. Several clinical syndromes have been described, including asymptomatic infection, mild-to-moderate viral-like illness, and severe disease with a fulminant course that sometimes results in death or a persistent relapsing illness. Concurrent infection with Lyme disease increases neither the number nor the duration of symptoms of babesiosis [30, 51]. It is unclear whether this is also true of concurrent babesiosis and human granulocytic anaplasmosis.

Asymptomatic Infection

Following transmission of the babesial parasite, the incubation period may last from 1 to 9 weeks [5, 8]. Many people who are infected with B. microti never experience symptoms, as suggested by the disparity between seroprevalence and the number of reported cases. The frequency of asymptomatic B. microti infection was derived from an epidemiologic study of babesiosis carried out on Block Island, Rhode Island [6]. About a third of babesial infections at this site were asymptomatic, including 19% (13 of 67) of adults and 40% (4 of 10) of children [6]. Asymptomatic infection may persist for months or years following resolution of symptomatic babesiosis [36]. It is uncertain whether patients experiencing asymptomatic babesial infection are at risk for any long-term complications. They may transmit the infection if they donate blood [33].

Mild-to-Moderate Illness

Most cases of B. microti infection consist of a mild to moderate viral-like illness. These cases typically begin with a gradual onset of malaise and fatigue followed by intermittent fever and one or more of the following: chills, sweats, headache, arthralgia, myalgia, anorexia, cough, and nausea (Table 1) [30, 52–54]. Less commonly noted are gastrointestinal symptoms, weight loss, conjunctival injection, and emotional lability [53–57]. On physical examination, fever is commonly observed and pallor, mild splenomegaly or hepatomegaly occasionally may be noted. The illness usually lasts for a week to months, occasionally with prolonged recovery that can last more than a year [30, 36, 53, 56, 57]. Parasitemia may continue even after the patient feels well and rarely may persist for more than two years after the initial episode [36].

Table 1: The most common symptoms of babesiosis caused by Babesia microti infection

Symptom	Percentage of outpatients (n = 41)	Percentage of inpatients (n = 173)	Percentage of all patients (n = 214)
Fever	68	89	85
Fatigue	78	79	79
Chills	39	68	63
Sweats	41	56	53
Headache	75	32	39
Myalgia	37	32	33
Anorexia	25	24	24
Cough	17	23	22
Arthralgia	31	17	18
Nausea	22	9	16

Outpatient cases are from Ruebush et al. [60] and Krause et al. [30]. Inpatient cases are from White et al. [54] and Hatcher et al. [52].

Severe Disease

Severe disease generally occurs in people with underlying immunosuppressive conditions that include HIV, malignancy, immunosuppressive medication, and splenectomy [50, 56, 58–60]. On physical examination, jaundice, retinal infarcts, or ecchymoses and petechiae may be noted [55, 58, 61]. The most common complications of severe babesiosis include acute respiratory failure, congestive heart failure, DIC, liver and renal failure, and splenic rupture [52]. A mortality rate of 5% was noted in a retrospective study of 136 patients experiencing B. microti infection on Long Island, New York, only one of whom was known to be immunocompromised [7]. In another study, the mortality rate among patients hospitalized for babesiosis was 9% [52]. The mortality rate is even higher among immunocompromised hosts. In a recent case-control study of 14 patients who were highly immunocompromised, 21% died and the remainder experienced a prolonged, relapsing course of illness, sometimes lasting more than a year, despite multiple courses of standard antibabesial therapy [59]. People 50 years of age and older also are more likely to experience severe babesiosis [52, 54, 62].

B. duncani Infection

Although studies of infection in hamsters suggest that B. duncani is more pathogenic than B. microti, the small number of reported B. duncani cases does not allow firm conclusions [32]. Of the nine reported cases of B. duncani, one died, one experienced pulmonary edema and renal insufficiency, and the remainder had a relatively mild clinical course or were asymptomatic [3, 39, 40, 42, 63]. Parasitemia ranged from 1% to 54%. Symptoms of B. duncani are similar to those of B. microti and consist of fever, chills, headache, sweats, myalgia, nausea, vomiting, diarrhea, dark urine, and fatigue.

B. divergens Infection

Nearly all 40 cases of B. divergens infection reported in Europe had been splenectomized and suffered a severe form of babesiosis [47–49]. Signs and symptoms begin 1 to 3 weeks after tick transmission and consist of high fever (40-41°C) with severe intravascular hemolysis that results in hemoglobinemia, hemoglobinuria, and jaundice. Headache, shaking chills, intense sweating, myalgia, and abdominal pain are common. More than half the cases experienced a rapid onset of renal failure and pulmonary edema. Ecchymoses, petechiae, congestive heart failure, and coma also have been reported. The illness generally is fulminant, lasting about a week and ending in death in more than a third of patients or in a prolonged convalescence.

B. venatorum (EU1) Infection

All three reported cases of B. venatorum infection had a history of Hodgkin's disease and had been splenectomized [12, 50]. One experienced mild babesiosis, whereas two had moderate-to-severe illness. In these two patients, babesiosis was concurrent with a relapse of nodular lymphocyte-predominant Hodgkin's lymphoma or with stage IIIA diffuse large B cell lymphoma. All three patients were admitted to the hospital and recovered after antibabesial therapy. One had a prolonged relapsing illness that eventually cleared. Peak parasitemia ranged from 1% to 30%. Symptoms included fever, dark urine, fatigue, chills, headache, confusion, jaundice, sweats, and shortness of breath.

DIAGNOSIS

The diagnosis of babesiosis should be considered in patients who live or travel in areas that are endemic for babesiosis and who experience a viral-like illness in the late spring, summer, or autumn (Table 2). As the symptoms and signs are relatively nonspecific, laboratory testing is required for diagnosis. In some cases, physicians may choose to obtain screening laboratory testing such as a CBC, platelet count, and liver enzymes before ordering specific diagnostic tests. Most cases of babesiosis are accompanied by some degree of hemolytic anemia with an elevated reticulocyte count. Thrombocytopenia is common. The leukocyte count usually is normal to slightly decreased. Elevated serum liver enzymes occur in about half the patients. Proteinuria and an elevated blood urea nitrogen and serum creatinine also may be noted. Specific laboratory tests that are used for the diagnosis of babesiosis are described below. Specific tests for concurrent Lyme disease and human granulocytic anaplasmosis should be performed in patients presenting with clinical manifestations that suggest coinfection, such as an erythema migrans type rash or neutropenia.

Table 2: Diagnosis of babesiosis

Epidemiology
– Residence in or travel to an area endemic for babesiosis
– Ixodes tick bite
– History of recent blood transfusion from a donor living or traveling in a Babesia endemic area
Symptoms
– Fever, fatigue, chills, sweats, headache, myalgia, anorexia, cough, arthralgia, nausea
– Less common: emotional lability and depression, hyperesthesia, sore throat, abdominal pain, conjunctival injection, photophobia, weight loss
Signs on physical examination
– Fever
– Splenomegaly, hepatomegaly, pallor
Common laboratory diagnostic procedures
– Identification of Babesia on Giemsa stained peripheral blood smears
– Amplification of Babesia DNA in blood using polymerase chain reaction
– Four-fold rise in Babesia antibody in acute or convalescent sera or identification of serum Babesia IgM antibody

Microscopic Identification

Specific diagnosis of babesiosis can be made by microscopic identification of the organism using Giemsa stains of thin blood smears [64, Figure 1]. Thick blood smears also may be performed but the babesial organisms are small and may be difficult to visualize. B. microti and other Babesia spp. are round, oval, or pear-shaped and have a blue cytoplasm with a red chromatin. The ring form is most common and can be mistaken for early stage ring forms of Plasmodium falciparum. Multiple thin blood smears should be examined when only a few erythrocytes are infected, particularly in the early stage of illness when most people seek medical attention. PCR and serology should be performed if only a few ring-like structures are observed. Parasitemia seldom exceeds 5% in normal hosts but may be as high as 85% in asplenic individuals [55]. B. divergens and related organisms often appear as paired piriforms in human red blood cells. Pairs of B. divergens and B. divergens-like organisms are located in a subcentral, central, or peripheral position [46]. B. venatorum are morphologically indistinguishable from B. divergens [12, 50]. The tetrad form, referred to as a Maltese cross, is pathognomonic of small Babesia spp. such as B. microti and B. duncani [3]. B. duncani display more tetrad forms than B. microti.

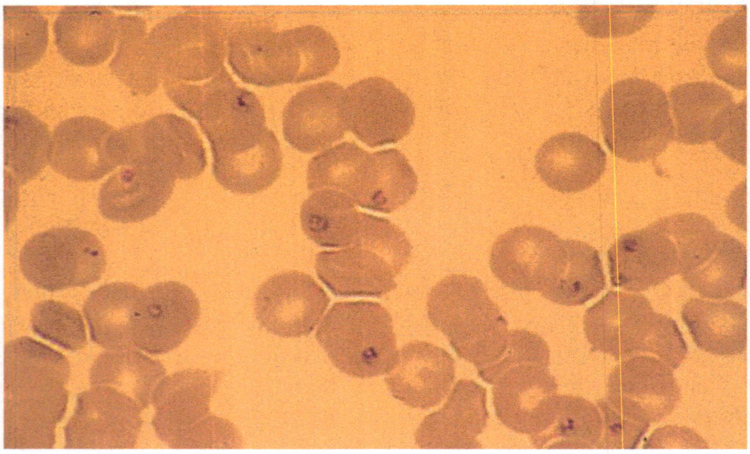

Figure 1: Ring forms of B. microti revealed by Giemsa staining of a human blood film (magnification 1000 x).

Polymerase Chain Reaction

The polymerase chain reaction (PCR) provides a highly sensitive and specific test for detecting Babesia DNA in blood and identifies the Babesia species [65, 66]. Rigorous precautions are required to avoid false positive results. PCR is recommended when parasites are not identified on blood smears but symptoms and history are suggestive of babesiosis. As with all Babesia specific tests, it should only be performed in laboratories that are experienced in such testing and meet the highest laboratory performance standards.

Serology

Babesial infection can be confirmed by serologic testing using the indirect immunofluorescent assay (IFA) [67, 68]. During the acute phase of B. microti illness, IgG titers usually exceed 1 : 1024 and decline to 1 : 64 or less within 8 to 12 months. Thus, IgG titers of 1 : 1024 or greater usually signify active or recent infection [69]. The detection of IgM is indicative of recent infection [67]. Although seroconversion occurs in virtually all immunocompetent individuals infected with B. microti, the diagnosis of active babesial infection based on serologic findings alone is suspect. Serology usually is not considered in cases attributed to B. divergens because the illness becomes fulminant before antibody can be detected. Sera from patients infected with B. divergens-like organisms or B. venatorum cross-react with antigen from B. divergens [41, 42, 63]. Sera from patients infected with B. duncani or related organisms do not crossreact with B. microti antigen [41, 42]. Sera from patients infected with one of several Babesia species may cross-react with antigen from Plasmodium species, but titers are almost always low (1 : 16 or lower).

Amplification of Babesia in Laboratory Animals

Babesia parasitemia can also be detected by injecting patient blood by the intravenous or intraperitoneal route into such laboratory animals as hamsters or gerbils [65]. This test is only available in a few research laboratories and is seldom useful for diagnosis. B. microti is easily detected in hamsters whereas B. duncani is often lethal in these animals [32]. This approach is not suited for rapid diagnosis, as Babesia usually do not appear in the blood of the laboratory animal until two to four weeks after inoculation.

TREATMENT

B. microti Infection

Mild-to-Moderate Disease

Most people infected with B. microti experience mild-to-moderate disease and can be successfully treated with a combination of atovaquone and azithromycin administered for 7 to 10 days [70, 71]. This combination was shown to be as effective as clindamycin and quinine, the first drug combination used in the treatment of babesiosis. The two regimens were directly compared in adults in a prospective, nonblinded randomized control trial [71]. While these drug combinations were similarly effective in clearing parasitemia and achieving resolution of symptoms, adverse effects were reported in 15% of subjects who received atovaquone and azithromycin compared with 72% of subjects who received clindamycin and quinine. The most common side effects associated with atovaquone and azithromycin were diarrhea and rash while those of clindamycin and quinine were tinnitus, hearing loss, and diarrhea. About a third of the subjects receiving clindamycin and quinine suffered from adverse reactions that were severe enough to require a decrease in dosage or discontinuing the medication. Only 2% of subjects taking atovaquone and azithromycin experienced such severe drug reactions. Although the atovaquone and azithromycin combination has not been studied in a controlled trial for pediatric use, cure has been achieved with use of this regimen in a child [72]. Clindamycin and quinine should be substituted for atovaquone and azithromycin when patients do not respond well to atovaquone and azithromycin.

Severe Disease

The combination of clindamycin (administered intravenously) and quinine given for 7 to 10 days is the treatment of choice for severe babesiosis. (Table 3) [70, 73]. Exchange red blood cell transfusion is indicated for all babesiosis patients experiencing heavy parasitemia (≥10%) or who have significant pulmonary, renal, or hepatic compromise [74–77]. Partial or complete exchange transfusion rapidly decreases parasite burden and removes toxic byproducts of Babesia infection.

Table 3: Treatment of babesiosis

Treatment	Dose	Frequency
Atovaquone and azithromycin		
Atovaquone	Adult: 750 mg	Every 12 hours
	Child: 20 mg/kg	Every 12 hours
	(maximum 750 mg/dose)	
Azithromycin	Adult: 500 to 1000 mg	On day 1
	250 to 1000 mg	On subsequent days
	Child: 10 mg/kg	On day 1
	(maximum 500 mg/dose)	
	5 mg/kg	On subsequent days
	(maximum 250 mg/dose)	
Clindamycin and quinine		

Clindamycin	Adult: 600 mg	Every 8 hours
	Child: 7–10 mg/kg	Every 6–8 hours
	(maximum 600 mg/dose)	
	Intravenous administration	
	Adult: 300–600 mg	Every 6 hours
	Child: 7–10 mg/kg	Every 6–8 hours
	(maximum 600 mg/dose)	
Quinine	Adult: 650 mg	Every 6–8 hours
	Child: 8 mg/kg	Every 8 hours
	(maximum 650 mg/dose)	

All antibiotics are administered by mouth unless otherwise specified. All doses are administered for 7 to 10 days except for persistent relapsing infection (see text). For immunocompromised patients experiencing babesiosis, successful outcome has been reported using atovaquone combined with higher doses of azithromycin (600–1000 mg per day) [78].

Complete or partial exchange transfusion should be considered for treatment of severe babesiosis.

Persistent Relapsing Disease

Babesial infection may persist and symptoms relapse in people with significant underlying immunosuppression despite standard combination antimicrobial therapy [59, 77]. Atovaquone-proguanil (250 mg–100 mg) was used to eradicate parasitemia in one such patient [77]. In a recent case-control study of chronic babesiosis in 14 highly immunocompromised patients, no single antimicrobial combination was uniformly superior to another in achieving resolution of infection [59]. Rather, cure was associated with duration of therapy for a minimum of six weeks and for at least two weeks after the last positive blood smear. Interestingly, the majority of case patients in the study had underlying B-cell lymphoma and had been treated with the anti-CD20 monoclonal antibody (Rituximab) prior to acute babesial infection, thereby dramatically impairing B-cell activity. It is important to recognize that a 7-to-10 day course of antibabesial therapy is sufficient for many immunocompromised patients. Thus, when acute babesiosis responds to a standard therapeutic course with resolution of symptoms and clearance of parasitemia on blood smear, no further treatment is required. Because immunosuppressed individuals are at increased risk for relapsing babesiosis, close clinical follow-up with repeat blood smears, Babesia PCR, and complete blood counts should be performed.

Asymptomatic Infection

In the unusual event that patients are identified with asymptomatic babesial infection, no treatment should be given unless parasitemia, as determined by blood smear or PCR, persists for longer than three months [70]. In this case, a one-week course of atovaquone and azithromycin should be considered. People who have positive serology, but negative blood smears and negative PCR should not be treated, as they likely have resolved the infection. Immunocompromised patients experiencing persistent asymptomatic parasitemia should have blood smears performed every month or two until they clear the infection.

B. duncani Infection

Recommended treatment consists of clindamycin and quinine [3, 39, 40, 42, 63]. Red cell exchange transfusion should be considered in the treatment of severe cases [41]. Renal insufficiency may require hemodialysis.

B. divergens and B. divergens-Like Infections

The morbidity and mortality rate of Babesia divergens infections are high and any such case should be considered a medical emergency [47, 49]. It is recommended that these infections be treated with exchange transfusion and clindamycin and quinine. One mild case of B. divergens infection was successfully treated with the combination of pentamidine and trimethoprim-sulfamethoxazole whereas another only required an abbreviated course of clindamycin and quinine (the quinine was stopped after 4 days) [79, 80]. In both cases, exchange transfusion was not needed. The Babesia divergens-like infections reported from Kentucky and Washington State were successfully treated with clindamycin and quinine or quinidine, but the case from Missouri died despite clindamycin and quinine therapy [4, 44, 45].

B. venatorum Infection

Of the three cases of B. venatorum infection, one cleared on clindamycin alone [12, 50]. The other two were given clindamycin and quinine. One of these patients was highly immunocompromised and relapsed after clindamycin and quinine was discontinued. He required a prolonged course of atovaquone and azithromycin followed by atovaquone alone for cure. In the third case, blood transfusion was given for massive hemolysis, and the infection eventually cleared following antimicrobial therapy.

PREVENTION

The use of multiple strategies is most likely to be effective for prevention of babesiosis. These include personal, residential, and community approaches [81–88]. One obvious personal protective measure is to avoid areas where ticks, mice, and deer are known to thrive, especially from May through October [84]. Immunocompromised people who are at increased risk of severe babesiosis need to avoid such areas. Anyone who may contact foliage in endemic sites should wear clothing that covers the lower part of the body, tuck cuffs of the trousers into stockings, and spray or impregnate clothing with permethrin (Permanone) [86]. DEET-containing products should be applied to the skin if legs remain uncovered. After travel through a high-risk area, a tick check should be performed and attached ticks should be removed as soon as possible by use of tweezers [84]. No data is available on the use of prophylactic antimicrobials after a tick bite to prevent babesiosis nor has a human babesiosis vaccine been developed.

Property modifications can help reduce tick exposure. These include keeping grass mowed, removing leaf litter at the edge of lawns, sealing stonewalls to decrease the number of mice, using plantings that do not attract deer, and fencing to keep deer away [84]. Acaracides can be applied to property, rodents (Damminix or fipronil), or deer (four poster device) [82, 84, 88]. Elimination of the deer population may sharply reduce the risk of babesiosis and other tick-borne infections. Within 3–5 years after deer were eliminated on Great Island off Cape Cod, Massachusetts, the density of I. scapularis ticks fell precipitously [87]. Currently, the Red Cross and other blood donation agencies prohibit people with a history of babesiosis from donating blood in order to prevent transfusion-related cases. Additional measures such as screening blood donors for silent Babesiainfection or inactivation of Babesia parasites in units of blood prior to transfusion have been considered but are not yet in use [89, 90].

ACKNOWLEDGEMENT

This review has been made possible thanks to the generous support of The Gordon and Llura Gund Foundation.

REFERENCES

1. V. Babes, "Sur l'hemoglobinurie bacterienne du boeuf," Comptes Rendus de l'Academie des Sciences, vol. 107, pp. 692–694, 1888.
2. Z. Skrabalo and Z. Deanovic, "Piroplasmosis in man; report of a case," Documenta de Medicina Geographica et Tropica, vol. 9, no. 1, pp. 11–16, 1957.
3. P. A. Conrad, A. M. Kjemtrup, R. A. Carreno, et al., "Description of Babesia duncani n.sp. (Apicomplexa: Babesiidae) from humans and its differentiation from other piroplasms," International Journal for Parasitology, vol. 36, no. 7, pp. 779–789, 2006.
4. B. L. Herwaldt, D. H. Persing, E. A. Précigout, et al., "A fatal case of babesiosis in Missouri: Identification of another piroplasm that infects humans," Annals of Internal Medicine, vol. 124, no. 7, pp. 643–650, 1996.
5. K.-P. Hunfeld, A. Hildebrandt, and J. S. Gray, "Babesiosis: recent insights into an ancient disease,"International Journal for Parasitology, vol. 38, no. 11, pp. 1219–1237, 2008.
6. P. J. Krause, K. McKay, J. Gadbaw, et al., "Increasing health burden of human babesiosis in endemic sites,"American Journal of Tropical Medicine and Hygiene, vol. 68, no. 4, pp. 431–436, 2003.
7. S. C. Meldrum, G. S. Birkhead, D. J. White, J. L. Benach, and D. L. Morse, "Human babesiosis in New York state: an epidemiological description of 136 cases," Clinical Infectious Diseases, vol. 15, no. 6, pp. 1019–1023, 1992.
8. E. Vannier, B. E. Gewurz, and P. J. Krause, "Human Babesiosis," Infectious Disease Clinics of North America, vol. 22, no. 3, pp. 469–488, 2008.
9. J. B. Bush, M. Isaacson, A. S. Mohamed, F. T. Potgieter, and D. T. de Waal, "Human babesiosis—a preliminary report of 2 suspected cases in South Africa," South African Medical Journal, vol. 78, no. 11, p. 699, 1990.
10. I. M. Foppa, P. J. Krause, A. Spielman, et al., "Entomologic and serologic evidence of zoonotic transmission of Babesia microti, eastern Switzerland," Emerging Infectious Diseases, vol. 8, no. 7, pp. 722–726, 2002.
11. A. Gorenflot, C. Bazin, and P. Ambroise-Thomas, "Human babesiosis. Treatment of severe forms," La Presse Médicale, vol. 16, no. 22, p. 1099, 1987.
12. B. L. Herwaldt, S. Cacciò, F. Gherlinzoni, et al., "Molecular characterization of a non-Babesia divergensorganism causing zoonotic babesiosis in Europe," Emerging Infectious Diseases, vol. 9, no. 8, pp. 942–948, 2003.
13. A. Hildebrandt, K.-P. Hunfeld, M. Baier, et al., "First confirmed autochthonous case of human Babesia microti infection in Europe," European Journal of Clinical Microbiology and Infectious Diseases, vol. 26, no. 8, pp. 595–601, 2007.
14. J.-Y. Kim, S.-H. Cho, H.-N. Joo, et al., "First case of human babesiosis in Korea: detection and characterization of a novel type of Babesia sp. (KO1) similar to ovine Babesia," Journal of Clinical Microbiology, vol. 45, no. 6, pp. 2084–2087, 2007.
15. A. Marathe, J. Tripathi, V. Handa, and V. Date, "Human babesiosis—a case report," Indian Journal of Medical Microbiology, vol. 23, no. 4, pp. 267–269, 2005.
16. L. Rios, G. Alvarez, and S. Blair, "Serological and parasitological study and report of the first case of human babesiosis in Colombia," Revista da Sociedade Brasileira de Medicina Tropical, vol. 36, no. 4, pp. 493–498, 2003.
17. C.-M. Shih, L.-P. Liu, W.-C. Chung, S.J. Ong, and C.-C. Wang, "Human babesiosis in Taiwan: asymptomatic infection with a Babesia microti-like organism in a Taiwanese woman," Journal of Clinical Microbiology, vol. 35, no. 2, pp. 450–454, 1997.
18. K. A. Western, G. D. Benson, N. N. Gleason, G. R. Healy, and M. G. Schultz, "Babesiosis in a Massachusetts resident," The New England Journal of Medicine, vol. 283, no. 16, pp. 854–856, 1970.
19. A. Spielman, M. L. Wilson, J. F. Levine, and J. Piesman, "Ecology of Ixodes dammini-borne human babesiosis and Lyme disease," Annual Review of Entomology, vol. 30, pp. 439–460, 1985.
20. S. E. Rodgers and T. N. Mather, "Human Babesia microti incidence and Ixodes scapularis distribution, Rhode Island, 1998–2004," Emerging Infectious Diseases, vol. 13, no. 4, pp. 633–635, 2007.
21. E. S. Eskow, P. J. Krause, A. Spielman, K. Freeman, and J. Aslanzadeh, "Southern extension of the range of

human babesiosis in the Eastern United States," Journal of Clinical Microbiology, vol. 37, no. 6, pp. 2051–2052, 1999.

22. S. J. Kogut, C. D. Thill, M. A. Prusinski, et al., "Babesia microti, upstate New York," Emerging Infectious Diseases, vol. 11, no. 3, pp. 476–478, 2005.
23. B. L. Herwaldt, P. C. McGovern, M. P. Gerwel, R. M. Easton, and R. R. MacGregor, "Endemic babesiosis in another eastern state: New Jersey," Emerging Infectious Diseases, vol. 9, no. 2, pp. 184–188, 2003.
24. M. K. Froberg, D. Dannen, N. Bernier, W.-J. Shieh, J. Guarner, and S. Zaki, "Case report: spontaneous splenic rupture during acute parasitemia of Babesia microti," Annals of Clinical and Laboratory Science, vol. 38, no. 4, pp. 390–392, 2008.
25. R. K. Pruthi, W. F. Marshall, J. C. Wiltsie, and D. H. Persing, "Human babesiosis," Mayo Clinic Proceedings, vol. 70, no. 9, pp. 853–862, 1995.
26. R. W. Steketee, M. R. Eckman, and E. C. Burgess, "Babesiosis in Wisconsin. A new focus of disease transmission," Journal of the American Medical Association, vol. 253, no. 18, pp. 2675–2678, 1985. ·
27. K. H. Berman, D. E. Blue, D. S. Smith, P. Y. Kwo, and S. Liangpunsakul, "Fatal case of babesiosis in postliver transplant patient," Transplantation, vol. 87, no. 3, pp. 452–453, 2009.
28. D. Blue, V. Graves, L. McCarthy, J. Cruz, S. Gregurek, and D. Smith, "Fatal transfusion-transmittedBabesia microti in the Midwest," Transfusion, vol. 49, no. 1, p. 8, 2009.
29. Q. Wei, M. Tsuji, A. Zamoto, et al., "Human babesiosis in Japan: isolation of Babesia microti-like parasites from an asymptomatic transfusion donor and from a rodent from an area where babesiosis is endemic,"Journal of Clinical Microbiology, vol. 39, no. 6, pp. 2178–2183, 2001.
30. P. J. Krause, S. R. Telford III, A. Spielman, et al., "Concurrent Lyme disease and babesiosis: evidence for increased severity and duration of illness," Journal of the American Medical Association, vol. 275, no. 21, pp. 1657–1660, 1996. ·
31. P. J. Krause, S. R. Telford III, R. Ryan, et al., "Geographical and temporal distribution of babesial infection in Connecticut," Journal of Clinical Microbiology, vol. 29, no. 1, pp. 1–4, 1991.
32. A. M. Kjemtrup and P. A. Conrad, "Human babesiosis: an emerging tick-borne disease," International Journal for Parasitology, vol. 30, no. 12-13, pp. 1323–1337, 2000. ·
33. D. A. Leiby, "Babesiosis and blood transfusion: flying under the radar," Vox Sanguinis, vol. 90, no. 3, pp. 157–165, 2006.
34. D. M. Gubernot, C. T. Lucey, K. C. Lee, G. B. Conley, L. G. Holness, and R. P. Wise, "Babesia infection through blood transfusions: reports received by the US Food and Drug Administration, 1997–2007,"Clinical Infectious Diseases, vol. 48, no. 1, pp. 25–30, 2009. · ·
35. J. V. Linden, S. J. Wong, F. K. Chu, G. B. Schmidt, and C. Bianco, "Transfusion-associated transmission of babesiosis in New York State," Transfusion, vol. 40, no. 3, pp. 285–289, 2000. ·
36. P. J. Krause, A. Spielman, S. R. Telford III, et al., "Persistent parasitemia after acute babesiosis," The New England Journal of Medicine, vol. 339, no. 3, pp. 160–165, 1998. ·
37. D. Esernio-Jenssen, P. G. Scimeca, J. L. Benach, and M. J. Tenenbaum, "Transplacental/perinatal babesiosis," Journal of Pediatrics, vol. 110, no. 4, pp. 570–572, 1987.
38. L. M. Fox, S. Wingerter, A. Ahmed, et al., "Neonatal babesiosis: case report and review of the literature,"Pediatric Infectious Disease Journal, vol. 25, no. 2, pp. 169–173, 2006.
39. B. L. Herwaldt, A. M. Kjemtrup, P. A. Conrad, et al., "Transfusion-transmitted babesiosis in Washington state: first reported case caused by a WA1-type parasite," Journal of Infectious Diseases, vol. 175, no. 5, pp. 1259–1262, 1997.
40. A. M. Kjemtrup, B. Lee, C. L. Fritz, C. Evans, M. Chervenak, and P. A. Conrad, "Investigation of transfusion transmission of a WA1-type babesial parasite to a premature infant in California,"Transfusion, vol. 42, no. 11, pp. 1482–1487, 2002.
41. D. H. Persing and P. A. Conrad, "Babesiosis: new insights from phylogenetic analysis," Infectious Agents and Disease, vol. 4, no. 4, pp. 182–195, 1995.
42. R. E. Quick, B. L. Herwaldt, J. W. Thomford, et al., "Babesiosis in Washington State: a new species of Babesia?" Annals of Internal Medicine, vol. 119, no. 4, pp. 284–290, 1993.
43. A. M. Kjemtrup, J. Thomford, T. Robinson, and P. A. Conrad, "Phylogenetic relationships of human and wildlife piroplasm isolates in the western United States inferred from the 18S nuclear small subunit RNA gene," Parasitology, vol. 120, no. 5, pp. 487–493, 2000. ·
44. J. F. Beattie, M. L. Michelson, and P. J. Holman, "Acute babesiosis caused by Babesia divergens in a resident of Kentucky," The New England Journal of Medicine, vol. 347, no. 9, pp. 697–698, 2002.
45. B. L. Herwaldt, G. de Bruyn, N. J. Pieniazek, et al., "Babesia divergens-like Infection, Washington State,"Emerging Infectious Diseases, vol. 10, no. 4, pp. 622–629, 2004.
46. P. J. Holman, "Phylogenetic and biologic evidence that Babesia divergens is not endemic in the United States," Annals of the New York Academy of Sciences, vol. 1081, pp. 518–525, 2006. · ·
47. A. Gorenflot, K. Moubri, E. Precigout, B. Carcy, and T. P. M. Schetters, "Human babesiosis," Annals of Tropical Medicine and Parasitology, vol. 92, no. 4, pp. 489–501, 1998. ·
48. A. Zintl, J. S. Gray, H. E. Skerrett, and G. Mulcahy, "Possible mechanisms underlying age-related resistance to bovine babesiosis," Parasite Immunology, vol. 27, no. 4, pp. 115–120, 2005. · ·
49. A. Zintl, G. Mulcahy, H. E. Skerrett, S. M. Taylor, and J. S. Gray, "Babesia divergens, a bovine blood parasite

of veterinary and zoonotic importance," Clinical Microbiology Reviews, vol. 16, no. 4, pp. 622–636, 2003.

50. K. Haselbarth, A. M. Tenter, V. Brade, G. Krieger, and K.-P. Hunfeld, "First case of human babesiosis in Germany—clinical presentation and molecular characterisation of the pathogen," International Journal of Medical Microbiology, vol. 297, no. 3, pp. 197–204, 2007.

51. P. J. Krause, K. McKay, C. A. Thompson, et al., "Disease-specific diagnosis of coinfecting tickborne zoonoses: babesiosis, human granulocytic ehrlichiosis, and Lyme disease," Clinical Infectious Diseases, vol. 34, no. 9, pp. 1184–1191, 2002.

52. J. C. Hatcher, P. D. Greenberg, J. Antique, and V. E. Jimenez-Lucho, "Severe babesiosis in Long Island: review of 34 cases and their complications," Clinical Infectious Diseases, vol. 32, no. 8, pp. 1117–1125, 2001.

53. T. K. Ruebush II, D. D. Juranek, and E. S. Chisholm, "Human babesiosis on Nantucket Island. Evidence for self-limited and subclinical infections," The New England Journal of Medicine, vol. 297, no. 15, pp. 825–827, 1977.

54. D. J. White, J. Talarico, H.-G. Chang, G. S. Birkhead, T. Heimberger, and D. L. Morse, "Human babesiosis in New York State: review of 139 hospitalized cases and analysis of prognostic factors," Archives of Internal Medicine, vol. 158, no. 19, pp. 2149–2154, 1998.

55. T. Sun, M. J. Tenenbaum, and J. Greenspan, "Morphologic and clinical observations in human infection with Babesia microti," Journal of Infectious Diseases, vol. 148, no. 2, pp. 239–248, 1983.

56. H. O. Mathewson, A. E. Anderson, and G. W. Hazard, "Self-limited babesiosis in a splenectomized child,"Pediatric Infectious Disease, vol. 3, no. 2, pp. 148–149, 1984.

57. J. M. Ortiz and R. C. Eagle Jr., "Ocular findings in human babesiosis (Nantucket fever)," American Journal of Ophthalmology, vol. 93, no. 3, pp. 307–311, 1982.

58. F. Rosner, M. H. Zarrabi, J. L. Benach, and G. S. Habicht, "Babesiosis in splenectomized adults. Review of 22 reported cases," American Journal of Medicine, vol. 76, no. 4, pp. 696–701, 1984.

59. P. J. Krause, B. E. Gewurz, D. Hill, et al., "Persistent and relapsing babesiosis in immunocompromised patients," Clinical Infectious Diseases, vol. 46, no. 3, pp. 370–376, 2008.

60. T. K. Ruebush II, P. B. Cassaday, and H. J. Marsh, "Human babesiosis on Nantucket Island: clinical features," Annals of Internal Medicine, vol. 86, no. 1, pp. 6–9, 1977.

61. C. P. Stowell, J. A. Gelfand, J.-A. O. Shepard, and A. Kratz, "Case 17-2007: a 25-year-old woman with relapsing fevers and recent onset of dyspnea," The New England Journal of Medicine, vol. 356, no. 22, pp. 2313–2319, 2007.

62. J. L. Benach and G. S. Habicht, "Clinical characteristics of human babesiosis," Journal of Infectious Diseases, vol. 144, no. 5, p. 481, 1981.

63. D. H. Persing, B. L. Herwaldt, C. Glaser, et al., "Infection with a Babesia-like organism in Northern California," The New England Journal of Medicine, vol. 332, no. 5, pp. 298–303, 1995.

64. G. R. Healy and T. K. Ruebush II, "Morphology of Babesia microti in human blood smears," American Journal of Clinical Pathology, vol. 73, no. 1, pp. 107–109, 1980.

65. P. J. Krause, S. R. Telford III, A. Spielman, et al., "Comparison of PCR with blood smear and inoculation of small animals for diagnosis of Babesia microti parasitemia," Journal of Clinical Microbiology, vol. 34, no. 11, pp. 2791–2794, 1996.

66. D. H. Persing, D. Mathiesen, W. F. Marshall, et al., "Detection of Babesia microti by polymerase chain reaction," Journal of Clinical Microbiology, vol. 30, no. 8, pp. 2097–2103, 1992.

67. P. J. Krause, R. Ryan, S. R. Telford III, D. Persing, and A. Spielman, "Efficacy of immunoglobulin M serodiagnostic test for rapid diagnosis of acute babesiosis," Journal of Clinical Microbiology, vol. 34, no. 8, pp. 2014–2016, 1996.

68. P. J. Krause, S. R. Telford III, R. Ryan, et al., "Diagnosis of babesiosis: evaluation of a serologic test for the detection of Babesia microti antibody," Journal of Infectious Diseases, vol. 169, no. 4, pp. 923–926, 1994.

69. T. K. Ruebush II, A. J. Sulzer, and G. R. Healy, "Development and persistence of antibody in persons infected with Babesia microti," American Journal of Tropical Medicine and Hygiene, vol. 30, no. 1, pp. 291–292, 1981.

70. G. P. Wormser, R. J. Dattwyler, E. D. Shapiro, et al., "The clinical assessments treatment, and prevention of lyme disease, human granulocytic anaplasmosis, and babesiosis: clinical practice guidelines by the Infectious Diseases Society of America," Clinical Infectious Diseases, vol. 43, no. 9, pp. 1089–1134, 2006.

71. P. J. Krause, T. Lepore, V. K. Sikand, et al., "Atovaquone and azithromycin for the treatment of babesiosis,"The New England Journal of Medicine, vol. 343, no. 20, pp. 1454–1458, 2000.

72. M. Raju, J. C. Salazar, H. Leopold, and P. J. Krause, "Atovaquone and azithromycin treatment for babesiosis in an infant," Pediatric Infectious Disease Journal, vol. 26, no. 2, pp. 181–183, 2007.

73. M. Wittner, K. S. Rowin, H. B. Tanowitz, et al., "Successful chemotherapy of transfusion babesiosis,"Annals of Internal Medicine, vol. 96, no. 5, pp. 601–604, 1982.

74. K. M. Cahill, J. L. Benach, L. M. Reich, et al., "Red cell exchange: treatment of babesiosis in a splenectomized patient," Transfusion, vol. 21, no. 2, pp. 193–198, 1981.

75. G. A. Jacoby, J. V. Hunt, K. S. Kosinski, et al., "Treatment of transfusion-transmitted babesiosis by exchange transfusion," The New England Journal of Medicine, vol. 303, no. 19, pp. 1098–1100, 1980.

76. V. I. Powell and K. Grima, "Exchange transfusion for malaria and babesia infection," Transfusion Medicine

Reviews, vol. 16, no. 3, pp. 239–250, 2002.

77. J. M. Vyas, S. R. Telford, and G. K. Robbins, "Treatment of refractory Babesia microti infection with atovaquone-proguanil in an HIV-infected patient: case report," Clinical Infectious Diseases, vol. 45, no. 12, pp. 1588–1590, 2007.

78. L. M. Weiss, M. Wittner, and H. B. Tanowitz, "The treatment of babesiosis," The New England Journal of Medicine, vol. 344, no. 10, p. 773, 2001.

79. D. Raoult, L. Soulayrol, B. Toga, H. Dumon, and P. Casanova, "Babesiosis, pentamidine, and cotrimoxazole," Annals of Internal Medicine, vol. 107, no. 6, p. 944, 1987.

80. E. Denes, J. P. Rogez, M. L. Darde, and P. Weinbreck, "Management of Babesia divergens babesiosis without a complete course of quinine treatment," European Journal of Clinical Microbiology and Infectious Diseases, vol. 18, no. 9, pp. 672–673, 1999. ·

81. E. B. Hayes and J. Piesman, "How can we prevent Lyme disease?" The New England Journal of Medicine, vol. 348, no. 24, pp. 2424–2430, 2003.

82. T. N. Mather, J. M. C. Ribeiro, and A. Spielman, "Lyme disease and babesiosis: acaricide focused on potentially infected ticks," American Journal of Tropical Medicine and Hygiene, vol. 36, no. 3, pp. 609–614, 1987.

83. G. R. Needham, "Evaluation of five popular methods for tick removal," Pediatrics, vol. 75, no. 6, pp. 997–1002, 1985.

84. K. C. Stafford III, Tick Management Handbook: An Integrated Guide for Homeowners, Pest Control Operators, and Public Health Officials for the Prevention of Tick-Associated Disease, The Connecticut Agricultural Experimental Station, New Haven, Conn, USA, 2007.

85. J. I. Tsao, J. T. Wootton, J. Bunikis, M. G. Luna, D. Fish, and A. G. Barbour, "An ecological approach to preventing human infection: vaccinating wild mouse reservoirs intervenes in the Lyme disease cycle,"Proceedings of the National Academy of Sciences of the United States of America, vol. 101, no. 52, pp. 18159–18164, 2004.

86. M. Vazquez, C. Muehlenbein, M. Cartter, E. B. Hayes, S. Ertel, and E. D. Shapiro, "Effectiveness of personal protective measures to prevent lyme disease," Emerging Infectious Diseases, vol. 14, no. 2, pp. 210–216, 2008.

87. M. L. Wilson, S. R. Telford III, J. Piesman, and A. Spielman, "Reduced abundance of immature Ixodes dammini (Acari: Ixodidae) following elimination of deer," Journal of Medical Entomology, vol. 25, no. 4, pp. 224–228, 1988.

88. D. Fish and J. E. Childs, "Community-Based Prevention of Lyme Disease and Other Tick-Borne Diseases Through Topical Application of Acaricide to White-Tailed Deer: Background and Rationale," Vector-Borne and Zoonotic Diseases, vol. 9, no. 4, pp. 357–364, 2009.

89. P. Grellier, R. Santus, E. Mouray, et al., "Photosensitized inactivation of Plasmodium falciparum- andBabesia divergens-infected erythrocytes in whole blood by lipophilic pheophorbide derivatives," Vox Sanguinis, vol. 72, no. 4, pp. 211–220, 1997.

90. B. Zavizion, M. Pereira, M. de Melo Jorge, et al., "Inactivation of protozoan parasites in red blood cells using INACTINE PEN110 chemistry," Transfusion, vol. 44, no. 5, pp. 731–738, 2004.

SECTION III: PARASITES OF SHEEP AND GOATS

CHAPTER 6

OCCURRENCE AND MOLECULAR CHARACTERIZATION OF GIARDIA DUODENALIS AND CRYPTOSPORIDIUM SPP. IN SHEEP AND GOATS REARED UNDER DAIRY HUSBANDRY SYSTEMS IN GREECE

Nikolaos Tzanidakis, Smaragda Sotiraki, Edwin Claerebout, Amimul Ehsan, Nikolaos Voutzourakis, Despoina Kostopoulou, Casaert Stijn, Jozef Vercruysse and Thomas Geurden

Keywords: Giardia, Cryptosporidium, Goat, Sheep, Dairy, Prevalence, Genotyping

INTRODUCTION

Giardia duodenalis and *Cryptosporidium* spp. are gastrointestinal protozoa that affect a wide range of mammals. Both parasites have a direct life cycle and are known to cause enteritis. In small ruminants, mainly young lambs and goat kids are infected. The prevalence of both parasites in small ruminants varies considerably between studies worldwide [13]. The most common clinical symptoms associated with *G. duodenalis* are the excretion of malodorous, loose to diarrhoeic faeces and impaired weight gain, whereas *Cryptosporidium* spp. infection can lead to severe diarrhoea, depression, anorexia and weight loss [1, 12]. Mortality has been associated with cryptosporidiosis, especially in animals with concurrent infections.

Since the initial claims on its potential public health relevance, eight genotypes or so-called assemblages have been identified within *G. duodenalis* [25]. Assemblage A and B are considered to be zoonotic genotypes, affecting both humans and small ruminants [1, 12, 16, 23], whereas Assemblage E is considered to be specific to hoofed livestock and has been found to be the most prevalent assemblage in lambs and goat kids [8, 12]. The genus *Cryptosporidium* consists of 20 species and more than 40 genotypes. In sheep, *C. parvum*, *C. xiaoi* and *C. ubiquitum* are most frequently identified [9, 12, 27, 29, 35, 41] whereas mainly *C. parvum* and to a lesser extent *C. xiaoi* has been reported in goats [9, 12, 35]. Due to the potential clinical and zoonotic relevance, there is a need to better understand the presence and abundance of both parasites in sheep and goat flocks.

The aim of this study was to estimate the prevalence of *G. duodenalis* and *Cryptosporidium* spp. infection in sheep and goat dairy farms in Greece. The small ruminant sector is very important in the Mediterranean basin from an economic, social and ecological point of view [5], especially in Greece with approximately 15 million sheep and goats which are kept traditionally for milk under low-input systems [20]. The most commonly applied farming systems practised in Greece can be categorized as extensive farming [43], and there is limited information on prevalence and especially molecular characterization of both parasites in these systems. The prevalence rates reported range from 33.3% to 49.6% for *G. duodenalis* and from 4.4% to 55% for *Cryptosporidium* spp. in sheep and goats [21, 32].

Citation: Tzanidakis N, Sotiraki S, Claerebout E, Ehsan A, Voutzourakis N, Kostopoulou D, Stijn C, Vercruysse J & Geurden T: Occurrence and molecular characterization of Giardia duodenalis and Cryptosporidium spp. in sheep and goats reared under dairy husbandry systems in Greece. Parasite, 2014,21, 45. DOI: http://dx.doi.org/10.1051/parasite/2014048.

MATERIALS AND METHODS

Study Design

The study was designed as a cross-sectional study in a high sheep and goat density area in Greece (i.e. the island of Crete where more than 1.5 million animals are kept). The farms enrolled in this survey were selected according to the following criteria: (a) type of animal on the farm (sheep, goats, or mixed sheep and goats), and (b) management practices applied ("intensive management system" where stocking rates are high and the young animals are reared indoors until weaning (30–40 days), and "extensive management system" where stocking rates are lower and young animals are reared with their mothers mostly on pasture). Each farm was visited on a single occasion in a 6-month period, and only animals between the age of 1 day and 10 weeks were considered for inclusion in the study. Sample size was calculated based on the number of expected births as an indicator of the number of animals on the farms: of the lambs, 5% of the expected births on each farm were sampled and of the goat kids, 10% of the expected births were sampled. Data on the type of water supply for the animals (public network supply, a private drill hole or natural well), the age of lambs or goat kids and the presence of diarrhoea were recorded.

Parasitological Examination

The faecal samples were examined in the laboratory using a quantitative immunofluorescence assay (IFA; Merifluor *Cryptosporidium/Giardia* kit; Meridian Diagnostics Inc.), as follows: 1 g of faeces was suspended in tap water and sieved three times through a layer of surgical gauze to withhold large debris. Sedimentation for at least 30 min was followed by discarding the supernatant. The remaining sediment was centrifuged at 3000 rpm for 5 min. The sediment was re-suspended in 1 mL of tap water. After thorough vortexing, an aliquot of 20 μL was applied onto an IFA slide. The samples, including a negative and positive control sample, were left to dry completely. After staining and incubating slides in a dark humidified chamber (for 30 min at room temperature), the entire slide was examined at 400× magnification under a fluorescence microscope. A sample was considered positive if at least one, clearly recognizable *Cryptosporidium* oocyst or *Giardia* cyst was identified. The number of (oo)cysts per gram of faeces was obtained by multiplying the total number of (oo) cysts on the slide by 50.

Molecular Characterization

Positive isolates for both parasites were selected for DNA extraction, using the QIAamp Stool Mini Kit (Qiagen), according to the manufacturer's instructions, incorporating an extended initial step of five freeze-thaw cycles (freezing in liquid nitrogen for 5 min and heating at 95 °C for 5 min) in the protocol to maximize (oo)cyst lesion. The selection of the positive isolates aimed to include at least one positive sample per farm.

For the amplification of the *Cryptosporidium* spp., the 18S ribosomal DNA (18S rDNA) gene PCR protocol was used (previously described in [40]), as well as a PCR targeting the 70 kDA heat shock protein (HSP70, described in [28]). Subgenotyping of the *C. parvum* positive samples was performed using the 60 kDa glycoprotein (gp60) gene [34]. *G. duodenalis* positive samples were characterized using the β-giardin gene [24], and the triose phosphate isomerase (TPI) gene [11]. Amplification products were visualized on 1.5% agarose gels with ethidium bromide. A positive and negative (PCR water) control sample was included in each PCR. PCR products were purified using the Qiaquick purification kit (Qiagen) and fully sequenced using the BigDye Terminator V3.1 Cycle Sequencing Kit (Applied Biosystems). Sequencing reactions were analysed on a 3100 Genetic Analyzer (Applied Biosystems) and assembled with Seqman II (DNASTAR, Madison, WI, USA). Sequences were compared with known sequences by BLAST-analysis against the NCBI database.

RESULTS

A total of 21 farms with either a sheep (n = 7) or goat (n = 7) flock, or a mixed sheep and goat flock (n = 7) were visited. On the majority of the farms (14/21) animals were reared under the intensive management system, whereas on 7 farms, goats and sheep were reared under the extensive management system (Table 1). In total, 684 faecal samples were examined, of which 429 samples were from lambs and 255 from goat kids. Mean lamb age was 5 weeks (range 4–8 weeks) and mean goat kid age was 6 weeks (range 4–9 weeks).

Table 1. Overview of the 21 farms included in the study, with the number of sheep and/or goats on the farms (N) and the type of management system (Sampled = number of animals sampled on each farm)

Farm identification number	Management system	Sheep		Goats	
		Number of animals	Sampled	Number of animals	Sampled
1	Intensive	203	17	0	0
7	Intensive	500	38	0	0
10	Intensive	450	29	0	0
11	Extensive	550	41	0	0
14	Extensive	170	13	0	0
16	Extensive	100	13	0	0
18	Extensive	750	34	0	0
2	Intensive	656	49	40	6

19	Extensive/intensive	400	24	40	8
4	Intensive	301	23	68	11
9	Intensive	500	38	85	14
3	Intensive	500	16	100	16
8	Intensive	680	51	174	28
12	Extensive	570	43	240	38
24	Extensive	0	0	190	15
22	Intensive	0	0	200	16
25	Intensive	0	0	210	17
27	Intensive	0	0	215	17
23	Intensive	0	0	250	20
26	Intensive	0	0	300	24
21	Intensive	0	0	315	25
	Total		429		255

The prevalence of *G. duodenalis* was 37.3% ($n = 160/429$) in lambs and 40.4% ($n = 103/255$) in goat kids. In total, 13 out of the 14 farms (92.9%) with a sheep flock, and 14 out of the 14 farms (100%) with a goat flock, were positive for *G. duodenalis* with a minimum of 4 positive samples on each positive farm. The prevalence of *Cryptosporidium* spp. oocysts was 5.1% ($n = 22/429$) in lambs and 7.1% ($n = 18/255$) in goat kids. In total, 8 out of the 14 farms (57.1%) with a sheep flock, and 7 out of the 14 farms (50.0%) with a goat flock, were positive with a minimum of 1 positive sample on each positive farm.

Intensity of *G. duodenalis* cyst excretion ranged from 50 to 800,000 cysts per gram (cpg) of faeces in lambs with an average of 48,989 cpg, and from 50 to 900,000 cpg for goat kids with an average of 94,053 cpg. The excretion level for *Cryptosporidium* oocysts was low in lambs with an average of 9143 oocysts per gram of faeces (range 200–31,900 opg), yet was high in goat kids with an average excretion of 47,744 opg (range 200–551,000 opg).

A minimum of 1 positive sample was selected for DNA extraction per farm for *G. duodenalis* and *Cryptosporidium* spp., respectively. In total, 71 samples yielded a positive amplicon for *G. duodenalis* (Table 2). The majority of the samples were typed as a mono-infection with the ruminant-specific assemblage E, both on the β-giardin gene and the TPI gene. Only a limited number of samples were typed as mixed assemblage A and E infections, both in lambs and in goat kids. For*Cryptosporidium*, 24 samples yielded a positive amplicon (Table 3). Three different *Cryptosporidium* species (*C. parvum*, *C. ubiquitum* and *C. xiaoi*) were identified, although *C. xiaoi* was not identified in lambs. The *C. parvum* positive samples were typed as subtype IId on the gp60 gene (IIdA4G2T14 and IIdA4G3T13).

Table 2. Results for molecular identification of *Giardia duodenalis* positive samples in goat kids and lambs, based on the B-giardin (= beta-giardin) or triose phosphate isomerase (TPI) gene (NA = no amplification; A = assemblage A; E = assemblage E; A + E = mixed infection with assemblage A and E)

Animal species	Number of samples	B-giardin			TPI			
		A	E	NA	A	E	A + E	NA
Goat kids	30	1	28	1	1	26	3	0
Lambs	41	1	35	5	1	35	3	2
Total	71	2	63	6	2	61	6	2

Table 3. Results for molecular identification of *Cryptosporidium* positive samples in goat kids and lambs

Animal species	Number of samples	*C. xiaoi*	*C. ubiquitum*	*C. parvum*
Goat kids	14	7	5	2 (IId)
Lambs	10	0	3	7 (IId)
Total	24	7	8	9

DISCUSSION

The present study illustrates that *G. duodenalis* is highly prevalent in both lambs and goat kids, as the parasite was detected in all but one of the sheep flocks and in all goat flocks. The high farm and animal prevalence is in line with previous studies in small ruminants in Europe [4, 13, 18]. The high *G. duodenalis* prevalence and the potential association with production losses [31, 44] require an appropriate level of awareness of this infection on those farms in terms of disease management and prevention of infection. In contrast to *G. duodenalis*, the prevalence of *Cryptosporidium* was lower than anticipated in both lambs and goat kids, probably due to the age range of the animals included in the present study. Nevertheless, the farm prevalence on the sheep (57.1%) and goat (50.0%) farms does suggest that *Cryptosporidium* is widespread and is a potential threat to the small ruminant population. In previous studies in Greece, *Cryptosporidium* has been associated with large outbreaks of diarrhoea in both sheep and goat flocks [14, 15, 37], similar to other major small ruminant rearing countries [6, 33].

Both for *G. duodenalis* and for *Cryptosporidium* spp. a potential public health threat has been suspected, based on the high prevalence of these parasites in small ruminants and on extrapolation of molecular insights from other animal species, such as cattle or companion animals. However, recent molecular data seem to suggest that small ruminants are mostly infected with non-zoonotic genotypes of *G. duodenalis* [12, 18, 38, 39, 46, 47] and *Cryptosporidium* spp. [38]. On the other hand, potentially zoonotic genotypes or species such as *G. duodenalis* assemblage A and B [1, 2, 12, 19, 26, 30, 41], *C. parvum* [3,6, 12, 22, 46], *C. hominis* [17], *C. meleagridis* [42] and *C. ubiquitum* [10, 12, 45] have been reported in small ruminants. Furthermore, the identification of potentially zoonotic genotypes does not necessarily imply that transmission occurs. Recently, host-associated populations of *C. parvum* have been described using a multi-locus genotyping (MLG) approach, and*C. parvum* populations found in goats were even found to differ from bovine and sheep MLGs [7]. Whether this is a true host-specific phenomenon or just a matter of the level of isolation and opportunities for out-crossing is still to be discussed. Nevertheless, the contradicting molecular findings illustrate the difficulty of evaluating a potential public health threat based solely on genetic data without considering the epidemiological background and transmission of infection. Direct transmission of *Cryptosporidium* infection through bottle feeding or petting of animals on educational farms has been described before [38], but is probably an occasional route of infection. Although there is no direct evidence of transmission of *Cryptosporidium*and *G. duodenalis* infections from small ruminants to the human population via contaminated water, it is considered a threat. Furthermore, the detection of both parasites in outbreaks and in water screening is not routine practice in most countries, and large waterborne outbreaks might go unnoticed. In a recent study in Spain, the prevalence of *Cryptosporidium* and*Giardia* in water was significantly higher in the inland area, with higher concentration of livestock and fewer water treatment plants [4], illustrating that a variety of factors define the odds for infection. In the specific study area on the island of Crete, only a limited number of water basins are used over the island to produce drinking water for the local population and for the tourist population in the summer. The pastures surrounding the drinking water basins are all grazed by small ruminants. Whether these conditions lead to a substantial public health threat will need to be evaluated further in a longitudinal study, including sampling of water.

In goats, a large proportion of the *Cryptosporidium* positive samples were typed as *C. xiaoi*, both on 18S and HSP-70. This is in agreement with previous studies in Spain [6] and France [36], yet contradicts the initial claim that *C. xiaoi* infections are largely restricted to sheep [9]. In the current study, *C. xiaoi* was found in goats from three different farms, of which 2 farms maintained a goat-only flock and 1 farm managed a mixed flock. This illustrates that, although the introduction in the goat flocks might be due to contact with infected sheep, a *C. xiaoi* infection is easily maintained in goats. As advocated by Fayer and Santin [9], further epidemiological data will be needed to confirm whether the reports of *C. xiaoi* in goats are incidental or a regularly observed finding.

In conclusion, a high animal and farm prevalence of *G. duodenalis*, and a high farm prevalence of *Cryptosporidium* spp. were detected in both lambs and goat kids. Although mainly non-zoonotic species were identified in the present study, the frequent contact and proximity of grazing grounds to the natural water sources used to produce drinking water in the study area warrant further investigation of the public health relevance of these infections.

ACKNOWLEDGMENTS

The authors would like to thank the farmers and research staff who participated in this study, with special thanks to Dr. Alexandros Stefanakis. The study was conducted within the framework of the COST Action FA0805 CAPARA. "*Goat-parasite interactions: from knowledge to control*".

REFERENCES

1. Aloisio F, Filippini G, Antenucci P, Lepri E, Pezzotti G, Caccio S-M, Pozio E. 2006. Severe weight loss in lambs infected with *Giardia duodenalis* assemblage B. Veterinary Parasitology, 142, 154–158.
2. Berrilli F, D'Alfonso R, Giangaspero A, Marangi M, Brandonisio O, Kaboré Y, Glé C, Cianfanelli C, Lauro R, Di Cave D. 2012. *Giardia duodenalis* genotypes and *Cryptosporidium* species in humans and domestic animals in Côte d'Ivoire: occurrence and evidence for environmental contamination. Transactions of the Royal Society of Tropical Medicine and Hygiene, 106, 191–195.
3. Cacciò SM, Sannella AR, Mariano V, Valentini S, Berti F, Tosini F, Pozio E. 2013. A rare *Cryptosporidium parvum*genotype associated with infection of lambs and zoonotic transmission in Italy. Veterinary Parasitology, 191, 128–131.
4. Castro-Hermida JA, García-Presedo I, Almeida A, González-Warleta M, Correia Da Costa JM, Mezo M. 2011.*Cryptosporidium* spp. and *Giardia duodenalis* in two areas of Galicia (NW Spain). Science of the Total Environment, 409, 2451–2459.
5. De Rancourt M, Fois N, Lavin MP, Tchakerian E, Vallerand F. 2006. Mediterranean sheep and goat production: an uncertain future. Small Ruminant Research, 62, 167–179.
6. Díaz P, Quílez J, Robinson G, Chalmers RM, Díez-Baños P, Morrondo P. 2010. Identification of *Cryptosporidium xiaoi* in diarrhoeic goat kids (*Capra hircus*) in Spain. Veterinary Parasitology, 172, 132–134.
7. Drumo R, Widmer G, Morrison LJ, Tait A, Grelloni V, D'Avino N, Pozio E, Cacciò SM. 2012. Evidence of host-associated populations of *Cryptosporidium parvum*

in Italy. Applied Environmental Microbiology, 78, 3523–3529.

8. Ey PL, Mansouri M, Kulda J, Nohynkova E, Monis PT, Andrews RH, Mayrhofer G. 1997. Genetic analysis of *Giardia* from hoofed farm animals reveals artiodactyls-specific and potentially zoonotic genotypes. Journal of Eukaryotic Microbiology, 44, 625–635.

9. Fayer R, Santin M. 2009. *Cryptosporidium xiaoi* n. sp. (Apicomplexa: *Cryptosporidiidae*) in sheep (*Ovis aries*). Veterinary Parasitology, 164, 192–200.

10. Fiuza VR, Cosendey RI, Frazão-Teixeira E, Santín M, Fayer R, de Oliveira FC. 2011. Molecular characterization of*Cryptosporidium* in Brazilian sheep. Veterinary Parasitology, 175, 360–362.

11. Geurden T, Geldhof P, Levecke B, Martens C, Berkvens D, Casaert S, Vercruysse J, Claerebout E. 2008. Mixed *Giardia duodenalis* assemblage A and E infections in calves. International Journal for Parasitology, 38, 259–264.

12. Geurden T, Thomas P, Casaert S, Vercruysse J, Claerebout E. 2008. Prevalence and molecular characterization of*Cryptosporidium* and *Giardia* in lambs and goat kids in Belgium. Veterinary Parasitology, 155, 142–145.

13. Geurden T, Vercruysse J, Claerebout E. 2010. Is *Giardia* a significant pathogen in production animals? Experimental Parasitology, 124, 98–106.

14. Giadinis ND, Panousis NK, Papadopoulos E, Antoniadou-Sotiriadou K, Karatzias H. 2006. The effects of halofuginone in cases of cryptosporidiosis in newborn lambs and kids in Greece. Proceedings of the 10th Greek Veterinary Congress, Athens. p. 195–196.

15. Giadinis N, Papadopoulos E, Panousis N, Papazahariadou M, Lafi SQ, Karatzias H. 2007. Effect of halofuginone lactate on treatment and prevention of lamb cryptosporidiosis: an extensive field trial. Journal of Veterinary Pharmacology and Therapeutics, 30, 578–582.

16. Giangaspero A, Paoletti B, Iorio R, Traversa D. 2005. Prevalence and molecular characterization of *Giardia duodenalis*from sheep in central Italy. Parasitology Research, 96, 32–37.

17. Giles M, Chalmers R, Pritchard G, Elwin K, Mueller-Doblies D, Clifton-Hadley F. 2009. *Cryptosporidium hominis* in a goat and a sheep in the UK. Veterinary Record, 164, 24–25.

18. Gómez-Muñoz MT, Navarro C, Garijo-Toledo MM, Dea-Ayuela MA, Fernández-Barredo S, Pérez-Gracia MT, Domínguez-Márquez MV, Borrás R. 2009. Occurrence and genotypes of *Giardia* isolated from lambs in Spain. Parasitology International, 58, 297–299.

19. Gómez-Muñoz MT, Cámara-Badenes C, Martínez-Herrero Mdel C, Dea-Ayuela MA, Pérez-Gracia MT, Fernández-Barredo S, Santín M, Fayer R. 2012. Multilocus genotyping of *Giardia duodenalis* in lambs from Spain reveals a high heterogeneity. Research in Veterinary Science, 93, 836–842.

20. Hadjigeorgiou I, Vallerand F, Tsimpoukas K, Zervas G. 2002. The socio-economics of sheep and goat farming in Greece and the implications for the future rural development. Options Méditerranéennes Series B, 39, 83–93.

21. Himonas CA, Antoniadou-Sotiriadou KS, Sotiraki ST, Papazahariadou MG. 1998. Intestinal protozoa of animals in Macedonia. Bulletin of the Hellenic Veterinary Medical Society, 49, 300–306.

22. Imre K, Luca C, Costache M, Sala C, Morar A, Morariu S, Ilie MS, Imre M, Dărăbuş G. 2013. Zoonotic *Cryptosporidium parvum* in Romanian newborn lambs (*Ovis aries*). Veterinary Parasitology, 191, 119–122.

23. Karanis P, Ey PL. 1998. Characterization of axenic isolates of *Giardia intestinalis* established from humans and animals in Germany. Parasitology Research, 84, 442–449.

24. Lalle M, Jimenez-Cardosa E, Cacciò SM, Pozio E. 2005. Genotyping of *Giardia duodenalis* from humans and dogs from Mexico using a beta-giardin nested polymerase chain reaction assay. Journal of Parasitology, 91, 203–205.

25. Lasek-Nesselquist E, Welch DM, Sogin ML. 2010. The identification of a new *Giardia duodenalis* assemblage in marine vertebrates and a preliminary analysis of *G. duodenalis* population biology in marine systems. International Journal for Parasitology, 40, 1063–1074.

26. Lim YA, Mahdy MA, Tan TK, Goh XT, Jex AR, Nolan MJ, Sharma RS, Gasser RB. 2013. First molecular characterization of *Giardia duodenalis* from goats in Malaysia. Molecular and Cellular Probes, 27, 28–31.

27. McLauchlin J, Amar C, Pedraza-Diaz S, Nichols GL. 2000. Molecular epidemiological analysis of *Cryptosporidium* spp. in the United Kingdom: Results of genotyping *Cryptosporidium* spp. in 1,705 faecal samples from humans and 105 faecal samples from livestock animals. Journal of Clinical Microbiology, 38, 3984–3990.

28. Morgan UM, Monis PT, Xiao L, Limor J, Sulaiman I, Raidal S, O'Donoghue P, Gasser R, Murray A, Fayer R, Blagburn BL, Lal AA, Thompson RC. 2001. Molecular and phylogenetic characterisation of *Cryptosporidium* from birds. International Journal for Parasitology, 31, 289–296.

29. Mueller-Doblies D, Giles M, Elwin K, Smith RP, Clifton-Hadley FC, Chalmers RM. 2008. Distribution of *Cryptosporidium*species in sheep in the UK. Veterinary Parasitology, 154, 214–219.

30. Nolan MJ, Jex AR, Pangasa A, Young ND, Campbell AJ, Stevens M, Gasser RB. 2010. Analysis of nucleotide variation within the triose-phosphate isomerase gene of *Giardia duodenalis* from sheep and its zoonotic implications. Electrophoresis, 31, 287–298.

31. Olson ME, McAllister TA, Deselliers L, Morck DW, Cheng KJ, Buret AG, Ceri H. 1995. Effects of giardiasis on production in a domestic ruminant (lamb) model. American Journal of Veterinary Research, 56, 1470–1474.

32. Panousis N, Diakou A, Giadinis N, Papadopoulos E, Karatzias H, Haralampidis S. 2008. Prevalence of *Cryptosporidium*infection in sheep flocks with a history

of lambs' diarrhoea. Revue de Médecine Vétérinaire, 159, 528–531.

33. Paraud C, Pors I, Chartier C. 2010. Evaluation of oral tilmicosin efficacy against severe cryptosporidiosis in neonatal kids under field conditions. Veterinary Parasitology, 170, 149–152.

34. Peng MM, Matos O, Gatei W, Das P, Stantic-Pavlinic M, Bern C, Sulaiman IM, Glaberman S, Lal AA, Xiao L. 2001. A comparison of *Cryptosporidium* subgenotypes from several geographic regions. Journal of Eukaryotic Microbiology Supplement, 48, 28S–31S.

35. Quilez J, Torres E, Chalmers RM, Hadfield SJ, Cacho E, Sanchez-Acedo C. 2008. *Cryptosporidium* Genotypes and subtypes in lambs and goat kids in Spain. Applied and Environmental Microbiology, 74, 6026–6031.

36. Rieux A, Paraud C, Pors I, Chartier C. 2013. Molecular characterization of *Cryptosporidium* spp. in pre-weaned kids in a dairy goat farm in western France. Veterinary Parasitology, 192, 268–272.

37. Robertson LJ. 2009. *Giardia* and *Cryptosporidium* infections in sheep and goats: a review of the potential for transmission to humans via environmental contamination. Epidemiology and Infection, 137, 913–921.

38. Robertson LJ, Gjerde BK, Hansen EF. 2010. The zoonotic potential of *Giardia* and *Cryptosporidium* in Norwegian sheep: a longitudinal investigation of 6 flocks of lambs. Veterinary Parasitology, 171, 140–145.

39. Ruiz A, Foronda P, Gonzalez JF, Guedes A, Abreu-Acosta N, Molina JM, Valladares B. 2008. Occurrence and genotype characterization of *Giardia duodenalis* in goat kids from the Canary Islands, Spain. Veterinary Parasitology, 154, 137–141.

40. Ryan UM, Bath C, Rovertson I, Read C, Elliot A, Mcinnes L, Traub R, Besier B. 2005. Sheep may not be an important zoonotic reservoir for *Cryptosporidium* and *Giardia* Parasites. Applied Environmental Microbiology, 71, 4992–4997.

41. Santin M, Trout JM, Fayer R. 2007. Prevalence and molecular characterization of *Cryptosporidium* and *Giardia* species and genotypes in sheep in Maryland. Veterinary Parasitology, 146, 17–24.

42. Silverlås C, Mattsson JG, Insulander M, Lebbad M. 2012. Zoonotic transmission of *Cryptosporidium meleagridis* on an organic Swedish farm. International Journal for Parasitology, 42, 963–967.

43. Stefanakis A, Volanis M, Zoiopoulos P, Hadjigeorgiou I. 2007. Assessing the potential benefits of technical intervention in evolving the semi-intensive dairy-sheep farms in Crete. Small Ruminant Research, 72, 66–72.

44. Sweeny JP, Robertson ID, Ryan UM, Jacobson C, Woodgate RG. 2011. Impacts of naturally acquired protozoa and strongylid nematode infections on growth and faecal attributes in lambs. Veterinary Parasitology, 184, 298–308.

45. Wang Y, Feng Y, Cui B, Jian F, Ning C, Wang R, Zhang L, Xiao L. 2010. Cervine genotype is the major *Cryptosporidium*genotype in sheep in China. Parasitology Research, 106, 341–347.

46. Yang R, Jacobson C, Gordon C, Ryan U. 2009. Prevalence and molecular characterisation of *Cryptosporidium* and*Giardia* species in pre-weaned sheep in Australia. Veterinary Parasitology, 161, 19–24.

47. Zhang W, Zhang X, Wang R, Liu A, Shen Y, Ling H, Cao J, Yang F, Zhang X, Zhang L. 2012. Genetic characterizations of *Giardia duodenalis* in sheep and goats in Heilongjiang Province, China and possibility of zoonotic transmission. PLoS Neglected Tropical Diseases, 6, e1826.

CHAPTER 7

PREVALENCE OF GASTROINTESTINAL HELMINTHS IN EXOTIC AND INDIGENOUS GOATS SLAUGHTERED IN SELECTED ABATTOIRS IN PORT HARCOURT, SOUTH-SOUTH, NIGERIA

Ovutor Owhoeli, Kingsley Elele, and Lebari Barine Gboeloh

INTRODUCTION

Ruminants, cattle, goats and sheep, represent an important source of animal protein in many countries of the world, supplying a good percentage of the daily meat and dairy products in cities and villages in such countries including Nigeria [1]. Apart from being the source of animal protein, their wastes are also very important in agriculture [1, 2]. These animals are used in special ceremonies such as wedding and burials in most parts of Nigeria. However, parasitic diseases coupled with inadequate management hampered the productive husbandry of these animals [2, 3].

Gastrointestinal parasitic infections are world-wide problem for both small and large-scale farmers, but their impact is greater in Sub-Saharan Africa due to the availability of a wide range of agroecological factors suitable for diversified hosts and parasite species [3]. Gastrointestinal parasites are known to be widespread in Nigeria [4, 5] and limit ruminant production in many areas of the country [5, 6]. The direct losses caused by these parasites are attributed to hyper-acuteness and death, premature slaughter, and rejection of some parts at meat inspection, whilst indirect losses include the reduction in productive potential such as decreased growth rate, weight loss, diarrhea, anorexia, and sometimes anaemia [7–9].

Helminths or worms cause a wide range of health problems to both man and animals [10]. Helminthiasis, in large part, is caused by members of the phyla Nematoda and Platyhelminthes [11]. Species belonging to both phyla occupy numerous niches within their mammalian hosts, ranging from intestinal lumen to intravascular and even intracellular sites [12]. They are responsible for substantial loss of productivity in the livestock industry. Their harmful effects on these animals range from gastroenteritis, anorexia, abdominal distention, diarrhoea, emaciation, and so forth; all of which result in serious economic losses to the farmer and the nation in general [13]. Similarly, they constitute a major impediment to efficient and profitable livestock production [14].

The prevalence of gastrointestinal helminths is related to the agroclimatic conditions like quantity and quality of pasture, temperature, humidity, and grazing behavior of the host [15]. However specific parasites may be distributed throughout the world; they have different impact according to production system, management, and geoclimatic conditions [11].

The information on the prevalence and distribution of various species of gastrointestinal parasites of cattle and goats kept by the nomadic Fulani's in Nigeria and those in Port

Citation: Ovutor Owhoeli, Kingsley Elele, and Lebari Barine Gboeloh, "Prevalence of Gastrointestinal Helminths in Exotic and Indigenous Goats Slaughtered in Selected Abattoirs in Port Harcourt, South-South, Nigeria,"Chinese Journal of Biology, vol. 2014, Article ID 435913, 8 pages, 2014. doi:10.1155/2014/435913.

Harcourt are important in the formulation of control strategies for the nomads and other farmers.

MATERIALS AND METHODS

Study Area

The study was conducted in Port Harcourt City, South-South, Nigeria. Obio/Akpor and Port Harcourt city Local governments are commonly referred to as Port Harcourt city. It is situated on the bonny River within the Niger Delta, South-South, Nigeria. The study area lies between latitude $4^0 40^1$ and $7^0 10^1$ to longitude $7^0 55^1$east of the Greenwich meridian. It is situated some 60 km from the open sea, which is immediately where the coastal marshes give way to the land of the interior. Four abattoirs were selected from Rumuodumaya: Ogbogoro, Eliozu, and Aluu communities in the study.

Collection of Faecal Samples

Faecal specimens were collected from goats in the four aforementioned community abattoirs and individual homes in the study area. Animals were usually slaughtered early in the morning between the hours of 6.30 am and 8.00 am daily for a period of ten months (May, 2008 to February, 2009). Faecal samples were randomly collected weekly from the intestines of slaughtered animals (exotic and indigenous). The samples were collected in clean labeled sterile vials, preserved in 10% formalin, and taken to the laboratory for microscopic examination.

Laboratory Examination

The formol-ether concentration technique [16] was used to analyze the samples. 1 g of stool sample was emulsified with 4 mL of 10% formol saline in a test tube. The mixture was filtered into a test tube using a cloth gauge and 3-4 mL of diethyl ether was added and it shaken vigorously and allowed to stand for two minutes. The mixture was then centrifuged at 1000 revolutions per minutes (1000 rpm) for 3 minutes. Using a glass rod, the faecal debris from the side of the tube was loosened and the tube was inverted to pour off the supernatants. The tube was returned to its original upright position and the fluid from the side of the tube allowed draining to the bottom. The deposit was mixed by tapping the tube with the finger and using a Pasteur pipette. A drop of the sediment was applied on a microscope slide, covered with a cover slip, and examined under the microscope using ×10 and ×40 objectives. Lugol's iodine was also used as a stain (Figures 1, 2, and 3).

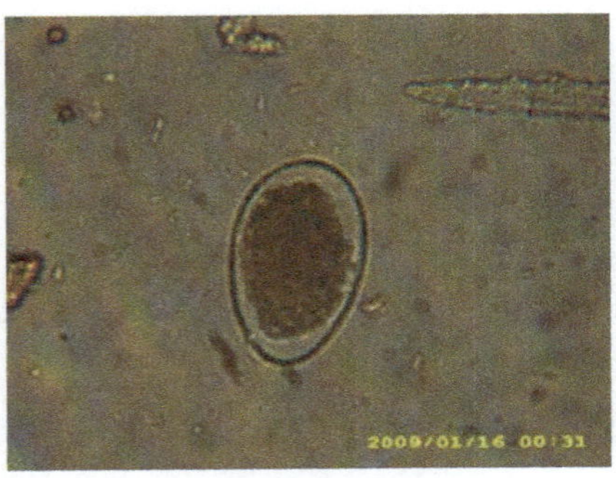

Ostertagia species

(a)

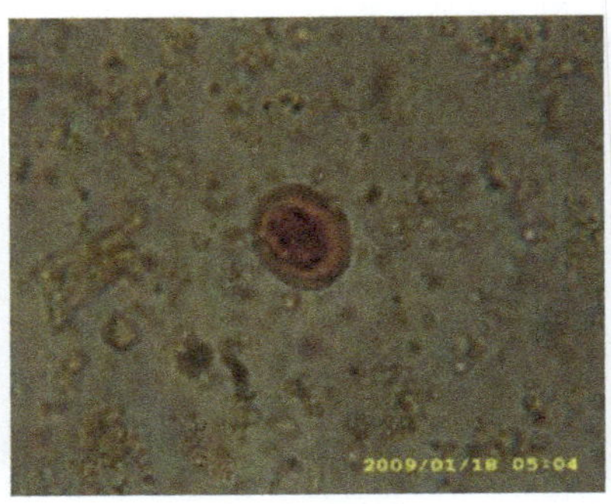

Ascaris species

(b)

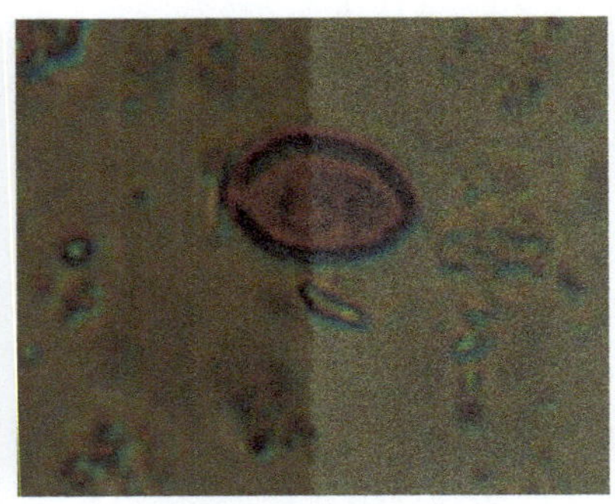

Trichuris species

(c)

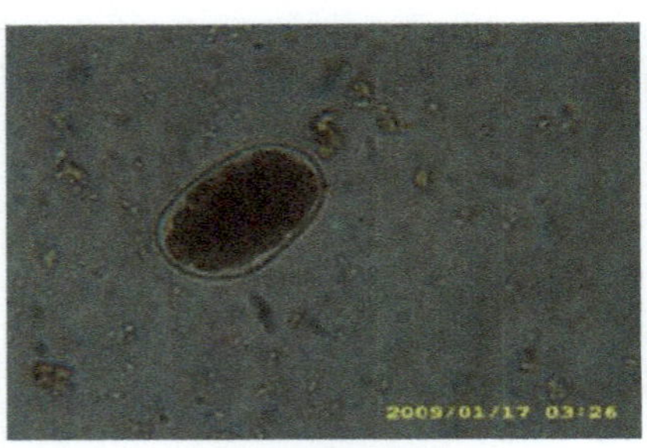

Chabertia species

(d)

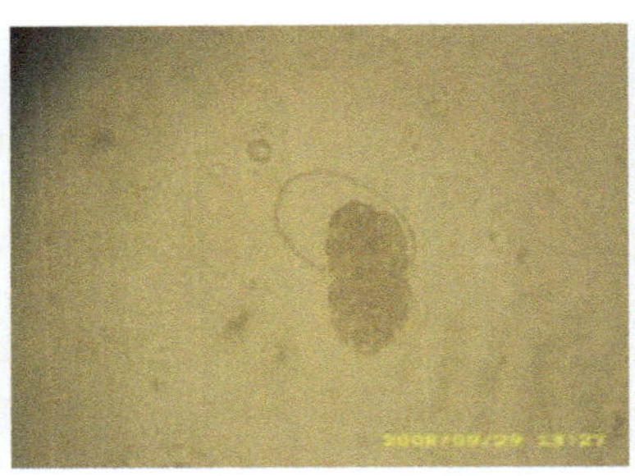

Hatching egg of *Chabertia* species

(e)

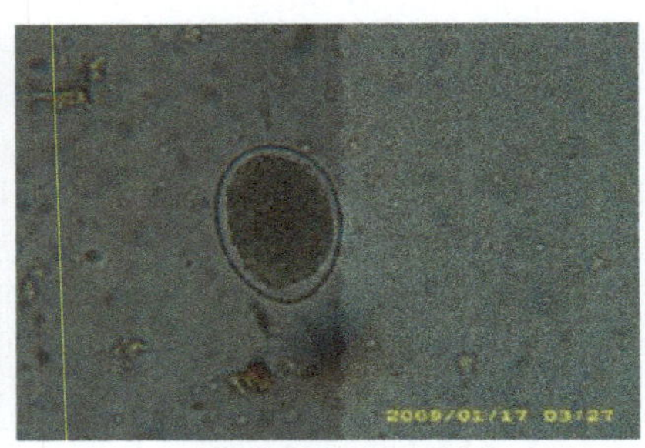

Haemonchus species

(f)

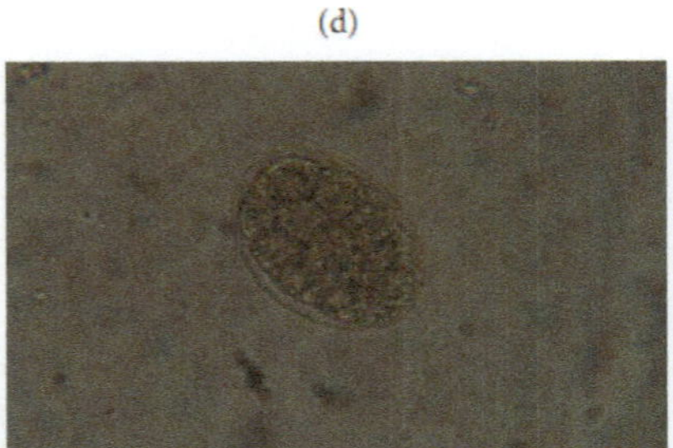

Bunostomum species

(g)

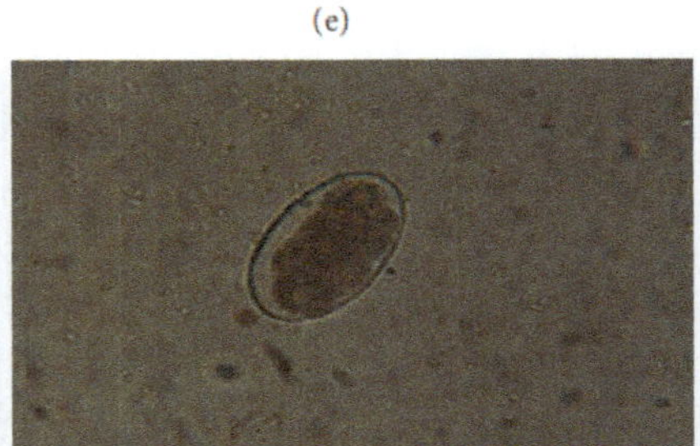

Trichostrongylus spp.

(h)

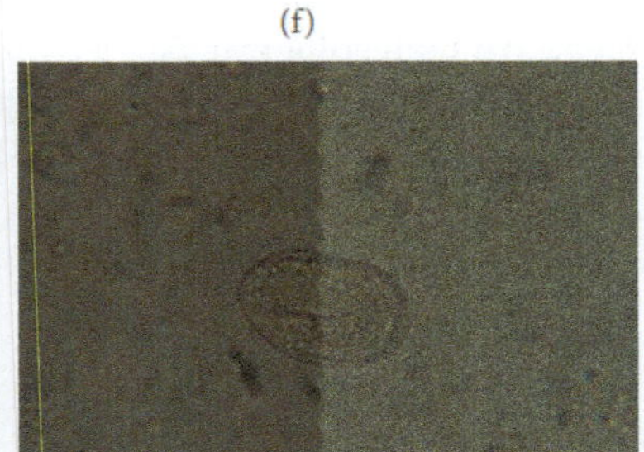

Strongyloides species

(i)

Figure 1: Eggs of Nematodes as seen under the ×40 objective of the microscope on slides stained with Lugol's iodine.

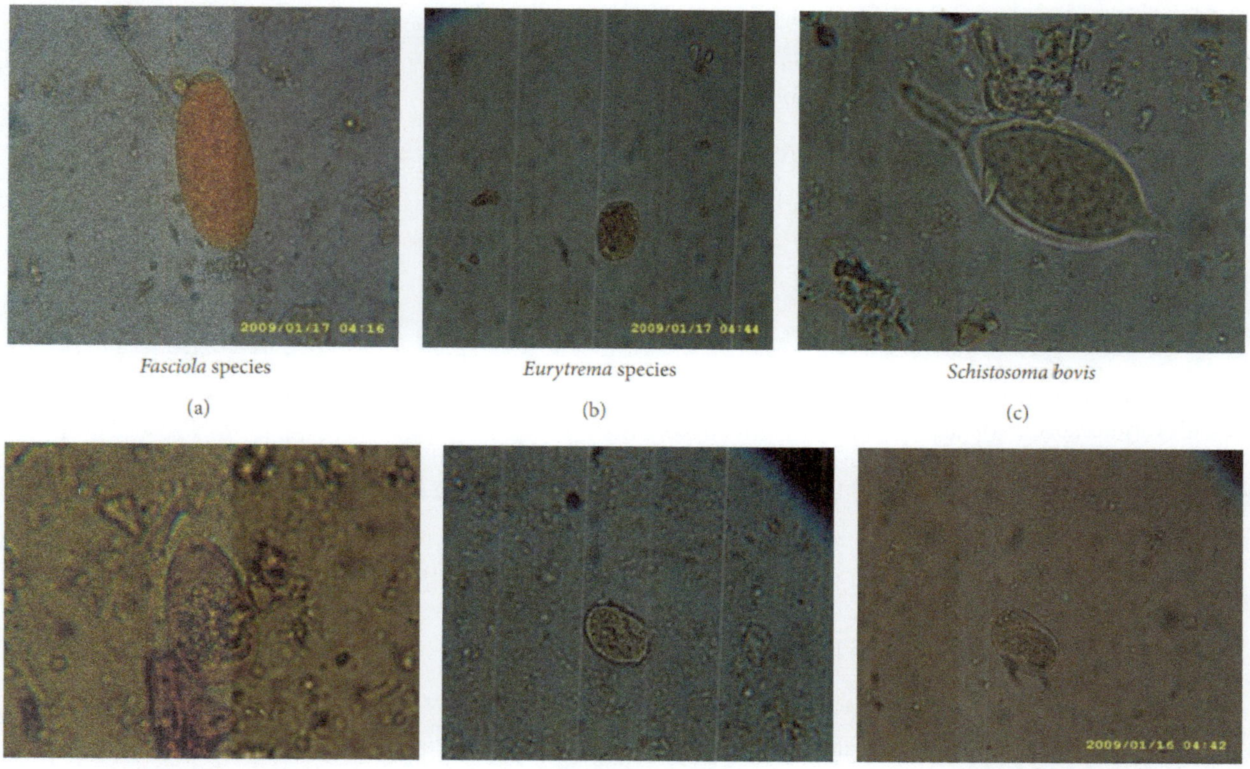

Fasciola species (a)

Eurytrema species (b)

Schistosoma bovis (c)

Gastrothylax species (d)

Schistosoma japonicum (e)

Dicrocoelium species (f)

Figure 2: Eggs of Trematodes as seen under the ×40 objective of the microscope on slides stained with Lugol's iodine.

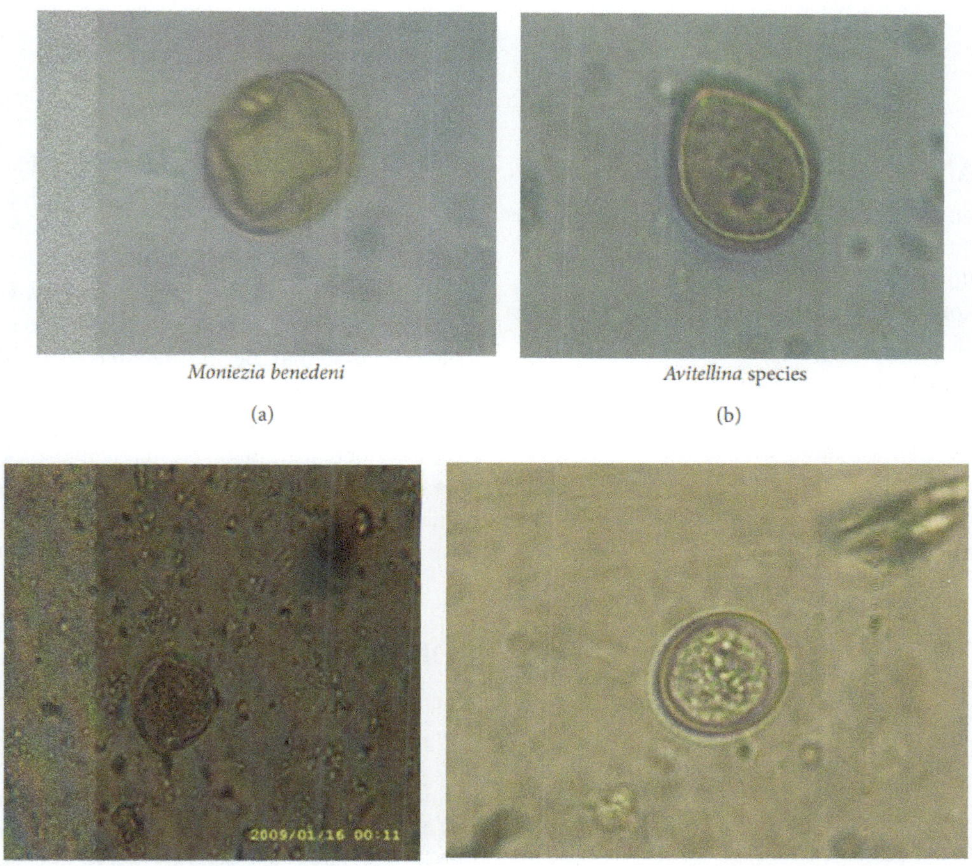

Moniezia benedeni (a)

Avitellina species (b)

Moniezia expansa (c)

Tenia species (d)

Figure 3: Eggs of Cestodes as seen under the ×40 objective of the microscope on slides stained with Lugol's iodine.

RESULTS

A total of 75 exotic goats were examined between the months of May and September 2010. Fifty-seven (57) were infected with various species of gastrointestinal helminths as follows (see Table 1).

Table 1: Species of helminths in exotic goats between the months of May 2008 and February 2009

	Parasite type					Nematodes					Cestodes				Trematodes		
Months	Numbers examined	Numbers infected	*Haemonchus*	*Strongyloides*	*Chabertia*	*Trichuris*	*Ostergia*	*Bunostomum*	*Trychostrongyloides*	*Ascaris*	*Tenia*	*Moniezia*	*Avitelina*	*Fasciola*	*Eurytrma*	Gastrotylax	*Schistosoma* spp	*Dicrocoelium*
May	13	9	2	0	1	0	1	0	0	1	0	1	0	2	0	1	0	0
June	17	14	4	2	1	0	0	1	0	1	1	1	1	1	0	1	0	1
July	16	13	3	0	1	1	2	1	0	0	0	3	0	1	0	1	0	0
August	15	11	2	1	1	1	0	1	1	0	1	0	0	1	0	1	0	1
September	14	10	2	1	1	0	1	0	0	0	0	2	1	2	0	1	0	0
Total	75	57 (76)	13 (17.3)	4 (5.3)	5 (6.6)	2 (2.6)	4 (5.3)	3 (4)	1 (1.3)	2 (2.6)	2 (2.6)	7 (9.3)	2 (2.6)	7 (9.3)	0	5 (6.6)	0	2 (2.6)

A total of 78 exotic goats were examined between the months of October 2010 and February 2011. Fifty-five (55) were infected with various species of gastrointestinal helminths as follows (see Table 2).

Table 2: Species of helminthes obtained between the months of October 2008 and February 2009 from exotic goats

	Parasite type					Nematodes					Cestodes				Trematodes		
Name of abattoir	Numbers examined	Numbers infected	*Haemonchus*	*Strongyloides*	*Chabertia*	*Trichuris*	*Ostergia*	*Bunostomum*	*Trychostrongyloides*	*Ascaris*	*Tenia*	*Moniezia*	*Avitelina*	*Fasciola*	*Eurytrma*	Gastrotylax	*Schistosoma* spp	*Dicrocoelium*
October	14	9	2	1	0	0	1	1	0	0	0	1	0	1	0	1	0	1
November	16	12	2	0	1	1	1	1	0	1	0	2	0	1	0	1	1	0
December	16	10	2	1	0	1	1	0	1	0	1	1	0	0	0	0	2	0
January	17	13	2	2	1	0	0	1	1	1	0	2	0	1	0	1	1	0
February	15	11	3	1	1	1	0	0	0	0	1	2	0	1	0	0	1	0
Total (%)	78	55 (70.5)	11 (17.1)	5 (6.4)	3 (3.8)	3 (3.8)	3 (3.8)	3 (3.8)	2 (2.5)	2 (2.5)	2 (2.5)	8 (10.2)	0	4 (5.1)	0	3 (3.8)	5 (6.4)	1 (1.2)

A total of 60 indigenous goats were examined in four communities during the period of study. Forty-nine (49) were infected with various species gastrointestinal helminthes as follows (see Table 3).

Table 3: Species of helminths obtained from indigenous goats

	Parasite type					Nematodes					Cestodes				Trematodes		
Name of abattoir	Numbers examined	Numbers infected	*Haemonchus*	*Strongyloides*	*Chabertia*	*Trichuris*	*Ostergia*	*Bunostomum*	*Trychostrongyloides*	*Ascaris*	*Tenia*	*Moniezia*	*Avitelina*	*Fasciola*	*Eurytrma*	Gastrotylax	*Schistosoma* spp	*Dicrocoelium*
Eliozu	15	10	3	2	2	0	1	0	0	2	1	0	0	1	0	1	0	1
Ogbogoro	15	14	3	2	0	0	1	0	1	2	0	1	0	2	1	0	0	0
Aluu	15	13	2	2	1	0	0	2	2	1	1	1	0	1	1	0	0	0
Rumuokoro	15	12	3	2	1	0	1	1	1	0	0	0	0	1	0	0	0	0
Total (%)	60	49 (81.6)	11 (18.3)	8 (13.3)	4 (6.6)	0	3 (5)	3 (5)	4 (6.6)	5 (8.3)	2 (3.3)	2 (3.3)	0	4 (6.6)	2 (3.3)	1 (1.6)	0	1 (1.6)

DISCUSSION AND CONCLUSION

The result of the study clearly indicates a high prevalence rate of gastrointestinal helminthes in cattle slaughtered in four selected abattoirs in Port Harcourt, namely, Eliozu, Ogbogoro, Rumuokoro, and Aluu abattoirs and various homes of indigenous people within the area.

The study revealed that 73.2% of the sampled exotic goats and 81.6% of indigenous goats were infected with various species of helminthes parasites. The goat slaughtered between May and September, 2009 had a prevalence rate of 76.0%, October 2009 and February, 2010 had a prevalence rate of 70.5%, while indigenous goat had 81.6% prevalence rate (see Tables 1 and 2, resp.). These results are consistent with findings of different researchers in the semiarid zone of North-Eastern and South-Eastern Nigeria [17–19].

The helminthes community isolated consisted of sixteen parasitic species, eight (8) nematodes (Haemonchus,Strongyloides, Chabertia, Trichuris, Ostertagia, Bunostomum, Trichostrongylus, and Ascaris), three (3) Cestodes (Taenia, Moniezia, and Avitellinium), and five (5) (Dicrocoelium, Fasciola, Eurytrema, Gastrothylax, andSchistosoma). Haemonchus species have the highest prevalence in all the positive samples. Fakae (1990) studies the epidemiology of helminthosis in ruminants under the traditional husbandry system in eastern Nigeria and reported prevalence of Haemonchus species as (87.1), higher than other helminthes species. It has been suggested that Haemonchus species can acquire resistance faster than any other gastrointestinal nematodes, likeTrichostrongylus, because of its high biotic potential [20]. The area of study shows how vulnerable workers in the abbatoir and people who consume the intestinal parts of the animals may be to infections especially to Taenia and Fasciola which are zoonotic and were observed in course of study. Globally, parasitic and other endemic diseases continue to be a major constraint on profitable livestock production. They are rarely associated with high mortality and easily identifiable clinical signs and their effects are usually characterized by lower outputs of animal products, by products, manure, and traction, all contributing to production and productivity losses.

CONCLUSION

In conclusion, various gastrointestinal parasites have been found in cattle in the study area. Hence, the high prevalence rate of helminthiasis in livestock needs to be checked periodically. Regular control measures should be practiced and farmers educated in the proper use of antihelminthiasis. Epidemiological facts suggest that high standard of sanitation in modern animal husbandry will prevent exposure of livestock to graze in deteriorated and environmentally polluted range lands will be effective in controlling disease.

RECOMMENDATION

The following recommendations will help in the prevention or reduction of helminth infections in the study area.

- There should be legislative control over slaughtering of goats and their distribution; the abbatoir workers should be properly trained on meat handling and zoonotic infections.
- Animals should be restricted to special areas of land provided by the government for grazing.
- The public should be enlightened on proper cooking of animal parts especially the intestine.
- A comprehensive approach should be adopted to ensure all inclusive meat inspection in the abattoirs before distribution to the public for consumption.

REFERENCES

1. C. O. Nwosu, P. P. Madu, and W. S. Richards, "Prevalence and seasonal changes in the population of gastrointestinal nematodes of small ruminants in the semi-arid zone of north-eastern Nigeria,"Veterinary Parasitology, vol. 144, no. 1-2, pp. 118–124, 2007. · ·
2. D. R. Nawathe, A. S. Sohael, and I. Umo, "Health management of a dairy herd on the Jos Plateau (Nigeria)," Bulletin of Animal Health and Production in Africa, vol. 33, pp. 199–205, 1985.
3. R. Fikru, S. Teshale, D. Reta, and K. Yosef, "Epidemiology of gastrointestinal parasites of ruminants in western Oromia, Ethiopia," International Journal of Applied Research in Veterinary Medicine, vol. 4, pp. 51–57, 2006.
4. J. P. Fabiyi, "Seasonal fluctuations of nematode infestations in goats in the savanna belt of Nigeria Bull,"Epizootic disease, vol. 21, pp. 227–286, 1973.
5. M. Eysker and R. A. Ogunsusi, "Observations on epidemiological and clinical aspects of gastrointestinal helminthiasis of sheep in northern Nigeria during the rainy season," Research in Veterinary Science, vol. 28, no. 1, pp. 58–62, 1980. ·
6. S. N. Chiejina, "The current status and priorities of research on the epidemiology and control helminth infections of ruminants in West Africa," in Proceedings of the 6th Symposium on Tropical Animal Health and Production, Helminth diseases of ruminants: diagnosis, epidemiology and control, 1995.
7. E. J. L. Soulsby, Helminths, Arthropods and Protozoa of Domestic Animals, The English Language Book Society and Bailliere Tindall, London, UK, 7th edition, 1986.
8. J. Nahed-Toral, Q. López-Tirado, G. Mendoza-Martínez, A. Aluja-Schunemann, and F. J. Trigo-Tavera, "Epidemiology of parasitosis in the Tzotzil sheep production system," Small Ruminant Research, vol. 49, no. 2, pp. 199–206, 2003. · ·
9. R. Gonzalez and A. C. Gonzalez, Alternatives For the Control of Gastrointestinal Nematodes in Sheep, Conf. EEPF Matanzas, Cuba, 2004.
10. D. G. Colley, P. T. LoVerde, and L. Savioli, "Infectious disease: medical helminthology in the 21st century," Science, vol. 293, no. 5534, pp. 1437–1438, 2001. · ·
11. M. W. Kennedy and W. Harnett, Eds., Parasitic Nematodes, CAB International, 2001.
12. D. T. J. Littlewood and R. A. Bray, Interrelationship of the Platyhelminthes, vol. 60, Taylor & Francis, London, UK, 2001.
13. A. U. Junaidu and S. G. Adamu, "Survey of Gastrointestinal helminth parasites of dogs of public health importance in Sokoto Metropolis," in Proceedings of the 22nd Annlual Conference of the Nigerian society for Animal Production, Abubaka Tafawa Balewa University Press, March 1997.
14. O. O. Akerejola, T. W. S. Van Veen, and C. O. Njoku, "Ovine and caprine diseases in Nigeria a review of economic losses," Bulletin of Animal Health and Production in Africa, vol. 27, no. 1, pp. 65–70, 1999.
15. R. A. Pal and M. Qayyum, "Prevalence of gastrointestinal nematodes of sheep and goats in upper Punjab," Pakistan Veterinary Journal, vol. 13, pp. 138–141, 1993.
16. K. Agyemang, R. H. Dwinger, D. A. Little, and G. J. Rowlands, Village N›Dama Cattle Production in West Africa: Six Years of Research in the Gambia, International Livestock Research Institute, Nairobi, Kenya, 1997.
17. B. M. Anene, E. O. Onyekwodiri, A. B. Chime, and S. M. Anika, "Gastrointestinal parasites in sheep and goats of southeastern Nigeria," Small Ruminant Research, vol. 13, no. 2, pp. 187–192, 1994. ·
18. B. M. Anene, E. O. Onyekwodiri, A. B. Chime, and S. M. Anika, "A survey of gastrointestinal parasites in cattle of southeastern Nigeria," Preventive Veterinary Medicine, vol. 20, no. 4, pp. 297–306, 1994. ·
19. B. B. Fakae, "The epidemiology of helminthosis in small ruminants under the traditional husbandry system in eastern Nigeria," Veterinary Research Communications, vol. 14, no. 5, pp. 381–391, 1990. · ·
20. B. B. Fakae and S. N. Chiejina, "The prevalence of concurrent trypanosome and gastrointestinal nematode infections in West African Dwarf sheep and goats in Nsukka area of eastern Nigeria,"Veterinary Parasitology, vol. 49, no. 2-4, pp. 313–318, 1993.

CHAPTER 8

GLOBAL CHANGE AND HELMINTH INFECTIONS IN GRAZING RUMINANTS IN EUROPE: IMPACTS, TRENDS AND SUSTAINABLE SOLUTIONS

Eric R. Morgan, Johannes Charlier, Guy Hendrickx, Annibale Biggeri, Dolores Catalan, Georg von Samson-Himmelstjerna, Janina Demeler, Elizabeth Müller, Jan van Dijk, Fiona Kenyon, Philip Skuce, Johan Höglund, Padraig O'Kiely, Bonny van Ranst, Theo de Waal, Laura Rinaldi, Giuseppe Cringoli, Hubertus Hertzberg, Paul Torgerson, Adrian Wolstenholme and Jozef Vercruysse

Keywords: Helminthoses; ruminants; diagnosis; control; infection risk; global change; climate change; anthelmintic resistance; risk management; spatio-temporal modelling; epidemiology; food security

IMPACT OF HELMINTH INFECTION ON THE SUSTAINABILITY AND EFFICIENCY OF LIVESTOCK FARMING

Livestock Farming As a Cornerstone of Society

Livestock farming is central to the sustainability of rural communities around the world, as well as being socially, economically and politically highly significant at national and international levels. In the European Union (EU), for instance, there are currently around 88 million cattle, 101 million sheep and 12 million goats [1]. Ongoing socioeconomic and climatic changes will increasingly emphasize the need for food security, obtained from sustainable intensification of agriculture [2]. It is inevitable that the production of meat and dairy products will also have to expand to meet the demands of increasing world population. Efficient ruminant livestock production is crucial to achieving this goal, especially in areas in which land is unsuitable for growing crops [3]. In this context, the competitiveness of livestock farming will largely depend on the degree to which this industry can achieve sustainable optimal production levels under changing environmental and socioeconomic pressures.

Costs to Economies and Animals

All grazing animals are exposed to helminth infections at pasture and any future intensification of pasture-based systems will likely increase the risk of helminth disease. Gastrointestinal nematodes (GIN) and liver fluke are the two major causes of lost productivity in ruminants, with lungworms also important in some situations. The economic costs of parasitic disease are currently difficult to quantify; however, some estimates exist within the scientific literature. For example, studies in the United Kingdom estimated the cost of parasitic nematodoses of sheep to be on the order of 99 million € per year [4], and in Switzerland, the cost of liver fluke disease has been estimated at 52 million € per year in cattle alone [5]. Within the EU as a whole, annual sales of anthelmintic drugs used to control these infections in ruminants have been estimated to be on the order of 400 million € [6]. It is likely that these figures only represent

Citation: Morgan, E.R.; Charlier, J.; Hendrickx, G.; Biggeri, A.; Catalan, D.; von Samson-Himmelstjerna, G.; Demeler, J.; Müller, E.; van Dijk, J.; Kenyon, F.; Skuce, P.; Höglund, J.; O'Kiely, P.; van Ranst, B.; de Waal, T.; Rinaldi, L.; Cringoli, G.; Hertzberg, H.; Torgerson, P.; Wolstenholme, A.; Vercruysse, J. Global Change and Helminth Infections in Grazing Ruminants in Europe: Impacts, Trends and Sustainable Solutions. Agriculture 2013, 3, 484-502. doi:10.3390/agriculture3030484.

the tip of the iceberg when it comes to calculating the true cost of livestock helminthoses endemic within the EU [7].

Parasitic gastroenteritis (PGE) in European cattle results principally from infections with *Ostertagia ostertagi* and *Cooperia oncophora* [8]. Although *Cooperia* is less pathogenic than *Ostertagia*, these parasite species usually occur together in the same host, with one contributing significantly to the pathogenic effect of the other. In European sheep and goats, *Teladorsagia circumcincta*, *Haemonchus contortus*, *Trichostrongylus* spp. and *Nematodirus* spp., parasitizing the intestine, are the most pathogenic GIN species, contributing significantly to PGE. Fasciolosis (liver fluke disease), caused by the trematode, *Fasciola hepatica*, is a worldwide infection of livestock, especially sheep and cattle, while lungworms in the genus *Dictyocaulus* cause significant disease in cattle and to a lesser extent in small ruminants. The main effect of all these infections is to reduce production efficiency, although under certain circumstances, mortalities can also be high: up to 20% with genera, such as*Haemonchus*, *Nematodirus* and *Fasciola* [9]. The major economic impact of parasitism is due to subclinical infections causing production losses. These costs have become increasingly important in the current economic climate with the low profit margins in the livestock sector.

At present, there is only a limited and fragmented understanding of the true costs of helminth parasitism, including costs associated with its control. This must be rectified if future control strategies are to be economically sensible and well integrated into farming systems. Recent advances in diagnostics, such as quantification of bulk milk anti-nematode antibodies, have enabled improved estimates of the production impacts of parasites in dairy herds and underpin optimized strategies for their control [10,11,12]. Further gains in understanding are likely to be made by comparing animal production in high and low intervention situations [13] and where anthelmintic efficacy fails. It is only by more fully characterizing and understanding the production impacts of parasites that future control can be optimized effectively.

INCREASED RISKS OF HELMINTH INFECTION IN LIVESTOCK DUE TO GLOBAL CHANGE

The Changing Environment

In recent years, sharp increases in helminth-associated disease frequency and intensity have been reported within the ruminant sector in some regions [14]. Climate warming, which in temperate regions tends to increase the developmental success of parasites, might be expected to increase pasture contamination with infective stages and may be one driver behind this trend. For example, there have already been reports of altered seasonal patterns of nematode and liver fluke infections in northern parts of the UK [15,16]. In Switzerland, unpublished data suggest that *H. contortus* transmission is occurring at higher altitudes than previously recorded, and in Sweden, transmission occurs near the Arctic Circle [17]. If these trends continue as predicted, European farmers may be faced with new and unfamiliar parasitological challenges that they are ill equipped to meet. However, the study of the effects of climate change on the endemic diseases of livestock is still in its infancy [18,19], and the effects of additional factors, such as altered land use, the emergence of anthelmintic resistance (AR) and farm management practices, have received little detailed attention [19]. Thus, attempts have been made to integrate the abundant knowledge of environmental, especially climatic, effects on parasite stages outside the livestock hosts into predictive mathematical models, especially focusing on selection for AR [20,21,22,23,24], and some have tried to predict future infection patterns [25]. However, the abundance and distribution of helminth infections of livestock is a complex and dynamic issue affected by a whole range of parameters, including those that could be classed as global changes (Figure 1). The situation is further complicated by interacting regional, seasonal and host-specific factors that influence disease and the fact that helminthoses are usually seen in animals that have concurrent multi-species infections. The fact that global change is much more than climate change alone must be acknowledged and incorporated more fully into future research approaches in this area.

The Importance of Anthelmintic Resistance

An equally important driver of increased disease and production loss due to helminths is likely to be treatment failure, which is being reported ever more frequently. The increasing occurrence of AR in helminth populations threatens the sustainability, as well as the efficiency of livestock production. Although there are a number of different approaches to the control of helminth parasitism in livestock, including nutritional, immunological and biological interventions [26], at present, effective control relies almost exclusively on effective anthelmintic drugs. Most of these compounds have broad-spectrum activity, *i.e.*, they kill all the common roundworm species (there are specific products effective against fluke), but effective control ultimately relies on multiple treatments each year. When first introduced, all these drugs were highly efficacious, but frequent and widespread use and misuse has resulted in the emergence of resistant parasite populations, such that AR is now a major global problem, especially (but not exclusively) in parasites of small ruminants [27], and is the greatest threat to the sustainable control of helminthoses in the short to medium term. Anthelmintic inefficacy and resistance has also become apparent in cattle, reported initially in the southern hemisphere [28,29,30], but more recently also within Europe [31,32].

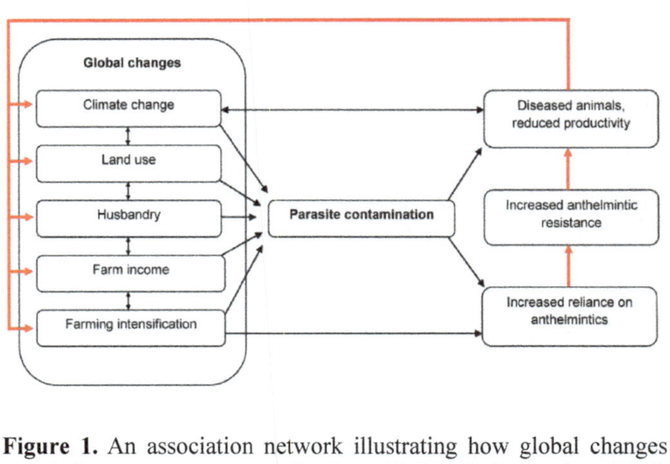

Figure 1. An association network illustrating how global changes may influence pasture contamination with helminth parasites. Black arrows represent positive enforcement, and those in red (bold) show potential associations arising from global change.

The problem of AR is compounded by the fact that many of these parasite populations are resistant to more than one class of anthelmintic [33,34] and that the prevalence of resistance is increasing inexorably in many regions [35]. Despite the recent introduction of two novel anthelmintic drug classes for sheep [36,37], the situation regarding the development and transmission of AR remains largely unaltered. Accordingly, there is an urgent need to reduce anthelmintic usage, while timing treatments optimally, taking into account global change-driven alterations in parasite seasonality. To maintain or, in some regions, regain control over these parasites, an improved understanding and quantification of the key mechanisms involved in their spatial and temporal prevalence is also paramount.

The Need for Increased Carbon Efficiency in Ruminant Farming

The increased prevalence of helminths, especially drug-resistant parasites, poses an even more pressing problem against a background of increasing pressure towards lowering the carbon footprint of ruminant livestock. Worldwide, ruminant livestock farming accounts for 70% of agricultural land use, occupies 30% of the ice-free surface of the planet and produces some 40% of the global agricultural Gross Domestic Product (GDP). Set against this, it is estimated to account for up to 18% of worldwide greenhouse gas emissions [38]. There is a new requirement for European livestock farming to become carbon emission efficiency-driven [39]. Animals emitting greenhouse gasses, while not growing or producing, because of illness, add significantly to a farm's carbon footprint; so, combating infectious and parasitic diseases on livestock farms is essential for any improvements in the carbon efficiency of production [40].

A particular issue regarding AR is that a response to increased infection pressure as a result of climate and other environmental change that relies on increased use of anthelmintic drugs will undermine the sustainability of control, as increased drug use selects more strongly for AR. As drug efficacy declines, production efficiency would be expected to decrease and greenhouse gas emissions per unit production, increase. This could trigger a positive feedback cycle, fuelling ongoing climate change and further increases in infection and its effects.

SCIENTIFIC PRIORITIES TO SUPPORT SUSTAINABLE HELMINTH CONTROL

The development and implementation of innovative, refined approaches to worm control, targeted at the appropriate regional scale, is a prerequisite for reducing the enormous burden helminth parasitism imposes upon ruminant livestock production. This goal can be supported by exploiting developments in high-throughput technologies coupled to novel diagnostics to identify sub-clinical infections within an affordable and flexible diagnostic capacity. However, the provision of innovative diagnostic tools to identify the species implicated in infections, and individual and/or herd/flock markers of helminthoses, are only the first steps in the process. To have real impact, new diagnostic capacity needs to integrate with decision support tools, such as measures of economic impact [11], predictive disease risk forecasting models and livestock management software. Statistically-based risk models of helminthoses that incorporate Geographical Information System (GIS)-based surveillance, as well as temporally explicit models predicting periods of high risk, could inform farm management responses to regional environmental, climatological, parasitological and sccioeconomic changes, and themselves depend on data generated from enhanced diagnostic capacity. In particular, optimizing intervention strategies, including extent and intensity of drug use to control worm infections, must be based on evidence. This requires accurate and efficiently collected information on levels of challenge, infection and production loss and integration of this information in such a way that optimal strategies can be devised. Scientific research can support this endeavour in four main fields: (1) diagnosis of helminthoses in livestock at the individual and herd level with specific attention to multi-species infections and the distribution of anthelmintic resistance; (2) prediction of the impact of global changes on the epidemiology of parasitic infections, as well as the distribution and spread of anthelmintic resistance; (3) explanation of current, and future predictions of, seasonal trends in helminth infections of grazing livestock; (4) strategies for the sustainable management of helminth infections in a changing landscape. The rationale for prioritizing these areas, and the scientific and technical challenges that they present, are discussed below.

Diagnosis

Many methods are already available for the diagnosis of helminth infections, clinical and sub-clinical disease and AR, but all have their weaknesses. The principal clinical signs, such as diarrhoea, anorexia and ill-thriftiness are common sequelae of many other infectious diseases and syndromes and, consequently, lack sensitivity and specificity. Many of the methods used to diagnose helminthoses can only be applied to individual animals and/or to hosts infected with one helminth species, with little or no capacity to deal with infections where multiple species are present. Current parasitological, immunological and molecular diagnostic technologies are often labor-intensive and, therefore, expensive, with limited application either on-farm or for large-scale surveillance.

Because helminthoses inevitably involve multiple parasite species, in order to ensure that the appropriate treatment is applied, it is important to identify the key species responsible for the signs of disease and/or production losses. Most routine helminth diagnoses rely on the detection of parasite stages (usually eggs) in faecal samples. Parasitological diagnoses offer the advantage of relatively low cost and can be conducted in non-specialized laboratories; however, the morphological identification of nematode eggs and larvae to the species (or even genus) level is difficult and requires experienced personnel [38]. In some circumstances, for example, treatment decisions based on increasing faecal nematode egg counts in grazing ruminants, specific identification is not a priority. However, control strategies that are truly directed at the major parasitic threats to health and production should be based on more detailed knowledge of these threats, including their economic impact.

Although species specificity is often more easily achievable through immunological detection, a major drawback with these approaches is that they do not necessarily indicate the presence of a currently active infection. A further complication is in obtaining suitable samples, since some tests require invasive procedures, such as blood sampling, which are not routine practices in sheep and cattle. Molecular genetic (Polymerase chain reaction, PCR-based) approaches have potential for this application, because they are sensitive and specific and can be applied to helminth parasite material [41], most notably, eggs and larvae extracted from faecal samples. To date, however, these approaches have tended to concentrate on single species and work best on material derived from single parasites [42,43], which requires considerable upstream processing. Real-time PCR and pyrosequencing approaches have also been developed in an attempt to provide quantitative information on species composition and show much promise, but more development work is required before validated molecular species identification tests can be made available [44,45].

AR is an additional complicating factor with regard to the diagnosis of helminthoses. Currently, the principal means of identifying AR *in vivo* is the faecal egg count reduction test (FECRT), based on a series of pre- and post-treatment individual egg counts. This test has limitations, not only because it is labour intensive, but also regarding the optimum sampling and counting criteria, especially in cattle, and can be confounded by over-dispersed parasite populations [46]. However, the FECRT is still a useful indicator of drug efficacy in the field, since samples can be submitted to diagnostic laboratories by post, but the test does still require simplification and further optimisation to encourage uptake by end-users. There are several *in vitro* bioassays available that examine the effects of differing drug concentrations on parasite behaviour and development, e.g., the egg hatch test (EHT), larval migration inhibition assay (LMIA), larval feeding inhibition assay (LFIA) and larval development test (LDT) [47]. These tests are useful for characterising single-species parasite isolates in the laboratory, but are not yet sufficiently standardised to be of use as routine diagnostic tests for resistance in the field. Moreover, they do not all work equally well with all available drug classes, e.g., the EHT can only be used to detect benzimidazole (BZ) resistance. Their utility is further compromised by the fact that different parasite species have their own inherent sensitivities to certain drugs, making the interpretation of test results from natural multi-species infections extremely difficult. Since AR has a genetic component, molecular (DNA-based) methods have great potential as putative diagnostic test systems here, too. However, this development requires validated genetic markers for resistance, and to date, this is only available for one drug class (the BZs) and not yet in all species [48]. Nonetheless, sensitive and accurate pyrosequencing assays have been published for the detection of BZ resistance-associated single nucleotide polymorphisms (SNPs) in *Haemonchus* and *Teladorsagia* [49,50] and have shown that BZ resistance allele frequencies correlate well with the outputs from FECRTs conducted in the field [51]. The search for resistance markers for the other drug classes has largely focused on candidate resistance genes, but has not been proven, to date, to be a fruitful exercise [52]. Although whole genome sequencing has the potential to reveal the genetic determinants of resistance, this approach is still very much in its infancy [53].

Cost and speed of reporting remain important barriers to the support of control with accurate diagnosis of helminth infection and disease. The use of emerging high-throughput immunological and molecular-based technologies offers the potential to reduce costs and offer diagnosis at a scale suitable for large-scale monitoring within Europe. The advent of microbead-based technologies has led to the development of a number of multiplex assay platforms, e.g., LUMINEX®, which permit multiple assays to be performed on the same samples and provide a range of versatile assay designs, including antibody/antigen, primer/probe and enzyme/substrate interactions [54,55,56,57,58]. The use of this platform allows the simultaneous determination of several parameters (in theory, up to 100; in practice, probably 10–20) from a single serum sample in a streamlined highly automatable workflow. This greatly enhances test/sample throughput and the efficiency of sample utilization, both prerequisites for effective surveillance and monitoring activities. Such methodologies are widely used in human diagnostic facilities, but, to date, have not been widely applied in veterinary parasitology. This platform is ideally suited for high-throughput Enzyme-linked immunosorbent assay (ELISA)-based test systems. Possible relevant parameters to be measured include not only circulating parasite antigen or anti-parasite specific antibodies [59,60,61], but also health indicators, such as markers of inflammation, e.g., acute phase proteins [62], and tissue damage, e.g., pepsinogen [63], for which validated assays already exist.

Multivalent platforms are suited to the incorporation of serological- and molecular-based tests. Prototype multiplex PCR-based molecular assays already exist for the detection of individual GIN species infecting sheep and cattle [43,44]. Such multiplex LUMINEX® assays have already been described for the detection of the protozoan pathogens, *Giardia* and*Cryptosporidium* spp., from faecal samples [64,65,66], but have not yet been developed or validated for helminth parasites. These high-throughput diagnostic platforms require considerable capital investment and experienced personnel to maintain the instruments and to run assays. There is still a need for relatively simple diagnostic tests that require little specialised equipment and that might, ultimately, have "pen-side" applications. Innovative approaches based on the recently developed loop-mediated isothermal amplification (LAMP) method show promise in this regard. This is a commercially available detection method to amplify nucleic acids and offers a rapid, accurate and cost-effective diagnosis of infectious diseases [67,68,69,70]. LAMP technology has the added advantage that it is not prone to inhibition by contaminants within faecal samples, as is the case with traditional PCR-based methods. These novel analytical platforms also have the potential to detect and quantify anthelmintic resistance-associated DNA polymorphisms in key parasite genera.

Spatial Epidemiology and Forecasting of Helminth Disease

More efficient targeting of anthelmintic-based control strategies can benefit not only from improved diagnosis, but also prediction of disease threats in space and time. In the ~50 years since the first epidemiologically-based helminth parasite model was published [71], a number of simplified models have been developed for both nematodes and trematodes [72]. However, simplified models often neglect crucial interactions, while those with a more realistic level of detail are usually over-parameterised, making it hard to interpret their output. Most existing models of disease and/or parasite ecology were not constructed against a background of global change and do not, therefore, include crucial factors, such as changing land use and farm management practices. Exclusion of such important drivers leads to a non-realistic output, which might help explain why such models have had a limited impact on parasite control in practice. The climate-based forecasting models previously developed for animal fasciolosis in different areas of Europe, Africa and the USA [73] also require further development to incorporate global change factors, including farm management practices, animal movements and climate change. Therefore, the more realistic models become by incorporating such factors, the less reliably their predictions can be extrapolated to other areas, circumstances and research or control questions. Efforts to model the dynamics and control of helminths in ruminants in other parts of the world [20,23] have value in highlighting general aspects of system dynamics, but ultimately, models for prediction and decision support in Europe should be constructed and validated in relation to local conditions [74]. Models will only be plausible to animal health advisors if shown to work well on the ground, and proper validation is vital if their use in decision support tools is to gain traction. An approach that builds local detail and variation onto a common, general framework for helminth-livestock interactions might, therefore, be a useful way forward.

Ultimately, both spatial and temporal models of parasite occurrence and abundance rely on solid data for their development and validation [75] and can, therefore, benefit from improved high-throughput diagnostics. The prohibitive costs and logistics of conducting extensive and repeated surveys of disease for purely descriptive information on distribution have led to an increased interest in computer-based geospatial technologies. Human and veterinary medicine has seen an increasing reliance on the application of geospatial tools—*i.e.*, GIS, Global Positioning System (GPS), satellite-based remote sensing (RS) and Virtual Globes (e.g., Google Earth™)—to study the spatial and temporal distribution of infectious and parasitic diseases and their vectors [76,77]. Health research based on geospatial tools is considered a timely approach in a changing environment to understand climatic-environmental-health linkages [78]. The application of spatial sampling strategies to animal diseases is relatively new, and the study of pathogen distribution and abundance at a geospatial scale has focused mainly on vector-borne diseases (VBD), mainly due to their direct link with the environment. As an example, 51% of the papers published by the journal, Geospatial Health [79], between 2005 and 2010 dealt with VBD, only 6% with non-vector transmitted helminths and 19% with trematode infections; however, the latter mainly pertain to schistosomes and, to a lesser extent, *Fasciola*. There therefore seems to be considerable scope for applying existing, as well as new geospatial approaches to understanding and predicting parasite distribution and disease risk in livestock. Important parameters, such as environmental factors and farm management, are also rarely taken into consideration when planning cross-sectional or longitudinal surveys for spatial modelling.

Predicting the Timing of Parasite Risk

Spatial variation in parasite disease risk enables the design of monitoring and intervention strategies that are locally appropriate, while also providing a systematic basis for assessing trends in risk as a result of global change. However, effective intervention against parasitic disease is temporally sensitive, relying on the coincidence of animal grazing with infective stage availability [80]. The timing of treatment and other actions, including grazing practice and diagnostic monitoring in support of targeted treatment strategies, is therefore very important to the outcome in terms of the reduction of disease challenge and selection for anthelmintic resistance. Moreover, one of the main effects of climate change on parasite epidemiology is likely to be the altered seasonal availability of infective stages [9,81]. For example, warmer temperatures appear to be reducing overwinter survival of GIN of sheep in the UK, but accelerating build-up of infection in summer, leading to decreases in recorded disease in spring, but increases in autumn [82]. Therefore, comprehensive modelling approaches should also consider temporal patterns of infection [83], for example, by building and populating mechanistic representations of the life-cycles of the major helminth species, with components that explicitly incorporate climatic stochasticity, forage availability and utilization and variation in farm management at the regional level. These can be extended to consider global change scenarios through variation in climate, farm systems and parasite biology, as well as, potentially, parasite adaptation. The extent to which parasite adaptation to changes in climate and management will affect their control has barely been considered in trichostrongyloids beyond drug resistance, with some exceptions [84]. The breadth of this approach and the specific consideration of the spatial scale over which important determinants of epidemiology act are crucial, not only to advancing existing scientific understanding of the processes involved [72], but also to practical application of modelling in support of disease control, in that explicit consideration of the timing of helminth transmission is needed to optimize control strategies. A future vision of mathematical and geospatial modelling for parasite control would combine temporal and spatial aspects, to provide forecasting and scenario analysis tools that are integrated at local, regional and global levels. These could be applied to on-farm decision making through decision support tools, to horizon-scanning for disease threats by industry and animal health authorities and to policy making at national and supra-national levels.

Validation of models with experimental and field data will be crucial to model plausibility. However, model exploration through scenario analysis is also essential to consider the possible effects of global change and, often, is impossible to validate fully, because scenarios will often go beyond the range of past or present experience. For the same reason, purely empirical approaches will be limited in their ability to demonstrate and predict the effects of global change: there is no controlled experiment possible to emulate the scope of global change on parasitism within farming systems as a whole. At the same time, limited standardization and centralization of parasitic disease data, and the many confounding factors in endemic disease surveillance, make it difficult to validate predictions of global change impacts on parasitic disease [82]. This explains the lack of well-documented, proven effects of global, including climate, change on disease incidence in livestock, which should not be taken to indicate the absence of such effects.

Sustainable Parasite Control

Ruminant production systems vary considerably, depending on social, economic and other environmental factors, such as soil, climate and farm structure. Predictable (and unpredictable) global changes will inevitably change the way these systems are operated [3]. These changes will also have both direct and indirect effects on helminth lifecycles (see above) and, thus, on the most appropriate preventative and remedial strategies required on farms.

Current chemically-based approaches to helminth control generally utilize frequent whole flock/herd treatments, even though these are known to lead to an increased rate of the development of anthelmintic resistance [85]. Additionally, there are societal concerns about the levels of chemicals present in food products. Although anthelmintic residue concentrations have been found to be very low in beef in Europe [86], concerns persist and underpin restrictions on anthelmintic use in livestock, especially in dairy cows [87]. In any event, the risk of AR is sufficiently serious that current chemical-based helminth control strategies can reasonably be deemed unsustainable unless considerably modified. Previous studies, reviewed in [85], have established proof-of-concept for *refugia*-based treatment strategies and have demonstrated the benefits of optimized anthelmintic usage in maintaining animal performance and drug efficacy, though mostly in small ruminants, rather than cattle. The ability to optimize treatments will likely change the way in which anthelmintics are used; they will only be given to those animals that actually need treatment, instead of, as is common practice now, treatment being given to all animals in a flock/herd simultaneously. Optimising drug treatments will slow the development of AR [88] and, thus, maximize the life of those anthelmintic families where resistance is known to be an issue and prolong the life expectancy of the two new sheep anthelmintic families, currently represented by monepantel [36] and derquantel [37]. Proof-of-concept studies so far published suggest that targeted whole-flock treatment or individual animal treatments are effective and pragmatic strategies for optimising anthelmintic use in Europe, as in a range of production systems across the world [63,85,89,90,91,92,93,94].

Targeted treatment (TT), *i.e.*, optimised whole flock/herd treatment, has been shown to be beneficial in controlling nematode infections, in both large and small ruminants. Targeted selective treatment (TST), *i.e.*, individual animal treatment, has been shown to reduce anthelmintic usage in small ruminants, whilst maintaining animal production and drug efficacy. However, to date, TST approaches have rarely been studied in cattle, and neither approach has been applied to liver fluke infections. The wide-scale uptake of these strategies can only be achieved with a full understanding of their potential costs and benefits; this has also not yet been properly evaluated, and the optimum balance between worm control and maintenance of efficacy in TST and Integrated Pest Control (IPC) programmes still needs to be identified. Current TT and TST strategies for small ruminants, for example, are most applicable for large-scale producers, because of the investment needed in efficient animal handling and performance monitoring systems. Indicators of the need to treat at the group or individual level, which are easily applicable within smaller scale enterprises, are needed.

In order to make it possible to integrate these new strategies into routine farm management practices, farmers (and their advisors) will need to fully understand the costs and benefits of these novel treatment strategies. Previous studies [85] showed that TT and TST strategies can reduce anthelmintic use and maintain drug efficacy; however, there may be some increased costs associated with the use of the new strategies (such as increased labor and the costs of new technology and diagnostics). The economic costs and benefits of these more sustainable treatment strategies, in the short and long term, have yet to be rigorously analyzed, with few specific studies [92], and the resulting uncertainty is perhaps the major obstacle to their adoption by livestock producers. This is compounded by the scarcity of hard data on the costs of anthelmintic resistance, as well as uncertainty regarding future access to new treatment compounds and their likely longevity in the face of selection for resistance.

Finally, to encourage the implementation of new treatment strategies into routine farm practices, decision support tools are needed. This is because targeted strategies are inherently more complex than universal protocol-based systems and must be flexible to differences in farm systems, climate and other context-specific factors [95]. Integration of decision support tools into pre-existing herd management software would help farmers to incorporate the ideas and approaches discussed above.

CONCLUSIONS

Anthelmintic resistance and global change are dominant factors underpinning current and future trends in parasitic disease in grazing ruminants. Climate warming acts on immature parasite stages outside the main host and could alter the level and timing of peak infection pressure. The way in which this translates to altered disease patterns is modified by many factors, including host immunity, grazing patterns and other farm management practices [96]. Meeting increased infection pressure with more frequent administration of anthelmintic drugs is unsustainable, due to rapid development of resistance in nematode and, probably, trematode populations. Therefore new approaches are required. Increasingly, the targeting of treatment at the group and individual level appears to be the only practical way forward for sustainable helminth control on farms. Much remains to be learned regarding the optimal design and implementation of such strategies in different contexts. We have outlined some of the challenges in this regard and identified key areas in which advances in science and technology can help to support effective and efficient strategies for maintaining productivity in the face of major future challenges. The adoption of improved parasite control practices is crucial for sustainable and efficient production from ruminants at pasture.

ACKNOWLEDGEMENTS

The authors are grateful for funding from EU FP7 project 288975 GLOWORM.

REFERENCES

1. FAOSTAT (2009). Available online: http://faostat.fao.org/ (accessed on 15 July 2013).
2. Baulcombe, D.; Crute, I.; Dunwell, J.; Gale, M.; Jones, J.; Pretty, J.; Sutherland, W.; Toulmin, C. *Reaping the Benefits—Science and the Sustainable Intensification of Global Agriculture*; Royal Society Policy Document: London, UK, 2009.
3. Chiotti, Q.P.; Johnston, T. Extending the boundaries of climate change research—A discussion on agriculture. *J. Rural Stud.* **1995**, *11*, 335–350.
4. Nieuwhof, G.J.; Bishop, S.C. Costs of the major endemic diseases in Great Britain and the potential benefits of reduction in disease impact. *Anim. Sci.* **2005**, *81*, 23–29.
5. Schweizer, G.; Braun, W.; Deplazes, D.; Torgerson, P.R. The economic effects of bovine fasciolosis in Switzerland. *Vet. Rec.* **2005**, *157*, 188–193.
6. Selzer, P.M. Preface. In *Antiparasitic and Antibacterial Drug Discovery. From Molecular Targets to Drug Candidates*; Wiley-Blackwell: Hoboken, USA, 2009; pp. 11–12.
7. Charlier, J.; Höglund, J.; von Samson-Himmelstjerna, G.; Dorny, P.; Vercruysse, J. Gastrointestinal nematode infections in adult dairy cattle: Impact on production, diagnosis and control. *Vet. Parasitol.* **2009**, *164*, 70–79.
8. Rehbein, S.; Baggott, D.G.; Johnson, E.G.; Kunkle, B.N.; Yazwinski, T.A.; Yoon, S.; Cramer, L.G.; Soll, M.D. Nematode burdens of pastured cattle treated once at turnout with eprinomectin extended-release injection. *Vet. Parasitol.* **2013**,*192*, 321–331.
9. Van Dijk, J.; Morgan, E.R. The influence of temperature on the development, hatching and survival of *Nematodirus battus* larvae. *Parasitology* **2008**, *135*, 269–283.
10. Mejia, M.E.; Perri, A.F.; Licoff, N.; Miglierina, M.M.; Cseh, S.; Ornstein, A.M.; Becu-Villalobos, D.; Lacau-Mengido, I.M. Comparison of three methods for gastrointestinal nematode diagnosis determination in grazing dairy cattle in relation to milk production. *Vet. Parasitol.* **2011**, *183*, 174–177.
11. Charlier, J.; van der Voort, M.; Hogeveen, H.; Vercruysse, J. ParaCalc®—A novel tool to evaluate the economic importance of worm infections on the dairy farm. *Vet. Parasitol.* **2012**, *184*, 204–211.
12. Charlier, J.; Levecke, B.; Devleesschauwer, B.; Vercruysse, J.; Hogeveen, H. The economic effects of whole-herd versus selective anthelmintic treatment strategies in dairy cows. *J. Dairy Sci.* **2012**, *95*, 2977–2987.
13. Mason, W.A.; Pomroy, W.E.; Lawrence, K.E.; Scott, I. The effect of repeated, four-weekly eprinomectin treatment on milk production in pasture-based, seasonally-calving dairy cattle. *Vet. Parasitol.* **2012**, *189*, 250–259.
14. Van Dijk, J.; Sargison, N.D.; Kenyon, F.; Skuce, P. Climate change and infectious disease: Helminthological challenge to farmed ruminants in temperate regions. Invited Review. *Animal* **2010**, *4*, 377–392.
15. Sargison, N.D.; Wilson, D.J.; Bartley, D.J.; Penny, C.D.; Jackson, F. Haemonchosis and teladorsagiosis in a Scottish sheep flock putatively associated with the over-wintering of hypobiotic fourth stage larvae. *Vet. Parasitol.* **2007**, *147*, 326–331.
16. Kenyon, F.; Sargison, N.D.; Skuce, P.J.; Jackson, F. Sheep helminth parasitic disease in South-Eastern Scotland arising as a possible consequence of climate change. *Vet. Parasitol.* **2009**, *163*, 293–297.
17. Lindqvist, A.; Ljungström, B.L.; Nilsson, O.; Waller, P.J. The dynamics, prevalence and impact of nematode infections in organically raised sheep in Sweden. *Acta Vet. Scand.* **2001**, *42*, 377–389.
18. De la Rocque, S.; Rioux, J.A.; Slingenbergh, J. Climate change: Effects on animal disease systems and implications for surveillance and control. *Rev. Sci. Tech. Int. Off. of Epizoot.* **2008**, *27*, 339–354.
19. Morgan, E.R.; Wall, R. Climate change and parasitic disease: Farmer mitigation? *Trends Parasitol.* **2009**, *7*, 308–313.
20. Leathwick, D.M.; Barlow, N.D.; Vlassoff, A. A model for nematodiasis in New Zealand lambs. *Int. J. Parasitol.* **1992**, *22*, 789–799.
21. Reynecke, D.P.; Waghorn, T.S.; Oliver, A.-M.B.; Miller, C.M.; Vlassoff, A.; Leathwick, D.M. Dynamics of the free-living stages of sheep intestinal parasites on pasture in the North Island of New Zealand. 2. Weather variables associated with development. *Vet. J.* **2011**, *59*, 287–292.
22. Leathwick, D.M.; Waghorn, T.S.; Miller, C.M.; Candy, P.M.; Oliver, A.-M.B. Managing anthelmintic resistance—Use of a combination anthelmintic and leaving some lambs untreated to slow the development of resistance to ivermectin.*Parasitology* **2012**, *187*, 285–294.
23. Dobson, R.J.; Barnes, E.H.; Tyrrell, K.L.; Hosking, B.C.; Larsen, J.W.A.; Besier, R.B.; Love, S.; Rolfe, P.F.; Bailey, J.N. A multi-species modelto assess the effect of refugia on worm control and anthelmintic resistance insheep grazing systems. *Aust. Vet. J.* **2011**, *89*, 200–208.
24. Laurenson, Y.C.S.M.; Bishop, S.C.; Forbes, A.B.; Kyriazakis, I. Modelling the short- and long-term impacts of drenching frequency and targeted selective treatment on the performance of grazing lambs and the emergence of anthelmintic resistance. *Parasitology* **2013**, *140*, 780–791.
25. Fox, N.J.; White, P.C.L.; McClean, C.J.; Marion, G.; Evans, A.; Hutchings, M.R. Predicting impacts of climate change on *Fasciola hepatica* risk. *PLoS One* **2011**, *6*, e16126.
26. Jackson, F.; Miller, J. Alternative approaches to control—Quo vadit? *Vet. Parasitol.* **2006**, *139*, 371–384.
27. Kaplan, R.M. Drug resistance in nematodes of veterinary importance: A status report. *Trends Parasitol.* **2004**, *20*, 477–481.
28. Familton, A.S.; Mason, P.; Coles, G.C. Anthelmintic-resistant *Cooperia* species in cattle. *Vet. Rec.* **2001**, *149*, 719–720.
29. Sangster, N.C.; Dobson, R.J. Anthelmintic Resistance.

In *The Biology of Nematodes*; Lee, D.L., Ed.; Taylor and Francis: London, UK, 2002; pp. 531–567.

30. Sutherland, I.A.; Leathwick, D.M. Anthelmintic resistance in nematode parasites of cattle—A global issue? *Trends Parasitol* **2010**, *27*, 176–181.

31. Demeler, J.; van Zeveren, A.M.; Kleinschmidt, N.; Vercruysse, J.; Höglund, J.; Koopmann, R.; Cabaret, J.; Claerebout, E.; Areskog, M.; von Samson-Himmelstjerna, G. Monitoring the efficacy of ivermectin and albendazole against gastro intestinal nematodes of cattle in Northern Europe. *Vet. Parasitol.* **2009**, *160*, 109–115.

32. El-Abdellati, A.; Charlier, J.; Geldhof, P.; Levecke, B.; Demeler, J.; von Samson-Himmelstjerna, G.; Claerebout, E.; Vercruysse, J. The use of a simplified faecal egg count reduction test for assessing anthelmintic efficacy on Belgian and German cattle farms. *Vet. Parasitol.* **2010**, *169*, 352–357.

33. Bartley, D.J.; Jackson, F.; Jackson, E.; Sargison, N. Characterisation of two triple resistant field isolates of *Teladorsagia*from Scottish lowland sheep farms. *Vet. Parasitol.* **2004**, *123*, 189–199.

34. Sargison, N.D.; Jackson, F.; Bartley, D.J.; Wilson, D.J.; Stenhouse, L.J.; Penny, C.D. Observations on the emergence of multiple anthelmintic resistance in sheep flocks in the south-east of Scotland. *Vet. Parasitol.* **2007**, *45*, 65–76.

35. Wolstenholme, A.J.; Fairweather, I.; Prichard, R.; von Samson-Himmelstjerna, G.; Sangster, N.; Nicholas, C. Drug resistance in veterinary helminths. *Trends Parasitol.* **2004**, *20*, 469–476.

36. Kaminsky, R.; Ducray, P.; Jung, M.; Clover, R.; Rufener, L.; Bouvier, J.; Weber, S.S.; Wenger, A.; Wieland-Berghausen, S.; Goebel, T.; *et al.* A new class of anthelmintics effective against drug-resistant nematodes. *Nature* **2008**, *452*, 176–180.

37. Little, P.R.; Hodges, A.; Watson, T.G.; Seed, J.A.; Maeder, S.J. Field efficacy and safety of an oral formulation of the novel combination anthelmintic, derquantel-abamectin, in sheep in New Zealand. *N. Z. Vet. J.* **2010**, *58*, 121–129.

38. Steinfeld, H.; Gerber, P.; Wassenaar, T.; Castel, V.; Rosales, M.; de Haan, C. *Livestock's Long Shadow: Environmental Issues and Options*; Report presented to the Food and Agricultural Organisation of the United Nations (FAO): Rome, Italy, 2006; p. 284.

39. Gill, M.; Smith, P.; Wilkinson, J.M. Mitigating climate change: The role of domestic livestock. *Animal* **2010**, *4*, 323–333.

40. Thornton, P.K. Livestock production: Recent trends, future prospects. *Philos. Trans. R. Soc. B Biol. Sci.* **2010**, *365*, 2853–2867.

41. Taylor, M.A.; Hunt, K.R.; Goodyear, K.L. Anthelmintic resistance detection methods. *Vet. Parasitol.* **2002**, *103*, 183–194.

42. Gasser, R.B.; Bott, N.J.; Chilton, N.B.; Hunt, P.; Beveridge, I. Toward practical, DNA-based diagnostic methods for parasitic nematodes of livestock—Bionomic and biotechnical implications. *Biotechnol. Adv.* **2008**, *26*, 325–334.

43. Zarlenga, D.S.; Chute, M.; Gasbarre, L.C.; Boyd, P.C. A multiplex PCR assay for differentiating economically important gastrointestinal nematodes of cattle. *Vet. Parasitol.* **2001**, *97*, 199–209.

44. Wimmer, B.; Craig, B.H.; Pilkington, J.G.; Pemberton, J.M. Non-invasive assessment of parasitic nematode species diversity in wild Soay sheep using molecular markers. *Int. J. Parasitol.* **2004**, *34*, 625–631.

45. Learmount, J.; Conyers, C.; Hird, H.; Morgan, C.; Craig, B.H.; von Samson-Himmelstjerna, G.; Taylor, M. Development and validation of real-time PCR methods for diagnosis of *Teladorsagia circumcincta* and *Haemonchus contortus* in sheep. *Vet. Parasitol.* **2009**, *166*, 268–274.

46. Dobson, R.J.; Sangster, N.C.; Besier, R.B.; Woodgate, R.G. Geometric means provide a biased efficacy result when conducting a faecal egg count reduction test (FECRT). *Vet. Parasitol.* **2009**, *161*, 162–167.

47. Coles, G.C.; Jackson, F.; Pomroy, W.E.; Prichard, R.K.; von Samson-Himmelstjerna, G.; Silvestre, A.; Taylor, M.A.; Vercruysse, J. The detection of anthelmintic resistance in nematodes of veterinary importance. *Vet. Parasitol.* **2006**, *136*, 167–185.

48. Von Samson-Himmelstjerna, G.; Blackhall, W.J.; McCarthy, J.S.; Skuce, P.J. Single nucleotide polymorphism (SNP) markers for benzimidazole resistance in veterinary nematodes. *Parasitology* **2007**, *134*, 1077–1086.

49. Von Samson-Himmelstjerna, G.; Walsh, T.K.; Donnan, A.A.; Carriere, S.; Jackson, F.; Skuce, P.J.; Rohn, K.; Wolstenholme, A.J. Molecular detection of benzimidazole resistance in *Haemonchus contortus* using real-time PCR and pyrosequencing. *Parasitology* **2009**, *136*, 349–358.

50. Skuce, P.J.; Stenhouse, L.; Jackson, F.; Hypsa, V.; Gilleard, J.S. Benzimidazole resistance allele haplotype diversity in United Kingdom isolates of *Teladorsagia circumcincta* supports a hypothesis of multiple origins of resistance by recurrent mutation. *Int. J. Parasitol.* **2010**, *40*, 1247–1255.

51. Höglund, J.; Gustaffson, K.; Ljungstrom, B.L.; Engstrom, A.; Donnan, A.A.; Skuce, P.J. Anthelmintic resistance in Swedish sheep flocks based on a comparison of the results from the faecal egg count reduction test and resistant allele frequencies of the beta-tubulin gene. *Vet. Parasitol.* **2009**, *161*, 60–68.

52. Beech, R.N.; Skuce, P.; Bartley, D.J.; Martin, R.J.; Prichard, R.K.; Gilleard, J.S. Anthelmintic resistance: Markers for resistance, or susceptibility? *Parasitology* **2010**, *138*, 160–174.

53. Gilleard, J.S. Understanding anthelmintic resistance: The need for genomics and genetics. *Int. J. Parasitol.* **2006**, *36*, 1227–1239.

54. Vignali, D.A.A. Multiplexed particle-based flow cytometric assays. *J. Immunol. Methods* **2000**, *243*, 243–255.

55. Pickering, J.W.; Martin, T.B.; Schroder, M.C.; Hill, H.R. Comparison of a multiplex flow cytometric assay with Enzyme-Linked Immunosorbent Assay for quantification of antibodies to Tetanus, Diphtheria and *Haemophilus influenza* Type b. *Clin. Diagn. Lab. Immunol.* **2002**, *9*, 872–876.

56. Dunbar, S.A.; Vander Zee, C.A.; Oliver, K.G.; Karem, K.L.; Jacobson, J.W. Quantitative, multiplexed detection of bacterial pathogens: DNA and protein applications of the Luminex LabMAPTM system. *J. Microbiol. Methods* **2003**, *53*, 245–252.

57. Morgan, E.R.; Varro, R.; Sepulveda, H.; Ember, J.A.; Apgar, J.; Wislon, J.; Lowe, L.; Chen, R.; Shivraj, L.; Agadir, A.; *et al.* Cytometric bead array: A multiplexed assay platform with applications in various areas of biology. *Clin. Immunol.***2004**, *110*, 252–266.

58. Dunbar, S.A. Application of Luminex xMAPTM technology for rapid, high-throughput multiplexed nucleic acid detection. *Clinia Chim. Acta* **2006**, *363*, 71–82.

59. Charlier, J.; Vercruysse, J.; Smith, J.; Vanderstichel, R.; Stryhn, H.; Claerebout, E.; Dohoo, I. Evaluation of anti-*Ostertagia ostertagi* antibodies in individual milk samples as decision parameter for selective anthelmintic treatment in dairy cows. *Prev. Vet. Med.* **2009**, *93*, 147–152.

60. McCann, C.M.; Baylis, M.; Williams, D.J.L. Seroprevalence and spatial distribution of *Fasciola hepatica*-infected dairy herds in England and Wales. *Vet. Rec.* **2010**, *166*, 612–617.

61. Andersen, U.V.; Howe, D.K.; Dangoudoubiyam, S.; Toft, N.; Reinemeyer, C.R.; Lyons, E.T.; Olsen, S.N.; Monrad, J.; Nejsum, P.; Nielsen, M.K. SvSXP: A *Strongylus vulgaris* antigen with potential for prepatent diagnosis. *Parasites Vectors***2013**, *6*, 84.

62. Ganheim, C.; Höglund, J.; Waller, P. Acute phase proteins in response to *Dictyocaulus viviparus* infection in calves.*Acta Vet. Scand.* **2004**, *45*, 79–86.

63. Charlier, J.; Dorny, P.; Levecke, B.; Demeler, J.; von Samson-Himmelstjerna, G.; Höglund, J.; Vercruysse, J. Serum pepsinogen levels to monitor gastrointestinal nematode infections in cattle revisited. *Res. Vet. Sci.* **2011**, *90*, 451–456.

64. Bandyopadhyay, K.; Kellar, K.L.; Moura, I.; Casaqui Carollo, M.C.; Graczyk, T.K.; Slemenda, S.; Johnston, S.P.; da Silva, A.J. Rapid microsphere assay for identification of *Cryptosporidium hominis* and *Cryptosporidium parvum* in stool and environmental samples. *J. Clin. Microbiol.* **2007**, *45*, 2835–2840.

65. Li, W.; Zhang, N.; Gong, P.; Cao, L.; Li, J.; Su, L.; Li, S.; Diao, Y.; Wu, K.; Li, L.; *et al.* A novel multiplex PCR coupled with Luminex assay for the simultaneous detection of Cryptosporidium spp., *Cryptosporidium parvum* and *Giardia duodenalis*. *Vet. Parasitol* **2010**, *173*, 11–18.

66. Stark, D.; Al-Qassab, S.E.; Barratt, J.L.; Stanley, K.; Roberts, T.; Marriott, D.; Harkness, J.; Ellis, J. An evaluation of a multiplex tandem real-time PCR for the detection of *Cryptosporidium* spp, *Dientamoeba fragilis*, *Entamoeba histolytica*, and *Giardia intestinalis* from clinical stool samples. *J. Clin. Microbiol.* **2010**, *49*, 257–262.

67. Iseki, H.; Alhassan, A.; Ohta, N.; Thekisoe, O.M.M.; Yokoyama, N.; Inoue, N.; Nambota, A.; Yasuda, J.; Igarashi, I. Development of a multiplex loop-mediated isothermal amplification (mLAMP) method for the simultaneous detection of bovine *Babesia* parasites. *J. Microbiol. Methods* **2007**, *71*, 281–287.

68. Parida, M.; Sannarangaiah, S.; Dash, P.K.; Rao, P.V.; Morita, K. Loop mediated isothermal amplification (LAMP): A new generation of innovative gene amplification technique; perspectives in clinical diagnosis of infectious diseases.*Rev. Med. Virol.* **2008**, *18*, 407–421.

69. Aonuma, H.; Yoshimura, A.; Perera, N.; Shinzawa, N.; Bando, H.; Oshiro, S.; Nelson, B.; Fukumoto, S.; Kanuka, H. Loop-mediated isothermal amplification applied to filarial parasites detection in the mosquito vectors: *Dirofilaria immitis* as a study model. *Parasites Vectors* **2009**, *2*, 15–21.

70. Mori, Y.; Notomi, T. Loop-mediated isothermal amplification (LAMP): A rapid, accurate and cost-effective diagnostic method for infectious diseases. *J. Infect. Chemother.* **2009**, *15*, 62–69.

71. Ollerenshaw, C.B.; Rowlands, W.T. A method of forecasting the incidence of fascioliasis in Anglesey. *Vet. Rec.* **1959**, *71*, 591–598.

72. Cornell, S. Modelling nematode populations: 20 years of progress. *Trends Parasitol.* **2005**, *21*, 542–545.

73. Fuentes, M.V. Remote sensing and climate data as a key for understanding fasciolosis transmission in the Andes: Review and update of an ongoing interdisciplinary project. *Geospat. Health* **2006**, *1*, 59–70.

74. Rose, H.; Wall, R. Modelling the impact of climate change on spatial patterns of disease risk: Sheep blowfly strike by*Lucilia sericata* in Great Britain. *Int. J. Parasitol.* **2011**, *41*, 739–746.

75. Biggeri, A.; Catelan, D.; Dreassi, E.; Rinaldi, L.; Musella, V.; Veneziano, V.; Cringoli, G. Multivariate spatially-structured variability of ovine helminth infections. *Geospat. Health* **2007**, *2*, 97–104.

76. Hendrickx, G.; Biesemans, J.; de Deken, R. The Use of GIS in Veterinary Parasitology. In *GIS and Spatial Analysis in Vet. Science*; Durr, P., Gatrell, A., Eds.; CABI Publishing: Wallingford, UK, 2004; pp. 145–176.

77. Rinaldi, L.; Musella, V.; Biggeri, A.; Cringoli, G. New insights into the application of geographical information systems and remote sensing in veterinary parasitology. *Geospat. Health* **2006**, *1*, 33–47.

78. Bergquist, R.; Rinaldi, L. Health research based on geospatial tools: A timely approach in a changing environment. *J. Helminthol.* **2010**, *84*, 1–11.

79. Geospatial health: Health applications in geospatial science. Available online http://www.geospatialhealth.unina.it(accessed on 11 August 2013).

80. Morgan, E.R.; Milner-Gulland, E.J.; Torgerson, P.R.; Medley, G.F. Ruminating on complexity: Macroparasites

of wildlife and livestock. *Trends Ecol. Evol.* **2004**, *19*, 181–188.

81. Morgan, E.R.; van Dijk, J. Climate and the epidemiology of gastrointestinal nematode infections of sheep in Europe. *Vet. Parasitol.* **2012**, *189*, 8–14.

82. Van Dijk, J.; David, G.P.; Baird, G.; Morgan, E.R. Back to the future: Developing hypotheses on the effects of climate change on ovine parasitic gastroenteritis from historical data. *Vet. Parasitol.* **2008**, *158*, 73–84.

83. Smith, G. Modeling of parasite populations—Gastrointestinal nematode models. *Vet. Parasitol.* **1994**, *54*, 127–143.

84. Van Dijk, J.; Morgan, E.R. Variation in the hatching behaviour of *Nematodirus battus*: Polymorphic bet hedging? *Int. J. Parasitol.* **2010**, *40*, 675–681.

85. Kenyon, F.; Greer, A.W.; Coles, G.C.; Cringoli, G.; Papadopoulos, E.; Cabaret, J.; Berrag, B.; Varady, M.; van Wyk, J.A.; Thomas, E.; *et al.* The role of targeted selective treatments in the development of refugia-based approaches to the control of gastrointestinal nematodes of small ruminants. *Vet. Parasitol.* **2009**, *164*, 3–11.

86. Cooper, K.M.; Whelan, M.; Kennedy, D.G.; Trigueros, G.; Cannavan, A.; Boon, P.E.; Wapperom, D.; Danaher, M. ProSafeBeef and anthelmintic drug residues-a case study in collaborative application of multi-analyte mass spectrometry to enhance consumer safety. *Anal. Bioanal. Chem.* **2012**, *404*, 1623–1630.

87. Imperiale, F.; Ortiz, P.; Cabrera, M.; Farias, C.; Sallovitz, J.M.; Iezzi, S.; Perez, J.; Alvarez, L.; Lanusse, C. Residual concentrations of the flukicidal compound triclabendazole in dairy cows' milk and cheese. *Food Addit. Contam. Part A Chem. Anal. Control Expo. Risk Assess.* **2011**, *28*, 438–445.

88. Greer, A.W.; Kenyon, F.; Bartley, D.J.; Jackson, E.B.; Gordon, Y.; Donnan, A.A.; McBean, D.W.; Jackson, F. Development and field evaluation of a decision support model for anthelmintic treatments as part of a targeted selective treatment (TST) regime in lambs. *Vet. Parasitol.* **2009**, *164*, 12–20.

89. Cringoli, G.; Rinaldi, L.; Veneziano, V.; Mezzino, L.; Vercruysse, J.; Jackson, F. Evaluation of targeted selective treatments in sheep in Italy: Effects on faecal worm egg count and milk production in four case studies. *Vet. Parasitol.* **2009**, *164*, 36–43.

90. Gallidis, E.; Papadopoulos, E.; Ptoches, S.; Arsenos, G. The use of targeted selective treatments against gastrointestinal nematodes in milking sheep and goats in Greece based on parasitological and performance criteria. *Vet. Parasitol.* **2009**, *164*, 53–58.

91. Höglund, J.; Morrison, D.A.; Charlier, J.; Dimander, S.; Larrson, A. Targeted selective treatments for gastrointestinal nematodes in first-season grazing cattle based on mid-season daily weight gains. *Vet. Parasitol.* **2009**, *164*, 80–88.

92. Leask, R.; van Wyk, J.A.; Thompson, P.N.; Bath, G.F. The effect of application of the FAMACHA© system on selected production parameters in sheep. *Small Rumin. Res.* **2013**, *110*, 1–8.

93. Gaba, S.; Cabaret, J.; Chylinski, C.; Sauve, C.; Cortet, J.; Silvestre, A. Can efficient management of sheep gastro-intestinal nematodes be based on random treatment? *Vet. Parasitol.* **2012**, *190*, 178–184.

94. Terrill, T.H.; Miller, J.E.; Burke, J.M.; Mosjidis, J.A.; Kaplan, R.M. Experiences with integrated concepts for the control of *Haemonchus contortus* in sheep and goats in the United States. *Vet. Parasitol.* **2012**, *186*, 28–37.

95. Van Wyk, J.A.; Reynecke, D.P. Blueprint for an automated specific decision support system for countering anthelmintic resistance in *Haemonchus* spp. at farm level. *Vet. Parasitol.* **2011**, *177*, 212–223.

96. Gauly, M.; Bollwein, H.; Breves, G.; Bruegemann, K.; Daenicke, S.; Das, G.; Demeler, J.; Hansen, H.; Isselstein, J.; Koenig, S.; *et al.* Future consequences and challenges for dairy cow production systems arising from climate change in Central Europe—A review. *Animal* **2013**, *7*, 843–859.

CHAPTER 9

SEROPREVALENCE AND RISK FACTORS FOR TOXOPLASMA GONDII IN SHEEP IN GROSSETO DISTRICT, TUSCANY, ITALY

Beniamino T Cenci-Goga, Antonio Ciampelli, Paola Sechi, Fabrizia Veronesi, Iolanda Moretta, Valentina Cambiotti and Peter N Thompson

Keywords: Toxoplasmosis, Sheep, Prevalence, Intra-cluster correlation coefficient, IFAT, Risk factors

BACKGROUND

Toxoplasma gondii is an intracellular protozoan parasite with felids as definitive hosts and a wide range of warm-blooded animals, including humans and domestic animals, as intermediate hosts [1, 2, 3]. Amongst food producing animals, sheep are the most susceptible to infection and T. gondii is an important cause of abortions and stillbirths [1]. Toxoplasmosis is a source of economic loss for sheep farmers and a danger for consumers, who can be infected by undercooked meat and untreated milk, with severe consequences mostly for pregnant women and immunocompromised individuals [2, 4, 5].

Sheep and goats are an important source of infected meat in southern European countries [6, 7]. Tachyzoites of T. gondii have also been detected in the milk of several intermediate hosts, including sheep, goats and cows [7]. Although the results of a recent study [8] demonstrate that, even with a low prevalence of infection in cattle, consumption of beef remains an important source of infection, lamb meat is an important risk factor, as determined by many case-control studies [9]. Seropositive sheep can be assumed to harbour large numbers of tissue cysts in their meat [10]. Sheep and lambs are usually kept on pasture and are therefore at risk of infection due to contamination of the environment with sporulated oocysts. If the environment is heavily contaminated with oocysts, infection prevalence can exceed 90% [5, 11]. This is of particular importance because tissue cysts have been found in many edible parts of sheep [12] and small ruminants are an important source of proteins (milk and meat) both in industrialized and developing countries. Considering the fact that in some countries raw or under-cooked lamb is considered an elite food, we can conclude that consumption of under-cooked lamb is an important risk factor for toxoplasmosis in humans. In countries where mutton is eaten well-cooked, the risk is much reduced [1].

Several studies have been conducted to establish the seroprevalence of T. gondii in sheep in different countries. Results range from 32.9% [13] to 80% [14] in Brazil, 84.5% in Serbia [15], 52.2% in Saudi Arabia [16], 29.1% in Iran [17], and 5.6% in South Africa [11]. In southern Italy, a cross-sectional study conducted in the Campania region found a seroprevalence of 28.5% in pastured sheep [18]. In addition, a study performed during the period 1999-2002 showed a seroprevalence of 28.4% in sheep in Sardinia, Italy [19]. Differences in seroprevalence between countries and regions may be due to different climatic and other risk factors as well as to differing cut-off values used to define seropositivity to the serological test [1, 20, 21]. Risk factors associated with infection are mainly related to animals (age, sex), rearing system, presence of cats on the farm, and farm management [11, 13, 15, 19, 22].

In an attempt to quantify the prevalence of T. gondii infection and further understand the potential risk posed to

Citation: Cenci-Goga et al.: Seroprevalence and risk factors for Toxoplasma gondii in sheep in Grosseto district, Tuscany, Italy. BMC Veterinary Research 2013 9:25. doi:10.1186/1746-6148-9-25.

humans in central Italy, a study was undertaken to determine seroprevalence and risk factors for T. gondiiinfection in sheep herds in Tuscany. This is the first time that such a study has been done in the region, therefore no data are available in literature.

METHODS

The research protocol for this study was approved by the council of the Dipartimento di Scienze Biopatologiche, no. 5, 28.09.2009

Study Population and Sample Size

Serum samples were collected from adult sheep (>18 months old) of the Sarda breed in dairy flocks in Grosseto district, Tuscany, Italy during May-June 2011. The study area extends from latitude 42.851078°N to 42.51902°N and from longitude 11.129635°E to 11.531657°E (Figure 1). The area is mainly hilly and the altitude of sampled farms ranged from 13 to 574 m above sea level. Sheep farming in Tuscany is very popular and the region has the fourth highest sheep population in Italy, the three highest being the islands of Sardinia and Sicily, and neighboring Lazio [23]. Grosseto district has approximately 730 sheep flocks and 122,000 sheep. None of the animals had ever been vaccinated against toxoplasmosis; indeed, such vaccination is not practiced in Italy.

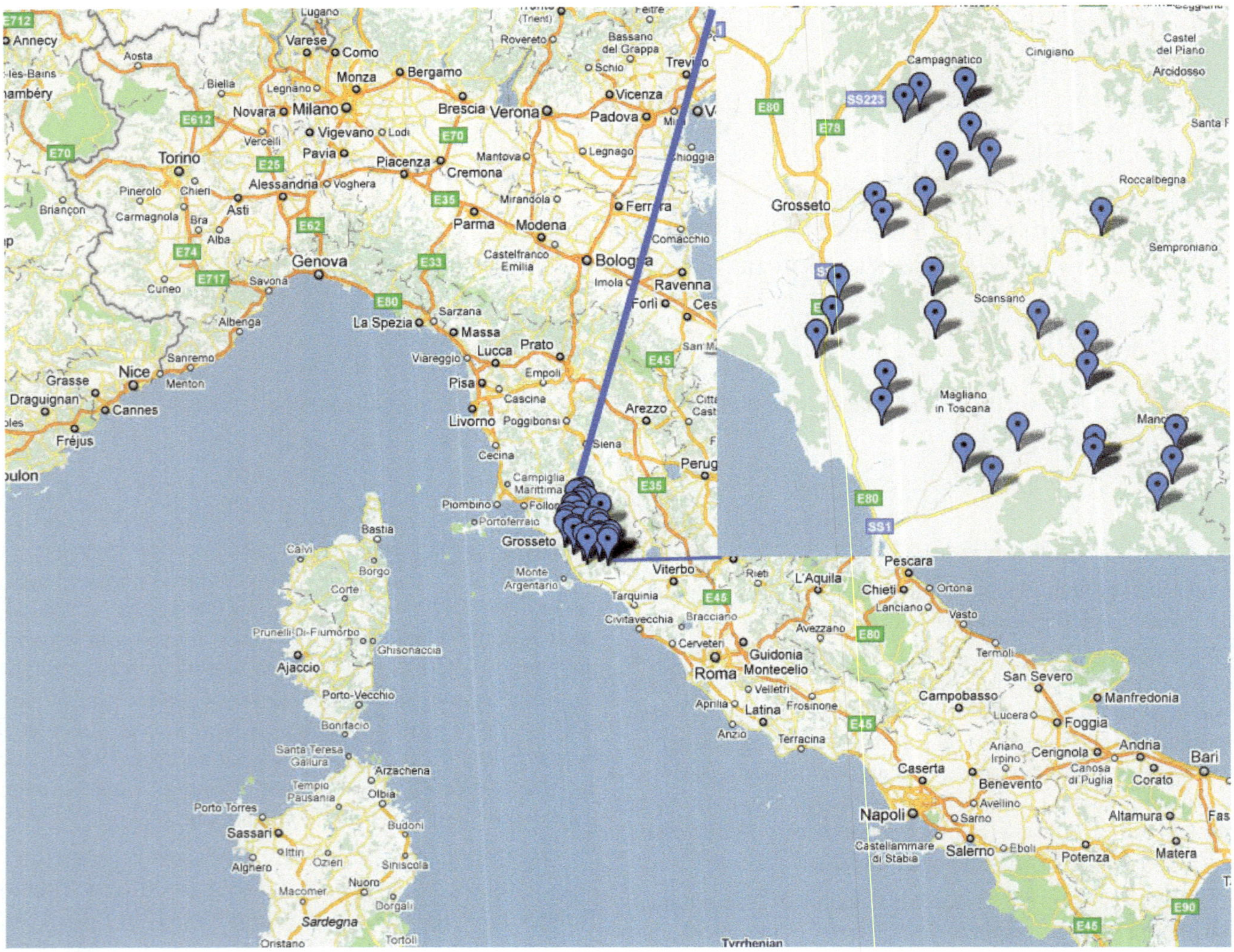

Figure 1: Study area and sampled farms.

Sample size was calculated using a 25% expected animal-level prevalence, 7.5% absolute error and 95% confidence level. This was adjusted for multi-stage sampling, in which an average of 20 animals per flock would be tested, using a conservative value for the intracluster correlation coefficient (ICC) of $\rho=0.20$ [24], which gave a required sample size of 620 animals in 31 flocks. This would also allow an estimate of flock-level seroprevalence of approximately 90% with 10% allowable error and 95% confidence. The flocks were selected using simple random sampling from a list of premise-identification numbers to ensure a representative sample of farms from the district. Within each selected flock, adult sheep (>18 months) were sampled by systematic random selection. Between 8 and 45 animals were selected per flock, approximately proportional to the total number of adult sheep present in the flock.

Questionnaire Data Collection

A questionnaire (Additional file 1 Audit form on rearing practices from 33 farms in Grosseto district, Tuscany, Italy.) was prepared to include questions on: rearing system (extensive: daily grazing in favorable weather conditions and returning to fold at night or daily grazing with possibility of shelter in bad weather; intensive: sheep housed day and night), water source (stagnant water source, e.g. pond or dam, used for sheep), separate water troughs and separate feeding troughs for young and adult animals, purchase of spare breeding animals, presence of resident and/or stray cats on the property, and access of cats to feed stores and water sources. The questionnaire was administered by the attending veterinarian at the time of blood sample collection and the veterinary practitioner, a co-author of this study, was always present during the interview.

Serology

Venous blood samples were collected from each selected animal and transferred to the laboratory on ice. After centrifugation (3000 rpm for 10 minutes), the sera were stored at -20°C until analysis [3]. Serum samples were analyzed using a commercial indirect immunofluorescence antibody assay (IFAT) to determine the presence of IgG antibodies against T. gondii. The serological test was performed according to the method of Camargo [25] using slides spotted with whole RH strain tachyzoites (Mega Cor Diagnostic, Horbranz, Austria) as antigens and fluorescein isothiocyanate-labelled rabbit anti-sheep IgG (whole molecule, Sigma-Aldrich, St Luis, MO, USA), diluted 1:100 in PBS plus 0.01% Evans blue, as conjugate. Sera were screened at 1:64 dilution (cut-off) and those testing positive were serially two-fold diluted to determine the end-point titre (the highest dilution of serum that gave a positive reaction). Positive and negative controls were included in each assay and the slides were examined under a fluorescence microscope (Olympus U-RFL-T) at 400 or 1000× magnification. Only a bright, linear, peripheral fluorescence of the tachyzoites was considered positive. Although the manufacturer claimed Se and Sp both to be >99%, we could not find independent confirmation of this, so for adjustment of apparent prevalence (see below) we used Se=80.4% and Sp=91.4%, reported elsewhere for another commercial IFAT [26].

Statistical Analysis

Within-flock seroprevalence for each farm, flock-level seroprevalence and exact binomial 95% confidence limits were calculated. The ICC (ρ), indicating the degree of clustering of seropositivity within flocks, was estimated by using a logistic model of individual animal test outcome, with a random effect for flock and no fixed effects, to obtain the flock random effect variance, σ_f^2, and then calculating $\rho=\sigma_f^2 / (\pi^2/3+\sigma_f^2)$, where $\pi^2/3$ is the variance of the logistic distribution [27]. Within each flock, sampling fraction was calculated as the proportion of animals >18 months that was sampled, and sampling weight was calculated as the inverse of the sampling fraction. Using the 'svy' commands in Stata 12, overall animal-level seroprevalence was calculated by weighting each individual's result by its sampling weight and the standard error was adjusted for clustering and weighting. Finally, animal-level prevalence estimates and confidence limits were adjusted for test sensitivity (80.4%) and specificity (91.4%) using the formula of Rogan and Gladen [28]: TP=(AP+Sp–1) / (Se+Sp–1), where TP=true prevalence, AP=apparent prevalence (after adjusting for sampling weight), Se=test sensitivity and Sp=test specificity.

The bivariable association between each potential risk factor and within-flock seroprevalence was assessed using a Poisson regression model of the number of seropositive animals in a herd with the number of animals tested as an exposure variable, i.e. ln(number tested) was included in the model with its coefficient constrained to 1. Variables associated with the outcome (P<0.20) were then entered into a multivariable Poisson model, with number tested as exposure, which was developed by backward elimination until all remaining variables were significant (P<0.05). All other variables were then re-tested in the model and retained if significant. Fit of the Poisson model was assessed using the Pearson goodness-of-fit test and dispersion parameter [27]. Finally, the corresponding negative binomial regression model of the number of seropositive animals in a herd was compared with the Poisson model using a likelihood ratio test. All analyses were done using Stata 12.1 (StataCorp, College Station, TX, U.S.A.).

RESULTS

Serum samples were collected from 630 sheep in 33 flocks and tested for antibodies to T. gondii by IFAT. Flock sizes ranged from 70 to 630 adult sheep (mean: 247; median: 210) and between 8 and 45 animals (mean: 19.1; median: 17) were tested per flock. Sampling fractions within flocks ranged from 0.059 to 0.135 (mean: 0.079; median: 0.075). Using a cut-off titre of 1:64, a total of 214/630 (34.0%) samples tested positive. Among the 214 reactive samples, 42 (19.6%) had a titre of 1:64, 36 (16.8%) of 1:128, 39 (18.2%) of 1:256, and 97 (45.3%) of 1:512 or above.

Overall animal-level seroprevalence in the district, adjusted for sampling weights and for test sensitivity and specificity, was 33.3% (95% CI: 24.8%, 42.7%). At least one seropositive animal was found in 32 of the 33 flocks tested, therefore the flock-level seroprevalence was estimated to be 97.0% (95% CI: 84.2%, 99.9%). In the positive flocks, median seroprevalence was 29.4% (interquartile range: 15.9%, 46.1%). The ICC (ρ) was estimated to be 0.211 (95% CI: 0.113, 0.360).

In the bivariable analysis of potential risk factors (Table 1), five variables (flock size, production system, stagnant water, resident cats, access of stray cats to water) were selected for inclusion in the multivariable Poisson model. The final Poisson model contained only two predictors (flock size and access of cats to water) but showed lack of fit (Pearson $\chi^2_{29\ df}$=48.0; P=0.015) and evidence of over dispersion (dispersion parameter=1.65, where >1 indicates over dispersion). Further, the likelihood ratio test comparing the corresponding negative binomial regression model with the Poisson model was marginally significant (P_{LRT}=0.052), therefore the negative binomial model was preferred. After re-testing each independent variable for significance, the final negative binomial model is shown in Table 2. Adjusted for the number tested, the number of seropositive animals in the flock decreased with increasing flock size (for >400 vs. <300 animals: count ratio (CR)=0.62; 95% CI: 0.41, 0.95; P=0.028). In addition, the number of seropositive animals was greater on farms where stray cats had access to animals' water (CR=1.54; 95% CI: 1.05, 2.26; P=0.027).

Table 1: Mean within-farm seroprevalence of Toxoplasma gondii in dairy sheep flocks and bivariable association with potential risk factors

Variable	**Level**	**Number of farms**	**Mean seroprevalence(%)**	***P*-value***
Size of flock	<300	14	42.4	<0.001
	300-400	10	33.5	
	>400	9	24.0	
Production system	Extensive	30	35.9	0.088
	Intensive	3	22.6	
Stagnant water used	No	21	31.3	0.05
	Yes	12	40.7	
Separate water trough for young and adult animals	No	29	33.7	0.587
	Yes	4	42.2	
Separate feed troughs for young and adult animals	No	10	31.3	0.948
	Yes	23	36.18	
Purchased breeding animals in last 5 years	No	3	22.7	0.481
	Yes	30	35.9	
Resident cats present on farm	No	10	28.4	0.122
	Yes	23	37.4	
Stray cats occur on farm	No	0	–	–
	Yes	33	34.7	
Access of stray cats to animal feed	No	7	32.4	0.715
	Yes	26	35.3	
Access of stray cats to animals' water	No	12	22.9	0.001
	Yes	21	41.4	

* From Poisson regression model with number tested as offset.

Table 2: Farm-level factors associated with number of animals seropositive to Toxoplasma gondii in 33 dairy sheep flocks: results of a negative binomial regression model

Variable	**Level**	**Count ratio**	**95%CI(CR)**	***P*-value**
Size of flock	<300	1*	–	–
	300-400	0.83	0.55, 1.26	0.377
	>400	0.62	0.41, 0.95	0.028
Access of stray cats to animals' water	No	1*	–	–
	Yes	1.54	1.05, 2.26	0.027
ln(number tested)	(exposure)	–	–	–

* Reference level.

DISCUSSION

There has been an increasing interest in recent years in the prevalence of T. gondii infection in small ruminants because of their role on the dissemination of the protozoan to man through direct contact or by consuming products of animal origin [1, 11, 14, 22, 29, 30, 31]. Although the average seroprevalence of T.gondii infection in sheep populations has long been estimated to be approximately 30% [32], very few studies have been conducted in Italy and little is known about the prevalence of T. gondii in many areas where sheep farming is an important element of the local economy. Lamb, mutton and sheep milk are important sources of human T. gondii infections, but actual data on the prevalence of T. gondii in sheep are scarce [1]. This study estimated the seroprevalence of T. gondii in dairy sheep in Tuscany, Italy, and investigated risk factors associated with the number of infected animals in a flock. The test of choice was a commercial indirect fluorescent antibody test (IFAT). Although the variability of the sensitivity and specificity depending on the Toxoplasma strain employed, and the subjectivity in interpreting the fluorescence reaction make it difficult to compare results between laboratories, the IFAT is simple to carry out and can easily be performed for large numbers of samples and several dilutions, even by inexpert lab technicians [1]. Data in the literature show some variability in sensitivity and specificity even in the same regions and in the same type of farm [26, 33,34]. A recent study [33] has revealed that there is poor agreement between IFAT and the modified agglutination test (MAT) in cat and dog sera. Moreover most surveys are performed on blood collected at the slaughterhouse after sticking, resulting in mixing of arterial and venous blood. The latter is required by good laboratory practice for serology, whereas the different pH and composition of arterial blood may influence the test sensitivity and specificity [35]. For our study we could not obtain reliable estimates of test sensitivity or specificity for the particular IFAT used, and therefore chose to use more conservative estimates from a different IFAT. However, with the high prevalence encountered in the study, the adjustment for test performance made very little change to the estimate and therefore did not materially influence our results.

In the present study, a 33.3% seroprevalence (95% CI: 24.8%, 42.7%) of T. gondii infection in sheep raised in the Grosseto district, Tuscany, Italy, was detected. When using multistage or cluster sampling, the standard error (SE) of the prevalence estimate is increased compared with simple random sampling of the same number of animals [8], and this should be taken into account when calculating a confidence interval for the prevalence estimate. In addition, when sampling fractions differ between clusters this should be adjusted for in calculating the point estimate of the prevalence. Ignoring the above adjustments, as well as the adjustment for test sensitivity and specificity, would have resulted in a seroprevalence estimate of 34.0% (95% CI: 30.3%, 37.8%). Our estimate of 33.3% (95% CI: 24.8%, 42.7%) therefore provides a more realistic measure of the precision of the study. The increase in SE with multi-stage sampling depends on the average number of units sampled from each cluster, as well as the ICC. The estimated ICC of $\rho=0.211$ indicates moderate clustering of infection within flocks and should be taken into account when calculating sample sizes for future surveys.

Comparison of our results with those of previous studies should be done with care since various assays have been used. Over a one year period following 31 abortions caused by T. gondii on a typical farm of 524 sheep in Italy, the prevalence of IgG positives ranged from 31.5% at the first sampling to 62.6% at the fourth sampling [36]. Authors [37] reported an overall seroprevalence of 51.3% in Sardinia using an ELISA test; seroprevalence increased significantly with age. In a cross-sectional serological survey to evaluate, irrespective of abortion, theT. gondii infection in pastured sheep from the Campania region of Southern Italy, 77.8% of the farms and 28.5% of the sheep tested positive [18]. In addition, the presence of T. gondii DNA was detected by PCR in 4/117 milk samples (3.4%). Analysis of sera from 1961 sheep, collected just before slaughtering from 62 farms in Sicily revealed a seroprevalence of 49.9% using a commercially available ELISA for Toxoplasma-specific IgG. Eighty-seven percent of the farms had at least one seropositive animal [38].

The worldwide seroprevalence of T. gondii infection in sheep was recently reviewed by Dubey [2]. Since then, seroprevalences of 44.1% have been reported in sheep from Grenada and Carriacou, West-Indies [39] and 18.6% in Sao Paulo, Brazil [40], using MAT. In a serological survey of T. gondii infection in adult breeding sheep in Great Britain, of the 3539 sera collected from 227 flocks, 74% were found to be positive for T. gondii specific antibody using latex agglutination [41]. Multilevel logistic modelling suggested that the likelihood of infection increased with age and this effect appeared to be amplified in animals vaccinated against T. gondii. The model also indicated that the odds of sheep being seropositive were increased on premises where cattle were also kept. These results suggest a high level of Toxoplasma infection in breeding sheep in Great Britain and provide further evidence to suggest that postnatal infection is more common than congenital infection in sheep.

The seroprevalence of more than 30% demonstrated in this study is therefore consistent with several previous reports [18, 19, 36], but lower than that reported by others [37, 38, 39, 41]. The variability of these results may be due to the differences in the age and management of the sampled animals, the environment and in the serological technique used [1, 34].

In the multivariable model, a strong positive association was found between within-farm seroprevalence of T.gondii and the access of cats to water given to animals, confirming that contact with feline species is important in the epidemiology of toxoplasmosis. The fact that cats, either resident or stray, were present on every farm could explain the high prevalence of T. gondii-specific antibodies observed in sheep in this study, due to elimination of oocysts by the cats and contamination of the environment. The strong association between seroprevalence and access of cats to water used by the sheep, but no association with access of cats to the feed store, suggests that contaminated water may be as important, if not more important a source of infection than contaminated feed. This supports the conclusion of a recent review paper [24] that waterborne transmission of T. gondii may be more common than previously thought. In a previous European study, the “use of surface water sources for drinking” was identified as a putative risk factor for T. gondii seropositivity in sheep [38].

In the initial bivariable analysis, but not in the multivariable analysis, there was an association between seroprevalence and the use of stagnant water, which may have been due to the fact that cats were more likely to have had access to stagnant water than to running water. As oocyst survival in soil for up to two years has been reported, any faecal material from infected cats will represent a hazard [1]. T. gondii oocysts survive in water (up to 54 months in cold water) so unfiltered water contaminated with T. gondii can lead to infection [42,43].

After adjusting for the number of sheep tested in the flock, as well as for confounding due to the other risk factors assessed, the number of seropositive animals in the flock was negatively associated with the size of the flock; seroprevalence was therefore higher in smaller flocks. Since all but three of the flocks in our study were classified as having an extensive management system, the association of this variable with seroprevalence could not be assessed. However, in our study area the farms with higher numbers of sheep tended to be more intensive, therefore the negative association between seroprevalence and flock size may have been due to unmeasured management or environmental factors related to degree of intensification. This would be consistent with the report of WNA van der Puije, et al. [44] that prevalence was higher in extensively managed sheep flocks. Possible reasons could be that some smaller, more extensively managed sheep flocks may have had more exposure to cats in the environment, or to contaminated stagnant pools (apart from their primary water source noted in the questionnaire). On the other hand, a recent sero-epidemiological study conducted in Greece [27] showed infection rates to be significantly higher in intensive rearing systems due to the higher exposure of animals to contaminated feed. In addition, farm facilities under intensive or semi-intensive conditions may provide shelter to various hosts of T. gondii (such as cats and rodents) which might be involved in the spread of infection [27].

No association with seropositivity was observed for the use of separate water and feed troughs for young and adult animals or for the purchase of spare breeding animals, supporting the prevailing view that direct sheep to sheep spread at lambing has not been proven and that transmission from rams at mating has been dismissed as a route of infection [2].

CONCLUSION

Based on the results obtained in this study, it can be concluded that small flock size and access of cats to drinking water are potential risk factors for Toxoplasma infection in sheep in the Grosseto district in Tuscany, Italy. Sheep could be an important source of T. gondii infection in humans, since we estimate that between 25% and 43% of sheep in the district are seropositive. Toxoplasmosis is also likely to be an important cause of abortion in sheep in the district. Control and prophylactic measures must be adopted to improve the rearing system and the implementation of health promoting programmes in a joint effort between sheep farmers, farmers' associations and veterinarians to inform about the means of transmission of the infection and for a better understanding of the disease.

ACKNOWLEDGMENTS

The authors thank all those colleagues who have helped in our on-going research projects, in particular Prof. Barend Louis Penzhorn and Dr Nada Abu Samra of the University of Pretoria, Faculty of Veterinary Science, Onderstepoort, South Africa; Dr Carlo Crotti and Dr Ludovico Renda, veterinary practitioners in Perugia, Italy, and Prof. Piergili Fioretti, University of Perugia, Italy. The authors also express sincere appreciation to members of Polyglot, Perugia, for a careful reading and comments on the article. The findings and conclusions in this paper are those of the authors and do not necessarily represent the views of the University of Perugia. Within the framework of the dottorato di ricerca «Sanità animale, produzioni zootecniche e sicurezza degli alimenti – XXVIII Ciclo» this research was supported by a grant from Fondazione Cassa di Risparmio di Perugia, Italy.

AUTHORS' CONTRIBUTIONS

The study idea was conceived by BCG. BCG, PS and AC participated in the design of the study. FV and IM participated in the acquisition of the laboratory data. AC collected serum samples with the attending veterinarians and helped administering the questionnaire. PT and VC provided previously acquired reference data. BCG and PT carried out the statistical analysis. Data interpretation was done by all authors. BCG and PT drafted the manuscript. All authors contributed to the critical revision of the manuscript for important intellectual content and have seen and approved the final draft.

REFERENCES

1. Cenci Goga BT, Rossitto PV, Sechi P, Mc Crindle CME, Cullor JS: Toxoplasma in animals, food and humans: an old parasite of new concern. Foodborne pathog dis. 2011, Vol. 8- n.7: 1-12.
2. Dubey JP: Toxoplasmosis in sheep - The last 20 years. Vet Parasitol. 2009, 163 (1-2): 1-14. 10.1016/j.vetpar.2009.02.026.
3. Urquart GM, Armour J, Duncan JL, Dunn AM, Jennings FW: Parassitologia veterinaria. 2nd edition. UTET, Milano, Italy, 2005.
4. Innes EA, Bartley PM, Buxton D, Katzer F: Ovine toxoplasmosis. Parasitology. 2009, 136 (14): 1887-1894. 10.1017/S0031182009991636.
5. Tenter AM, Heckeroth A, Weiss LM: Toxoplasma gondi, from animals to humans. Int J Parasitol. 2000, 30 (12–13): 1217-1258.
6. Clancy R, Ren Z, Turton J, Pang G, Wettstein A: Molecular evidence for Mycobacterium avium subspecies paratuberculosis (MAP) in Crohn's disease correlates with enhanced TNF-alpha secretion. Digestive Liver Dis. 2007, 39: 445-451. 10.1016/j.dld.2006.12.006. 5, May, 2007
7. Tenter AM: Toxoplasma gondii in animals used for human consumption. Memorias do Instituto Oswaldo Cruz. 2009, 104: 364-369. 10.1590/S0074-02762009000200033.
8. Opsteegh M, Prickaerts S, Frankena K, Evers EG: A quantitative microbial risk assessment for meatborne Toxoplasma gondii infection in The Netherlands. Int J Food Microbiol. 2011, 150 (2–3): 103-114.
9. Anonymous: Toxoplasmose: état des connaisances et évaluation du risque lié à l'alimentation. In AFSSA - Report of the Afssa working group "Toxoplasma gondii", University of Pretoria. 2005, http://www.afssa.fr/Documents/MIC-Ra-Toxoplasmose.pdf.
10. Dubey JP, Jones JL: Toxoplasma gondii infection in humans and animals in the United States. Int J Parasitol. 2008, 38 (11): 1257-1278. 10.1016/j.ijpara.2008.03.007.
11. Samra NA, Mc Crindle CM, Penzhorn BL, Cenci Goga BT: Seroprevalence of toxoplasmosis in sheep in South Africa. JS AfrVet Assoc. 2007, 78 (3): 116-120.
12. Dubey JP, Kirkbride CA: Enzootic toxoplasmosis in sheep in North-Central United-States. J Parasitol. 1989, 75 (5): 673-676. 10.2307/3283047.
13. Pinheiro JJW, Mota RA, da Fonseca Oliveira AA, Faria EB, Gondim LFP, da Silva AV, Anderlini GA: Prevalence and risk factors associated to infection by Toxoplasma gondii in ovine in the state of alagoas, Brazil. Parasitol Res. 2009, 105: 709-715. 10.1007/s00436-009-1472-3.
14. Rossi GF, Cabral DD, Ribeiro DP, Pajuaba AC, Correa RR, Moreira RQ, Mineo TW, Mineo JR, Silva DA: Evaluation ofToxoplasma gondii and neospora caninum

infections in sheep from Uberlandia, minas gerais state, Brazil, by different serological methods. Vet Parasitol. 2011, 175 (3–4): 252-259.

15. Klun I, Djurkovic O, Katic-Radivojevic S, Nikolic A: Cross-sectional survey on Toxoplasma gondii infection in cattle, sheep and pigs in Serbia: seroprevalence and risk factors. Vet Parasitol. 2006, 135: 121-131. 10.1016/j.vetpar.2005.08.010.

16. Sanad MM, Al Ghabban AJ: Serological survey on toxoplasmosis among slaughtered sheep and goats in Tabouk, Saudi Arabia. J Egypt Soc Parasitol. 2007, 37 (1): 329-340.

17. Bonyadian M, Hematzade F, Manuchehri K: Seroprevalence of antibodies to Toxoplasma gondii in sheep in center of Iran. Pak J Biol Sci. 2007, 10 (18): 3228-3230.

18. Fusco G, Rinaldi L, Guarino A, Proroga YT, Pesce A, de Giuseppina M, Cringoli G: Toxoplasma gondii in sheep from the Campania region (Italy). Vet Parasitol. 2007, 149 (3-4): 271-274. 10.1016/j.vetpar.2007.07.020.

19. Masala G, Porcu R, Madau L, Tanda A, Ilba B, Satta G, Tola S: Survey of ovine and caprine toxoplasmosis by IFAT and PCR assays in Sardinia, Italy. Vet Parasitol. 2003, 117 (1-2): 15-21. 10.1016/j.vetpar.2003.07.012.

20. Cenci Goga BT: Toxoplasmosi negli animali, negli alimenti e nell'uomo. Una sfida per il medico veterinario – prima parte. Praxis veterinaria. 2009, Vol. xxx- n.3: 7-15.

21. Cenci Goga BT: Toxoplasmosi negli animali, negli alimenti e nell'uomo. Una sfida per il medico veterinario – seconda parte. Praxis veterinaria. 2009, Vol. xxx- n.4: 7-12.

22. Lopes WD, Santos TR, da Silva Rdos S, Rossanese WM, de Souza FA, de Faria Rogrigues JD, de Mendonça RP, Soares VE, Costa AJ: Seroprevalence and risk factors for Toxoplasma gondii in sheep raised in the jabotical microregion, Sao Paulo State, Brazil. Res Vet Sci. 2010, 88 (1): 104-106. 10.1016/j.rvsc.2009.06.006.

23. Anonymous: Anagrafe nazionale zootecnica - statistiche. 2012, http://www.izs.it/IZS.

24. Otte M, Gumm I: Intra-cluster correlation coefficients of 20 infections calculated from the results of cluster-sample surveys. Prev Vet Med. 1997, 31: 147-150. 10.1016/S0167-5877(96)01108-7.

25. Camargo ME: Introdução às técnicas de imunofluorescência. Revista Brasileira de Patologia Cĺi nica. 1974, 10: 143-171.

26. Shaapan RM, El-Nawawi FA, Tawfik MAA: Sensitivity and specificity of various serological tests for the detection ofToxoplasma gondii infection in naturally infected sheep. Vet Parasitol. 2008, 153 (3–4): 359-362.

27. Dohoo IRMW, Stryhn H: Veterinary epidemiologic research. 2nd edition. Charlottetown: VER Inc, 2009.

28. Rogan W, Gladen B: Estimating prevalence from the results of a screening test. Am J Epidemiol. 1978, 107: 71-76.

29. Alvarado-Esquivel C, García-Machado C, Alvarado-Esquivel D, Vitela-Corrales J, Villena I, Dubey JP: Seroprevalence ofToxoplasma gondii infection in domestic sheep in Durango state, Mexico. J Parasitol. 2012, 98 (2): 271-273. 10.1645/GE-2958.1.

30. Opsteegh M, Teunis P, Mensink M, Züchner L, Lothar Z, Titilincu A, Langelaar M, van der Giessen J: Evaluation of ELISA test characteristics and estimation of Toxoplasma gondii seroprevalence in Dutch sheep using mixture models. Prevent Veterinary Med. 2010, 96 (3-4): 232-240. 10.1016/j.prevetmed.2010.06.009.

31. Ueno TE, Gonçalves VS, Heinemann MB, Dilli TL, Akimoto BM, de Souza SL, Gennari SM, Soares RM: Prevalence of Toxoplasma gondii and neospora caninum infections in sheep from federal district, central region of Brazil. Trop Anim Health Prod. 2009, 41 (4): 547-552. 10.1007/s11250-008-9220-8.

32. Blewett DA: The epidemiology of ovine toxoplasmosis. I. The interpretation of data for the prevalence of antibody in sheep and other host species. Br Vet J. 1983, 139: 537-545.

33. Macrì G, Sala M, Linder A, Pettirossi N, Scarpulla M: Comparison of indirect fluorescent antibody test and modified agglutination test for detecting Toxoplasma gondii immunoglobulin G antibodies in dog and cat. Parasitol Res. 2009, 105 (1): 35-40. 10.1007/s00436-009-1358-4.

34. Piergili Fioretti D: Problematiche e limiti dei metodi convenzionali ed innovativi nella diagnosi di Toxoplasmosi nell'uomo e negli animali. Parassitologia. 2004, 46: 177-181.

35. Anonymous: Single-use containers for venous blood specimen collection. ISO. 1995, 6710: 1995.

36. Zedda MT, Rolesu S, Pau S, Rosati I, Ledda S, Satta G, Patta C, Masala G: Epidemiological study of Toxoplasma gondii infection in ovine breeding. Zoonoses and Public Health. 2010, 57 (7–8): e102-e108.

37. Natale A, Porqueddu M, Capelli G, Mocci G, Marras A, Sanna Coccone GN, Garippa G, Scala A: Sero-epidemiological update on sheep toxoplasmosis in Sardinia, Italy. Parassitologia. 2007, 49 (4): 235-238.

38. Vesco G, Buffolano W, La Chiusa S, Mancuso G, Caracappa S, Chianca A, Villari S, Currò V, Liga F, Petersen E: Toxoplasma gondii infections in sheep in Sicily, southern Italy. Vet Parasitol. 2007, 146 (1,Äì2): 3-8.

39. Chikweto A, Kumthekar S, Tiwari K, Nyack B, Deokar MS, Stratton G, Macpherson CNL, Sharma RN, Dubey JP: Seroprevalence of Toxoplasma gondii in pigs, sheep, goats, and cattle from Grenada and carriacou, west Indies. J Parasitol. 2011, 97 (5): 950-951. 10.1645/GE-2811.1.

40. Langoni H, Greca Júnior H, Guimarães FF, Ullmann LS, Gaio FC, Uehara RS, Rosa EP, Amorim RM, Da Silva RC: Serological profile of Toxoplasma gondii and neospora caninum infection in commercial sheep from Sào Paulo State, Brazil. Vet Parasitol. 2011, 177 (1–2): 50-54.

41. Hutchinson JP, Wear AR, Lambton SL, Smith RP, Pritchard GC: Survey to determine the seroprevalence of Toxoplasma gondii infection in British sheep flocks. Vet

Rec. 2011, 169 (22): 582-10.1136/vr.d5764.

42. Dubey JP, Beattie CP: Toxoplasmosis of animals and Man. 1988, CRC Press, Boca Raton, FL, USA

43. Dubey JP: Toxoplasma gondii oocyst survival under defined temperatures. J Parasitol. 1998, 84 (4): 862-865. 10.2307/3284606.

44. van der Puije WNA, Bosompem KM, Canacoo EA, Wastling JM, Akanmori BD: The prevalence of anti-Toxoplasma gondii antibodies in Ghanaian sheep and goats. Acta Trop. 2000, 76 (1): 21-26. 10.1016/S0001-706X(00)00084-X.

CHAPTER 10

GENETIC CHARACTERIZATIONS OF GIARDIA DUODENALIS IN SHEEP AND GOATS IN HEILONGJIANG PROVINCE, CHINA AND POSSIBILITY OF ZOONOTIC TRANSMISSION

Weizhe Zhang, Xiaoli Zhang, Rongjun Wang, Aiqin Liu, Yujuan Shen, Hong Ling, Jianping Cao, Fengkun Yang, Xiaoyun Zhang, Longxian Zhang

INTRODUCTION

Giardia duodenalis (syn. Giardia lamblia, Giardia intestinalis) is one of the most common protozoa in humans and animals. Giardiasis of humans and animals has a wide spectrum of clinical signs, including the onset of diarrhea, abdominal pain, bloating, vomiting, nausea and/or weight loss. The parasite can lead to growth and development retardation of children, even in asymptomatic cases [1], and is also of significant clinical and economic importance in livestock and pet animals [2]–[4].

To date, molecular data revealed the presence of seven assemblages (A to G) within G. duodenalis based on genetic analysis and host specificity. In a recent study, assemblage H has been described in marine vertebrates [5]. Among them, assemblages A and B have the widest host range. They both have the ability to infect humans and a variety of mammals, including livestock, dogs, cats and wildlife [6], [7]. Assemblages C, D, E, F and G seem to be host specific for nonhuman species. However, assemblages C, D, E and F have been isolated from humans, but at a very low prevalence [7].

Outbreaks of human giardiasis are most frequently waterborne and caused by contamination of drinking water, although other routes have also been described [8], [9]. G. duodenalis is one of the most common pathogens in water-associated outbreaks of parasitic protozoan diseases, accounting for 40.6% (132/325) out of total outbreaks [10]. The sources of contamination of water supplies may come from humans, farm animals and wildlife. Due to the lack of data of transmission dynamics between humans and animals, the role of animals in the spread of infections remains unclear. Contact with farm animals has been pointed out as a risk factor of human infection of G. duodenalis in case control studies [11], [12]. The previous report of an outbreak of sheep giardiasis with the death of some animals in Central Italy is of concern for sheep farmers [3].

Years of epidemiological data have documented the occurrence of G. duodenalis infection in sheep and goats, indicating a wide range in prevalence from 1.5% to 55.6% in sheep and from 12.3% to 42.2% in goats [13]. Studies using molecular analysis have confirmed the presence of assemblages A, B and E of G. duodenalis in sheep and goats. Assemblage E was the major genotype in sheep/goats in most countries, with assemblage A being occasionally detected in Australia, Sweden, the USA, Belgium, and Spain and with assemblage B being occasionally detected in Norway and Spain [14]–[21]. In a study in Australia, assemblage A is the most common subtype in sheep [22]. Interestingly, only G. duodenalis assemblages A and B have been reported in sheep in Italy, with an absence of assemblage E [3], [23].

In China, there are no reports about the investigations and genotyping data of sheep and goat giardiasis so far. China has

Citation: Zhang W, Zhang X, Wang R, Liu A, Shen Y, Ling H, et al. (2012) Genetic Characterizations of Giardia duodenalis in Sheep and Goats in Heilongjiang Province, China and Possibility of Zoonotic Transmission. PLoS Negl Trop Dis 6(9): e1826. doi:10.1371/journal.pntd.0001826

one of the largest populations of sheep and goat flocks [24]. To understand the prevalence and distribution of G. duodenalis in sheep and goats in China, a survey of G. duodenalis was conducted in sheep and goats in Heilongjiang Province, and thetpi gene sequences of G. duodenalis isolates were analyzed for genetic characterization and assessment of the potential of zoonotic transmission at both genotyping and subtyping levels.

MATERIALS AND METHODS

Ethics Statement

Before beginning work on the study, we contacted the farm owners and obtained their permission to have their animals involved. During specimen collection, all animal work followed guidelines in accordance with the Regulations for the Administration of Affairs Concerning Experimental Animals, and approved by the Animal Ethical Committee of Harbin Medical University.

Specimen Collection

A total of 678 fecal specimens (539 from sheep and 139 from goats) were randomly collected on six farms within Heilongjiang Province, China in a two-year survey from October 2009 to November 2011 (Table 1). The specimens were taken directly from the rectum of each animal with sterile plastic gloves. For each animal, the sampling date, species, ages and the identification number were recorded. Their ages ranged from one month to four years. The specimens were transported to the laboratory in a cool box and then stored at 4°C and processed within two days of collection. Each fecal specimen was directly used to smear three slides for iodine wet mount staining. Wet smears were examined for the presence of G. duodenalis cysts by light field microscopy at 400× magnification. All G. duodenalis-positive specimens were stored in 2.5% potassium dichromate solution at 4°C before DNA extraction.

Table 1. Prevalence and assemblage distribution of G. duodenalis on six farms of sheep and goats in Heilongjiang Province

Farm	Animal species	No. of Positive/No. of Examined (%)					No. of *G. duodenalis* assemblages A, B and E
		Age group (month)					
		<2	3–6	7–11	>12	Total	
Farm1	sheep	4/15 (26.7)	5/54 (9.3)	1/21 (4.8)	1/46 (2.2)	11/136 (8.1)	E(9)
Farm2	sheep	2/11 (18.2)	2/41 (4.9)	1/29 (3.4)	0/23 (0)	5/104 (4.8)	A(1), B(2)
Farm3	sheep	1/6 (16.7)	2/33 (6.1)	2/41 (4.9)	0/10 (0)	5/90(5.6)	E(4)
Farm4	sheep	2/13 (15.4)	4/42 (9.5)	3/58 (5.2)	1/35 (2.9)	10/148 (6.8)	A(3), E(6)
Farm5	sheep	0/8 (0)	0/22 (0)	0/13 (0)	0/18 (0)	0/61 (0)	
Farm6	goat	2/19 (10.5)	1/21 (4.8)	1/48 (2.1)	0/51 (0)	4/139 (2.9)	E(4)
Total		11/72 (15.3)	14/233 (6.0)	8/220 (3.6)	2/183 (1.1)	34/678 (5.0)	A(4), B(2), E(23)

doi:10.1371/journal.pntd.0001826.t001

DNA Extraction

G. duodenalis-positive fecal specimens were washed four times with distilled water to remove potassium dichromate from the solution. Genomic DNA was directly extracted from approximately 200 mg of the fecal pellet using a QIAamp DNA Stool Mini Kit (QIAgen, Hilden, Germany) according to manufacturer's instruction. DNA was eluted in 200 μL of AE elution buffer and DNA preparation was stored at −20°C prior to use in PCR analysis.

G. duodenalis Genotyping and Subtyping

G. duodenalis isolates were genotyped and subtyped at the tpi locus using a nested PCR which amplifies an approximately 530-bp fragment as previously described [25]. All secondary PCR products were purified and directly sequenced. Each DNA preparation was analyzed at least twice by PCR. Genotypes and subtypes of G. duodenalis isolates were identified by analyzing and comparing the tpi gene sequences obtained in the present study with those published in GenBank.

DNA Sequence Analysis

All secondary PCR products were sequenced with secondary PCR primers on an ABI PRISM™ 3730 DNA Analyzer (Applied Biosystems, USA), using a BigDye Terminator v3.1 Cycle Sequencing kit (Applied Biosystems, USA). Accuracy of the sequencing data was confirmed by sequencing in both directions and a new PCR product once more if necessary for some isolates. Nucleotide sequences obtained in the present study were aligned with each other and reference sequences downloaded from GenBank and analyzed using Clustal X 1.83.

RESULTS

Prevalence of *G. duodenalis*

678 fecal specimens were examined by microscopy after iodine staining. 34 of which were positive for G. duodenalis cysts. The average prevalence of G. duodenalis infection was 5.0% (34/678), with 5.6% (30/539) for the sheep versus 2.9% (4/139) for the goats. With the exception of Farm 5 where G. duodenalis infection was absent, the parasite was detected on the other five farms (Table 1).

Assemblage Distribution of *G. duodenalis*

PCR products were obtained from 32 of 34 G. duodenalis -positive specimens. However, only 29 were successfully sequenced at the tpi locus. The sequences obtained were aligned with reference sequences and identified as three G. duodenalis assemblages: 13.8% (4/29) for assemblage A, 6.9% (2/29) for assemblage B and 79.3% (23/29) for assemblage E.

Assemblage E was not only the most prevalent but also the most widespread in the investigated areas, accounting for assemblage E on four farms, assemblage A on two farms and assemblage B on only one farm (Table 1).

Genetic Diversity of Assemblages A, B and E

Sequence analysis of the tpi gene of G. duodenalis revealed the presence of two subtypes out of four assemblages A isolates. Three assemblage A isolates belonged to subtype AI (JQ928711), which had 100% similarity with the human-derived subtype AI sequences from Malaysia (HQ836660), France (FJ560569), the USA (EF688031 to EF688043), Peru (EF688038, EF688039), Australia (EF688031, EF688034), Israel (EF688040), Egypt (EF688036) and Henan of China (GU564274 to GU564276). It was also identical to subtype AI sequences from animals, including sheep in Australia (GQ444447), cattle (EF654693, AY655704) in the USA, and cats (AB569393) in Japan. The remaining one was a novel subtype of assemblage A (JQ928710), having four, four and five base differences compared to AI, AII and AIII, respectively (Table 2). The genetic variations led to our proposal of the designation of subtype AIV. The same sequences have been found in human-derived assemblage A isolates from Sweden (GQ329677, GQ329678) and Western Sahara (EU041756), and cat-derived assemblage A isolates (AB569394, AB569398) from Japan. In the present study, two sequences of assemblage B were identical to each other at the tpi locus (JQ928712) and had 100% homology with those from dairy cattle (JN162353), rabbits (HQ397719) and wastewater (HQ603781) in the investigated areas.

Table 2. Variations in the TPI nucleotide sequences among subtypes of G. duodenalis assemblage A in sheep and goats in Heilongjiang Province

Sequence	Nucleotide at position							Accession no. in GenBank
	Subtype	28	41	92	102	210	370	
Ref sequences	AI	T	G	T	T	A	C	GU564274
	AII	T	G	T	C	A	T	GU564277
	AIII	T	G	C	T	A	C	EF654695
This study	AI	T	G	T	T	A	C	JQ928711
	AIV	C	A	T	C	G	C	JQ928710

doi:10.1371/journal.pntd.0001826.t002

The intra-genotypic diversity of G. duodenalis assemblage E was observed in the present study. Seven representative sequences (JQ928713 to JQ928717, JQ951964, JQ951965) were obtained out of 23 tpi gene sequences. They were respectively named as subtypes E-I to E-VII for convenient description, with one to four base variations noted at nine different nucleotide sites (Table 3) using the AY655706 as a reference sequence. The same sequences have been described, with subtype E-I (n=9) having been found in cattle (AY655706, EF654682, AY228646, JN162347), and subtype E-II (n=2) in sheep (GQ444461). The remaining five subtypes (E-III to E-VII) were never identical to any reported assemblage E subtypes and all of them had a low frequency, accounting for 13.0% (3/23) for E-IV and EVII, and 8.7% (2/23) for EIII, E-V and E-VI.

Table 3. Variations in the TPI nucleotide sequences among subtypes of G. duodenalis of assemblage E in sheep and goats in Heilongjiang Province

Subtype (No.)	Nucleotide at position									Accession no. in GenBank
	45	78	82	108	262	303	430	441	469	
Ref sequence	T	T	A	C	T	T	A	G	G	AY655706
E-I(9)	T	T	A	C	T	T	A	G	G	JQ928713
E-II(2)	T	T	G	C	T	T	A	A	G	JQ928714
E-III(2)	C	G	A	T	T	T	G	G	G	JQ928715
E-IV(3)	C	T	G	C	T	T	A	G	G	JQ928716
E-V(2)	T	T	G	C	C	T	A	A	G	JQ928717
E-VI(2)	T	T	A	C	T	T	A	G	A	JQ951964
E-VII(3)	T	T	A	C	T	C	A	G	G	JQ951965

doi:10.1371/journal.pntd.0001826.t003

In the present study, even on some individual farms, we also observed the widespread occurrence of intra-genetic diversity of assemblage E at the tpi locus. At least two subtypes have been found on four farms for 23 isolates of assemblage E. For assemblage A, two subtypes representing four isolates have been found on Farm 2 and Farm 4, respectively (Table 4).

Table 4. G. duodenalis genotypes and subtypes identified in sheep and goats on farms in Heilongjiang Province

Farm	No. of Positive	Subtype (No.)		
		Assemblage A	Assemblage B	Assemblage E
Farm1	9			E-I(5), E-II(2), E-III(2)
Farm2	3	AIV(1)	B*(2)	
Farm3	4			E-I(2), E-VI(2)
Farm4	9	AI(3)		E-IV(3), E-VII(3)
Farm5	0			
Farm6	4			E-I(2), E-V(2)
Total	29	AI(3), AIV(1)	B*(2)	E-I(9), E-II(2), E-III(2), E-IV(3), E-V(2), E-VI(2),E-VII(3)

*There is no clear subtyping in assemblage B currently.
doi:10.1371/journal.pntd.0001826.t004

DISCUSSION

The present study is the first to report the occurrence and genetic characterization of G. duodenalis in sheep and goats in China. The average infection rate for sheep would be 5.6% versus 2.9% for the goats, which was lower than those reported worldwide except in Italy (1.5%) [13]. Infection rates of G. duodenalis were noticed to be inversely associated with the age of animals, with the highest infection rate (17.0%) in lambs and (10.5%) in goat kids. There were an apparent declining infection rates with the increasing age of the animals (Table 1). Young animals were more susceptible to opportunistic parasites than adults. Thus, in the limited epidemiological studies of giardiasis of sheep and goats, the majority focused on the occurrence of G. duodenalis in lambs and goat kids. In a longitudinal study of lambs in Norway, overall prevalence of G. duodenalis was 23.0% at the first sampling and 31.0% at the second sampling [19]. In Belgium, the prevalence was 25.5% in lambs and 35.8% in goat kids [14]. A 42.0% infection rate of G. duodenalis was reported in (one to three)-month-old lambs in Spain[20]. In fact, infection rates are complicated and are often related to many factors, including detection methods, health status and age of the animals, size and structure of specimens, management system, geographical and seasonal differences [14]. Due to the lack of related epidemiological data on giardiasis of animals in the investigated areas, we could not give the reasons for the low prevalence in addition to the low sensitivity of morphological methods and the relative small number of specimens examined from less than two-month-old lambs and goat kids compared to other age groups in the present study. Four out of five sheep farms and the one goat farm had G. duodenalis infected animals, and infection rates ranged from 2.9% to 8.1% (Table 1). Farm 5 was not contaminated by G. duodenalis. This might be related to strict sanitation management with the farm being built newly.

Currently, PCR-based molecular analysis techniques (DNA sequencing of PCR products and PCR-RFLP) have been developed and used to identify G. duodenalis-positive isolates [26]. Among the numerous target genes (such as the SSU rRNA, gdh, tpi, ef1α, bg, and variant surface protein [vsp] genes), tpi gene was frequently used to differentiate G. duodenalis at genotype and subtype levels because of the highest genetic heterogeneity at the locus [27]. In the present study, 29 partial tpi gene sequences were obtained, with 13.8% (4/29),6.9%(2/29) and 79.3% (23/29) for assemblages A, B and E, respectively. Assemblage E was detected on four farms, whereas assemblages A and B were detected on two farms and one farm, respectively (Table 1). Assemblage E was more prevalent and widespread than assemblages A and B in sheep and goats in the present study. Similar results were also commonly seen in sheep/goats, respectively in Belgium, Australia, Sweden, the USA, Norway, Spain and Mexico, where molecular epidemiological data have showed that assemblage E constituted the majority of G. duodenalis-positive specimens (percentages from 60.7% to 100%) [14]–[21], [28], [29]. Assemblage E seems to have apparent host preference. Molecular epidemiological data showed that assemblage E is the most common in cattle and pig in addition to sheep and goats[13]. The present results implied that sheep and goats in the investigated areas have been infected with assemblage E and posed a threat to other susceptible animals, including uninfected sheep and goats, cattle and pigs. Assemblage E might be less risky to humans based on the fact that it has only been isolated from three Egyptians [30]. It has been reported that G. duodenalis infections have an effect on growth and performance of animals, and most of relationship studies are only at the species level of G. duodenalis [31]. A recent study demonstrated that lambs infected with G. duodenalis could lead to decreased hot carcase weights and dressing percentage of sheep [32]. Up to date, no information is obtained on clinical symptoms of animal giardiasis resulting from assemblage E.

Sequence analysis of the tpi gene of G. duodenalis revealed the presence of seven subtypes out of 23 assemblage E isolates. The most common subtype E-I (39.1%; 9/23) showed 100% similarity with the cattle-derived assemblage E sequences in our investigated areas (JN162347) and the USA (AY655706, EF654682, AY228646). Subtype E-II (8.7%; 2/23) had the same nucleotide sequence as the isolate of G. duodenalis from an Australian sheep (GQ444447). Subtypes E-I and E-II appeared to have no differences in geographical distribution. The remaining five novel subtypes (E-III to E-VII) have never been reported before and might represent endemic genetic characterizations of assemblage E in the investigated areas. In addition to high polymorphism observed within assemblage E in sheep and goats at the tpilocus in the present and previous studies [29], intra-genotype variations of assemblage E were also described in the animals at the bg locus [14], [20], [29]. A high level of genetic diversity within assemblage E has also been reported in cattle based on the tpi gene [27], [33].

It is generally considered that assemblages A and B are infrequently detected in sheep and goats. However, there are exceptions appearing in a few studies of sheep and goat giardiasis, with assemblage A being found to be a common genotype besides assemblage E [14], [17],[18]. Even in an Australian study, assemblage A was found to be more prevalent than assemblage E in sheep [22]. More surprisingly, assemblage A isolates have been identified from Italian sheep with the absence of assemblages B and E [23]. For assemblage B, so far, there have only been four reports involved in sheep and goats, with three in sheep [3], [19], [21]and one in goats [34]. The low occurrence of assemblages A and B in sheep and goats as well as in cattle may be related to the predominance of assemblage E in these animals, for they have to compete with the more common assemblage E.

In the present study, four assemblage A isolates (13.8%; 4/29), representing two subtypes, were detected from the G. duodenalis-positive specimens. Three of them were identified as subtype AI, showing 100% homology with each other as well as the subtype AI tpi gene sequences from humans (Table 5) and some animals [22], [27], [35], [36]. The remaining one isolate was a novel subtype of assemblage A, which was designated as subtype AIV based on the base variations compared to subtypes AI, AII and AIII, respectively (Table 2). The same sequences have been obtained from humans in Sweden and Western Sahara (Table 5), and cats in Japan [36]. Currently, three subtypes AI, AII and AIII constitute the overwhelming majority of assemblage A isolates, and all of them appear to have different host preferences. Subtype AI is mostly found in animals and occasionally in humans; subtype AII commonly infects humans and was sometimes seen in animals; subtype AIII circulated in wildlife, but it has been seen in a few humans based on the bg gene [5]. Two tpi gene sequences of assemblage B isolates in the present study had 100% homology with each other and was identical to those obtained from dairy cattle, rabbits and wastewater in the investigated areas [33], [37], [38]. The same sequence has never been reported before in human and animal cases in other countries or areas. This may be of characteristic geographical distributions.

Table 5. Homology analyses of sheep/goat-derived isolates of assemblages A and B with human-derived isolates

Country	Ref	Host	No. of isolates characterized	Loci amplified	Assemblage (subtype)	Accession No.	Accession No. of human-derived isolates[b] (country)
Australia	[22]	Sheep	26	TPI	A (AI)	GQ444447	EF688042-43(USA), EF688041(Puerto Rico), EF688040(Israel), EF688036(Egypt), EF688038-39(Peru), EF688031,34(Australia), GU564274-76(China), HQ836660(Malaysia)
		Sheep	1	TPI	A	GQ444448	No
		Sheep	1	TPI	A	GQ444449	No
		Sheep	1	TPI	A	GQ444450	No
		Sheep	1	TPI	A	GQ444451	No
unspecified	unpublished	sheep	unspecified	GDH	A (AI)	JF958092	AB569385(Japan), EU594662(Cuba), EF685702(USA), GQ502960(Uganda), GQ168944(Australia), GQ329674(Sweden), HM748043(Thailand), JF917089(Iran), JF918516 and JF918453(India)
Belgium	[14]	Sheep	2	BG	A (AII)	EU642896	GU396696 and FJ009208(Poland), HM165227(Sweden)
	[14]	Goat	6	BG	A (AII)	EU642897	No
USA	[16]	Sheep	1	SSU rDNA	A	AY655700[a]	AY826204-05(Holland)
Italy	[23]	Sheep	5	GDH	A (AI)	M84604[a]	No
				BG	A (AI)	M36728[a]	No
Spain	[20]	Sheep	1	BG	A (AI)	EU726988	No
Norway	[19]	Sheep	1	BG	B	GQ337974	No
China	This study	Sheep	1	TPI	A (AIV)	JQ928710	EU041756(Western Sahara), GQ329677-78(Sweden)
			3	TPI	A (AI)	JQ928711	EF688031, 34(Australia), EF688036(Egypt), EF688038, 39 (Peru), EF688040(Israel), EF688041(Puerto Rico), EF688042-43(USA), J560569(France), GU564274-76(China), HQ836660(Malaysia)
			2	TPI	B	JQ928712	No

Note:
[a]Accession Nos indicating that sheep-derived isolates have 100% homology with the sequences of instead of their own.
[b]All the human-derived isolates having 100% homology with sheep/goat-derived isolates of assemblages A and B.
doi:10.1371/journal.pntd.0001826.t005

Although no human giardiasis cases were reported in the investigated areas, the molecular epidemiological data worldwide can help us to assess the possibility of zoonotic giardiasis caused by sheep and goats. To date, at least 52 sheep-/goat-derived isolates of assemblages A and B have been obtained based on tpi, gdh, bg and SSU rRNA genes. Among 14 representative sequences of assemblage A obtained from 49 isolates, six sequences show 100% homology with those derived from humans. Even in Australia and China, the same sequences of assemblage AI have been seen in both humans and sheep (Table 5). Thus, there might be the large possibility of cross-species transmission of assemblage AI between sheep and humans due to the similar genetic backgrounds of assemblage AI. However, what portion of human subtype AI infections attributable to zoonotic transmission is still unclear. The role that sheep and goats may play in the epidemiology of human giardiasis remains controversial. Some studies do not support sheep and goats as an important reservoir mainly based on the fact that G. duodenalis assemblage E is the predominant genotype in these animals in most countries and areas [15], [19], [29]. Up to date, few epidemiological studies have assessed the importance of zoonotic transmission of G. duodenalis. An assessment of zoonotic transmission had better come from the dynamics data of giardiasis between humans and animals in the same household or localized focus of endemicity.

In conclusion, the findings above provide the first report on sheep and goat giardiasis in China. Percentages and genetic characteristics of G. duodenalis assemblages in Heilongjiang Province seem to be different from other countries or areas and may represent the endemicity of G. duodenalis. The fact that the sequences of subtypes AI and AIV in the present study have also been described in human-derived G. duodenalis isolates implies the sheep infected with assemblage A posed a serious threat to local inhabitants and are of public health importance. The unique finding of the tpi gene sequence of assemblage B in different hosts (cattle, rabbits and sheep) and environmental specimen (wastewater) in the investigated areas may reflect characteristic geographical distribution. The transmission dynamic of assemblages A and B, and the burden of human giardiasis caused by animals need to be assessed by systematic molecular epidemiological investigations of humans and animals in the future.

AUTHOR CONTRIBUTIONS

Conceived and designed the experiments: AL LZ WZ. Performed the experiments: WZ Xiaoli Zhang AL. Analyzed the data: RW Xiaoyun Zhang WZ. Contributed reagents/materials/analysis tools: YS JC LZ HL FY. Wrote the paper: WZ AL.

REFERENCES

1. Prado MS, Cairncross S, Strina A, Barreto ML, Oliveira-Assis AM, et al. (2005) Asymptomatic giardiasis and growth in young children; a longitudinal study in Salvador, Brazil. Parasitology 131: 51–56. doi: 10.1017/s0031182005007353
2. Olson ME, O'Handley RM, Ralston BJ, McAllister TA, Thompson RC (2004) Update on Cryptosporidium and Giardia infections in cattle. Trends Parasitol 20: 185–191. doi: 10.1016/j.pt.2004.01.015
3. Aloisio F, Filippini G, Antenucci P, Lepri E, Pezzotti G, et al. (2006) Severe weight loss in lambs infected with Giardia duodenalis assemblage B. Vet Parasitol 142: 154–158. doi: 10.1016/j.vetpar.2006.06.023
4. View Article PubMed/NCBI Google Scholar
5. Thompson RC, Palmer CS, O'Handley R (2008) The public health and clinical significance of Giardia and Cryptosporidium in domestic animals. Vet J 177: 18–25. doi: 10.1016/j.tvjl.2007.09.022
6. Lasek-Nesselquist E, Welch DM, Sogin ML (2010) The identification of a new Giardia duodenalis assemblage in marine vertebrates and a preliminary analysis of G. duodenalis population biology in marine systems. Int J Parasitol 40: 1063–1074. doi: 10.1016/j.ijpara.2010.02.015
7. Xiao L, Fayer R (2008) Molecular characterisation of species and genotypes of Cryptosporidium and Giardia and assessment of zoonotic transmission. Int J Parasitol 38: 1239–1255. doi: 10.1016/j.ijpara.2008.03.006
8. Sprong H, Caccio SM, van der Giessen JW (2009) Identification of zoonotic genotypes of Giardia duodenalis. PLoS Negl Trop Dis 3: e558. doi: 10.1371/journal.pntd.0000558
9. Eisenberg JN, Brookhart MA, Rice G, Brown M, Colford JM Jr (2002) Disease transmission models for public health decision making: analysis of epidemic and endemic conditions caused by waterborne pathogens. Environ Health Perspect 110: 783–790. doi: 10.1289/ehp.02110783
10. Thompson RC (2000) Giardiasis as a re-emerging infectious disease and its zoonotic potential. Int J Parasitol 30: 1259–1267. doi: 10.1016/s0020-7519(00)00127-2
11. Karanis P, Kourenti C, Smith H (2007) Waterborne transmission of protozoan parasites: a worldwide review of outbreaks and lessons learnt. J Water Health 5: 1–38. doi: 10.2166/wh.2006.002
12. Hoque ME, Hope VT, Kjellstrom T, Scragg R, Lay-Yee R (2002) Risk of giardiasis in Aucklanders: a case-control study. Int J Infect Dis 6: 191–197. doi: 10.1016/s1201-9712(02)90110-4
13. Hoque ME, Hope VT, Scragg R, Kjellstrom T (2003) Children at risk of giardiasis in Auckland: a case-control analysis. Epidemiol Infect 131: 655–662. doi: 10.1017/s0950268803008598
14. Feng Y, Xiao L (2011) Zoonotic potential and molecular epidemiology of Giardia species and giardiasis. Clin Microbiol Rev 24: 110–140. doi: 10.1128/cmr.00033-10
15. Geurden T, Thomas P, Casaert S, Vercruysse J, Claerebout E (2008) Prevalence and molecular characterisation of Cryptosporidium and Giardia in lambs and goat kids in Belgium. Vet Parasitol 155: 142–145. doi: 10.1016/j.vetpar.2008.05.002
16. Ryan UM, Bath C, Robertson I, Read C, Elliot A, et al. (2005) Sheep may not be an important zoonotic reservoir for Cryptosporidium and Giardia parasites. Appl Environ Microbiol 71: 4992–4997. doi: 10.1128/aem.71.9.4992-4997.2005
17. Santín M, Trout JM, Fayer R (2007) Prevalence and molecular characterization of Cryptosporidium and Giardia species and genotypes in sheep in Maryland. Vet Parasitol 146: 17–24. doi: 10.1016/j.vetpar.2007.01.010
18. Yang R, Jacobson C, Gordon C, Ryan U (2009) Prevalence and molecular characterisation of Cryptosporidium and Giardia species in preweaned sheep in Australia. Vet Parasitol 161: 19–24. doi: 10.1016/j.vetpar.2008.12.021
19. Lebbad M, Mattsson JG, Christensson B, Ljungström B, Backhans A, et al. (2010) From mouse to moose: multilocus genotyping of Giardia isolates from various animal species. Vet Parasitol 168: 231–239. doi: 10.1016/j.vetpar.2009.11.003
20. Robertson LJ, Gjerde BK, Furuseth Hansen E (2010) The zoonotic potential of Giardia and Cryptosporidium in Norwegian sheep: a longitudinal investigation of 6 flocks of lambs. Vet Parasitol 171: 140–145. doi: 10.1016/j.vetpar.2010.03.014
21. Gómez-Muñoz MT, Navarro C, Garijo-Toledo MM, Dea-Ayuela MA, Fernández-Barredo S, et al. (2009) Occurrence and genotypes of Giardia isolated from

lambs in Spain. Parasitol Int 58: 297–299. doi: 10.1016/j.parint.2009.06.005

22. Castro-Hermida JA, Almeida AM, Gonzalez-Warleta JM, Correia da Costa C, Rumbo-Lorenzo, et al (2007) Occurrence of Cryptosporidium parvum and Giardia duodenalis in healthy adult domestic ruminants. Parasitol Res 101: 1443–1448. doi: 10.1007/s00436-007-0624-6
23. Nolan MJ, Jex AR, Pangasa A, Young ND, Campbell AJ, et al. (2010) Analysis of nucleotide variation within the triose-phosphate isomerase gene of Giardia duodenalis from sheep and its zoonotic implications. Electrophoresis 31: 287–298. doi: 10.1002/elps.200900480
24. Giangaspero A, Paoletti B, Iorio R, Traversa D (2005) Prevalence and molecular characterization of Giardia duodenalis from sheep in central Italy. Parasitol Res 96: 32–37. doi: 10.1007/s00436-005-1317-7
25. Robertson LJ (2009) Giardia and Cryptosporidium infections in sheep and goats: a review of the potential for transmission to humans via environmental contamination. Epidemiol Infect 137: 913–921. doi: 10.1017/s0950268809002295
26. Sulaiman IM, Fayer R, Bern C, Gilman RH, Trout JM, et al. (2003) Triosephosphate isomerase gene characterization and potential zoonotic transmission of Giardia duodenalis. Emerg Infect Dis 9: 1444–1452. doi: 10.3201/eid0911.030084
27. Wielinga CM, Thompson RC (2007) Comparative evaluation of Giardia duodenalis sequence data. Parasitology 134: 1795–821. doi: 10.1017/s0031182007003071
28. Feng Y, Ortega Y, Cama V, Terrel J, Xiao L (2008) High intragenotypic diversity of Giardia duodenalis in dairy cattle on three farms. Parasitol Res 103: 87–92. doi: 10.1007/s00436-008-0932-5
29. Di Giovanni GD, Betancourt WQ, Hernandez J, Assadian NW, Flores Margez JP, et al. (2006) Investigation of potential zooanthroponotic transmission of cryptosporidiosis and giardiasis through agricultural use of reclaimed wastewater. Int J Environ Health Res 16: 405–418. doi: 10.1080/09603120601095100
30. Ruiz A, Foronda P, González JF, Guedes A, Abreu-Acosta N, et al. (2008) Occurrence and genotype characterization of Giardia duodenalis in goat kids from the Canary Islands, Spain. Vet Parasitol 154: 137–141. doi: 10.1016/j.vetpar.2008.03.003
31. Foronda P, Bargues MD, Abreu-Acosta N, Periago MV, Valero MA, et al. (2008) Identification of genotypes of Giardia intestinalis of human isolates in Egypt. Parasitol Res 103: 1171–1181. doi: 10.1007/s00436-008-1113-2
32. O'Handley RM, Olson ME (2006) Giardiasis and cryptosporidiosis in ruminants. Vet Clin North Am Food Anim Pract 22: 623–643. doi: 10.1016/j.cvfa.2006.07.002
33. Sweeny JP, Ryan UM, Robertson ID, Jacobson C (2011) Cryptosporidium and Giardia associated with reduced lamb carcase productivity. Vet Parasitol 182: 127–139. doi: 10.1016/j.vetpar.2011.05.050
34. Liu A, Zhang X, Zhang L, Wang R, Li X, et al. (2012) Occurrence of bovine giardiasis and endemic genetic characterization of Giardia duodenalis isolates in Heilongjiang Province, in the Northeast of China. 11: 655–61. doi: 10.1007/s00436-012-2883-0
35. Berrilli F, D'Alfonso R, Giangaspero A, Marangi M, Brandonisio O, et al. (2012) Giardia duodenalis genotypes and Cryptosporidium species in humans and domestic animals in Côte d'Ivoire: occurrence and evidence for environmental contamination. Trans R Soc Trop Med Hyg 106: 191–195. doi: 10.1016/j.trstmh.2011.12.005
36. Trout JM, Santín M, Greiner E, Fayer R (2004) Prevalence of Giardia duodenalis genotypes in pre-weaned dairy calves. Vet Parasitol 124: 179–186. doi: 10.1016/j.vetpar.2004.07.010
37. Suzuki J, Murata R, Kobayashi S, Sadamasu K, Kai A, et al. (2011) Risk of human infection with Giardia duodenalis from cats in Japan and genotyping of the isolates to assess the route of infection in cats. Parasitology 138: 493–500. doi: 10.1017/s0031182010001459
38. Zhang W, Shen Y, Wang R, Liu A, Ling H, et al. (2012) Cryptosporidium cuniculus and Giardia duodenalis in Rabbits: Genetic Diversity and Possible Zoonotic Transmission. PLoS One 7: e31262. doi: 10.1371/journal.pone.0031262
39. Liu A, Ji H, Wang E, Liu J, Xiao L, et al. (2011) Molecular identification and distribution of Cryptosporidium and Giardia duodenalis in raw urban wastewater in Harbin, China. Parasitol Res 109: 913–918. doi: 10.1007/s00436-011-2333-4

CHAPTER 11

WORM CONTROL PRACTICE AGAINST GASTRO-INTESTINAL PARASITES IN NORWEGIAN SHEEP AND GOAT FLOCKS

Atle VM Domke, Christophe Chartier, Bjørn Gjerde, Nils Leine, Synnøve Vatn, Olav Østerås and Snorre Stuen

BACKGROUND

Nematode parasitic disease remains one of the greatest limiting factors in successful, sustainable ruminant livestock production worldwide. Currently, the control of nematode infections still relies mainly on the use of effective anthelmintics, which often represent the simpler, safer and cheaper option [1]. However, anthelmintic-resistant (AR) nematodes are now recognized as an important threat to the productivity and welfare of sheep in many parts of the world, including Europe [2]. The profitability and sustainability of the goat industry are also seriously threatened by rapid development of AR [3].

Twenty years ago, AR was a devastating problem only of the Southern Hemisphere, but now it has been recognized as a global concern. In some countries of Northern Europe, resistance to benzimidazoles has been found in up to 80% of the goat flocks, even in a context of a rather limited drenching frequency [4], and resistance to two, or even all three, major classes of anthelmintics has been recorded for goats in France and for sheep in Scotland [5, 6, 7]. However, the situation may be different in some other European countries such as Sweden, Germany and Slovakia, where AR have been detected years ago at a rather low frequency [8, 9,10]. Different situations may also be encountered regarding the nematode species involved and the intensity of infection. Severe clinical reports of AR in small ruminants with very high worm burdens have been made with *Haemonchus contortus*, especially in tropical areas, whereas subclinical cases were more frequently described with the common abomasal (*Teladorsagia circumcincta*) and intestinal (*Trichostrongylus colubriformis*) worms under temperate areas. However, although less severe than under the tropics, drug resistance issue is in the UK considered a threat to the economical sustainability of sheep production [11].

In Norway, only benzimidazoles and macrocyclic lactones are licenced for use in sheep and goats. The release of the amino-acetonitrile derivative (AAD) drug, monepantel, in 2010 represents the first new anthelmintic class since the launch of ivermectin in the early 1980s for use in sheep, but this drug is not yet licenced in Norway.

The AR situation in Norway is, however, not well documented. Only sporadic cases of AR in small ruminant flocks have so far been reported in Norway [12].

The main factors for selection for anthelmintic resistance are:

- the application of anthelmintics in a situation where parasites have a small refugia [13, 14],
- a high treatment frequency [15],
- under-dosing [16, 17], and
- the use of the same anthelmintic class over several years [17].

Citation: Domke et al.: Worm control practice against gastro-intestinal parasites in Norwegian sheep and goat flocks. Acta Veterinaria Scandinavica 2011 53:29. doi:10.1186/1751-0147-53-29.

These factors, alone or in combination, together with certain types of farm management can accelerate the development of AR [1, 18, 19].

Norway has a great variability in climatic and geographical conditions, which influences the farm management. The inland and northern areas have an alpine climate in contrast to the subalpine climate in the coastal lowland area [20]. There is approximately one million winter fed sheep in Norway, with an average flock size of 66 animals [21]. Ewes and lambs are normally put on fenced spring pastures one or more weeks after lambing. After a few weeks, the ewes and lambs are moved to common rangeland pastures in the mountains or forests. The densities of sheep on mountain pastures in Norway vary between 10 and 80 animals per km^2 [22]. It is estimated that more than 2/3 of all sheep are moved to grazing on mountain or forest pastures from June-July until August-September [23]. In contrast, dairy goats, which in Norway represent a total number of approximately 40 000 animals older than one year, with an average flock size of 83 animals, are normally on pastures close to the farm during the whole grazing period [21]. However, in some areas of Norway the use of mountain dairy farming during summer is still practiced [24]. In addition, there are approximately 4000 fiber (non-dairy) goats in Norway with an average flock size of 6.5 animals.

Surveys based on questionnaires regarding worm control practices in small ruminants in Europe have previously been done in Denmark [25, 26], the United Kingdom [27, 28, 29, 30], France [31] and the Slovak Republic[32]. In Norway, a similar survey has not been performed. The aim of the present study was therefore to improve our knowledge about the worm control practices in small ruminant flocks in Norway. The objective was to focus more specifically on the anthelmintic usage and to examine to what extent the risk practices for developing AR were encountered in these flocks.

METHODS

Questionnaire

In the autumn of 2007, a questionnaire was sent to Norwegian sheep and goat farmers in order to collect information concerning which gastrointestinal parasite control measures had been used during 2005-2007, such as pastures management, deworming practices and the use of anthelmintics. The flocks were selected from the Norwegian governmental list of farms that apply for production subsidies [21]. Before this, two small pilot studies with a limited number of farmers involved were performed in order to avoid misunderstandings and misinterpretations of the final questionnaire. The questionnaire was comprised in two sections. The first section was related to main characteristics of the farm management such as flock size, breed, grazing conditions and housing time. The second section was dedicated to the use of pastures and the anthelmintic parasite control practice. Questions regarding clinical signs linked to parasitism, time and reason for anthelmintic treatment, anthelmintic products used in the years 2005 to 2007, dose determination, mode of application and the source of information regarding worm control, were included.

Selection Procedures

Flocks were selected from the three main areas of small ruminant farming; i.e., Rogaland, Hordaland, Sogn og Fjordane and Møre og Romsdal counties in western Norway (the coastal area), Hedmark, Oppland and Telemark counties in south-eastern Norway (the inland area), and Nordland and Troms counties in northern Norway (the northern area) (Figure 1). These three areas also represent the main types of grazing and farm management in Norway. In each area, flocks from a minimum of three municipalities were selected.

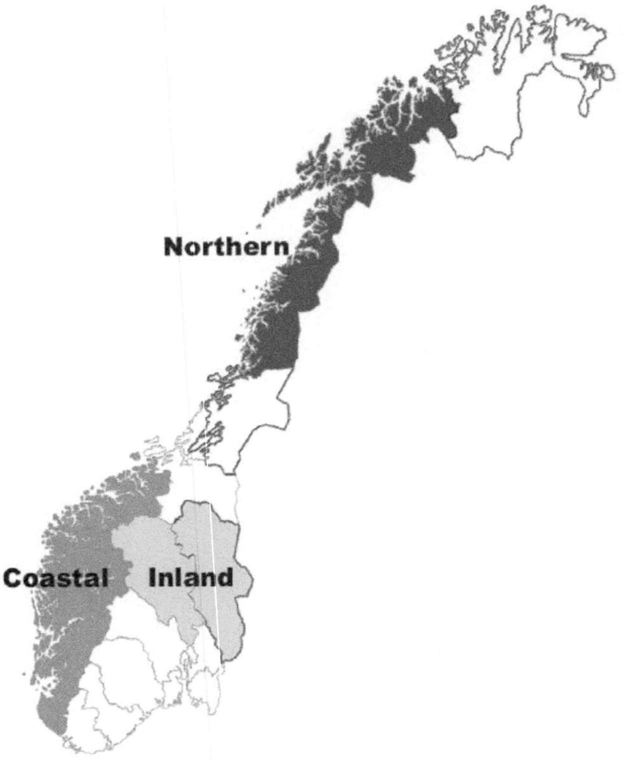

Figure 1: Map of Norway showing the three geographical areas represented in the survey.

Only sheep farms with a flock size larger than 20 winterfed ewes were included, i.e., 9.8% of the total number of flocks with more than 20 ewes in Norway [21]. A total of 1145 sheep flocks were randomly selected, including 522 flocks with a flock size of 20-100 ewes (selection rate of 5%) and 623 flocks with more than 100 ewes (selection rate of 50%). In addition, dairy goat farms with more than 24 goats and fiber goat (non-dairy) flocks with more than 6 goats were included. In total, 379 farms with dairy goats and 73 farms with fiber goats were selected, representing 100% of all goat farms fulfilling the inclusion criteria. The questionnaire was not anonymous. Farmers that did not respond to the questionnaire within one month, were reminded once.

Statistical Analysis

SPSS (SPSS Inc. Chicago, Version 16.0) and Excel 2003 (Microsoft Inc.) were used for statistical calculations. The Kruskal-Wallis ANOVA was used for calculating the significant differences regarding number of anthelmintic treatments in different areas of Norway. Chi-square analyses were used for group differences using SAS (SAS Institute Inc., Cary, NC).

RESULTS

A total of 825 questionnaires (51.6%) were returned, representing 587 sheep flocks (51.3% of those selected) and 238 goat flocks (52.6%). These flocks represented 74472 winter fed sheep, 20466 dairy goats and 262 fiber goats. All sheep flocks were considered together, independent of flock size. Fiber goats were represented in 14 (5.9%) of the goat flocks and were grouped together with the dairy goats in the calculations. Seventy (8.5%) of the flocks had both sheep and goats, but each of these was treated as either a sheep or a goat flock in the survey.

Sheep Flocks

General Information

The three main sheep breeds represented in the sampled farms were: the Norwegian White Sheep ("Norsk Kvit Sau") with 76.2% of all sheep flocks, the Old Norwegian Short Tail ("Spelsau") with 11.4% of the flocks, and the Norwegian Feral Sheep ("Villsau") with 4.2% of the flocks (data not shown). This distribution reflects the Norwegian sheep population well [21]. Lambs together with their ewes were turned out on pasture in April/May in the coastal area and in May/June in the northern and inland area. Average lamb age at turnout was 2-3 weeks (Table 1). Lambs had a grazing period lasting 6-8 months in the coastal area and 6-7 months in the inland and northern areas. During the summer period, 68.5% of the sheep flocks used a mountain or forest pasture. In 68.6% of the sheep flocks, grazing together with cattle both at home pasture and on the mountain/forest pasture were practiced, while less than 4% of the sheep flocks co-grazed with goats only. The local veterinarian (56.0%), agriculture magazines (22.2%) and other farmers (18.9%) were the three most important sources of information regarding worm control practice (data not shown).

Table 1: General management characteristics of Norwegian sheep and goat flocks in present survey

	Sheep	Goats
Number of flocks (%)	587 (100)	238 (100)
Mean flock size (± SD) (range)	126.3 ± 74.4 (20-500)	95.0 ± 45.1 (12-300)
Number of farms with organic farming (%)	29 (5.2%)	18 (7.6%)
Mean turn out time on pasture	Early May	Mid-May
Mean range of age in lambs/kids at turn out (weeks)	2 - 3	>12
Mean housing time	Late September	Mid-September
Practicing dose-and-move (percentage)	212 (35.8)	5 (2.1)

Drenching Time

In 57.4% of the flocks the timing and frequency of the anthelmintic treatments against gastro-intestinal parasites were based only on previously established routines and experience, together with regularity and when housing the animals (Table 2). The dose and move strategy was practiced in 33.2% of the sheep flocks.

Table 2: Main determination of time and routines for anthelmintics drenching in Norwegian sheep and goat flocks (frequency and percentage)

			Sheep		Goats	
			n	%	n	%
Determination of treatment time	Sheep flocks (*n* = 587)	Pasture rotation	195	33.2		
		Only at housing	51	8.7		
		Faecal egg count	0	0.0		
		Clinical signs/scouring	4	0.7		
		Combination[a]	337	57.4		
	Goat flocks (*n* = 235)	Non lactating period			199	84.7

		Pasturing			21	8.9
		Faecal egg count			1	0.4
		No treatment			14	6.0
Calculation or estimation of weight		Individual weight	12	2.1	1	0.8
		Weighing (heaviest animal)	35	6.2	2	1.7
		Weighting (mean sized animal)	69	12.2	5	4.1
		Visual appraisal	444	78.6	103	85.1
		No estimation[b]	5	0.9	10	8.3
		Total	565		121	
Control of drenching gun		1 per flock treatment	225	41.4	94	51.9
		2 per flock treatment	90	16.6	11	6.1
		>2 per flock treatment	81	14.9	7	3.9
		Never	147	27.1	69	38.1
		Total	543		181	

[a] Combination: Treatment time based on previously established routines and experience, together with regularity and housing.

[b]done by veterinarian.

Dose-Estimation

In 78.6% of the sheep flocks the anthelmintic dose was determined by visual appraisal of the weight of the heaviest lamb or ewe before the start of the drenching operation. In 27.1% of the sheep flocks, the farmers never checked the accuracy of their drench guns when giving their animals an anthelmintic treatment.

Drenching Frequency

The mean yearly drenching rate in lambs and ewes were 2.5 ± 1.7 and 1.9 ± 1.1, respectively (Table 3). The mean drenching rate of lambs in the coastal, inland and northern area was 3.4, 2.0 and 1.3 times per year, respectively. For ewes the drenching rates in the same areas were 2.2, 1.6 and 1.5 times per year, respectively. In 8.7% of the sheep flocks, the treatment against gastro-intestinal parasites was given only at housing in the autumn (Table 2). In contrast, in ten flocks (1.7%) the number of annual treatments for lambs was ≥7. Nine of these ten flocks were located in Rogaland County. In the coastal area, lambs were treated more than three times per year in 45.9% of the flocks (Table 3). This was a significantly higher number of treatments compared to the two other areas ($p < 0.001$).

Table 3: Distribution of flocks according to the annual number of treatments against gastro-intestinal parasites in lambs and ewes in the different areas (percentage) of Norway

Number of treatments		n	Coastal	Inland	Northern	Total
Lambs	1	144	13.9[a]	33.0	47.6	26.5
	2	174	19.5[a]	44.3	47.6	32.0
	3	87	20.7[a]	14.7	3.6	16.0
	>3	139	45.9[a]	8.0	1.2	25.5
	Mean[b]		3.4	2.0	1.3	2.5
Ewes	1	202	24.3	38.9	51.0	36.4
	2	246	44.7	52.2	43.8	44.3
	3	72	20.4[a]	6.7	5.2	13.0
	>3	35	10.6[a]	2.2	0.0	6.3
	Mean		2.2[a]	1.6	1.5	1.9

The mean number is also calculated for each area.

[a] superscripts indicate $p < 0.001$ (Kruskal-Wallis) between this area compared with the other areas in the same line.

[b] superscripts indicate $p < 0.001$ (Kruskal-Wallis) between all three areas.

Similarly, for ewes, the proportion of flocks with more than three treatments per year in the coastal, inland and northern area was 10.6%, 2.2% and 0.0%, respectively. The use of benzimidazoles in sheep flocks decreased significantly ($p < 0.001$) from 73.5% of the flocks in 2005 to 64.9% in 2007. During the same period, there was a significant increase ($p < 0.001$) in the use of macrocyclic lactones in the sheep flocks from 14.3% of the flocks to 23.4% (Table 4). Five sheep flocks used no anthelmintic treatment at all during the period 2005-2007.

Table 4: Type of anthelmintics used during 2005 - 2007 in sheep and goat flocks in Norway (percentage)

Type of anthelmintics	Sheep			Goat		
	2005	2006	2007	2005	2006	2007
	n = 551	*n* = 561	*n* = 587	*n* = 205	*n* = 203	*n* = 189
Benzimidazoles (BZ)	73.5[a]	66.3[a]	64.9[a]	51.3[a]	46.6[a]	42.3
Macrocyclic lactones (ML)	14.3[b]	21.1[b]	23.4[b]	32.9[b]	36.0[b]	39.1
Tetrahydropyrimidines (THP)**	4.4	2.1	0.9	-	-	-
BZ + ML	6.7	9.4	9.7	7.9	8.1	8.3
No treatment	1.1	1.1	1.1	7.9	9.3	10.3
Total	100	100	100	100	100	100

[a, b] different superscripts in the same column indicate a significant difference ($p < 0.001$, Kruskal-Wallis) between BZ and ML within the years.

**In the anthelmintic class Tetrahydropyrimidines only the label «Exhelm®, Pfizer, (Morantel)» was used. This class has not been registered in Norway after 2006.

Drug Alternation

The proportion of farms using both benzimidazoles and macrocyclic lactones the same year was significantly higher ($p < 0.001$) in the coastal area compared to the inland and northern area (Table 5). The two anthelmintics were used alternately and not at the same time. More flocks choose macrocyclic lactones in the inland and northern area than in the coastal area. The use increased from 15.5% and 16.0% of the flocks in the inland and northern area, respectively, in 2005 to 29.4% and 28.0% of the flocks in 2007. In the period 2005 - 2007, 46.3% of the sheep flocks never changed the anthelmintic class, whereas 16.8% of the flocks changed the anthelmintic class two times or more.

Table 5: Type of anthelmintics used in the different areas during 2005 - 2007 in sheep flocks (percentage) in Norway (see also Table 4)

Area	Year	BZ	ML	THP	BZ/ML	No treatment
Coastal	2005	71.9	13.6	2.2	11.4[a]	0.9
	2006	65.9	15.1	2.2	16.4[a]	0.4
	2007	65.2	18.5	0.0	15.9[a]	0.4
Inland	2005	73.8	15.5	7.1	2.4 [b]	1.2
	2006	62.9	24.7	5.6	5.6 [b]	1.1
	2007	62.4	29.4	1.2	9.3 [b]	1.2
Northern	2005	74.5	16.0	6.4	3.2 [b]	0.0
	2006	66.0	30.9	1.1	2.1 [b]	0.0
	2007	71.0	28.0	0.0	1.1 [b]	0.0

[a,b] $p < 0.001$(Chi-Square) between coastal area compared with inland and northern area regarding use of both BZ and MLs for a given year.

Goat Flocks

General Information

In the dairy herds, the Norwegian dairy goat was the only breed present. Kashmir and Angora were the two most common fiber goat breeds. The time of turnout was mainly in Mid-May (90.3% of the flocks), with an average grazing period of five to six months (Table 1). The main kidding period was from December to March, and 89.4% of the kids were two months or older at turn out. Co-grazing with cattle or sheep was practiced by 74.6% of the flocks (data not shown).

Drenching Time and Frequency

On 84.7% of the dairy goat farms, the anthelmintic was administered during the dry period (Table 2). The yearly mean drenching rate in both kids and adult goats was one time per year. However, in 2007 10.3% of the goat flocks did not receive any anthelmintic treatment at all.

Dose-Estimation

To determine the anthelmintic dose, 85.1% of the goat farms used visual appraisal of weight for a common weight estimation for the entire flock. In 8.3% of the goat flocks, the anthelmintics were administered by a veterinarian using a subcutaneous injection of macrocyclic lactones. However, there was no information regarding what kind of weight estimation that had been used in these flocks. In 38.1% of the goat flocks, the farmers never checked the accuracy of their drench gun.

Drug Alternation

Benzimidazoles were the most common anthelmintic class used in goats (Table 4). The proportion of flocks using macrocyclic lactones increased from 32.9% in 2005, to 39.1% in 2007. In the same time period, the number of goat flocks using no anthelmintic treatment increased from 7.9% to 10.3% (Table 4). There were no differences between the three areas regarding the use of different anthelmintic classes or combinations in the goat flocks.

DISCUSSION

In the present study, the response rate was above 50%. The response rate for sheep flocks were 42.7% in flocks with 20-100 ewes, and 58.7% in flocks with more than 100 ewes. Compared to the total number of sheep flocks in Norway, flocks with less than 100 winter fed ewes were underrepresented. Similar surveys have been based on a lower response rate, ranging from 15% to 24% [16, 25, 28].

Drenching Time

The maintenance of a pool of susceptible parasites not exposed to the drug as free-living stages in the environment or as adults in un-drenched animals, i.e., worms in *refugia*, seems to play an important role in the prevention of anthelmintic resistance in ruminants [13]. The apparent usefulness of maintaining worms in*refugia* influence the different ways of controlling the gastrointestinal nematode population in grazing livestock. In the sheep and goat flocks in this survey, the decision to use anthelmintics was not evidence-based using clinical indicators such as scouring or weight loss or coproscopical examinations, and thus no targeted selective treatment was performed. Actually, in 57.4% of the sheep flocks, the main triggering factors for treating was weather and climatic observations during the grazing season, pasture management and the experience from earlier years, and the whole group of animals (young or adults) was treated. In general, the anthelmintic treatment seemed to have been based mainly on established routines that in previous years had given an apparently economical and sustainable livestock production.

In the present study, 35.8% of the sheep farmers combined the anthelmintic treatment with a change of pasture, i.e., a dose-and-move strategy. Such practices were especially used for ewes and lambs before transporting them to the common grazing areas in the forest or mountains during the summer months. The dose-and-move strategy in small ruminant flocks has also been noticed as a common practice in other European countries [25, 31, 32, 33]. However, moving drenched sheep onto pastures with a low level of parasite contamination increases the risk for AR [34, 35]. The role of the mountain and forest pastures as potential *refugia* for the gastrointestinal nematodes is thus a key question. Indeed, the cold and long winter period, which probably allows a limited survival of overwintering infective larvae, in combination with anthelmintic treatment prior to moving the animals, might represent a significant selective pressure on the worm population [36, 37]. Only *Teladorsagia circumcincta* and *Nematodirus battus* among the most pathogenic nematodes are regarded as being capable of overwintering on pasture in Norway [38]. However, the low animal density decreases the probability of finding a new host for the nematodes on mountain pasture. The duration from September until June next year, when the animals are re-entering these pastures contribute to decrease the worm burden [39]. On the other hand, some nematode populations, such as *Haemonchus contortus*, are unable to survive as overwintering larvae under Nordic conditions and refugia as free-living stages from year to year may be considered as virtual [40]. This epidemiological trait of *H. contortus* has led to consider a possible eradication of this worm from farms by treating all the animals when housing with an anthelmintic drug achieving a high efficacy against inhibited larvae [40]. In our work, anthelmintic treatment was given to ewes either at housing or during the housing period in 66% of the sheep flocks. As far as *H. contortus* is concerned, this practice represents a real threat for AR to emerge.

Under-Dosing

A poor drenching practice can result in under-dosing of a drug and select for AR [41, 42]. Not only incorrect estimation of animal live-weight, but also incorrect calibration of drench guns can cause under-dosing. To ensure a correct dose, one has to estimate the weight as accurately as possible [2], preferably by an individual weighing of each animal. Weighing the heaviest animal before drenching all animals with a slightly over-calculated dose can also be considered as an appropriate way to ensure correct anthelmintic dose.

In 78.6% of the sheep flocks, visual appraisal of weight based on knowledge and experience was used for calculating the anthelmintic dose. In the goat flocks, 85.1% used visual appraisal for weight estimation. Similar results were found in Slovakia and France, where visual weight estimation was used in 87.8% and 100.0% of the small ruminant flocks, respectively [31, 32]. If weighing each animal or only the heaviest animals, were considered as the only acceptable method for calculating the dose, only 8.3% of the sheep flocks and 2.5% of the goat flocks in our survey had an appropriate dose calculation.

The present study showed that 90% of the anthelmintics used in sheep and goat farming in Norway were administrated orally. It is known that the efficacy of oral drenches, in particular benzimidazoles, depends partly on the extent of oesophageal groove closure, and that this partial or complete rumen bypass is a very frequent phenomenon at least in goats [43]. The issue regarding the use of specific anthelmintic dose rates for goats was not investigated in this survey. However, earlier studies have shown that goats metabolize anthelmintics faster than sheep, in particular as regards the benzimidazoles, and this has led to an advice of using higher anthelmintic dose rates for goat compared to sheep [44]. In Norway, only fenbendazole (Panacur vet., Intervet) has been licenced for goats, and then at the same dose rate as for sheep (5 mg/kg). This dose is clearly inappropriate for goats [45]. As a result, in some countries such as France, specific recommendations have been added in 2008 in the "Summary of Product Characteristics" of several benzimidazole compounds (Chartier, personal communication). In Norway, the use of the sheep dose for goats seems most common (Leine, personal communication). Eprinomectin (Eprinex vet, Merial) has been used by goat farmers the last years although this product has been licenced only for cattle in Norway.

In addition, the drench gun was never controlled in 27.1% of the sheep flocks and in 38.1% of the goat flocks. An inaccurate drench gun may also contribute to under-dosing of the anthelmintics [46].

Frequency

A high treatment frequency is considered as a major risk factor for the development of anthelmintic resistance [47, 48, 49]. The mean drenching rates in lambs and ewes in Norway was 2.5 and 1.9 times per year, respectively. These figures are of a similar magnitude to those reported elsewhere in northern Europe. Thus, in Denmark, Maingi et al. reported a mean drenching rate in lambs and ewes of 1.9 and 2.3 per year, respectively [25]. In Scotland and England, the mean drenching rate ranged from 2.2 to 4.4 annual treatments per lamb, respectively [28, 50]. However, in the present work, the drenching frequency in lambs and ewes was significantly higher in the coastal area (3.4 and 2.2, respectively) than in the inland and northern area.

It is unknown if the high drenching frequency in the coastal area could be a sign of a higher parasite challenge or of anthelmintic resistance. High treatment frequency may be due to the longer grazing season and a more favourable environment for larval development and survival in the coastal area. Recent reports from the UK indicates that *H. contortus* and *T. circumcincta* are able to establish further north than earlier reported [51]. In Norway, the coastal areas have a similar climate as found in Scotland and England and represent a more favourable location for nematode infections compared to northern areas. There is also a prolonged grazing period near the farm on cultivated pastures in the coastal area compared to the inland and northern area [52]. Normally, the animal stocking rate on the cultivated pastures in the coastal area is high in the spring compared with the inland and northern area [53]. However, since the treatment frequency is not based on clinical signs or laboratory examinations, the necessity of frequent drenching has to be elucidated.

Drug Alternation

In 83.2% of the total number of sheep and goat flocks, no changes of anthelmintic class were done in the investigated period. Benzimidazoles (BZ) were the major anthelmintic class used in sheep and goat flocks (Table 4). However, there was a slight increase in the use of macrocyclic lactones (ML) in all areas. In general, the change to MLs use was more dominant in sheep flocks in the inland and northern areas. The recent emphasis on drug alternation from Norwegian animal health organizations can have resulted in an increased use of MLs. Other reasons for the increased use of MLs can be their persistent activity and their better efficacy on inhibited larval stages of gastrointestinal nematodes. MLs also have an effect on ectoparasites and the conveniences of using pour-on products, e.g. eprinomectin. This probably explains the common use of MLs in goat flocks compared to sheep flocks. A reduced drug efficacy could also lead to a change of anthelmintic drug class. So far, only sporadic cases of AR in small ruminant flocks have been reported in Norway [12]. Thus none of the farmers in the survey have reported reduced anthelmintic effect.

Norway Compared with other European Countries

The worm control management and use of anthelmintics in Norway do not fundamentally differ from general practices in Denmark, France, Slovakia and the UK [25, 28, 29, 31, 32]. To some extent, inaccurate dose calculations and a dose-and-move strategy seem to occur in all these countries. However, as a result of having only two anthelmintic classes on the marked in Norway, drench alternation is not a common practice. Regarding the drenching frequency, our results in lambs are similar to what have been reported from UK. [28]. In contrast, the common use of mountain and forest pasture during the summer months combined with a low stocking rate is probably the main peculiarity of Norwegian sheep farming.

CONCLUSIONS

The present study has shown that the anthelmintic drenching routines used in small ruminants in Norway may contribute to the development of AR. Over 90% of the sheep and goat flocks had insufficient weight estimation for calculating correct anthelmintic dose. This combined with few farmers controlling their drench gun represents a high risk for under-dosing anthelmintics in these flocks. A high risk was also suggested by a high treatment frequency, especially in lambs in the coastal area, a lack of anthelmintic class rotation and a common use of a dose-and-move practice. The early detection of AR may be quite difficult [50, 54]. In order to avoid or slow down the emergence of AR, correct use of anthelmintics, on-farm information of gastrointestinal parasite burdens and knowledge regarding how to maintain parasites in *refugia* have to be implemented in the worm control management. This includes focus on dose rate, anthelmintic class alternation, treatment frequency, stocking rate and new treatment strategies, such as targeted (selective) treatment in combination with faecal egg counts. Giving the farmers the right information regarding worm control is a key stone in preventing anthelmintic resistance. Since the distribution of anthelmintic resistant nematodes in Norway is unknown a national surveillance program for AR detection should be established.

ACKNOWLEDGEMENTS AND FUNDING

Thanks to all the farmers who responded to the questionnaire. Thanks to Katrine Sægrov at the Norwegian School of Veterinary Science (Høyland Field Station) for her assistance with the questionnaire. We also thank the Norwegian Goat Health Service, Animalia by the Norwegian Sheep Health Service, the Norwegian School of Veterinary Science and the Norwegian Research Council for financial support.

AUTHORS' CONTRIBUTIONS

AVMD, CC, BG, NL, SV, OØ and SS initiated and designed the study. AVMD performed the questionnaire and recorded the data. AVMD and OØ performed the statistical analysis. AVMD and SS drafted the manuscript. All authors read and approved the manuscript.

REFERENCES

1. Jackson: Worm control in sheep in the future. Small Rum Res. 2009, 86: 40-45. 10.1016/j.smallrumres.2009.09.015.
2. Waller PJ: Anthelmintic resistance. Vet Parasitol. 1997, 72: 391-412. 10.1016/S0304-4017(97)00107-6.
3. Watson TG, Hosking BC: Evidence for multiple anthelmintic resistance in two nematode parasite genera on a Saanen goat dairy. N Z Vet J. 1990, 38: 50-10.1080/00480169.1990.35615.
4. Chartier C, Soubirac F, Pors I, Silvestre A, Hubert J, Couquet C, Cabaret J: Prevalence of anthelmintic resistance in gastrointestinal nematodes of dairy goats under extensive management conditions in southwestern France. J Helminthol. 2001, 75: 325-330.
5. Sargison N, Scott P, Jackson F: Multiple anthelmintic resistance in sheep. Vet Rec. 2001, 149: 778-779.
6. Bartley D, Jackson F, Coop RL, Jackson E, Johnston K, Mitchell GB: Anthelmintic-resistant nematodes in sheep in Scotland. Vet Rec. 2001, 149: 94-95.
7. Paraud C, Kulo A, Pors I, Chartier C: Resistance of goat nematodes to multiple anthelmintics on a farm in France. Vet Rec. 2009, 164: 563-564. 10.1136/vr.164.18.563.
8. Várady M, Corba J, Cernanská : A survey on anthelmintic resistance in nematode parasites of sheep in the Slovak Republic. Vet Parasitol. 2006, 135: 39-45. 10.1016/j.vetpar.2005.09.001.
9. Scheuerle MC, Mahling M, Pfister K: Anthelminthic resistance of Haemonchus contortus in small ruminants in Switzerland and Southern Germany. Wien Klin Wochenschr. 2009, 121: 46-49. 10.1007/s00508-009-1235-2.
10. Höglund J, Gustafsson K, Ljungström BL, Engström A, Donnan A, Skuce P: Anthelmintic resistance in Swedish sheep flocks based on a comparison of the results from the faecal egg count reduction test and resistant allele frequencies of the beta-tubulin gene. Vet Parasitol. 2009, 161: 60-68. 10.1016/j.vetpar.2008.12.001.
11. Sargison ND: Pharmaceutical control of endoparasitic helminth infections in sheep. Vet. Clin. North Am Food Anim Pract. 2011, 27: 139-156. 10.1016/j.cvfa.2010.10.014.
12. Vatn S, Myklebust O, Stuen S: Resistente parasitter hos sau? Resultat fra et lite prosjekt i Rogaland. Prakisnytt. 2005, 3: 12-14.
13. van Wyk JA: Refugia--overlooked as perhaps the most potent factor concerning the development of anthelmintic resistance. Onderstepoort J Vet Res. 2001, 68: 55-67.
14. Martin PJ, Le Jambre LF, Claxton JH: The impact of refugia on the development of thiabendazole resistance in Haemonchus contortus. Int J Parasitol. 1981, 11: 35-41. 10.1016/0020-7519(81)90023-0.
15. Chartier C, Pors I, Hubert J, Rocheteau D, Benoit C, Bernard N: Prevalence of anthelmintic resistant nematodes in sheep and goats in Western France. Small Rum Res. 1998, 29: 33-41. 10.1016/S0921-4488(97)00116-8.
16. Maingi N, Bjørn H, Thamsborg SM, Bøgh HO, Nansen P: A survey of anthelmintic resistance in nematode parasites of goats in Denmark. Vet Parasitol. 1996, 66: 53-66. 10.1016/S0304-4017(96)01006-0.
17. Sargison ND, Jackson F, Bartley DJ, Wilson DJ, Stenhouse LJ, Penny CD: Observations on the emergence of multiple anthelmintic resistance in sheep flocks in the south-east of Scotland. Vet Parasitol. 2007, 145: 65-76. 10.1016/j.vetpar.2006.10.024.
18. Jackson F, Coop RL: The development of anthelmintic resistance in sheep nematodes. Parasitology. 2000, 120: 95-107. 10.1017/S0031182099005740.
19. Jabbar A, Iqbal Z, Kerboeuf D, Muhammad G, Khan MN, Afaq M: Anthelmintic resistance: The state of play revisited. Life Sciences. 2006, 79: 2413-2431. 10.1016/j.lfs.2006.08.010.
20. Austrheim G, Asheim LJ, Bjarnason G, Feilberg J, Fosaa AM, Holand O, Jonsdottir IS, Jonsdottir IS, Magnusson B, Mortensen LE: Sheep grazing in the North-Atlantic region. A long term perspective on managment, resource economy and ecology. 2008, NTNU
21. NAA: Norwegian Agricultural Authority. 2007
22. Mysterud A, Stenseth NC, Yoccoz NG, Langvatn R, Steinheim G: Nonlinear effects of large-scale climatic variability on wild and domestic herbivores. Nature. 2001, 410: 1096-1099. 10.1038/35074099.
23. Vatn S: The sheep industry in the Nordic countries. Small Rum Res. 2009, 86: 80-83. 10.1016/j.smallrumres.2009.09.023.
24. Nedkvitne JJ, Garmo T, Staaland H: Beitedyr i kulturlandskap. 1995, Landbruksforlaget
25. Maingi N, Bjørn H, Thamsborg SM, Dangolla A, Kyvsgaard NC: Worm control practices on sheep farms

in Denmark and implications for the development of anthelmintic resistance. Vet. Parasitol. 1996, 66: 39-52. 10.1016/S0304-4017(96)01005-9.

26. Maingi N, Bjørn H, Thamsborg SM, Dangolla A, Kyvsgaard NC: A questionnaire survey of nematode parasite control practices on goat farms in Denmark. Vet Parasitol. 1996, 66: 25-37. 10.1016/S0304-4017(96)01004-7.
27. Gettinby G, Armour J, Bairden K, Plenderleith R: A survey by questionnaire of parasitic worm control in cattle and sheep at the Glasgow University Lanark practice. Vet Rec. 1987, 121: 487-490. 10.1136/vr.121.21.487.
28. Coles GC: Nematode control practices and anthelmintic resistance on British sheep farms. Vet Rec. 1997, 141: 91-93. 10.1136/vr.141.4.91.
29. Fraser DE, Hunt PJ, Skinner RJ, Coles GC: Survey of parasite control on sheep farms in south-west England. Vet Rec. 2006, 158: 55-57. 10.1136/vr.158.2.55.
30. Morgan ER, Coles GC: Nematode control practices on sheep farms following an information campaign aiming to delay anthelmintic resistance. Vet Rec. 2010, 166: 301-303. 10.1136/vr.b4772.
31. Hoste H, Chartier C, Etter E, Goudeau C, Soubirac F, Lefrileux Y: A questionnaire survey on the practices adopted to control gastrointestinal nematode parasitism in dairy goat farms in France. Vet Res Commun. 2000, 24: 459-469. 10.1023/A:1006499522154.
32. Cernanská D, Várady M, Cudeková P, Corba J: Worm control practices on sheep farms in the Slovak Republic. Vet Parasitol. 2008, 154: 270-276. 10.1016/j.vetpar.2008.03.026.
33. Boa ME, Thamsborg SM, Kassuku AA, Bøgh HO: Comparison of worm control strategies in grazing sheep in Denmark. Acta Vet Scand. 2001, 42: 57-69. 10.1186/1751-0147-42-57.
34. Waghorn TS, Miller CM, Oliver A-MB, Leathwick DM: Drench-and-shift is a high-risk practice in the absence of refugia. N Z Vet J. 2009, 57: 359-363. 10.1080/00480169.2009.64723.
35. Kenyon : The role of targeted selective treatments in the development of refugia-based approaches to the control of gastrointestinal nematodes of small ruminants. Vet Parasitol. 2009, 164: 3-11. 10.1016/j.vetpar.2009.04.015.
36. Tharaldsen J: The epidemiology of trichostrongylid infections in young cattle in Norway. Acta Vet Scand Suppl. 1976, 1-21.
37. Lindqvist A, Ljungström BL, Nilsson O, Waller PJ: The dynamics, prevalence and impact of nematode infections in organically raised sheep in Sweden. Acta Vet Scand. 2001, 42: 377-389. 10.1186/1751-0147-42-377.
38. Gjerde B: Parasitter hos sau (Sheep parasites). 2009
39. Helle O: The survival of nematodes and cestodes of sheep in the pasture during the winter in eastern Norway. Acta Vet Scand. 1971, 12: 504-512.
40. Waller PJ, Rydzik A, Ljungström BL, Törnquist M: Towards the eradication of Haemonchus contortus from sheep flocks in Sweden. Vet Parasitol. 2006, 136: 367-372. 10.1016/j.vetpar.2005.11.017.
41. Smith G, Grenfell BT, Isham V, Cornell S: Anthelmintic resistance revisited: under-dosing, chemoprophylactic strategies, and mating probabilities. Int J Parasitol. 1999, 29: 77-91. 10.1016/S0020-7519(98)00186-6.
42. Wolstenholme AJ, Fairweather I, Prichard R, von Samson-Himmelstjerna G, Sangster NC: Drug resistance in veterinary helminths. Trends Parasitol. 2004, 20: 469-476. 10.1016/j.pt.2004.07.010.
43. Prichard RK, Hennessy DR: Effect of oesophageal groove closure on the pharmacokinetic behaviour and efficacy of oxfendazole in sheep. Res Vet Sci. 1981, 30: 22-27.
44. Chartier C: Résistance des strongles gastro-intestinaux au thiophanate chez la chèvre angora. Le Point vétérinaire. 1993, 25: 357-360.
45. Short CR, Barker SA, Hsieh LC, Ou SP, Davis LE, Koritz G, Neff-Davis CA, Bevill RF, Munsiff IJ, Sharma GC: Disposition of fenbendazole in the goat. Am J Vet Res. 1987, 48: 811-815.
46. Jackson F: Anthelmintic resistance--the state of play. Br Vet J. 1993, 149: 123-138.
47. Hong C, Hunt KR, Coles GC: Occurrence of anthelmintic resistant nematodes on sheep farms in England and goat farms in England and Wales. Vet Rec. 1996, 139: 83-86. 10.1136/vr.139.4.83.
48. Van Wyk JA, Stenson MO, Van der Merwe JS, Vorster RJ, Viljoen PG: Anthelmintic resistance in South Africa: surveys indicate an extremely serious situation in sheep and goat farming. Onderstepoort J Vet Res. 1999, 66: 273-284.
49. Waller PJ: The development of anthelmintic resistance in ruminant livestock. Acta Tropica. 1994, 56: 233-243. 10.1016/0001-706X(94)90065-5.
50. Bartley DJ, Jackson E, Johnston K, Coop RL, Mitchell GBB, Sales J, Jackson F: A survey of anthelmintic resistant nematode parasites in Scottish sheep flocks. Vet Parasitol. 2003, 117: 61-71. 10.1016/j.vetpar.2003.07.023.
51. Kenyon F, Sargison ND, Skuce PJ, Jackson F: Sheep helminth parasitic disease in south eastern Scotland arising as a possible consequence of climate change. Vet Parasitol. 2009, 163: 293-297. 10.1016/j.vetpar.2009.03.027.
52. Skurdal E: Rangeland grazing - management and practice. 1997, Oslo: Landbruksforlaget
53. Asheim LJ, Mysterud I: The Norwegian sheep farming production system. Proceedings of the Symposium of the Sub-Network on Production Systems of the FAO-CIHEAM Inter-Regional Cooperative Research and Development Network on Sheep and Goats. 1999
54. Martin P, Anderson N, Jarrett R: Detecting benzimidazole resistance with faecal egg count reduction tests and in vitro assays. Aust Vet J. 1989, 66: 236-240. 10.1111/j.1751-0813.1989.tb13578.x.

CHAPTER 12

A STUDY ON THE DETERMINATION OF RISK FACTORS ASSOCIATED WITH BABESIOSIS AND PREVALENCE OF BABESIA SP., BY PCR AMPLIFICATION, IN SMALL RUMINANTS FROM SOUTHERN PUNJAB (PAKISTAN)

F. Iqbal, M. Fatima, S. Shahnawaz, M. Naeem, R.S. Shaikh, M. Ali, A.S. Shaikh, M. Aktas and M. Ali

Keywords: Sheep / goats / PCR amplification / *Babesia* sp

INTRODUCTION

Babesiosis is a parasitic infection due to the multiplication of *Babesia* sp. in erythrocytes (Levine, 1985; Piesman, 1987). Genus *Babesia* consists of group of intracellular parasites with around hundred species. Clinical signs of disease caused by *Babesia*, babesiosis, are variable including fever, icterus, hemoglubinuria and anemia in the host (Uilenberg, 2001; Yakhchali & Hossein 2006). These tick borne parasites infect a wide variety of vertebrate hosts including small ruminants (sheep and goat) and cattle (Persing & Conrad, 1995). In Pakistan ticks belonging to *Haemophysalis* sp. and *Hyalomma* sp. are involved in the transmission of various piroplasms to small and large ruminants (Rehman *et al.*, 2004).

The economic losses due to babesiosis in sheep and goat production are significant in tropical and subtropical areas (Mehlhorn & Schein, 1984; Bai *et al.*, 2002) and remain an important impediment to meat and milk production because infected animals exhibit high parasitemia and mortality (Caracappa, 1999). Babesiosis in domesticated small ruminants is due to at least three species *Babesia motasi*, *Babesia crassa* and *Babesia ovis* (Friedhoff, 1988). *Babesia ovis* is pathogenic especially in sheep and its case-fatality in susceptible hosts range from 30 to 50 % in field infections (Hashemi-Fesharki, 1997). It leads to significant losses among small ruminants due to its drastic effect on hemobiotic system (Radostits *et al.*, 2000).

The diagnosis of small ruminant piroplasmosis is based on the microscopic examination of Giemsa stained blood smears and clinical symptoms in acute cases. After acute

Citation: F. Iqbal, M. Fatima, S. Shahnawaz, M. Naeem, R.S. Shaikh, M. Ali, A.S. Shaikh, M. Aktas and M. Ali, "A study on the determination of risk factors associated with babesiosis and prevalence of Babesia sp., by PCR amplification, in small ruminants from Southern Punjab (Pakistan)," DOI: http://dx.doi.org/10.1051/parasite/2011183229.

infections, recovered animals frequently sustain sub clinical infections, which are microscopically undetectable (Calder *et al.*, 1996). They can be considered as a source of infection for the potential vector causing natural transmission of the disease. Serological methods are frequently employed in determining sub clinical infections. However, serology for detecting carrier state lack specificity and sensitivity, especially for infection status (Passos*et al.*, 1998). Therefore, DNA amplification methods, which are more sensitive and specific than other conventional methods may facilitate and use a powerful tool for the diagnosis of babesiosis (Aktas *et al.*, 2005, Altay *et al.*, 2005, Nagore *et al.*, 2004).

The aim of the present study was to optimize a specific, reliable and sensitive molecular tool, the polymerase chain reaction (PCR), for the detection of *Babesia* sp. in blood of small ruminants as parasite cannot easily be diagnosed by examination of stained blood film and negative microscopic examination does not exclude the possibility of infection. The objective of this pilot study is to provide baseline data regarding the prevalenece of *Babesia* sp. and risk factors involved in the spread of babesiosis in southern Punjab as to our knowledge, this parasite has never been reported in Pakistan.

MATERIALS AND METHODS

Whole blood samples were collected from 107 clinically healthy small ruminants (40 sheep, 67 goats) from randomly selected herds from seven districts (Multan, Muzaffar Garh, Layyah, Dera Ghazi Khan, Khanewal, Vehari and Bahawalnagar) in the important livestock production regions of Southern Punjab (Fig. 1). Blood of 10 % animals from each herd was sampled from jugular vein in Eppendorf tubes and preserved by adding few drops of 0.5 M EDTA. Data on the characteristics of animals (species, gender, age, tick presence or absence, prior treatment for babesiosis) and the herd (location, size, species of animals, dogs associated with the herds, presence of ticks on dogs associated with the herds) was collected through questionnaires completed by the investigators on the spot during sample collection in order to calculate the risk factors involve in the spread of babesiosis. All the experiments were approved by the research and ethic committee of Bahauddin Zakariya University Multan, Pakistan.

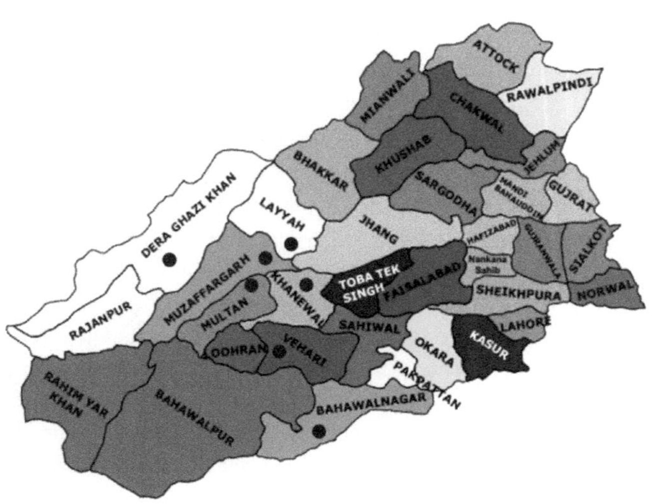

Figure 1. Map of Punjab. Sampling sites in southern Punjab are marked with circles.

Inorganic method of DNA extraction was used following Shaikh *et al.* (2005). The quality of the DNA extract in regard to purity and integrity was assessed with optical density counts at 260/280 nm and submerged gel electrophoresis. A pair of oligonucleotide primers was used to amplify the 146 bp region of 18S rRNA gene of *Babesia* sp. (Nucleotide sequence data reported in this paper are available in GenBank, EMBL and DDBJ databases under accession numbers AY150058, AY534883, AY150061, AY048113) following Theodoropoulos *et al.* (2006).

PCR was performed in 50 μl of a mixture containing about 500 ng of template DNA, 1X PCR buffer, 10 pmol of each primer, 0.2 mM of dNTPs, 1.5 mM MgCl2, 1 % betaine solution and 1 U of Taq DNA polymerase (Vivantis, UK). Remaining volume was adjusted with double distilled water. PCR amplification was obtained after 35 cycles. Each cycle consisted of a denaturing step of 1 min at 95 C, an annealing step of 1 min at 56 C and an extension step of 1 min at 72 C. Distilled water and *Babesia* sp. DNA (previously isolated from naturally infected sheep, GenBank accession no. AY998123) were used in each test as negative and positive controls, respectively. Ten microliters of the amplification products were visualized on 2 % agarose gel stained with ethidium bromide and observed under UV illumination.

For statistical purposes animals were grouped into two age categories: less than 1-year and more than 1-yearold. Herds were divided into two size categories: herds composed of 1-15 and herds with more than 15 animals. Also, herds were divided according to their composition into three categories: herds with sheep only, herds with goat only and herds containing both sheep and goats. The tick burden of sheep, goats and dogs associated with the herds was also scored. Association between the presence (positive and negative blood samples) of *Babesia* and the various parameters, *i.e.* herd location, herd size, species, gender and age of animal, herd composition, presence or absence of ticks on sheep and goats, presence or absence of ticks on dogs associated with the herd was assessed by contingency table analysis using the Fisher's exact test (for 2×2 tables). Statistical package Mini Tab (Version 16) was used for statistical analysis.

RESULTS AND DISCUSSION

Results of PCR amplification revealed that 36 out of 107 sampled sheep and goats were positive for *Babesia* sp. 20 sheep and 16 goat blood samples were parasite positive. The parasite prevalence varied between 18 % (Dera Ghazi Khan district) to 60 % (Layyah district). Sampling sites, total number of samples collected and positive sample along with prevalence details are mentioned in Table I. Table II presents the prevalence of *Babesia* sp. in sheep and goats in relation to the parameters describing the characteristics of the animals while Table III shows the characteristics of herds associated with the incidence of babesiosis.

Table 1. Sampling sites along with the total number of samples collected (N) from each district. Prevalence of parasite is given in parenthesis

	Babesia ovis		
District	**N**	**Positive**	**Negative**
Dera Ghazi Khan	38	7 (18%)	31 (82%)
Bahawalnagar	5	1 (20%)	4 (80%)
Multan	18	4 (22%)	14 (78%)
Khanewal	3	1 (33%)	2 (67%)
Muzaffar Garh	13	5 (38%)	89 (62%)
Vehari	5	2 (40%)	3 (60%)
Layyah	25	15 (60%)	10 (40%)
Total Animals (Sheep and Goat)	107	36 (34)	71 (66)
Sheep	40	20 (50%)	20 (50%)
Goat	67	16 (24%)	51 (76%)

Table 2. Association between parasite prevalence in goats and sheep and the studied parameters describing animal characters

				Babesia ovis		
Animal Type		**Parameter**	**No. of samples**	**Positive**	**Negative**	**P-value**
Sheep and Goat	Sex	Male	37	20 (54%)	17 (46%)	0.009
		Female	70	16 (23%)	54 (77%)	**
	Age	> 1 year	72	17 (24%)	55 (76%)	0.01
		< 1 year	35	19 (61%)	16 (39%)	**
	Tick burden	No tick	96	31 (32%)	65 (68%)	0.522
		One or more ticks	11	5 (45%)	6 (55%)	NS
Sheep	Sex	Male	20	15 (75%)	5 (25%)	0.71
		Female	20	5 (25%)	15 (75%)	NS
	Age	> 1 year	20	6 (30%)	14 (70%)	0.67
		< 1 year	20	14 (70%)	6 (30%)	NS
	Tick burden	No tick	33	18 (55%)	15 (45%)	0.07
		One or more ticks	7	2 (28%)	5 (72%)	NS
Goat	Sex	Male	17	5 (29%)	12 (71%)	0.528
		Female	50	11 (22%)	39 (78%)	NS
	Age	> 1 year	52	11 (21%)	41 (79%)	0.326
		< 1 year	15	5 (33%)	10 (67%)	NS
	Tick burden	No tick	62	13 (21%)	49 (79%)	0.083
		One or more ticks	5	3 (60%)	2 (40%)	NS

Probability of Fisher Exact test is mentioned for each parameter: NS = non significant (P > 0.05); ** = significant (P < 0.01).

Table 3. Association between parasite prevalence in sheep and goats and the studied parameters describing animal and herd characters

			Babesia ovis		
	Parameter	**No. of samples**	**Positive**	**Negative**	**P-value**
Size of herd	1-15	72	17 (24%)	56 (76%)	0.007
	15-30	35	18 (51%)	16 (49%)	**
Herd composition	Goat only	51	14 (27%)	37 (73%)	0.022
	Sheep only	18	4 (22%)	14 (78%)	*

	Sheep and goat together	38	17 (45%)	21 (55%)	
Association of dog with the herd	Dog absent	76	17 (22%)	59 (78%)	0.003
	Dog present	31	18 (58%)	13 (42%)	**
Tick burden on dog	No	76	19 (25%)	57 (75%)	0.011
	Yes	31	17 (55%)	14 (45%)	*

Probability of Fisher Exact test is mention for each parameter except herd composition where ANOVA is applied: NS = non significant (P > 0.05); * = least significant (P < 0.05); ** = significant (P < 0.01).

DNA amplification by PCR is a sensitive and specific tool as compared to other conventional methods (blood smear formation and serological studies) for the diagnosis of babesiosis (Aktas *et al.*, 2005; Altay *et al.*, 2005; Nagore *et al.*, 2004). The small subunit (SSU) 18S rRNA gene is one of the most important markers for PCR based detection of several parasites including*Babesia* sp. as it is part of the ribosomal functional core and is exposed to similar selective forces in all living beings (Criado-Fornelio *et al.*, 2003).

In the present study, among 107 sampled animals 36 (34 %) were positive for *Babesia* sp., which shows the high prevalence of this parasite in southern districts of Punjab. The results indicated that male sheep and goats (54 %) were more infected than females (23 %). This association between gender and parasite prevalence was statistically significant (P = 0.009) (Table II). Our results are contradictory to Theodoropoulos *et al.* (2006) who reported 17 % prevalence of *Babesia ovis* in female sheep and goats in Greece but they did not find any infected male. Our results demonstrated that animals less than one year old (61 %) were more affected with parasite as compared to older animals (Table II) and this association was statistically significant (P = 0.01) indicating that probably the animals develop immunity against parasite with age. Similar finding were reported by Razmi *et al.* (2003).

We also observed an association, although statistically non significant (P = 0.522), between tick burden and parasite prevalence 45 % of the sampled animals having tick present on them were positive for *Babesia* sp. (Table II) confirming the previous findings by Theodoropoulos *et al.* (2006) and. (Atlay *et al.* 2005) that ticks are involved in the spread of babesiosis.

Among the characters of herds, we observed that herds having more than 15 animals were more affected (P = 0.007) with the parasite (51 %) than herds composed of less than 15 animals (Table III). Also herd consisting of both sheep and goat had more *Babesia* sp. positive animals (P = 0.022) than herds containing sheep or goats only (Table III). Our results coincide with the findings of Theodoropoulos *et al.* (2006) indicating that over crowding of animals is a potential risk factor for the spread of babesiosis.

Results indicated that the presence of dog was a primary source of tick transmission (58 %) to small ruminants as the herds with dogs had higher prevalence of parasite (P = 0.003) than those without dogs (Table III). Also herds having dogs with tick burden had 55 % infected animals indicating that the vector, ticks, might have reached the small ruminants through dogs. This association between tick burdens on dog and parasite prevalence was statistically significant (P = 0.011) complementing the finding of Theodoropoulos *et al.* (2006).

Sheep were more susceptible for babesiosis than goats in the present study. The prevalence of *Babesia* sp. in sheep was 50 % as compared to 24 % infected goats (Table I). Friedhoff (1997) had reported that *Babesia* sp. causes diseases exclusively in sheep and rarely in goats. Moreover, males and sheep less than one year old sheep were more affected as compared to female and sheep older than one year but all these associations were statistically non significant (Table II). Our results coincide with the findings of Friedhoff (1997) that younger sheep are more prone to parasites due to developing immune system. Analysis of the data from sampled goats revealed similar findings as in sheep (Table II).

There is hardly any report on the prevalence of babesiosis in ruminants of Pakistan. To our knowledge this is the first report describing the survey on ovine babesiosis in small ruminants through PCR amplification in southern Punjab. High prevalence of *Babesia* sp. indicates that other species of this genus might be existing as well. In the present study, all 107 small ruminants were raised locally indicating that the babesiosis is endemic in this region. A major reason for high prevalence of parasite in southern Punjab could be the poor hygienic conditions and poverty especially in small towns and villages. In many cases, veterinarians are not available for the help and guidance of livestock owners. By generating the public awareness regarding the risk factors, the prevalence of piroplasms can be significantly decreased resulting in better health and output of sheep and goats.

ACKNOWLEDGMENTS

This study was sponsored by Research and External Linkages Division, Bahauddin Zakariya University, Multan (Pakistan). The investigators are grateful to all the veterinarians for their help in blood sample collection.

REFERENCES

1. Aktas M., Altay K. & Dumanli N. Development of a polymerase chain reaction method for diagnosis of *Babesia ovis*infection in sheep and goats. Veterinary Parasitology, 2005, 133, 277–281.
2. Altay K., Dumanli N., Holman P.J. & Aktas M. Detection of *Theileria ovis* in naturally infected sheep by nested PCR. Veterinary Parasitology, 2005, 127, 99–104.
3. Bai Q., Liu G., Liu D., Ren J. & Li X. Isolation and preliminary characterization of large *Babesia* sp. from sheep and goats in the eastern part of Gansu Province. China Parasitology Research, 2002, 88, 16–21.
4. Calder J.A., Reddy G.R., Chieves L., Courney C.H., Littell R., Livengood J.R., Norval R.A., Smith G. & Dame J.B. Monitoring *Babesia bovis* infection in cattle by using PCR-based test. Journal of Clinical Microbiology, 1996, 34, 2748–2755.

5. Caracappa S. Livestock production and animal health in Sicily Italy. Parasitology, 1999, 41, 17–23.

6. Cariado-Fornelio A., Martinez M.A., Bulinga S.A. & Barba-Carretero J.C. Molecular studies on *Babesia, Theileria* and*Hepatozoon* in Southern Europe Part 1 Epizootological aspects. Veterinary Parasitology, 2003, 113, 189–201.

7. Friedhoff K.T. Transmission of *Babesia, in* Babesiosis of domestic animals and man. Ristic M. (ed.), CRC Press, Boca Raton, Florida, 1988, 23–52.

8. Friedhoff K.T. Tick-borne diseases of sheep and goats caused by *Babesia, Theileria* or *Anaplasma* spp. Parasitology, 1997, 39, 99–109.

9. Hashemi-Fesharki R. Tick-borne diseases of sheep and goats and their related vectors in Iran. Parasitology, 1997, 39, 115–117.

10. Levine N.D. Veterinary Protozoology. Iowa State University Press, Ames,.1985, 24–41.

11. Mehlhorn H. & Schein E. The piroplasms: life cycle and sexual stages. Advances in Parasitology, 1984, 23, 37–103.

12. Nagore D., García-Sanmartín J., García-Pérez A.L., Juste R.A. & Hurtado A. Identification, genetic diversity and prevalence of *Theileria* and *Babesia* species in sheep population from Northern Spain. International Journal of Parasitology, 2004, 34, 1059–1067.

13. Passos L.M., Bell-Sakyi L. & Brown C.G. Immunochemical characterization of *in vitro* culture-derived antigens of*Babesia bovis* and *Babesia bigemina*. Veterinary Parasitology, 1998, 76, 239–249.

14. Persing D.H. & Conrad P.A. Babesiosis: new insights from phylogenetic analysis. Infectious Agents Diseases, 1995, 4, 182–195.

15. Piesman J. Emerging tick-borne diseases in temperate climates. Parasitology Today, 1987, 3, 197–199.

16. Radostits O.M., Gay C.C., Blood D.C. & Hinchcliff K.M. Veterinary Medicine. WH Sounders, London,.2000, 134–142.

17. Razmi G.R., Naghibi A., Aslani M.R., Dastjerdi K. & Hossieni H. An epidemiological study on *Babesia* infection in small ruminants in Mashhad suburb, Khorasan province, Iran. Small Ruminant Research, 2003, 50, 39–44.

18. Rehman W.U., Khan I.A., Qureshi A.H. & Hussain S. Prevalence of different species of Ixodidae (hard ticks) in Rawalpindi and Islamabad. Pakistan Journal of Medical Science, 2004, 43, 42–46.

19. Shaikh R.S., Ramzan K., Nazil S., Sattar S., Khan S.N., Riazuddin S., Ahmed Z.M. & Friedman T.B. A new locus for non syndromic deafness DFNB51 maps to chromosome 11p 13-p12. American Journal of Medical Genetics A, 2005, 138, 392–395.

20. Theodoropoulos G., Gazouli M., Ikonomopoulos J.A., Kantzoura V. & Kominakis A. Determination of prevalence and risk factors of infection with *Babesia* in small ruminants from Greece by polymerase chain reaction amplification. Veterinary Parasitology, 2006, 135, 99–104.

21. Uilenberg G. Babesiosis, *in:* Encyclopedia of artropod-transmitted infection of man and domesticated animals. Wallingford M.W. (ed.), CABI Publishing, UK, 2001, 122–144.

22. Yakhchali M. & Hossein A. Prevalence and ectoparasites fauna of sheep and goats flocks in Urmia suburb Iran. Veterinarski Arhiv, 2006, 76, 431–442.

SECTION IV: PARASITES OF HORSES AND DONKEYS

CHAPTER 13

RISK FACTORS ASSOCIATED WITH THE OCCURRENCE OF GASTROINTESTINAL HELMINTHS AMONG INDIGENOUS DONKEYS (EQUUS ASINUS) IN NORTHEASTERN NIGERIA

Saleh Mohammed Jajere, Jallailudeen Rabana Lawal, Amina Mohammed Bello, Yakaka Wakil, Usman Aliyu Turaki and Ibrahim Waziri

INTRODUCTION

Donkeys (Equus asinus) are among the early-domesticated equines that have been a beast of burden for thousands of years [1]. Currently, there are about 44 million donkeys distributed throughout the world [2]. In Africa, the donkey population is estimated at 13 million [3]. Despite the increase in mechanization throughout the world, donkeys still have a prominent position in the agricultural systems of many developing countries [4–6]. Donkeys represent an important aspect of small holder farming system especially in rural communities and hamlets, where there exist poor road networks or even nonexisting roads; they are used for conveying people, goods, and farm inputs and outputs to and from farms [7, 8]. Unfortunately, Donkeys are left malnourished and underfed, subjected to different conditions of hardships like maltreatment, poor management conditions, and overladen [9].

Citation: Saleh Mohammed Jajere, Jallailudeen Rabana Lawal, Amina Mohammed Bello, Yakaka Wakil, Usman Aliyu Turaki, and Ibrahim Waziri, "Risk Factors Associated with the Occurrence of Gastrointestinal Helminths among Indigenous Donkeys (Equus asinus) in Northeastern Nigeria," Scientifica, vol. 2016, Article ID 3735210, 7 pages, 2016. doi:10.1155/2016/3735210.

Donkey still remains one of the most underappreciated animals and an important draught one, serving a key role in the agricultural economy of the developing world including Africa [10, 11]. They are often engaged in work for long hours and when set free, they are left to browse and feed on less nutritive garbage. This has been linked with potential negative effect especially on their welfare and health status [12, 13].

Donkeys like other domesticated animals are vulnerable to parasitic, bacterial, fungal, and viral diseases [14,15]. Among parasitic diseases are the haemoparasites such as babesiosis, trypanosomiasis, and gastrointestinal helminthosis, which are considered silent killers of the animal [16–19]. Donkeys are hosts to a variety of gastrointestinal tract parasites of the family Strongylidae, commonly called Strongyle nematodes or Strongyles[20]. The most common gastrointestinal parasites of donkeys include large and small Strongyles, Ascaris, pinworms (Oxyuris equi), Gasterophilus, lung worms, and fluke and tape worms which are by far the commonly encountered parasites in most veterinary parasitological examinations of donkeys [6, 14, 21, 22]. Some of these gastrointestinal tract parasites, especially Strongyles, are active bloodsuckers; where there is heavy parasitic burden, the commonly encountered manifestations are anaemia, weakness, emaciation, and sometimes colic and diarrhea [23]. The intestinal mucosa is damaged where the worms attach themselves and suck blood. These parasites usually deprive their host animals of sufficient and adequate absorption of digestive nutrients, which in the long run lead to retarded growth and impaired productivity, reduced work output, discomfort, and pains and sometimes death ensued [24, 25]. The various degrees of damage caused by the gastrointestinal parasites of donkeys depend on factors such as the species affected and nutritional and immune status of the animal [25].

Although many studies were conducted on the prevalence and risk factors associated with gastrointestinal parasitism in horses in northeastern Nigeria, there are few researches on the risk factors, epidemiology, and prevalence of gastrointestinal parasites among indigenous donkeys (Equus asinus) in the region. Moreover, the huge numbers and increasing importance of donkeys in the economy of the semiarid zone of Nigeria particularly seen in hamlets and rural communities where these animals are used for variety of purposes including transporting people and farming inputs and outputs, make them important in these communities. Therefore, this study was designed to determine the prevalence and associated risk factors of gastrointestinal helminths among working donkeys in northeastern Nigeria. It is expected to provide baseline epidemiological data on prevalence and risk factors for which further research would be conducted in elucidating gastrointestinal helminthoses among indigenous donkeys in the region.

MATERIALS AND METHODS

Study Areas

This study was conducted in some parts of three provinces of the northeastern Nigeria comprising Bauchi, Yobe, and Gombe states. Gombe state, a multiethnic city, is located in the northeastern zone of Nigeria, with Gombe city as its capital. It is located at latitudes 9°30′ and 12°30′N and longitudes 8°45′ and 11°45′E. It shares common borders with Borno, Bauchi, Yobe, Taraba, and Adamawa states due to its location within the expansive savannah zone. The state has an area of 20,265 km^2 and an estimated population of 2,353,000 people as of 2006. Gombe state has two distinct climates, rainy season spanning from April to October and dry season spanning from November to March with an average rainfall of 850 mm (https://en.wikipedia.org/wiki/Gombe_State).

Bauchi state is located in the northeastern zone of Nigeria at latitudes 9°3′ and 12°3′N and longitudes 8°50′ and 11°E. It has a total landmass of 49,119 km^2 and an estimated human population of 4,653,066 as of 2006 census. The state shares border with seven states, namely, Taraba and Plateau state to the south, Yobe and Gombe state to the east, Kano and Jigawa state to the north, and Kaduna state to the west. The state has two distinctive kinds of vegetation: the Sudan savannah covering the entire southern part and Sahel savannah from the middle of the state as you go from the southern to the northern part of the state. Majority of the northern part is sandy, while the southern part is mountainous resulting from continuation of the Jos plateau. The rainfall ranges from 700 mm in the northern part to 1300 mm per annum seen in the southern part of the state. Rain starts early from April in the southern part, which is heavier and lasts longer. However, in contrast, rain starts lately around June or July and lasts shorter (https://en.wikipedia.org/wiki/Bauchi_State).

Yobe state is located in the arid zone of northeastern Nigeria within latitude 11°5′ north and longitude 13°10′ east. It has an estimated human population of 2,757,000 as of 2011 and covers a land mass area of 45,502 km^2. Damaturu is its capital city. The state shares an international border with Diffa and Zinder regions of the Niger Republic to the north. In addition, it shares border with Nigerian states of Bauchi, Borno, Gombe, and Jigawa. It lies within the dry savanna belt. The climate is mostly dry and hot throughout the year with milder climate seen in the southern part of the state. The short rainy season starts lately around June and ends in September.

Study Design, Baseline Characteristics, and Sample Collection

Cross-sectional study was conducted on six hundred randomly selected indigenous donkeys from Bauchi ($n = 200$), Gombe ($n = 200$), and Yobe states ($n = 200$) in northeastern Nigeria. The sample comprises 364 males and 236 females: 103 young, 416 adult, and 81 older Donkeys. Faecal samples were collected, while data on sex, age, body condition scoring, season of the year, and so forth were also recorded accordingly. Random faecal samples were collected directly from the rectum of the donkeys after a well physical restrained technique by owners and voluntary veterinary attendants (especially the temperamental animals) using sterilized disposable hand gloves. About 10 grams of fresh faecal samples was collected. Some faecal samples were also collected from donkeys with previous history of medications. Each sample was labeled with necessary information and then kept in icebox and immediately transported to parasitology diagnostic laboratory for examination. Other relevant information on management systems was also noted at the time of sampling.

Age and Body Condition Estimation

The age was determined using birth records gathered from information obtained from the owners' and dentition characteristics [26] and this was categorized as young (<12 months) ($n = 103$), adult (>1 year) ($n = 416$), and old (>6 years) ($n = 81$). These age classifications were described elsewhere [27–29]. The body condition scoring was based on the criteria of NEWC [30] and body condition of animals was classified into poor, medium (moderate), and good.

Faecal Analysis and Coprology

Samples were kept in refrigerator at 4°C when immediate processing was not possible but processed within 48 hrs. Some samples were held using 10% formalin solution. Parasitological examination was carried out by direct smear, sedimentation, and flotation techniques, following the standard procedures for the screening of parasites and microscopic examination (10x and 40x objectives) as described by Soulsby [31]. Identification of the helminth parasite eggs in the faeces of the donkeys was evaluated using the coprological flotation and sedimentation techniques [32]. The flotation fluid used in the present study was supersaturated solution of sodium chloride (NaCl) salt prepared in the laboratory.

Data Analysis

The raw data were cross-tabulated initially using Microsoft Office Excel version 2011 to obtain proportions and prevalence of infection. This was later imported into SPSS statistical software version 22 for chi-square analysis and Fisher's exact test in order to determine the strength of association between the dependent and independent variables. The association is considered significant at $p < 0.05$.

RESULTS AND DISCUSSION

An overall prevalence of 98.3% was obtained (Table 1), of which 78.3%, 40.3%, and 17.5% were, respectively, from Strongyle spp., Parascaris equorum, and Oxyuris equi (Table 2). Based on the study areas, prevalence of gastrointestinal helminthosis ranged from 99.0% observed in both Yobe and Gombe states to 97% in Bauchi state. Infection rates were not statistically significant across the study areas ($p > 0.05$). The infection burden with the nematodes was manifested in both single and mixed infections (Table 3)

Table 1: Risk factors associated with the occurrence of gastrointestinal helminthosis in northeastern Nigeria

Risk factors	**Number of donkeys sampled**	**Number of positives**	**Prevalence (%)**	value
Age				
Young (<12 mo)	103	103	100.0	
Adult (>1 yr)	416	407	97.8	0.292
Old (>6 yrs)	81	80	98.8	
Sex				
Male	364	357	98.1	0.542
Female	236	233	98.7	
Body condition score				
Thin	355	355	100.0	
Medium	150	150	100.0	
Fat	95	85	89.5	<0.001
Settlement				
Urban	120	110	91.6	<0.001
Rural	480	480	100	
Season				
Rainy	300	298	99.3	
Dry	300	292	97.3	0.056
Anthelminthic medication history				
Dewormed	31	21	67.7	<0.001
Not dewormed	569	569	100	
Management system				
Poor	517	517	100	
Moderate	52	52	100	
Good	31	21	67.7	<0.001
Overall	*600*	*590*	*98.3*	

Management system (feeding, shelter, healthcare, welfare, etc.).

Table 2: Prevalence of gastrointestinal nematode parasite of donkeys (Equus asinus) in northeastern Nigeria ($n = 600$)

Parasites encountered	**Number of positives**	**Prevalence % (95% CI)**
Strongyle	470	78.3 (75.00–81.60)
Parascaris equorum	242	40.3 (36.38–44.22)
Oxyuris equi	150	17.5 (14.46–20.54)

*Statistically significant at $p < 0.05$.

Table 3: The relative proportion of gastrointestinal nematode parasites of donkeys (Equus asinus) in northeastern Nigeria

Nematodes	Number of positives	Relative frequency (%)
Strongyle	282	47.8
Parascaris equorum	88	14.9
Oxyuris equi	32	5.4
Strongyle + Parascaris equorum	115	19.5
Strongyle + Oxyuris equi	34	5.8
Strongyle + Parascaris equorum + Oxyuris equi	39	6.6
Overall	590	100

The relative frequency of single infection ranged from 47.8% seen in Strongyle to 5.4% as seen in Oxyuris equi, while it ranges from 19.5% in Strongyle + Parascaris equorum to 5.8% seen in Strongyle + Oxyuris equi in the mixed infection (Table 3). The age-, season-, sex-specific prevalence rates were similar across each of these categories and were not statistically significant (Table 1). However, donkeys sampled from rural areas, not previously dewormed, with thin body condition score and raised under poor management systems had high infection rates and were significantly associated with the risks of gastrointestinal helminthosis ($p < 0.001$) (Table 1). Table 4 presents the distribution of the gastrointestinal nematodes of indigenous donkeys with the occurrence of Strongyle eggs significantly higher compared with the other nematodes encountered.

Table 4: Burden of helminth infection according to the risk factors among donkeys (Equus asinus) in northeastern Nigeria

Risk factors ()	% distribution of helminths based on species					
	Strongyle	Parascaris equorum	Oxyuris equi	Strongyle + P. equorum	Strongyle + O. equi	Strongyle + P. equorum + O. equi
Age						
Young (<12 mo) (103)	47 (45.6)	14 (13.6)	8 (7.8)	22 (21.4)	4 (3.9)	8 (7.8)
Adult (>1 yr) (407)	197 (47.4)	62 (14.9)	17 (4.1)	80 (19.2)	26 (6.3)	25 (6.0)
Old (>6 yrs) (80)	38 (46.9)	12 (14.8)	7 (8.6)	13 (16.0)	4 (4.9)	6 (7.4)
Sex						
Male (357)	172 (47.3)	56 (15.4)	16 (4.4)	68 (18.7)	21 (5.8)	24 (6.6)
Female (233)	110 (46.6)	32 (13.6)	16 (6.8)	47 (9.9)	13 (5.5)	15 (6.4)
BCS						
Thin (355)	161 (45.4)	59 (16.6)	17 (4.8)	75 (21.1)	20 (5.6)	23 (6.5)
Medium (150)	78 (52.0)	19 (12.7)	9 (6.0)	25 (16.7)	9 (6.0)	10 (6.7)
Fat (85)	43 (45.3)	10 (10.5)	6 (6.3)	15 (15.8)	5 (5.3)	6 (6.3)
Settlement						
Urban (110)	52 (43.3)	14 (11.7)	8 (6.7)	23 (19.2)	6 (5.0)	7 (5.8)
Rural (480)	230 (47.9)	74 (15.4)	24 (5.0)	92 (19.2)	28 (5.8)	32 (6.7)
Season						
Rainy (298)	147 (49.0)	41 (13.7)	14 (4.7)	50 (16.7)	18 (6.0)	28 (9.3)
Dry (292)	135 (45.0)	47 (15.7)	18 (6.0)	65 (21.7)	16 (5.3)	11 (3.7)
Anthelminthic history						
Dewormed (21)	12 (38.7)	4 (12.9)	0 (0.0)	3 (9.7)	2 (6.5)	0 (0.0)
Not dewormed (569)	270 (47.5)	84 (14.8)	32 (5.6)	112 (19.7)	32 (5.6)	39 (6.9)
Management system						
Poor (517)	245 (47.4)	73 (14.1)	25 (4.8)	107 (20.7)	31 (6.0)	36 (7.0)

Moderate (52)	25 (48.1)	11 (21.2)	7 (13.5)	5 (9.6)	1 (1.9)	3 (5.8)
Good (21)	12 (38.7)	4 (12.9)	0 (0.0)	3 (9.7)	2 (6.5)	0 (0.0)

[a]Statistically significant at $p < 0.05$.

[b]BCS: body condition score.

Parasitic helminths continue to be the major constraints affecting the health and working performance of donkeys worldwide. They cause various degrees of damage depending on the species and nutritional and the immune status of the donkey. They decrease the performance and productivity through reduction of body weight or retarded weight gain and even death in acute cases. The overall prevalence of helminth parasites among donkeys reported is 98.3% (Table 1), which agrees with reports by Ayele et al. [28], Ibrahim et al. [14], and Wannas et al. [33] who reported respective prevalence of 98.2%, 96.9%, and 100% in Dugda Bora District, southern Ethiopia, and Al Diwaniyah Governorate, respectively. However, it is relatively lower than 90%, 86.5%, 75.9%, and 55.7% prevalence rates as reported by Samuel et al. [6], Parsani et al. [9], Getachew et al. [34], and Muhammad et al. [35] in Kombolcha Town, North Gujarat, Ethiopia, and Pakistan, respectively. These differences might be connected with factors such as variations in sample sizes, sampling periods, deworming strategy, accessibility to veterinary clinics, and methods employed for sample analysis, which may affect the prevalence rate. This may also be partly explained by the nutritional status of donkeys in the respective study areas, management systems, and environmental factors that can influence the level of immunity to infection and manifestation of the parasitic infections. In the present study, Strongyle, Parascaris equorum, and Oxyuris equi were reported with respective prevalence of 78.3%, 40.3%, and 17.5% (Table 2). Several studies highlighted the significance of these nematodes as important gastrointestinal parasites of donkeys [6, 13, 14, 20, 36, 37].

Considering a single gastrointestinal nematode infection, Strongyle spp. egg was prevalent and dominant and the most encountered nematode species examined from all samples collected from the study areas (Table 3). This agrees with previous studies by Saeed et al. [38], Wannas et al. [33], Mezgebu et al. [25], and Tesfu et al. [37] which further explained the predomination of Strongyle egg with prevalence rates of 58.5%, 57.14%, and 66.67%, respectively, over Parascaris spp. eggs. In the current study, Oxyuris equi with prevalence rate of 5.5% was in accord with the study of Ayele et al. [28] and Umur and Açici [24], where both reported rates of 6% and 6.45%, respectively. However, Yoseph et al. [29] and Ibrahim et al. [14] reported respective rates of 32.4% and 31.8% of Oxyuris equi in their study. This could probably be due to influence of climatic conditions on the dynamics of egg expulsion [39]. The relative frequency for the occurrence of mixed infection in the present study agrees with similar study by Samuel et al. [6].

Age-specific prevalence rates revealed a slightly higher rate among young donkeys (Table 1). This agrees with the study by Regassa and Yimer [36] and Tesfu et al. [37], which reported high prevalence of gastrointestinal nematodes in younger donkeys as compared to the adult age groups. This might be associated with apparent inability of the younger age groups to develop adequate acquired immunity predisposing them to high risks of severe infection with gastrointestinal nematode parasite when compared with adult donkeys. Higher infection rates and more severe infections reflect lack of immunity in younger population [40].

Sex was not significantly associated with infection rates, as both sexes share equal chances of acquiring nematode infection, because they are reared and grazed on the same pasture without sex discrimination. It could also result from decreased infection resistance at the time of parturition and during early lactation. The periparturient relaxation of resistance to gastrointestinal nematode infection has been reported in the female donkeys [40].

Body condition score was significantly associated with infection rates (Table 1). Donkeys with poor body condition score were significantly associated with high parasitic activities in their gastrointestinal tracts depriving them of adequate absorption and assimilation of digested nutrients resulting in emaciation and cachexia. Similarly, Ayele et al. [28], Ibrahim et al. [14], Worku and Afera [21], Tesfu et al. [37], and Samuel et al. [6] all reported that the body condition score is a reliable indicator of parasitic burden and can serve as a useful indicator used to identify donkeys that require an immediate attention for anthelminthic remedies.

Mean egg counts were high among donkeys from rural areas compared with those from urban settlements (Table 1). Donkeys in the rural areas are subjected to prolonged working time, exposed to harsh environmental temperature, and overloaded without adequate observation of their welfare. Donkeys in rural areas are generally malnourished and underfed, left to graze after hard labor on dry poorly nutritive pastures especially during the dry season, without any supplementation with essential nutrients that will improve their health status. Consequently, they become immunosuppressive and therefore vulnerable to infection with helminthic parasites. In addition, most of these rural areas lack veterinary facilities or clinics for routine medical attention to these donkeys [11, 13, 25].

Donkeys with no history of recent deworming had significantly high mean egg counts compared with those routinely dewormed. This implies that routine deworming of donkeys with effective anthelminthic will reduce egg burden, thereby safe-guarding the animals from nematode infections. Muhammad et al. [35] reported respective 73.21% and 96.42% mean reduction in number of eggs per gram of faeces on days 7 and 14 after medication with an efficacious anthelminthic. Binev et al. [41] and Seri et al. [42] also reported 96% and 100% elimination of nematodes egg burden in donkeys after day 14 after treatment, respectively.

Low mean egg counts were observed in donkeys reared under good management systems provided with good feed, watering, and veterinary attention as compared with those reared under poor management conditions. Animals reared under a good management system tend to possess strong immunity and demonstrate resistance to infectious diseases [11, 22, 43].

In conclusion, gastrointestinal helminth parasites are endemic among the indigenous donkeys of northeastern Nigeria, with Strongyle as frequently encountered compared with the other nematodes (Tables 2 and 4). Therefore, it is recommended that donkey owners be trained on how to improve on the management systems, especially as regards provision of adequate nutritional supplements to donkeys so that they can have good body condition that will in the long run confers some level of resistance against helminths infection. Donkeys should be well fed and served with fresh clean water following hard labor. All newly introduced donkeys into the herd meant for restocking or breeding purposes must be quarantined, properly screened, and treated to prevent environmental contamination with helminth parasites. Further studies are recommended on the impact of parasitic infections on the health status, working efficiency, reproductive efficiency, draftability, and longevity of donkeys.

ACKNOWLEDGMENTS

The authors wish to express their gratitude to the Ministry of Animal Husbandry and Nomadic Affairs, Gombe state, Nigeria, for sponsoring this research work. The authors are equally grateful to all the technical staff of the Research Laboratory, Department of Biological Science, Federal University Kashere, Gombe, Veterinary Medicine Laboratory, Department of Veterinary Medicine, and Parasitology Research Laboratory, Department of Veterinary Microbiology and Parasitology, University of Maiduguri, Nigeria, for their technical assistance throughout the period of this research.

REFERENCES

1. C. Saul, L. Siefert, and J. Opuda-Asibo, "Disease and health problems of donkeys: a case study from eastern Uganda," in Proceedings of the International Animal Traction Network for Eastern and Southern Africa (ATNESA '97), Debre Zeit, Ethiopia, May 1997.
2. P. Starkey and M. Starkey, "Regional and world trends in donkey populations," in Donkeys, People and Development. A Resource Book of the Animal Traction Network for Eastern and Southern Africa, P. Starkey and D. Fielding, Eds., pp. 10–21, ACP-EU Technical Centre for Agricultural and Rural Cooperation (CTA), Wageningen, The Netherlands, 2004.
3. P. Starkey and M. Starkey, "Regional and world trends in donkey populations," in Proceedings of the Animal Traction Network for Eastern and Southern Africa Improving Donkey Utilization and Management, pp. 230–237, ATENSA, Debre Zeit, Ethiopia, May 1997.
4. E. Mwenya and G. Tandkeib, "History and utilization of donkey in Namibia," in Donkeys, People and Development. A Resource Book of the Animal Traction Network for Eastern and Southern Africa, P. Starkey and D. Fielding, Eds., pp. 172–174, ACP-EU Technical Center for Agricultural and Rural Cooperation (CTA), Wageningen, The Netherlands, 2004.
5. G. B. Shrikhande, S. G. Rewatkar, S. S. Deshmukh, D. K. Maske, and Y. M. Raghorte, "The incidence of helminth parasites in donkeys," Veterinary World, vol. 2, no. 6, p. 224, 2009.
6. E. Samuel, A. Ashenafi, M. Natnael, and B. Shiret, "Prevalence of gastro intestinal nematode parasitic infections of horses and donkeys in and around Kombolcha town," American-Eurasian Journal of Scientific Research, vol. 10, no. 4, pp. 228–234, 2015.
7. F. Regassa, R. Dhuguma, T. Sorry, and M. Bzunesh, "Prevalence of equine gastro-intestinal parasite in western high lands of Oromia, Ethiopia," Bulletin of Animal Health and Production Africa, no. 53, pp. 161–166, 2005.
8. Y. T. Hailu and H. T. Ashenafi, "Epidemiological study on gastrointestinal helminths of horses in arsi-bale highlands of Oromiya region, Ethiopia, Addis Ababa University, College of Veterinary Medicine and Agriculture," Ethiopian Veterinary Journal, vol. 17, no. 2, pp. 51–62, 2013.
9. H. Parsani, R. Momin, A. Lateef, and H. Das, "Studies on gastro-intestinal helminths of Equus acinus in North Gujarat, India," Egyptian Journal of Biology, vol. 15, no. 1, 2013.
10. O. Fred and K. Pascal, Extension Approaches to Improving the Welfare of Working Equines, Kenya Network for Dissemination of Agricultural Technologies (KENDAT), Nairobi, Kenya, 2006.
11. M. I. Ahmed, A. N. Tijjani, and A. R. Mustapha, "Survey for common diseases and management practices of donkeys (Equus asinus) in Borno, State Nigeria," Nigerian Veterinary Journal, vol. 29, no. 3, pp. 1–5, 2008.
12. S. Mekuria and R. Abebe, "Observation on major welfare problems of equine in Meskan district, Southern Ethiopia," Livestock Research for Rural Development, vol. 22, no. 3, 2010.
13. B. Bogale, Z. Sisay, and M. Chanie, "Strongyle nematode infections of donkeys and mules in and around Bahirdar, Northwest Ethiopia," Global Veterinaria, vol. 9, no. 4, pp. 497–501, 2012.
14. N. Ibrahim, T. Berhanu, B. Deressa, and T. Tolosa, "Survey of prevalence of helminth parasites of donkeys in and around Hawassa town, Southern Ethiopia," Global Veterinaria, vol. 6, no. 3, pp. 223–227, 2011.
15. D. Sumbria, L. D. Singla, A. Sharma, A. D. Moudgil, and M. S. Bal, "Equine trypanosomosis in central and western Punjab: prevalence, haemato-biochemical response and associated risk factors," Acta Tropica, vol. 138, pp. 44–50, 2014.
16. R. Ravindran, J. R. Rao, A. K. Mishra et al., "Trypanosoma evansi in camels, donkeys and dogs in India: comparison of PCR and light microscopy for detection—short communication," Veterinarski Arhiv, vol. 78, no. 1, pp. 89–94, 2008.
17. E. S. Siham, M. A. Abdalla, O. B. Amel, and M. A. Rabab, "Investigation of major diseases affecting donkeys (Equus asinus) in Khartoum State-Sudan," in Proceedings of the 13th Scientific Conference, Faculty of Veterinary Medicine, Assiut University, Assiut, Egypt, 2008.
18. B. Mekibib, M. Manegerew, A. Tadesse et al., "Prevalence of haemoparasites and associated risk

factors in working donkeys in Adigudem and Kwiha Districts of Tigray Region, Northern Ethiopia," Journal of Animal and Veterinary Advances, vol. 9, no. 17, pp. 2249–2255, 2010. ·

19. H. Bedada and S. Dagnachew, "Study on the prevalence of donkey trypanosomosis in Awi zone northwest Ethiopia," Ethiopian Veterinary Journal, vol. 16, no. 2, pp. 65–76, 2012. ·
20. A. Gizachew and D. Ayana, "Study on strongyles and parascaris parasites population in working donkeys of central Shoa, Ethiopia," Livestock Research for Rural Development, vol. 22, pp. 1–5, 2010.
21. S. Worku and B. Afera, "Prevalence of equine nematodes in and around Kombolcha South Wollo, Ethiopia," Revista Electrónica de Veterinaria, no. 13, pp. 1–13, 2012.
22. J. Atawalna, B. O. Emikpe, E. K. Sallah, W. Shaibu, and R. D. Folitse, "The health problems, gastrointestinal and blood parasites commonly associated with donkeys in the upper east Region of Ghana," African Journal of Biomedical Research, vol. 18, no. 1, pp. 37–41, 2015. ·
23. F. A. Burden, N. Du Toit, M. Hernandez-Gil, O. Prado-Ortiz, and A. F. Trawford, "Selected health and management issues facing working donkeys presented for veterinary treatment in rural Mexico: some possible risk factors and potential intervention strategies," Tropical Animal Health and Production, vol. 42, no. 4, pp. 597–605, 2010. ·
24. Ş. Umur and M. Açici, "A survey on helminth infections of equines in the Central Black Sea region, Turkey," Turkish Journal of Veterinary and Animal Sciences, vol. 33, no. 5, pp. 373–378, 2009. ·
25. T. Mezgebu, K. Tafess, and F. Tamiru, "Prevalence of gastrointestinal parasites of horses and donkeys in and around Gondar Town, Ethiopia," Open Journal of Veterinary Medicine, vol. 3, no. 6, pp. 267–272, 2013.
26. M. Crane, "Medical," in The professional Hand Books of the Donkey, E. D. Svendsen, Ed., pp. 29–31, Whittet Books Limitted, London, UK, 3rd edition, 1997.
27. E. D. Svendsen, Parasites Abroad. The Professional Hand Book of the Donkey, Whittet Books Limited, London, UK, 3rd edition, 1997.
28. G. Ayele, G. Feseha, E. Bojia, and A. Joe, "Prevalence of gastro-intestinal parasites of donkeys in Dugda Bora District, Ethiopia," Livestock Research for Rural Development, vol. 18, no. 10, 2006.
29. S. Yoseph, G. Feseha, and W. Abebe, "Survey on helminthosis of equines in Wonchi, Ethiopia," Journal of Ethiopian Veterinary Association, no. 5, pp. 47–61, 2001.
30. National Equine Welfare Council (NEWC), "Equine industry welfare guidelines compendium for horses, ponies and donkeys," in Body Condition Scoring of Horses and Donkeys, pp. 28–29, 2nd edition, 2005.
31. E. T. L. Soulsby, Helimenthes, Arthropods and Protozoa of Domestic Animals, Bailliere Tindall, London, UK, 7th edition, 1992.
32. Ministry of Agricultural Fisheries (MAFF), "Manual of veterinary laboratory techniques," Technical Bulletin 18, Ministry of Agricultural Fisheries (MAFF), London, UK, 1979.
33. H. Y. Wannas, K. A. Dawood, and G. A. Gassem, "Prevalence of gastro-intestinal parasites in horses and donkeys in al diwaniyah governorate," AL-Qadisiya Journal of Veterinary and Medical Science, vol. 11, no. 1, pp. 148–155, 2012.
34. M. Getachew, A. Trawford, G. Feseha, and S. W. J. Reid, "Gastrointestinal parasites of working donkeys of Ethiopia," Global Veterinaria, vol. 6, no. 3, pp. 223–227, 2011.
35. W. Muhammad, S. K. Muhammad, Z. D. Aneela et al., "Prevalence of gastrointestinal parasites, chemotherapy and haematology of strongylosis in donkeys of District Lahore, Pakistan," International Journal of Current Microbiololgy and Applied Sciences, vol. 3, no. 7, pp. 198–207, 2014.
36. A. Regassa and E. Yimer, "Gastrointestinal parasites of equine in South Wollo zone, North Eastern Ethiopia," Global Veterinaria, vol. 11, no. 6, pp. 824–830, 2013.
37. N. Tesfu, B. Asrade, R. Abebe, and S. Kasaye, "Prevalence and risk factors of gastrointestinal nematode parasites of horse and donkeys in hawassa town, ethiopia," Journal of Veterinary Science & Technology, vol. 5, no. 5, 2014.
38. K. Saeed, Z. Qadir, K. Ashraf, and N. Ahmad, "Role of intrinsic and extrinsic epidemiological factors on strongylosis in horses," Journal of Animal and Plant Sciences, vol. 20, no. 4, pp. 277–280, 2010.
39. T. A. Kuzmina, Y. I. Kuzmin, and V. A. Kharchenko, "Field study on the survival, migration and overwintering of infective larvae of horse strongyles on pasture in central Ukraine," Veterinary Parasitology, vol. 141, no. 3-4, pp. 264–272, 2006. ·
40. G. M. Urquhart, J. Armour, J. L. Duncan, A. M. Dunn, and F. W. Jennings, Veterinary Parasitology, The Faculty of Veterinary Medicine, University of Glasgow Scotland, 2nd edition, 1996.
41. R. Binev, Z. Kirkova, J. Nikolov et al., "Efficacy of parenteral administration of ivermectin in the control of strongylidosis in donkeys," Journal of the South African Veterinary Association, vol. 76, no. 4, pp. 214–216, 2005.
42. H. I. Seri, A. D. Abakar, A. A. Ismail, and T. A. Tigani, "Efficacy of Ivermectin in an injectable formulation against gastrointestinal nematodes of donkeys (Equus asinus)," Veterinary Archives, vol. 75, no. 4, pp. 369–374, 2005.
43. A. Sow, K. M. Kalandi, N. P. Ndiaye, A. Bathily, and G. J. Sawadogo, "Clinical and biochemical parameters of Burkinabese local donkey breeds," International Research Journal of Biochemistry and Bioinformatics, vol. 2, no. 4, pp. 84–89, 2012.

CHAPTER 14

MOLECULAR EPIDEMIOLOGY OF THEILERIA EQUI IN HORSES AND THEIR ASSOCIATION WITH POSSIBLE TICK VECTORS IN THE STATE OF RIO DE JANEIRO, BRAZIL

Maristela Peckle, Marcus S. Pires, Tiago M. dos Santos, Erica C. R. Roier, Claudia B. da Silva, Joice A. R. Vilela, Huarrisson A. Santos, Carlos L. Massard

INTRODUCTION

Equine theileriosis is a disease caused by an intra-erythrocytic protozoan Theileria equi(Laveran 1901) (Mehlhorn and Schein 1998) and is characterized by fever, anemia, jaundice, hepatomegaly, splenomegaly, and hemoglobinuria. However, most infected animals became asymptomatic carriers, acting as a source of infection for tick vectors (De Waal 1992). In these animals, a low parasitemia level often precludes microscopic diagnosis by Giemsa-stained blood smears (Böse et al. 1995).

The worldwide problem of equine piroplasmosis is considered the main impediment to the international movement of horses because positive or seropositive animals are denied either entry for sports competitions or final export into several countries considered free of the disease (Knowles 1996; Friedhoff 1990).

The biological agent transmission occurs via the inoculation of sporozoites in horses by a tick vector. To date, ten tick species from three distinct genera (Dermacentor, Rhipicephalus, and Hyalomma) have been identified in T. equi transmission (Mehlhorn and Schein 1998). Until now in the Americas, Dermacentor variabilis and Rhipicephalus microplus (Canestrini 1887) have been tick species identified as transmitters of T. equi in experimental conditions (Stiller and Coan 1995; Guimarães et al. 1998a; Ueti et al. 2005; Ueti et al. 2008). In Latin America, horses are regularly infested with three species of ticks: Dermacentor nitens, Rhipicephalus microplus, and Amblyomma cajennense (Borges and Leite 1998; Labruna et al. 2001; Da Costa Pereira et al. 2005). R. microplus has been implicated as a vector (Guimarães et al. 1998a, b; Ueti et al. 2005), but it is a monoxenic tick, and T. equi transovarial transmission has not yet been reported. Thus, its epidemiological importance has been questioned. The role of D. nitensin the transmission of T. equi has not been reported (Denning 1988). In addition to biological transmission, congenital and iatrogenic forms of transmission have been observed (Tenter and Friedhoff 1986; Allsopp et al. 2007; Santos et al. 2008).

Theileria equi remains in the infected animal body for years and possibly throughout the animal's life (Mehlhorn and Schein 1998). Thus, the real-time polymerase chain reaction (qPCR), which is highly sensitive and specific, is a molecular technique that can be used to quantify the actual circulation of the agent in the studied area, in addition to allowing the quantification and investigation of circulating strains. Few studies have been conducted using molecular tools to investigate the epidemiological aspects of equine theileriosis in Brazil.

This study aimed to detect T. equi in horses and ticks by qPCR and to relate the variables about the host, environment and potential tick vectors to the presence of T. equi DNA in horses domiciled in the Seropedica and Petropolis municipalities of the state of Rio de Janeiro, Brazil.

Citation: Peckle, M., Pires, M.S., dos Santos, T.M. et al., "Molecular epidemiology of Theileria equi in horses and their association with possible tick vectors in the state of Rio de Janeiro, Brazil," Parasitol Res (2013) 112: 2017. doi:10.1007/s00436-013-3360-0.

MATERIALS AND METHODS

Sampling

From January to May 2009, 30 properties with horses in the Seropedica and Petropolis municipalities of the state of Rio de Janeiro, Brazil, were analyzed. The sampling was calculated according to an equation described by Sampaio (2002), and the collection was performed by convenience in the studied area, with an assumed expected frequency of 59 % (Heim et al.2007), an error of 5 % and an accuracy of 9 %. Blood samples were collected from 314 horses (n=173 in Petropolis and n=141 in Seropedica), and 300 samples were collected from ticks on these horses.

After the horse owners consented to the procedure, the animals were inspected for the presence of ticks, and the infestation level was assessed, followed by the collection of ticks. The blood samples were collected by jugular venipuncture and placed under vacuum in sterile tubes containing ethylenediamine tetraacetic acid (EDTA) anticoagulant.

An average of ten tick specimens in various developmental stages was collected from the different body parts of each infested animal. The taxonomic identification was based on the dichotomous keys of Aragão and Fonseca (1961) and Barros-Battesti et al. (2006). After identification, these specimens were stored in polypropylene tubes containing isopropyl alcohol according to the species, developmental stage, and sexual dimorphism. The infestation level of the ticks on the horses was measured subjectively based on the observation of adult tick specimens on the horses, categorized, and sorted into two infestation levels (absent/low or moderate/high) according to Labruna et al. (2001).

Epidemiological Questionnaire

To assess the possible factors associated with infection by T. equi in the horses, a semi-structured questionnaire about the horses and the breeding and property management characteristics was administered to the owners. The factors investigated by the questionnaire were organized as follows: municipalities of Seropedica (low-altitude regions, less than 400 m in elevation) or Petropolis (high-altitude regions, more than 400 m in elevation); satisfactory or unsatisfactory zootechnical and sanitary management (Santos et al. 2011); presence or absence of ticks on animals; horses bred in close contact with cattle (cattle and horses shared the same pasture or were located close in proximity) or without contact with cattle; confined breeding system (confined system: animals had no access to outside areas and were restricted to the bay) or semi-confined/extensive system (limited access or total access to pasture areas); activities of the horses (sport/exhibition; work/walk or recreation; reproduction); gender (male or female); age (≤ 2 years old or >2 years old); racial definition (breeded horses or mixed-breed horses).

DNA Extraction

The extraction of deoxyribonucleic acid (DNA) from the blood samples was performed from 300 μL of blood using the Wizard® Genomic DNA Purification kit according to manufacturer's recommendations.

For the DNA extraction from the tick samples, the specimens corresponding to each developmental stage were macerated in pools (nymphs=ten copies; larvae=ten copies; not engorged females=two copies; males=three copies), with the exception of the engorged females, which were macerated individually. After this step, genomic DNA was extracted based on the protocol for genomic DNA extraction according to Ferreira and Grattapaglia (1998). Each group of 11 samples had a control sample containing ultrapure water to rule out contamination during DNA extraction.

The DNA samples were resuspended in 200 μL of Tris–EDTA, quantified using the spectrophotometer Nanodrop ND-2000®, standardized at a concentration of 60 ng/μL and stored at −20 °C until use.

Real-Time PCR Assay

The detection of T. equi DNA was performed using a TaqMan PCR system in a Real-Time StepOne Plus® instrument to amplify the 81-bp fragment of the 18S rRNA gene. The assay used the Be18SF (5′-GCGGTGTTTCGGTGATTCATA-3′) and Be18SR (5′-TGATAGGTCAGAAACTTGAATGATACATC-3′) primer set and a fluorescent hydrolysis probe, Be18SP (5′-AAATTAGCGAATCGCATGGCTT-3′), which was labeled at the 5' end with the reporter dye 6-carboxyfluorescein and the 3' end with the quencher dye 6-carboxy-tetramethylrhodamine (Kim et al. 2008). The reactions were performed in duplicate on different plates with a final volume of 12 μL, which contained: 1X TaqMan® Universal PCR Master Mix, 450 nM of each primer, the 250 nM of hydrolysis probe and 180 ng of total DNA.

The thermocycling conditions were 50 °C for 2 min, 95 °C for 10 min, and 45 cycles at 95 °C for 20 s, followed by 55 °C for 1 min (Kim et al. 2008). The quantification cycle (C_q) was standardized between plates and was manually allocated three cycles after the fluorescence base. Samples with C_q values less than or equal to 40 cycles were considered positive.

The analytical sensitivity of the assay was determined by evaluating the serial decimal dilutions of the 18S rRNA gene of T. equi cloned into the plasmid pGEM-T® Easy Vector System. The sensitivity of the real-time PCR was evaluated with and without the addition of 1 μL of DNA from an uninfected blood sample and the addition of 1 μL DNA from an uninfected tick. The concentration and purity of the plasmid DNA were measured by spectrophotometer Nanodrop ND-2000®. The concentration of the plasmid DNA was the basis for calculating the plasmid number. For determining the analytical sensitivity of the qPCR, a curve was created using five points, which were plotted as the number of copies of plasmid based on C_q values. The number of copies ranged from 3×10^4 to 3, and four separate dilutions were performed for each point on the curve.

Statistical Analysis

The horses' positivity for T. equi, as determined by qPCR, was examined for association with epidemiological questionnaire variables using the chi-squared or Fisher's exact tests at a 20 % significance level.

Among the independent variables that were statistically significant ($p<0.20$) in the bivariate analysis, the Spearman correlation test was applied to check the collinearity and to eliminate highly correlated variables from the logistic regression model. In this test, the independent variables with $p<0.05$ and $\rho<0.6$ were included in the multiple logistic regression model. Among the two highly correlated variables ($p<0,05$ and $\rho\geq 0,6$), the one most biologically important was kept in the model.

A multiple logistic regression model was performed with the dependent variable (horses with molecular positivity for T. equi), which was dichotomous (negative=0, positive=1), as a function of the independent variables presented in the epidemiological questionnaire, at a 5 % level of significance.

In the tick samples, the presence of the infectious agent DNA was evaluated according to the species collected (using the genus, evolutionary stage, and the studied municipalities) by the chi-squared or Fisher's exact tests at a 5 % significance level.

For the verification of the isolated effect of the presence of a tick variable on the presence of T.equi DNA in horses, a logistic regression model was established using a qualitative dichotomous variable (absence=0 or presence=1) for each tick species in relation to the presence of T. equi DNA in the horses. Based on these results, another simple logistic regression model was created to evaluate the level of A. cajennense infestation according to the presence of T. equi DNA in the animals. This tick infestation level was a qualitative and dichotomous variable (absent/low=0 or moderate/high=1) (Labruna et al. 2001).

All final logistic regression models were analyzed by a likelihood ratio. Statistical analyses were performed using the R programming package within the graphical interface R-Studio (Development Core Team 2010, http://www.r-project.org).

RESULTS

The analytical sensitivity of the qPCR technique was evaluated using a known number of copies of the vector-insert. The detection limit of the technique was three copies of the plasmid containing the 18S rRNA gene. The determination coefficient of four replications of five dilutions tested in the standard curve was 99 %, with varying C_q 22.64±0.15 cycles in the first dilution (3×10^4 copies of plasmid) to 35.73±0.38 cycles in last dilution (three copies of the plasmid) (Figure 1). No significant difference ($p>0.05$) in analytical sensitivity when 1 µL of uninfected equine blood and tick DNA was added to the PCR. The curves show the same slope during the exponential phase of the amplification reaction demonstrating the efficiency of 97.65 %, even a point with few targets (Figure 2).

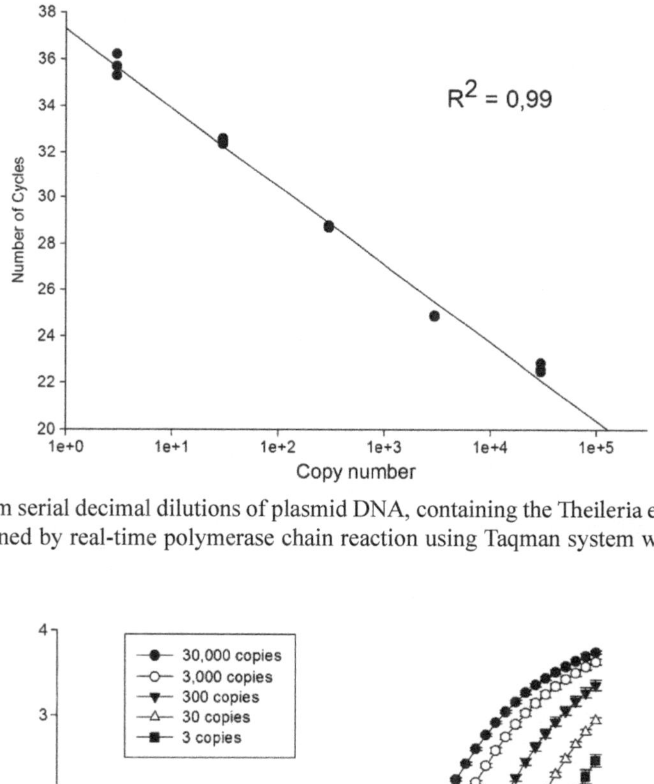

Figure 1: Standard curve plotted from serial decimal dilutions of plasmid DNA, containing the Theileria equi 18S rRNA gene (~1,600 bp). The quantification cycle (C_q) value obtained by real-time polymerase chain reaction using Taqman system was plotted as a function of the initial number of plasmid copies.

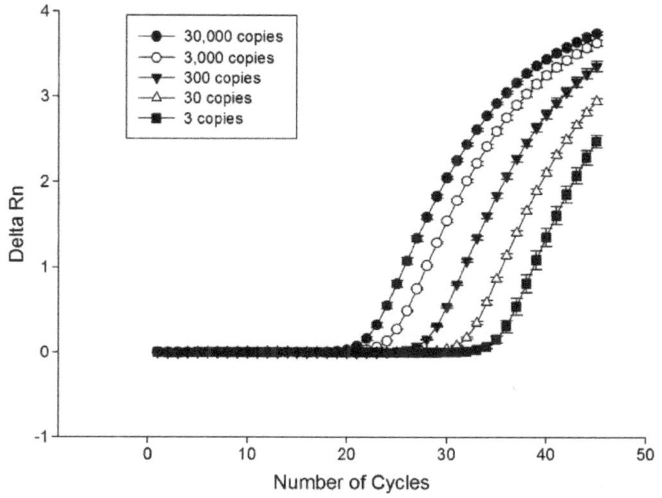

Figure 2: Real-time polymerase chain reaction analytical sensitivity, showing the amplification curves of plasmid DNA, containing the Theileria equi 18S rRNA gene (~1,600 bp), in serial dilutions (3–30,000 copies).

Of the equine analyzed samples, 81 % (n=253/314) exhibited fragmented amplification of the 81 bp of the 18S rRNA gene specific for T. equi by qPCR. With regard to the analyzed cities, 91 % (n=128/141) of the horses in Seropedica were considered positive for T. equi, significantly higher ($p<0.001$) than the percentage of positive horses in Petropolis (72 %, n=125/173) (Table 1).

Table 1: Bivariate and multivariate analysis of factors associated to Theileria equi infection in horses, by real-time PCR, according to animal characteristics, locality, zootechnical and sanitary management, contact with cattle, animals activity, breeding systems, ticks infestation in Petropolis and Seropedica municipalities, Rio de Janeiro, Brazil

Characteristic of the animals and management	**Real-time PCR**		**Bivariate**		**Multivariate**		
	Number of animals sampled	**Positives (%)**	χ^2	***P***	***P***	**OR**	**CI 95 %**
Gender							
Male	194	80.00	0.003	0.956	–	–	–
Female	120	80.93					
Age							
≤2 years	42	78.57	0.020	0.887	–	–	–
>2 years	272	80.88					
Racial definition							
Mixed breed	140	83.57	0.444	0.505	–	–	–
Defined breed	174	78.16					
Locality							
Petropolis (>400 m)	173	72.25	15.870	0.000	–[a]		
Seropedica (<400 m)	141	90.78			0.39	–	0.6–3.2
Zootechnical and sanitary management							
Satisfactory	150	66.67	33.803	0.000[b]	–	–	–
Unsatisfactory	164	93.29					
Contact with cattle							
No	218	77.06	4.900	0.027	–[a]		
Yes	96	88.54			0.48	–	0.2–1.8
Activity							
Sport/exposition	118	61.02	46.200	0.000	–[a]		
Work/walk	127	92.13			0.00	5.75	2.2–14.4
Reproduction	69	92.75			0.02	3.85	1.3–11.5
Breeding system							
Confined	19	78.95	–	0.970[c]	–	–	–
Extensive/semi-extensive	295	78.64					
Ticks infestation							
No	153	67.97	28.713	0.000	–[a]		
Yes	161	92.55			0.03	2.63	1.1–6.2
Animals' origin							
Inside property	98	84.69	1.186	0.276	–	–	–
Outside property	216	78.70					

χ^2 value of chi-square test, P p value, OR odds ratio, CI confidence interval

[a]Category reference

[b]Removed from the multivariate analysis due to collinearity verified by Spearman test

[c]Fisher's exact test

The variables inherent to equines, such as gender, racial definition, and age, were not associated with T. equi positivity ($p>0.20$). However, with regard to variables related to ownership and breeding, municipality ($p<0.0001$), property management ($p<0.00001$), tick infestation of the animals ($p<0.0001$), the horses in contact with cattle ($p=0.027$), and the equine activity on-property ($p<0.0001$) were associated with the presence of T. equi DNA in the samples ($p<0.20$) (Table 1).

In the logistic regression model, only the equine activity on-property ($p<0.00001$) and tick infestation ($p=0.02$) were associated with T. equi infection. The property management variable ($p<0.00001$) was removed from the multivariate analysis because it presented collinearity with the variable for the ticks infestation ($p<0.00001$ and $\rho=0.6$).

Compared with the horses that had activities related to sports or exhibition, the horses with activities related to work (draft animals in agriculture, riding animals for cattle handling) or walking (people transportation and recreation) were 5.75 times (CI, 2.3–14.4) more likely to be infected by T. equi. The horses with reproductive activity were 3.8 times (CI, 1.3–11.5) more likely to have the infection. Horses with an infestation of ticks were 2.6 times (CI, 1.1–6.2) more likely to present T. equi DNA.

Tick infestations were identified in 51.3 % (n=161/314) of the evaluated horses. A. cajennense and D. nitens were found on these infected horses with frequencies of 47.8 % (n=150/314) and 31.8 % (n=100/314), respectively. Infestation with these two tick species was identified in 28.3 % (n=89/314) of the evaluated horses. Among the 300 collected ticks, 63.7 % (n=191/300) were identified as A. cajennense and 34.7 % (n=104/300) as D. nitens. The ticks were primarily adults (n=274/300, 91.3 %), followed by nymphs (n=21/300, 7 %) and larvae (n=5/300, 1.7 %). The specimens collected at an immature stage of development were identified taxonomically as larvae Ixodida. In relation to the ticks' gender, 61 % (n=183/300) were identified as females and 30.3 % (n=91/300) as males.

Regarding the detection of T. equi DNA in the evaluated ticks, 7.7 % (n=23/300) of the ticks were positive. Furthermore, 9.9 % (n=19/191) of the A. cajennense and 3.8 % of the D. nitens(n=4/104) had amplified the 81-bp fragment from the T. equi 18S rRNA gene, with no statistically significant difference ($p=0.07$) between the species (Table 2). Nevertheless, it is noteworthy that although not significantly different in frequency, the A. cajennense samples were 2.6 times more likely to be considered positive for T. equi than the D. nitens samples. TheT. equi DNA fragment was not detected in the nymphs (n=0/21) or larvae (n=0/5) samples. The males were significantly more likely ($p<0.05$) to be positive for T. equi (15.4 %, n=14/91) than the females (4.9 %, n=9/183). The males were more likely ($p<0.05$) to be positive for T.equi (18.2 %, n=12/66) than the A. cajennense females (5.8 %, n=7/121). However, the D.nitens males (8 %, n=2/25) and females (3.2 %, n=2/62) did not significantly differ ($p>0.05$) in their positivity for T. equi (Table 2).

Table 2: Bivariate analysis of factors associated to Theileria equi infection in tick samples, by real-time PCR, according to samples characteristics, as locality, identified species, developmental stage, and tick gender in the state of Rio de Janeiro, Brazil

Tick samples characteristics	**Real-time PCR**		**Bivariate**	
	Number of animals sampled	**Positives (%)**	χ^2	***P***
Altitude				
<400 m (Seropedica)	238	6.69	–	0.28[a]
>400 m (Petropolis)	62	11.29		
Species				
Amblyomma cajennense	191	9.95	3.96	0.07[a]
Dermacentor nitens	104	3.85		
Developmental stage				
Adults	274	8.39	2.36	0.31
Nymphs	21	0.00		
Larvae	5	0.00		
Gender				
Male	91	15.38	11.77	0.00
Female	183	4.92		
Amblyomma cajennense				
Male	66	18.18	7.78	0.02
Female	121	5.79		
Nymphs	4	0.00		
Dermacentor nitens				

Male	25	8.00	1.91	0.38
Female	62	3.23		
Nymphs	17	0.00		

χ^2 value of chi-square test, P p value

[a]Fisher's exact test

The logistic regression model, which was applied to the tick species in relation to the presence ofT. equi DNA in the horses, indicated that the horses infested with A. cajennense were four times more likely to harbor T. equi (Table 3). Using a simple logistic regression model to evaluate the A. cajennense infestation level in comparison with the animals' positivity, the horses with moderate to high infestation were 2.7 times more likely to have T. equi DNA than the horses with low-level or no A. cajennense infestation (Table 4).

Table 3: Multivariate analysis of Theileria equi positivity in horses by real-time PCR, in relation to the tick species observed on animals in the state of Rio de Janeiro, Brazil

Ticks	Real-time PCR		Multivariate		
	Number of animals sampled	**Positives (%)**	***P***	**OR**	**CI**
Amblyomma cajennense					
Yes	150	92.7	0.00	4.10	(1.8–9.1)
No	164	69.5	–[a]	–	–
Dermacentor nitens					
Yes	100	93.0	0.18	–	–
No	214	74.8	–[a]	–	–

P p value, OR odds ratio, CI confidence interval

[a]Category reference

Table 4: Simple logistic regression model to evaluate the Amblyomma cajennense infestation level in comparison with the animals′ positivity for Theileria equi in the state of Rio de Janeiro, Brazil

Amblyomma cajennense	Real-time PCR		Logistic regression		
	Number of animals sampled	**Positives (%)**	***P***	**OR**	**CI**
Infestation level					
Moderate/many	74	90.5	0.01	2.77	(1.2–6.4)
None/few	240	77.5	–[a]	–	–

P p value, OR odds ratio, CI confidence interval

[a]Category reference

DISCUSSION

This epidemiological study reinforces the endemic character that equine theileriosis assumes in Brazil (Pfeifer-Barbosa et al. 1995; Heuchert et al. 1999; Golynski et al. 2008; Kerber et al. 2009; Santos et al. 2011). In addition, this study highlights the possible factors relevant to properties, breed management, and animal characteristics that are associated with T. equi presence in horses. It also demonstrates the importance of epidemiology as a vector research tool to understand the possible role of other tick species in addition to R. microplus in the transmission and spread of T. equi in Brazil.

The high frequency of T. equi among the horses in the studied municipalities is in agreement with several serological studies conducted in areas located near the studied municipalities (Pfeifer-Barbosa et al. 1995; Santos et al. 2011). However, importantly, this study detected T.equi DNA using qPCR, a highly sensitive and specific technique used in many molecular epidemiology investigations (Monis et al. 2005).

The municipality of Seropedica, which is located in the low-altitude region of the state of Rio de Janeiro, has a semi-humid tropical climate, with an annual average temperature of approximately 24 °C. In contrast, the municipality of Petropolis, which is located in the high-altitude region of the state, has a tropical climate and an annual average temperature of approximately 16 °C, with winter temperatures that may reach 0 °C. The conditions encountered by tick vectors in high-altitude cities such as Petropolis are less favorable for their development and reproduction, which contributed to the lower tick infestation and the lower frequency of T.equi infection in the horses in that location (Davey and Cooksey 1989; Chacón et al. 2003). Furthermore, management conditions and the quality of the properties found in Petropolis are better than those of properties in Seropedica.

According to the bivariate analysis, the T. equi positivity of the horses bred in close contact with cattle was significantly different from the T. equi positivity of the horses bred in the absence of cattle. This observation suggests a possible involvement of R. microplus on the epidemiological chain of equine theileriosis in the studied region. Experimental studies indicate that R.microplus is capable of being infected and is capable of transmitting the equine theileriosis agent when feeding on horses chronically infected or with an acute infection of T. equi(Guimarães et al. 1998a, b; Stiller et al. 2002; Ueti et al. 2008). Furthermore, horses with an infestation of R. microplus have been observed in areas where cattle graze (Bittencourt 1990; Labruna et al. 2001). However, it is unlikely that R. microplus plays an important role in the equine theileriosis enzootic cycle in the studied region because this study found no horses infested by this tick species. Perhaps other forms of transmission or other arthropods may be involved in maintaining the high level of the disease observed in the studied area.

The horses activities related to work, walking, and reproduction were factors that determined the infection with T. equi. This finding was observed by Abutarbush et al. (2012), in which the animals used for work showed a higher frequency of T. equi positivity, which differed significantly from other variables, such as the animals raised for practicing polo, running, jumping, reproduction, and exposure. These findings may also be related to the activities that the horse exerts on the property, where in many cases, the animals with work or walking activities also move into large pasture perimeters and increase their chances of infestation by potential tick vectors. Furthermore, animals with work, walking, and reproduction activities often live on properties that have poor management (Santos et al. 2011; Heuchert et al. 1999), are in close contact with cattle in pastures infested by different tick species (Heuchert et al.1999), and have a grazing habit (Abutarbush et al. 2012; Nizoli et al. 2008), so they are at increased risk of contact with tick vectors. In our study, we observed that animals destined for sports and exposure activities receive management considered ideal for these types of breeding, with appropriate zootechnical buildings where the animals receive balanced meals, systematic veterinary care, and sanitary control; thus, they are at decreased risk of tick vector infestation.

The experimental transmission of T. equi is associated with Rhipicephalus ticks (Guimarães et al. 1998a, b; Stiller and Coan 1995; De Waal 1992; Ueti et al. 2005). However, to date, there are no reports that demonstrate the truly natural vector of this etiologic agent of importance in horses worldwide. Studies suggest that the species A. cajennense can act as a natural vector (Scoles et al. 2011; Kerber et al. 2009) of this agent because of its increased dispersion and predilection for horses. Nevertheless, in an experimental study conducted by Ribeiro et al. (2011), T. equi infection was not observed in A. cajennense that fed on horses with an acute or chronic infection. This study demonstrated that A. cajennense is associated with the presence ofT. equi DNA in horses, but the participation of A. cajennense as a natural vector remains unclear. Thus, the high frequency of A. cajennense infestation among the horses may be considered a confounding factor in the epidemiological analysis. In support of this confounding factor are studies demonstrating that T. equi can be transmitted congenitally in equines (Santos et al. 2008), making vector investigation through epidemiological analysis difficult. However, in a study conducted in Texas in the USA, Scoles et al. (2011) found that A. cajennense was capable of becoming naturally infected by T. equi and was able to experimentally transmit it when feeding on infection-free horses, demonstrating that T. equi can be transmitted in an interstadial way by this tick species.

In this study, A. cajennense males were significantly more likely than females to have T. equiDNA. The A. cajennense males are able to feed on various hosts during their lifecycle, increasing their chances of becoming infected with T. equi, and they survive for long fasting periods (Serra-Freire 1982; Oliveira et al. 2003). These characteristics make them important transmitters of etiologic agents in animals and humans.

The high frequency of T. equi in horses in Brazil and around the world suggests that the natural vector is abundant among the animals, is common in all locations where horse breeding occurs, and is capable of transmitting T. equi from an infected animal to a susceptible one. Therefore, epidemiologically, A. cajennense could be a suitable vector in the studied area because it requires three hosts to complete its life cycle, is distributed throughout the Americas, and seems to prefer horses as the hosts for all parasitic stages (Aragão 1936; Oliveira et al. 2000). In this study, the horses infested with A. cajennense at moderate or high levels were more likely to be infected with T. equi, corroborating previous findings.

The qPCR technique was an excellent tool for epidemiological hemoparasite investigation because T. equi has a chronic nature in the equine organism. Infestation by ticks and animal activities are factors associated with T. equi infection in the studied region. Among the investigated ticks, A. cajennense was the species epidemiologically regarded as a potential biological vector of this piroplasma under natural conditions in the studied area.

ACKNOWLEDGMENTS

The authors thank the owners of the animals used in the study, due to availability, trust, and patience. This research was supported by National Council for Scientific and Technological Development (CNPq) of Brazil, 'Carlos Chagas Filho' Foundation for Research Support of the State of Rio de Janeiro (FAPERJ), and Coordination of Improvement of Higher Education Personnel (CAPES) funds. The authors are also grateful for the statistical assistance provided by Professor Wagner Tassinari (Mathematics Department at Universidade Federal Rural do Rio de Janeiro).

REFERENCES

1. Abutarbush SM, Alqawasmeh DM, Mukbel RM, Al-Majali AM (2012) Equine Babesiosis: seroprevalence, risk factors and comparison of different diagnostic methods in Jordan. Transbound Emerg Dis 59:72–78. doi:10.1111/j.1865-1682.2011.01244.x
2. Allsopp MTEP, Lewis BD, Penzhorn BL (2007) Molecular evidence for transplacental transmission of Theileria equi from carrier mares to their apparently healthy foals. Vet Parasitol 148:130–136. doi:10.1016/j.vetpar.2007.05.017
3. Aragão H (1936) Ixodidas brasileiros e de alguns paizes limitrophes. Mem Inst Oswaldo Cruz 31:759–843.

doi:10.1590/S0074-02761936000400004

4. Aragão H, Fonseca F (1961) Notas de Ixodologia. VIII lista e chave para os representantes para a fauna ixodológica brasileira. Mem Inst Oswaldo Cruz 59:115–129. doi:10.1590/S0074-02761961000200001
5. Barros-Battesti DM, Arzua M, Bechara GH (2006) Carrapatos de Importância Médico-Veterinária da Região Neotropical: Um guia ilustrado para identificação de espécies. VOX/ICTTD-3/BUTANTAN,São Paulo
6. Bittencourt AJ (1990) Boophilus microplus (Canestrini, 1887): (Infestações artificiais, biologia da fase não parasitária e prevalências em caprinos e equinos). Dissertation, Universidade Federal Rural do Rio de Janeiro
7. Böse R, Jorgensen WK, Dalgliesh RJ, Friehoff KT, De Vos AJ (1995) Current state and future trends in the diagnosis of babesiosis. Vet Parasitol 57:61–74. doi:10.1016/0304-4017(94)03111-9
8. Borges LMF, Leite RC (1998) Ixodological populations of the ears of equines in Minas Gerais and Bahia, Brazil. Braz J Vet Anim Sci 50:87–89
9. Chacón SC, Correia PG, Barbieri FS, Daemon E, Faccini JLH (2003) Efeito de três temperaturas constantes sobre a fase não parasitária de Amblyomma cajennense (Fabricius, 1787) (Acari: ixodidae). Braz J Vet Parasitol 12:13–20
10. Da Costa Pereira MAV, Massard CL, Faccini JLH, Siqueira LFG (2005) Variação da sorotitulação ao teste de Fixação de Complemento para Babesia equi e Babesia caballi em equinos da região Serrana do Rio de Janeiro. Ars Vet 21:338–343
11. Davey RB, Cooksey LM (1989) Effects of prolonged exposure at low temperature on Boophilus microplus (Acari: Ixodidae). J Med Entomol 26:407–410
12. De Waal DT (1992) Equine piroplasmosis: a review. Br Vet J 148:6–14. doi:10.1016/0007-1935(92)90061-5
13. Denning F (1988) Unsuccessful attempts at transmission of Babesia equi by Anocentor nitensand Amblyomma cajennense. Dissertation, Hannover Veterinary College.
14. Ferreira ME, Grattapaglia D (1998) Introdução ao uso de marcadores moleculares em análise genética. EMBRAPA-CENARGEN, Brasil
15. FriedhoffKT, TenterAM, MullerI(1990)Haemoparasites of equines: impact on international trade of horses. Rev Sci Tech 9:1187–1194
16. Golynski AA, Fernandes KR, Baldani CD, Golynski AL, Madeiro AS, Machado RZ, Botteon PTL, Massard CL (2008) Estudo soroepidemiológico da Babesia equi em equinos do estado do Rio Grande do Sul, Brasil, determinado pelos testes de imunofluorescência indireta e Elisa. Braz J Vet Parasitol 17:317–321. doi:10.1590/S1984-29612010000100001
17. Guimarães AM, Lima JD, Ribeiro MFB, Camargos ERS, Bozzi IA (1998a) Ultrastructure of sporogony in Babesia equi in salivary glands of adult female Boophilus microplus ticks. Parasitol Res 60:69–74. doi:10.1007/s004360050359
18. Guimarães AM, Lima JD, Ribeiro MFB (1998b) Sporogony and experimental transmission ofBabesia equi by Boophilus microplus. Parasitol Res 84:323–327. doi:10.1007/s004360050404
19. Heim A, Passos LF, Ribeiro MFB, Costa-Júnior L, Bastos CV, Cabral DD, Hirzmann J, Pfister K (2007) Detection and molecular characterization of Babesia caballi and Theileria equi isolates from endemic areas of Brazil. Parasitol Re 102:63–68. doi:10.1007/s00436-007-0726-1
20. Heuchert CMS, Giulli V, Athaide DF, Böse R, Friedhoff KT (1999) Seroepidemiologic studies onBabesia equi and Babesia caballi infections in Brazil. Vet Parasitol 85:1–11. doi:10.1016/S0304-4017(99)00108-9
21. Kerber CE, Labruna MB, Ferreira F, De Waal DT, Knowles DP, Gennari SM (2009) Prevalence of equine Piroplasmosis and its association with tick infestation in the state of São Paulo, Brazil. Braz J Vet Parasitol 18:1–8. doi:10.4322/rbpv.01804001
22. Kim C, Blanco LBC, Alhassan A, Iseki H, Yokoyama N, Xuan X, Igarashi I (2008) Diagnostic real-time PCR assay for the quantitative detection of Theileria equi from equine blood samples. Vet Parasitol 151:158–163. doi:10.1016/j.vetpar.2007.10.023
23. Knowles D Jr (1996) Equine babesiosis (Piroplasmosis): a problem in the international movement of horses. Br Vet J 52:123–126
24. Labruna MB, Kerber CE, Ferreira F, Faccini JLH, De Waal DT, Genari SN (2001) Risk factors to tick infestations and their occurrence on horses in the state of São Paulo, Brazil. Vet Parasitol 97:1–14. doi:10.1016/S0304-4017(01)00387-9
25. Mehlhorn H, Schein E (1998) Redescription of Babesia equi Laveran, 1901 as Theileria equiMehlhorn, Schein 1998. Parasitol Res 84:467–475. doi:10.1007/s004360050431
26. Monis PT, Giglio S, Keegan AR, Thompson RCA (2005) Emerging technologies for the detection and genetic characterization of protozoan parasites. Trends Parasitol 21:340–346. doi:10.1016/j.pt.2005.05.012
27. Nizoli LQ, Götze MM, Félix SR, Silva SS, Nogueira CEW (2008) Frequency of seropositive equines for Theileria equi in the southern Rio Grande do Sul State, Brazil. Parasitol Latinoam 63:46–50. doi:10.4067/S0717-77122008000100008
28. Oliveira PR, Borges LMF, Leite RC, Freitas CMV (2003) Seasonal dynamics of the Cayenne tick,Amblyomma cajennense on horses in Brazil. Med Vet Entomol 17:412–416. doi:10.1111/j.1365-2915.2003.00459.x
29. Oliveira PR, Borges LMF, Lopes CML, Leite RC (2000) Population dynamics of the free-living stages of Amblyomma cajennense (Fabricius, 1787) (Acari: Ixodidae) on pastures of Pedro Leopoldo, Minas Gerais State, Brazil. Vet Parasitol 92:295–301. doi:10.1016/S0304-4017(00)00322-8
30. Pfeifer-Barbosa IB, Bose R, Peymann B, Friedhoff KT (1995) Epidemiological aspects of equine babesioses in a herd of horses in Brazil. Vet Parasitol 58:1–8. doi:10.1016/0304-4017(94)00704-G

31. R Development Core Team (2010) R: a language and environment for statistical computing. R Fundation for Statistical Computing, Vienna, Austria. http://www.r-projetc.org. Accessed 31 jan 2010

32. Ribeiro MFB, Silveira JAG, Bastos CV (2011) Failure of the Amblyomma cajennense nymph to become infected by Theileria equi after feeding on acute or chronically infected horses. Exp Parasitol 128:324–327. doi:10.1016/j.exppara.2011.03.016

33. Sampaio IBM (2002) Estatística aplicada à experimentação animal. FEPMVZ, Belo Horizonte

34. Santos TM, Santos HA, Massard CL (2008) Diagnóstico molecular de babesiose congênita em potros neonatos no estado do Rio de Janeiro, Brasil. Braz J Vet Parasitol 17:348–350. doi:10.1590/S1984-29612010000100001

35. Santos TM, Roier ECR, Santos HA, Pires MS, Vilela JAR, Moraes LMB, Almeida FQ, Baldani CD, Machado RZ, Massard CL (2011) Factors associated to Theileria equi in equids of two microregions from Rio de Janeiro, Brazil. Braz J Vet Parasitol 20:235–241. doi:10.1590/S1984-29612011000300011

36. Scoles GA, Hutcheson HJ, Schlater JL, Hennager SG, Pelzel AM, Knowles PD (2011) Equine piroplasmosis associated with Amblyomma cajennense ticks, Texas, USA. Emerg Infect 17:1903–1905. doi:10.3201/eid1710.101182

37. Serra-Freire NM (1982) Epidemiologia de Amblyomma cajennense: Ocorrência estacional e comportamento dos estágios não parasitários em pastagens do Estado do Rio de Janeiro. Arq Univ Fed Rural Rio Jan 5:187–193

38. Stiller D, Coan ME (1995) Recent developments in elucidating tick vector relationships for anaplasmosis and equine piroplasmosis. Vet Parasitol 57:97–108. doi:10.1016/0304-4017(94)03114-C

39. Stiller D, Goff WL, Johnson LW, Knowles DP (2002) Dermacentor variabilis and Boophilus microplus (Acari: Ixodidae): experimental vectors of Babesia equi to equids. J Med Entomol 39:667–670. doi:10.1603/0022-2585-39.4.667

40. Tenter AM, Friedhoff KT (1986) Serodiagnosis of experimental and natural Babesia equi and B.caballi infections. Vet Parasitol 20:49–61. doi:10.1016/0304-4017(86)90092-0

41. Ueti WM, Palmer GH, Kappmeyer LS, Statfield M, Scoles GA, Knowles PD (2005) Ability of vector tick Boophilus microplus to acquire and transmit Babesia equi following feeding on chronically infected horses with low-level parasitemia. J Clin Microbiol 43:3755–3759. doi:10.1128/JCM.43.8.3755-3759.2005

42. Ueti WM, Palmer GH, Scoles GA, Kappmeyer LS, Knowles PD (2008) Persistently infected horses are reservoirs for intrastadial tick-borne transmission of the apicomplexan parasiteBabesia equi. Infect Immun 76:3525–3529. doi:10.1128/IAI.00251-08

CHAPTER 15

PREVALENCE OF ANTIBODIES TO LEISHMANIA INFANTUM AND TOXOPLASMA GONDII IN HORSES FROM THE NORTH OF PORTUGAL

Ana Patrícia Lopes, Susana Sousa, JP Dubey, Ana J Ribeiro , Ricardo Silvestre, Mário Cotovio, Henk DFH Schallig, Luís Cardoso and Anabela Cordeiro-da-Silva

Keywords: Antibodies, Horses, Leishmania infantum, Portugal, Toxoplasma gondii

FINDINGS

Protozoan parasites *Leishmania* spp. and *Toxoplasma gondii* are agents of zoonotic diseases with considerable importance worldwide [1, 2]. Leishmaniosis caused by *Leishmania infantum* (syn. *Leishmania chagasi*) is endemic in the Mediterranean basin (including Portugal), the Americas, and Asia. Dogs are the main reservoir of the parasite, which is transmitted among animals and to humans by phlebotomine sand flies [3]. Infection with *L. infantum* in humans may cause severe visceral or mild cutaneous clinical outcomes, while canine leishmaniosis is a relatively frequent chronic viscerocutaneous and even fatal illness [4]. Cases of presumed autochthonous cutaneous leishmaniosis in horses have been sporadically reported from southern [5] and Central Europe [6].

Toxoplasmosis can be the cause of morbidity and mortality in congenitally infected children and imunocompromised people [1]. Felids are the only recognized definitive hosts of the parasite, while a large variety of mammals, including human beings and horses, serve as intermediate hosts. The consumption of improperly cooked infected horse meat can be a risk to human health, sometimes with serious consequences [7]. Recently, public attention has been drawn to adulteration of beef with horse meat in Europe.

The present study aimed at estimating the seroprevalences of *L. infantum* and *T. gondii* in horses from the north of Portugal, since no information is available on these zoonotic agents among the regional equine population.

Between November 2008 and July 2010, blood from 173 horses living in the north of Portugal was collected from a jugular vein into EDTA tubes and plasma stored at -25°C until use. Information on gender, age, type of housing and ability (Table 1) was obtained by filling in a questionnaire. The average age was 9.3 years (standard deviation: 5.8 years). Based on physical examination and clinical history, horses were considered as sick if they had fever, anorexia and/or intolerance to exercise. Those animals with no detectable clinical signs were regarded as apparently healthy (Table 1). This study was approved by the University of Trás-os-Montes e Alto Douro Veterinary Teaching Hospital ethical committee as complying with the Portuguese legislation for the protection of animals (Law no. 92/1995, 12 September).

Citation: Lopes et al.: Prevalence of antibodies to Leishmania infantum and Toxoplasma gondii in horses from the north of Portugal. Parasites & Vectors 2013 6:178. doi:10.1186/1756-3305-6-178.

Table 1: Seropositivity among horses from the north of Portugal to *Leishmania infantum* and *Toxoplasma gondii* by gender, age group, type of housing, ability and clinical status

	Animals tested (n)	**Relative distribution (%)**	***L. infantum*-seropositive**		***T. gondii*-seropositive**	
			(n)	**(%)**	**(n)**	**(%)**
Gender						
Female	78	45.1	3	3.8	11	14.1
Male	30	17.3	2	6.7	1	3.3
Gelding	65	37.6	2	3.1	11	16.9
Age (years)						
1.5–6	48	27.7	3	6.3	5	10.4
7–612	76	43.9	1	1.3	8	10.5
13–630	49	28.3	3	6.1	10	20.4
Housing						
Indoors	73	42.2	3	4.1	6	8.2
Mixed/outdoors	99	57.2	4	4.0	17	17.2
Not determined	1	0.6	0	0.0	0	0.0
Ability						
Recreation	109	63.0	7	6.4	14	12.8
Farming	30	17.3	0	0.0	4	13.3
Sports	30	17.3	0	0.0	5	16.7
Not determined	4	2.3	0	0.0	0	0.0
Clinical status						
Apparently healthy	148	85.5	5	3.4	21	14.2
Sick	14	8.1	2	14.3	2	14.3
Not determined	11	6.4	0	0.0	0	0.0
Total	**173**	**100**	7	**4.0**	**23**	**13.3**

The direct agglutination test (DAT) for titration of immunoglobulin G (IgG) antibodies specific to *Leishmania* followed the general procedures described by Schallig *et al.* [8], using a standard freeze-dried antigen at a concentration of 5×10^7 promastigotes/ml (KIT Biomedical Research, Amsterdam, The Netherlands). Twofold dilution series ranging from 1:25 to 1:1600 were tested. Results obtained with the DAT are expressed as an antibody titre, i.e. the reciprocal of the highest dilution at which agglutination (large diffuse blue mats) is still clearly visible after 18 h incubation at room temperature. Plasma from a horse from the north of Portugal with cutaneous leishmaniosis (J. Elias and col., personal communication) and a DAT titre of 200 was used as positive control. Plasma from another horse (DAT titre<25) that lived in a non-endemic region was used as negative control. To maximize specificity and sensitivity of the DAT, a cut-off titre of 200 was chosen for seropositivity.

The plasma samples were tested for IgG antibodies to *T. gondii* with a modified agglutination test (MAT) commercial kit (Toxo-Screen DA®, bioMérieux, Lyon, France) following the manufacturer's instructions. Sera were analysed at the dilutions of 1:20, 1:40, 1:80 and 1:160. Positive and negative controls supplied with the kit were included in each plate. MAT positive results had visible agglutination (at least one half of the well's diameter) after 5–18 h of incubation at room temperature. A cut-off titre of 20 (2 IU/ml in relation to a WHO international reference serum) was chosen to maximize both sensitivity and specificity of the test [9, 10].

Chi-square or Fisher's exact tests were used to compare percentages, including positivity levels among categories of the same independent variables (i.e. gender, age, type of housing, ability and clinical status) and total prevalences of antibodies to each one of the two agents. Exact binomial test established confidence intervals (CI) for the totals, with a 95% confidence level. Analyses were carried out using StatLib and SPSS 11.5 software for Windows, with a probability (p) value <0.05 regarded as statistically significant [11].

Table 1 summarizes results. The seven (4.0%; 95% CI: 1.6–8.2) horses seropositive to *L. infantum* had titres of 200 (n=5), 800 (n=1) and≥1600 (n=1). The 166 horses seronegative to *L. infantum* had titres of<25 (n=156), 25 (n=2) and 50 (n=8). The 23 (13.3%; 95% CI: 8.6–19.3) horses seropositive to *T. gondii* had titres of 20 (n=13), 40 (n=5), 80 (n=3) and≥160 (n=2). No horse was simultaneously seropositive to *L. infantum* and *T. gondii*.

This is the first epidemiological investigation on equine *Leishmania* and *T. gondii* infections in the north of Portugal, a region where both agents have previously been found to be endemic in other hosts species [12,13]. A higher level of exposure to *T. gondii* in comparison with *L. infantum* has been revealed in horses from northern Portugal, but gender, age, type of housing, ability and clinical status had no significant influence on the seropositivity to both parasites. The fact that no horse was simultaneously seropositive to *L. infantum* and*T. gondii* is a good indicator of the high specificity of the direct agglutination tests under use (i.e. the DAT and MAT).

Also by using the DAT, seroprevalences of *Leishmania* in dogs from the north of Portugal have been shown to range from less than 5% [14] to approximately 20% [12]. In domestic cats from this region prevalence found by means of the same serological test was 1.9% [15]. This is the first report of the DAT being used to investigate *Leishmania* infection in horses in Europe.

To the best of our knowledge, in Portugal only two clinical cases of equine cutaneous leishmaniosis have been reported: one from the north (J. Elias and col., personal communication) and the other one from the south-central region of Lisbon [16]. As previously observed in dogs, cats and humans, in areas of endemicity, the prevalence of subclinical *Leishmania* infection in horses is considerably higher than that of the disease [2, 15,17].

In northern Portugal, out of 57 female *Phlebotomus ariasi* and *Phlebotomus perniciosus*, 38.6% were found to have fed on humans, 19.3% on dogs, 12.3% on chicken and 29.8% on other species, but no sand flies were detected with equine blood [18]. Nevertheless, in Spain *P. perniciosus* has been shown to feed on horses [19], a fact that does not exclude equines from taking part in the epidemiology of *L. infantum*.

Worldwide seroprevalences of *T. gondii* in horses were summarized by Dubey and Beattie [20] and Dubey [1]. In general, seroprevalence in horses is lower than in other livestock species and prevalences were higher in domestic than in wild horses [1]. The MAT titre that should be considered specific for the detection of antibodies to *T. gondii* in horses is unknown because only a few attempts have been made to isolate viable *T. gondii* from naturally exposed horses. Judging from results obtained with other species, a MAT titer of 20 is considered specific for the detection of antibodies to *T. gondii*. In the present study, 10 of the 23 seropositive horses had a titre of 40 or higher. Viable *T. gondii* was isolated from horses even with a very low titer of 4 in the Sabin Feldman dye test and horses experimentally infected with *T. gondii* oocysts do develop high MAT titres [9].

Horses are considered clinically resistant to toxoplasmosis and there are no confirmed cases of clinical toxoplasmosis in these animals [1]. The results of the present study indicate that horses in the north of Portugal are exposed to *T. gondii* and so their tissues might harbour parasitic cysts. The voluntary consumption of horse meat by people is not a common habit in Portugal, but the risk of *T. gondii* transmission from horses to humans should not be neglected due to the recent contamination of beef with horse meat noticed in Europe. Infections with *T. gondii* are common in food animals and humans in northern Portugal [13,21].

CONCLUSIONS

In conclusion, horses are commonly exposed to and may be infected with *L. infantum* and *T. gondii* in areas where these zoonotic parasites are endemic, such as the north of Portugal. The degree of involvement of horses in the specific transmission of these agents to other hosts including humans is yet to be defined at the local level. However, in any case should equine infections with *L. infantum* or *T. gondii* be underestimated, respectively, as a potential cause of disease for horses themselves and as a risk to public health.

ACKNOWLEDGEMENTS

The authors would like to thank Dr. José M. Maia for collecting and characterizing samples from horses. This work was funded by FEDER funds through the Operational Competitiveness Programme – COMPETE and by National funds through FCT – Fundação para a Ciência e a Tecnologia under the project FCOMP-01-0124-FEDER-014658 (PTDC/CVT/110732/2009). RS was supported by Programa Ciência, financed by Programa Operacional Potencial Humano – Quadro de Referência Estratégica Nacional – Tipologia 4.2 – Promocão do Emprego Científico, cofunded by Fundo Social Europeu and national funding from the Ministry of Science, Technology and Higher Education.

AUTHORS' CONTRIBUTIONS

APL participated in serological testing and data analysis and drafted the manuscript; SS participated in serological testing and data analysis; JPD, RS, HDFHS and ACdS provided conceptual advice and reviewed the manuscript; AJR and MC collected samples and clinical data; LC participated in data analysis, helped to draft and revised the manuscript. All authors read and approved the final manuscript.

REFERENCES

1. Dubey JP: Toxoplasmosis of Animals and Humans. 2010, Boca Raton: CRC Press, 2
2. WHO: WHO Technical Report Series 949. Control of the Leishmaniases. 2010, Geneva: World Health Organization
3. Palatnik-de-Sousa CB, Day MJ: One Health: The global challenge of epidemic and endemic leishmaniasis. Parasit Vectors. 2011, 4: 197-10.1186/1756-3305-4-197.
4. Solano-Gallego L, Miró G, Koutinas A, Cardoso L, Pennisi MG, Ferrer L, Bourdeau P, Oliva G, Baneth G: LeishVet guidelines for the practical management of canine leishmaniosis. Parasit Vectors. 2011, 4: 86-10.1186/1756-3305-4-86.
5. Solano-Gallego L, Fernández-Bellon H, Serra R, Gállego M, Ramis A, Fondevila D, Ferrer L: Cutaneous leishmaniosis in three horses in Spain. Equine Vet J. 2003, 35: 320-323.
6. Müller N, Welle M, Lobsiger L, Stoffel MH, Boghenbor KK, Hilbe M, Gottstein B, Frey CF, Geyer C, Von Bomhard W: Occurrence of *Leishmania* sp. in cutaneous lesions of horses in Central Europe. Vet Parasitol. 2009, 166: 346-351. 10.1016/j.vetpar.2009.09.001.
7. Pomares C, Ajzenberg D, Bornard L, Bernardin G, Hasseine L, Dardé M-L, Marty P: Toxoplasmosis and horse meat, France. Emerg Infect Dis. 2011, 17: 1327-1328. 10.3201/eid1707.101642.

8. Schallig HDFH, Schoone GJ, Beijer EGM, Kroon CCM, Hommers M, Özbel Y, Özensoy S, da Silva ES, Cardoso LM, da Silva ED: Development of a fast agglutination screening test (FAST) for the detection of anti-*Leishmania* antibodies in dogs. Vet Parasitol. 2002, 109: 1-8. 10.1016/S0304-4017(02)00268-6.
9. Dubey JP, Desmonts G: Serological responses of equids fed *Toxoplasma gondii* oocysts. Equine Vet J. 1987, 19: 337-339. 10.1111/j.2042-3306.1987.tb01426.x.
10. Boughattas S, Bergaoui R, Essid R, Aoun K, Bouratbine A: Seroprevalence of *Toxoplasma gondii* infection among horses in Tunisia. Parasit Vectors. 2011, 4: 218-10.1186/1756-3305-4-218.
11. Petrie A, Watson P: Statistics for Veterinary and Animal Science. 2006, Oxford: Blackwell Publishing, 2
12. Sousa S, Lopes AP, Cardoso L, Silvestre R, Schallig H, Reed SG, Cordeiro da Silva A: Seroepidemiological survey of*Leishmania infantum* infection in dogs from northeastern Portugal. Acta Trop. 2011, 120: 82-87. 10.1016/j.actatropica.2011.06.003.
13. Lopes AP, Dubey JP, Neto F, Rodrigues A, Martins T, Rodrigues M, Cardoso L: Seroprevalence of *Toxoplasma gondii*infection in cattle, sheep, goats and pigs from the North of Portugal for human consumption. Vet Parasitol. 2013, 193: 266-269. 10.1016/j.vetpar.2012.12.001.
14. Cardoso L, Mendão C, Madeira de Carvalho L: Prevalence of *Dirofilaria immitis*, *Ehrlichia canis*, *Borrelia burgdorferi*sensu lato, *Anaplasma* spp. and *Leishmania infantum* in apparently healthy and CVBD-suspect dogs in Portugal – a national serological study. Parasit Vectors. 2012, 5: 62-10.1186/1756-3305-5-62.
15. Cardoso L, Lopes AP, Sherry K, Schallig H, Solano-Gallego L: Low seroprevalence of *Leishmania infantum* infection in cats from northern Portugal based on DAT and ELISA. Vet Parasitol. 2010, 174: 37-42. 10.1016/j.vetpar.2010.08.022.
16. Rolão N, Martins MJ, João A, Campino L: Equine infection with *Leishmania* in Portugal. Parasite. 2005, 12: 183-186. 10.1051/parasite/2005122183.
17. Fernández-Bellon H, Solano-Gallego L, Bardagí M, Alberola J, Ramis A, Ferrer L: Immune response to *Leishmania infantum* in healthy horses in Spain. Vet Parasitol. 2006, 135: 181-185. 10.1016/j.vetpar.2005.09.007.
18. Alves-Pires C, Novo MT, Sousa CA: Os flebótomos de Portugal. VII – Preferências hemáticas dos flebótomos (*Diptera, Psychodidae*) da região do Alto Douro. Bol Soc Port Entomol. 1992, 3: 607-613.
19. De Colmenares M, Portús M, Botet J, Dobaño C, Gállego M, Wolff M, Seguí G: Identification of blood meals of*Phlebotomus perniciosus* (Diptera: Psychodidae) in Spain by a competitive enzyme-linked immunosorbent assay biotin/avidin method. J Med Entomol. 1995, 32: 229-233.
20. Dubey JP, Beattie CP: Toxoplasmosis of Animals and Man. 1988, Boca Raton: CRC Press
21. Lopes AP, Dubey JP, Moutinho O, Gargaté MJ, Vilares A, Rodrigues M, Cardoso L: Seroepidemiology of *Toxoplasma gondii*infection in women from the North of Portugal in their childbearing years. Epidemiol Infect. 2012, 31: 1-6.

CHAPTER 16 SEROPREVALENCE OF TOXOPLASMA GONDII IN HORSES AND DONKEYS IN YUNNAN PROVINCE, SOUTHWESTERN CHINA

Qiang Miao, Xi Wang, Li-Na She, Ya-Ting Fan, Fei-Zhou Yuan, Jian-Fa Yang, Xing-Quan Zhu and Feng-Cai Zou

BACKGROUND

Toxoplasma gondii is an important zoonotic parasite, which can infect humans and almost all warm-blood animals, with a worldwide distribution [1, 2, 3, 4, 5]. Toxoplasmosis is not only of great importance for livestock and causes huge economic loss to the livestock industry, it is also a public health problem owing to its transmission to humans by ingestion of uncooked meat containing tissue cysts, or consuming food or drink contaminated with oocysts, or accidental ingestion of sporulated oocysts from the environment [1, 2, 3, 4, 5]. Although *T. gondii* infection rarely displays obvious clinical symptoms in adults, it may lead to severe consequences in an immunodeficient person such as an AIDS patient, and infection in pregnant women may lead to abortion, still birth, or other serious congenital consequences in newborns [1, 2, 3].

Horses and donkeys are important and useful animals to humans in many ways, such as sport competitions, police work, carriage, and so on. Horse and donkey meat are also the popular and delicate food for people worldwide. Infection of *T. gondii* is subclinical in horses, atypical clinical signs includes fever, ataxia, retinal degeneration and encephalomyelitis, and abortion or stillbirth in pregnant equids. Human toxoplasmosis cases associated with consumption of horse meat have been reported in some countries [6, 7].

Yunnan Horse and Yunnan Donkey are fine equine breeds in China, they play very important roles in agriculture and tourism, and meat of horse and donkey are considered as special delicacy dishes in local restaurants in Yunnan Province. However, data on horse and donkey infection with *T. gondii* is limited in southwestern China. The objective of the present survey was to examine the seroprevalence of *T. gondii*infection in horses and donkeys in Yunnan Province, southwestern China, and the results would provide fundamental data for prevention and control of *T. gondii* infection in equine animals, and also will provide base-line information on potential risk factors associated with public health.

METHODS

Ethics Statement

The collection of serum samples from equids in the present study was consented by owners of equids, and all horses and donkeys were handled in strict accordance with good animal practice according to the Animal Ethics Procedures and Guidelines of the People's Republic of China.

Sampled Regions

The serum samples were collected from Diqing, Lijiang, Dehong, Baoshan, Yuxi and Zhaotong prefectures and municipalities of Yunnan Province, southwestern China (Figure 1).

Citation: Miao et al.: Seroprevalence of Toxoplasma gondii in horses and donkeys in Yunnan Province, Southwestern China. Parasites & Vectors 2013 6:168. doi:10.1186/1756-3305-6-168.

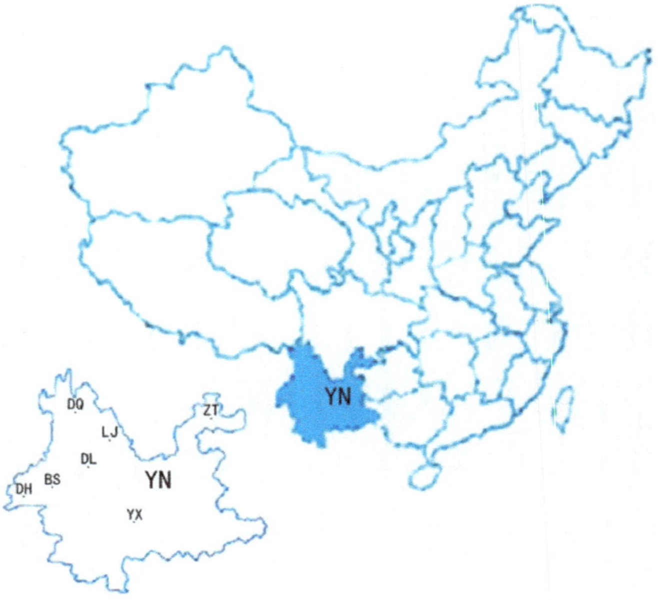

Figure 1: Map showing Yunnan Province (YN), shadowed in southwestern China, where horse and donkey serum samples were collected for detection of *Toxoplasma gondii* antibodies. The specific locations of sampling areas were marked in the enlarged map of Yunnan Province (YN), including Diqing state (DQ), Lijiang City (LJ), Dali state (DL), Baoshan city (BS), Dehong state (DH), Yuxi City (YX) and Zhaotong City (ZT).

Blood Samples

A total of 399 blood samples (266 from horses and 133 from donkeys) were collected via jugular vein of animals in 2012 in Yunnan Province. Whenever possible, data regarding species/ breed, geographic origin, age and gender of each animal were collected. The ages of animals were classified into four categories according to their growth cycle: foal ($0<yr\leq1$, 73 samples), adolescent ($1<yr\leq5$, 108 samples), middle age ($5<yr\leq10$, 138 samples) and elderly age ($yr>10$, 80 samples), 190 were males and 209 were females. All samples were sent to the laboratory in Kunming and centrifuged (3,000 rpm) for 5 min, and the serum samples were kept at −20°C until assayed for antibodies to *T. gondii*.

Serological Assay

Antibodies to *T. gondii* were detected in serum samples by an indirect hemagglutination antibody (IHA) test using a commercially available kit (Veterinary Research Institute, Jiangsu Academy of Agricultural Sciences, Nanjing, China) according to the recommended protocol of the manufacturer for the detection of antibodies to *T. gondii* in animals. The serum sample was considered as positive when a layer of agglutinated erythrocytes was observed in wells with dilutions of 1:64 or higher.

Statistical Analysis

Statistical analysis of *T. gondii* seroprevalence in different regions, ages and genders of animals were performed using Generalized Lineal Model (GLM) test in the SPSS software (Release 18.0 standard version, SPSS Inc., Chicago, Illinois), and $P<0.05$ was considered statistically significant.

RESULTS AND DISCUSSION

108 of 399 examined equids were seropositive for *T. gondii* antibodies, the overall seroprevalence was 27.1%, and the seroprevalence ranged from 18.8% in Dehong to 37.5% in Diqing. 81 (30.5%) of the examined horses and 27 (20.3%) of the examined donkeys were seropositive, but the difference was not statistically significant ($P>0.05$). The antibody titers were 1:64 in 38 horses and 13 donkeys, 1:128 in 20 horses and 5 donkeys, 1:256 in 13 horses and 2 donkeys, 1:512 in 2 horses and 1 donkey, 1:1024 in 8 horses and 6 donkeys. Seroprevalence in male and female equids was 27.4% and 26.8%, respectively, and the difference was not statistically significant ($P>0.05$). Seroprevalence in animals of four different age groups were not significantly different ($P>0.05$) (Table 1).

Table 1: Seroprevalence of *Toxoplasma gondii* infection in equids in Yunnan province, southwestern China

Factor	Category	Sample size	Positive no.	Positive no. in different titers				
			(Seroprevalence %)	1:64	1:128	1:256	1:512	1:1024
Species	Horse	266	81 (30.5)	38	20	13	2	8
	Donkey	133	27 (20.3)	13	5	2	1	6
Age	$0<yr\leq1$	73	24 (32.9)	12	5	3	1	3
(year)	$1<yr\leq5$	108	34 (31.5)	14	5	9	2	4
	$5<yr\leq10$	138	29 (21)	12	11	2	0	4
	$yr>10$	80	21 (26.3)	13	4	1	0	3

Gender	Male	190	52 (27.4)	25	12	6	1	8
	Female	209	56 (26.8)	26	13	9	2	6
Regions	Diqing	16	6 (37.5)	0	1	2	0	3
	Lijiang	83	23 (27.7)	16	7	0	0	0
	Dali	116	36 (31)	31	5	0	0	0
	Baoshan	39	9 (23.1)	2	5	2	0	0
	Dehong	16	3 (18.8)	1	1	1	0	0
	Yuxi	93	20 (21.5)	1	5	2	1	11
	Zhaotong	36	11 (30.6)	0	1	8	2	0
	Total	399	108 (27.1)	51	25	15	3	14

Under natural conditions, *T. gondii* seroprevalence in horses may vary from 0% to 90% [8]. In the present study, the overall average *Toxoplasma* seroprevalence was 27.1% in horses and donkeys in Yunnan Province, which was the highest among reported studies in China [9, 10, 11, 12, 13, 14, 15, 16, 17, 18, 19, 20] (Table 2). *T.gondii* seroprevalence in horses was 30.5% in this survey, which was the second highest so far reported in the world. Previously reported *T. gondii* seroprevalence in horses were: 31.6% in Saudi Arabia by DT [21], 28.8% in Iran by MAT [22], 25% in Egypt by ELISA [23], 17.7% in Tunisa by MAT [24], 11.6% in Brazil by IFAT [25], 10.8% in Spain by MAT [26], 7.2% in Turkey by DT [27], 6.9% in North America by MAT [6], 6.1% in Mexico by MAT [28], 2.6% in South Korea by IFAT [29], and 1% in Sweden by DAT [30].

Table 2: Seroprevalence of *Toxoplasma gondii* infection in equids in China

Species	Provinces	No. tested	Prevalence (%)	Serological test	Cut-off value	Time tested	References
Horses	Liaoning	711	25	MAT[a]	1:25	2012	[9]
	Sichuan	242	4.55	IHA[b]	1:64	1982	[10]
	Liaoning	76	1.32	IHA	1:64	1989-1990	[11]
	Shangdong	147	0	IHA	1:64	1991-1993	[12]
	Gansu	149	2.7	IHA	1:64	unknown	[13]
	Qinghai	100	6	IHA	1:64	2000	[14]
	Xinjiang	60	0	IHA	1:64	unknown	[15]
	Hebei	43	2.33	IHA	1:64	unknown	[16]
Donkeys	Liaoning	738	23.6	MAT	1:25	2012	[9]
	Shangdong	17	5.88	IHA	1:64	1991-1993	[12]
	Xinjiang	30	0	IHA	1:64	unknown	[15]
	Hebei	33	26.06	IHA	1:64	unknown	[16]
Equids*	Ningxia	945	0.95	IHA	1:64	unknown	[17]
	Shanxi	1108	0.09	IHA	1:64	1986	[18]
	Henan	230	0.43	IHA	1:64	1988-1993	[19]
	Guangdong	149	2.7	IHA	1:64	1982	[20]

* Data for horses and donkeys were not separately reported in these references.

[a] MAT: Modified Agglutination test.

[b] IHA: Indirect Haemagglutination test.

The different seroprevalence results may due to differences in hygiene conditions, climates, and the prevalence of *T. gondii* in cats, as well as the sensitivity of the serological methods. Our preliminary survey showed that the prevalence of *T. gondii* oocysts in the faeces of stray cats in Yunnan was 25.6% (unpublished data), indicating a high risk as a source of *T. gondii* infection for equids, other animals and humans. In the present study, we used IHA to detect antibodies to *T. gondii* in horse and donkey serum samples because IHA is considered one of the most sensitive and specific serological methods for detecting *T. gondii* antibodies in equids, other animals and humans [31, 32, 33, 34, 35], and it have been extensively used in China (Table 2, [32,33, 34, 35]). The cutoff value of 1:64 was used according to the national standard (GB/T 18448.2-2008) of China for detection of *T. gondii* antibodies in humans and animals.

Due to the population size of donkeys in Yunnan Province, the sampled number (No = 133) of donkeys in the present study was small, and the results of the present survey may not reflect the accurate *T. gondii* seroprevalence in donkeys. Nevertheless, the present investigation revealed that horses and donkeys in Yunnan Province had a high *T. gondii* seroprevalence, indicating a potential threat to public health in this province, which is one of the most famous tourist destinations in China.

CONCLUSIONS

The results of the present study indicate that *T. gondii* seroprevalence in horses and donkeys in Yunnan Province is quite high, consumption of horse or donkey meat is likely to be a risk factor for human infection with *T. gondii*. Therefore, it is imperative to take prevention and control measures to reduce *T. gondii*prevalence in equine animals in this province.

ACKNOWLEDGEMENTS

This work was supported by the Yunnan Provincial Program for Introducing High-level Scientists (Grant No. 2009CI125).

AUTHORS' CONTRIBUTIONS

FCZ and XQZ conceived and designed the study, and critically revised the manuscript. QM, XW, and JFY performed the experiments, analyzed the data and drafted the manuscript, NLS, FZY and YTF helped in study design, study implementation and manuscript revision. All authors read and approved the final manuscript.

REFERENCES

1. Dubey JP: Toxoplasmosis of Animals and Humans. 2010, Boca Raton, Florida: CRC Press, 313-2
2. Tenter AM, Heckeroth AR, Weiss LM: *Toxoplasma gondii*: from animals to humans. Int J Parasitol. 2000, 30: 1217-1258. 10.1016/S0020-7519(00)00124-7.
3. Zhou P, Chen Z, Li HL, Zheng H, He S, Lin RQ, Zhu XQ: *Toxoplasma gondii* infection in humans in China. Parasit Vectors. 2011, 4: 165-10.1186/1756-3305-4-165.
4. Chen J, Xu MJ, Zhou DH, Song HQ, Wang CR, Zhu XQ: Canine and feline parasitic zoonoses in China. Parasit Vectors. 2012, 5: 152-10.1186/1756-3305-5-152.
5. Nardoni S, Angelici MC, Mugnaini L, Mancianti F: Prevalence of *Toxoplasma gondii* infection in *Myocastor coypus* in a protected Italian wetland. Parasit Vectors. 2011, 4: 240-10.1186/1756-3305-4-240.
6. Dubey JP, Thulliez P, Romand S, Kwok OC, Shen SK, Gamble HR: Serologic prevalence of *Toxoplasma gondii* in horses slaughtered for food in North America. Vet Parasitol. 1999, 86: 235-238. 10.1016/S0304-4017(99)00148-X.
7. Pomares C, Ajzenberg D, Bornard L, Bernardin G, Hasseine L, Darde ML, Marty P: Toxoplasmosis and horse meat, France. Emerg Infect Dis. 2011, 17: 1327-1328. 10.3201/eid1707.101642.
8. Tassi P: *Toxoplasma gondii* infection in horses. A review. Parassitologia. 2007, 49: 7-15.
9. Yang N, Mu MY, Yuan GM, Zhang GX, Li HK, He JB: Seroprevalence of *Toxoplasma gondii* in slaughtered horses and donkeys in Liaoning province, northeastern China. Parasit Vectors. 2013, 6: 140-10.1186/1756-3305-6-140.
10. Ling CW, Wang PD: Investigation report of *Toxoplasma gondii* antibodies to horse and mule in Sichuan region. J Vet Sci Technol. 1984, 4: 32-34. In Chinese
11. Ge LM, Song LH, Chen FY, Wang M, Yu XJ, Yu YH, Zhao QQ, Lin RH: Investigation of *Toxoplasma gondii* infection in humans and animals in Dalian City. Chin J Zoonoses. 1991, 5: 34-In Chinese
12. Fu B, Wang ZM: Epidemiological investigation of toxoplasmosis in Shandong Province. Chin J Parasit Dis Cont. 1995, 8: 205-207. In Chinese
13. Zhang DL, Niu ZW: Epidemiological investigation of toxoplasmosis in humans and livestock in Tianzhu region. Gansu J Anim Vet Sci. 1998, 28: 20-21. In Chinese
14. Gao LY, Yang K, Chen DT: Seroprevalence of *Toxoplasma gondii* infection in horse in Tianjun region. Chin J Anim Quarantine. 2001, 18: 38-In Chinese
15. Bai WS, Chen Y, Ba LT, Mai MT: Investigation of toxoplasmosis in livestock in Aksu district usig serological method. Chin J Vet Parasitol. 2002, 2: 29-30. In Chinese
16. Cui P, Fang SF, Wu ZY, Wu BQ: Epidemiological survey of toxoplasmosis in livestock in Hebei Province. Chin J Vet Sci Technol. 2004, 34: 33-34. In Chinese
17. Zhang QQ, Xu WP, Wang XQ, Chen YM, Liu W, Ma JW, Li GD, Du CB, Wang Z: Seroepidemiological survey of toxoplasmosis in livestock and poultry in Ningxia. Chin J Vet Sci Technol. 1987, 6: 22-24. In Chinese
18. Bian QH, Bai JY, Su DS, Liu BS, Liu XF: Seroepidemiological survey of toxoplasmosis in humans and livestock in Shanxi, Gansu, Ningxia and Qinghai. Chin J Vet Sci Technol. 1988, 1: 17-19. In Chinese
19. Feng XR, Wang SR: Serological investigation report of *Toxoplasma gondii* among livestock in Henan Province. J China Agricultural University. 1998, 2: 172-173. In Chinese
20. Zhang WD: Preliminary Investigation of *Toxoplasma gondii* antibodies in livestock in South China. Chin J Zoonoses. 1986, 2: 55-In Chinese
21. Alanazi AD, Alyousif MS: Prevalence of antibodies to *Toxoplasma gondii* in horses in Riyadh Province, Saudi Arabia. J Parasitol. 2011, 5: 943-945.
22. Hajialilo E, Ziaali N, Harandi MF, Saraei M, Hajialilo M: Prevanlence of anti-Toxoplasma gondii antibodies in sport horses from Qazvin, Iran. Trop Anim Health Prod. 2010, 42: 1321-1322. 10.1007/s11250-010-9576-4.
23. Haridy FM, Shoukry NM, Hassan AA, Morsy TA: ELISA-seroprevalence of *Toxoplasma gondii* in draught horses in Greater Cairo, Egypt. J Egypt Soc Parasitol. 2009, 3: 821-826.
24. Boughattas S, Bergaoui R, Essid R, Aoun K, Bouratbine A: Seroprevalence of *Toxoplasma gondii* infection among horses in Tunisia. Parasit Vectors. 2011, 4: 218-10.1186/1756-3305-4-218.
25. Evers F, Garcia JL, Navarro IT, Zulpo DL, Nino BD, Ewald MP, Pagliari S, Almeida JC, Freire RL: Diagnosis and isolation of*Toxoplasma gondii* in horses from Brazilian slaughterhouses. Rev Bras Parasitol Vet. 2013, doi.org/10.1590

26. García-Bocanegra I, Cabezón O, Arenas-Montes A, Carbonero A, Dubey JP, Perea A: Almería S:Seroprevalence of Toxoplasma gondii in equids from southern Spain. Parasitol Int. 2012, 3: 421-424.

27. Karatepe B, Babür C, Karatepe M, Kılıc S: Seroprevalence of toxoplasmosis in horses in Niğde Province of Turkey. Trop Anim Health Prod. 2010, 42: 385-389. 10.1007/s11250-009-9430-8.

28. Alvarado-Esquivel C, Rodríguez-Peña S, Villena I, Dubey JP: Seroprevalence of *Toxoplasma gondii* infection in domestic horses in Durango State, Mexico. J Parasitol. 2012, 5: 944-945.

29. Gupta GD, Lakritz J, Kim JH, Kim DY, Kim JK, Marsh AE: Seroprevalence of *Neospora*, *Toxoplasma gondii* and *Sarcocystis neurona* antibodies in horses from Jeju island, South Korea. Vet Parasitol. 2002, 106: 193-201. 10.1016/S0304-4017(02)00064-X.

30. Jakubek EB, Lunde NA, Uggla A: Seroprevalence of *Toxoplasma gondii* and *Neospora* sp. Infections in Swedish horses. Vet Parasitol. 2006, 138: 194-199. 10.1016/j.vetpar.2006.02.002.

31. Dubey JP, Thulliez P, Weigel RM, Andrews CD, Lind P, Powell EC: Sensitivity and specificity of various serologic tests for detection of *Toxoplasma gondii* infection in naturally infected sows. Am J Vet Res. 1995, 56: 1030-1036.

32. Zou FC, Sun XT, Li B, Xie YJ, Zhao GH, Duan G, Zhu XQ: Seroprevalence of *Toxoplasma gondii* in pigs in Southwestern China. Parasitol Int. 2009, 58: 306-307. 10.1016/j.parint.2009.06.002.

33. Wang CR, Qiu JH, Gao JF, Liu LM, Wang C, Liu Q, Yan C, Zhu XQ: Seroprevalence of *Toxoplasma gondii* infection in sheep and goats in northeastern China. Small Ruminant Res. 2011, 97: 130-133. 10.1016/j.smallrumres.2011.02.009.

34. Qiu JH, Wang CR, Zhang X, Sheng ZH, Chang QC, Zhao Q, Wu SM, Zou FC, Zhu XQ: Seroprevalence of *Toxoplasma gondii*in cattle and dairy cows in Northeast China. Foodborne Pathogen Dis. 2012, 9: 579-582. 10.1089/fpd.2011.1104.

35. Chang QC, Zheng X, Qiu JH, Wang CR, Zhu XQ: Seroprevalence of *Toxoplasma gondii* infection in fattening pigs in Northeast China. J Parasitol. 2013, 99: 544-545. 10.1645/12-102.1.

CHAPTER 17

INTRINSIC FACTORS INFLUENCING THE INFECTION BY HELMINTH PARASITES IN HORSES UNDER AN OCEANIC CLIMATE AREA (NW SPAIN)

I. Francisco, M. Arias, F. J. Cortiñas, R. Francisco, E. Mochales, V. Dacal, J. L. Suárez, J. Uriarte, P. Morrondo, R. Sánchez-Andrade, P. Díez-Baños, andA. Paz-Silva

INTRODUCTION

The horse industry is increasing because of its diversity, and involves business, sport, gaming, entertainment, or recreation. The raising of horses plays a significant role, due to the high number of animals for leisure, which has generated several direct jobs, such as those needed for handling and the sanity of the animals.

Nowadays, horses are being used in wild pastures and countries for the forest management, utilizing unwanted vegetation for production. For this reason, this industry deserves the attention of the general public and the governments also. This new situation requires more information about the sanitary status of these animals, and the appropriate measures for ensuring the horses are in an adequate fitness condition. Among the diseases affecting horses, helminth infections are much extended [1].

An oceanic climate (also called marine west coast climate and maritime climate) is the climate typically found along the west coasts at the middle latitudes of all the world's continents and in southeastern Australia. Oceanic climates are characterized by a narrower annual range of temperatures than are encountered in other places at a comparable latitude and do not have the extremely dry summers of Mediterranean climates. Under those conditions, survival of parasitology resistant forms is enhanced, enabling thus the possibility for infection throughout the year.

Several investigations have shown the effect of some factors on the infection by parasites in horses. Osterman Lind et al. [2] and Larsen et al. [3] observed the highest output of strongyle eggs in animals aged 2-3 years from Sweden. Bucknell et al. [4] reported that in Australia cyathostomes were more prevalent in young horses, and P. equorum was found exclusively in horses less than 2 years of age, and the highest mean intensity of infection forAnoplocephala perfoliata was in those horses. Lyons et al. [5] obtained similar results in equids from Kentucky (USA). Nevertheless, there is a lack of knowledge about the influence of breed or sex on the infection by helminth parasites in horses from oceanic climate areas.

This study reports the effect of various intrinsic factors (breed, age, sex) on the equine infection by helminth parasites. Fecal samples were individually collected form 418 horses in an oceanic climate area (NW Spain) and analyzed by the coprological flotation, sedimentation, and migration techniques. Coprocultures were also done to identify the main strongylid genera affecting the horses.

MATERIAL AND METHODS

Horses

Between April and September 2007, fecal samples from the rectum of 418 horses from NW Spain were collected. According to the breed, four groups were established (Table 1): Spanish Sport Horse (SSH), Spanish Pure Breed (SPB), English Pure Breed (EPB) and the autochthonous Pura Raza Galega (PRG). By considering the age, horses were divided into three groups: G-1 (<3 years old), G-2 (3–10), and G-3 (>10) (Table 1).

Citation: I. Francisco, M. Arias, F. J. Cortiñas, et al., "Intrinsic Factors Influencing the Infection by Helminth Parasites in Horses under an Oceanic Climate Area (NW Spain)," Journal of Parasitology Research, vol. 2009, Article ID 616173, 5 pages, 2009. doi:10.1155/2009/616173.

Table 1: Distribution of the fecal samples from horses under an oceanic climate area (NW Spain) according to their breed, sex, and age

	Female				Male				Total
Breed	Age (years)								
	<3	3–10	>10	Total	<3	3–10	>10	Total	
CDE	4	8	7	19	3	4	2	9	28
PRE	1	6	5	12	3	2	5	10	22
PSI	15	40	20	75	3	5	0	8	83
PRG	40	129	55	224	16	37	8	61	285
Total	60	183	87	330	25	48	15	88	418

Study Design

Although some interesting information about horses management as hygienic conditions, treatment history, and so forth would be helpful to explain the results, it was not possible to achieve in many cases, so we decided not to include it in the current paper. Many samples were collected from horses under an extensive management, and ask those questions to the owners was not possible.

For that reason, the impossibility for ensuring the collection of all data belonging to the total population limited us to the analysis of the factors possibly involved in the infection of equines by helminth parasites. The factors we analyzed corresponded to parameters which can be observed and measured for us in all cases.

The influence of climatic conditions on the dynamics of egg expulsion has been reported [6]. Nevertheless, by considering that the main goal in the current work was to gain more information about the presence of helminth infection in horses and the difficulty in taking more than one fecal sample from each animal in several cases, the data presented here must be comprehended as a coprological survey.

Coprological Analysis

The observation of parasitic forms in the feces of the horses was evaluated by using the coprological flotation, sedimentation, and migration techniques [7]. Five grams of each fecal sample were processed (in duplicate) by the flotation, sedimentation, and migratory techniques [8], with a sensitivity of 10 eggs per gram of feces (EPG).

The laboratory technician conducting the microscope analysis was also blinded to the study design of the selection of the stool specimens.

Genera Identification

Since it is not possible to distinguish strongyle eggs of different species morphologically, fecal samples are cultured for 10–14 days at 20–25°C to allow the development of L3s, which may be collected by means of the Baermann procedure [6, 9]. Genera were identified according to Lichtenfels [10].

Statistical Analysis

By taking account that the egg elimination is not normally distributed, statistical analysis was done by means of the nonparametric Kruskal-Wallis and Mann-Whitney U two-sided tests ($\alpha = 0.05$), and significant differences were considered when $p< .05$. The descriptive parameters were the EPG quartiles 1, 2, and 3. All tests were done using SPSS for Windows (14.1).

Prevalences were expressed as the percentage and the 95% Confidence Interval (CI).

The existence of correlation among the different parameters was assessed by using nonparametric Spearman's rank correlation test.

RESULTS

Identification of Helminth Parasites

Eggs from gastrointestinal nematoda and cestoda were observed in the feces of the horses. No eggs from trematoda or lungworm larvae were obtained.

The analysis of the gastrointestinal eggs showed that the horses were parasitized by Parascaris equorum, Strongyles, and Oxyuris equi. By means of the coprocultures, we identified Cyathostominea and Gyalocephalusspp (small strongyles) and Strongylus and Triodontophorus (large strongyles).

No differences in the genera of strongyles identified according to breed, age, or sex were recorded.

Prevalence of Helminth Parasites

Eighty nine percent (95% CI 86, 92) of the samples had gastrointestinal eggs and 1% (0, 2) cestoda. The prevalence of horses passing Parascaris eggs by feces was 11% (8, 14), 88% (85, 91) strongyles, and 3% (1, 5) oxyurids.

As drawn in Table 2, the highest prevalence of parascariosis was obtained in the youngest animals, English Pure Blood horses and females. No Parascaris eggs were observed in Sport Spanish Horse animals. Significant differences were obtained by considering the age, breed, and sex of the animals.

Table 2: Prevalences of helminth parasites in 418 horses from an oceanic climate area (NW Spain). Results are expressed as the percentage and the 95% Confidence Interval (CI). Spanish Sport Horse (SSH), Spanish Pure Breed (SPB), English Pure Breed (EPB), autochthonous Pura Raza Galega (PRG)

		Ascarids	Strongyles	Oxyurids	Cestoda
Age	<3	22	93	1	0
		(18, 26)	(90, 96)	(0, 2)	
	3–10	6	91	2	2
		(4, 8)	(88, 94)	(1, 3)	(1, 3)
	>10	12	81	6	1
		(9, 15)	(77, 85)	(4, 8)	(0, 2)
	$\chi 2$	15.842	8.732	5.584	2.228
	p	0.001	0.0013	0.061	0.328
Breed	SSH	0	0	0	0
	SPB	5	19	0	0
		(3, 7)	(15, 23)		
	EPB	34	98	5	1
		(29, 39)	(97, 99)	(3, 7)	(0, 2)
	PRG	5	100	2	2
		(3, 7)		(1, 3)	(1, 3)
	$\chi 2$	64.960	366.936	2.87	0.976
	p	0.001	0.001	0.412	0.807
Sex	Male	12	90	3	2
		(9, 15)	(87, 93)	(1, 5)	(1, 3)
	Female	2	84	0	0
		(1, 3)	(80, 88)		
	$\chi 2$	7.244	3.333	2.799	1.508
	p	0.007	0.068	0.094	0.219

The prevalence of strongyles was higher in G-1 and G-2, horses belonging to the autochthonous PRG breed and females. No positive cases were recorded in the Sport Spanish horses. Significant differences were observed by taking into account the age and the breed of the animals.

Table 2 reflects that the greatest percentage of horses with oxyurids corresponded to the oldest animals (G-3), English Pure Blood, and females. No eggs were observed in males or in SSH animals.

Finally, the highest prevalence of horses passing cestode eggs by feces was obtained in the equids from the G-2 (3–10 years), autochthonous (PRG), and females, although these differences were not significant.

Spearman's rank test showed a statistical negative correlation between the age of the horses and the prevalence of ascarids and strongyles ($r = -0.141$, $p = 0.005$ and $r = -0.143$, $p = 0.004$, resp.). Likewise, a weak and positive correlation between age and prevalence of pinworms was matched ($r = 0.113, 0.023$).

Intensity of Infection

The results of the egg-excretion are summarized in Table 3. The highest number of Parascaris eggs was observed in the foals, autochthonous horses (PRG), and males. The Kruskal-Wallis test showed significant differences according to the age of the animals.

Table 3: Helminth eggs per gram of feces (EPG) in 418 horses from an oceanic climate area (NW Spain). Spanish Sport Horse (SSH), Spanish Pure Breed (SPB), English Pure Breed (EPB); autochthonous Pura Raza Galega (PRG). Results are expressed as EPG quartiles 1, 2, and 3 (Q1, Q2, and Q3, resp.)

		Statistics	Ascarids	Strongyles	Oxyurids	Cestoda
Age	<3	Q1	0	100	350	
		Q2	50	400	350	
		Q3	137	775	350	
	3–10	Q1	0	100	112	50
		Q2	0	380	150	50
		Q3	50	750	3225	150
	>10	Q1	0	100	100	50
		Q2	0	200	100	50
		Q3	50	500	325	50
		$\chi2$	14.781	10.500	1.560	0.2
		p	0.001	0.005	0.458	0.655
Breed	SSH	Q1				
		Q2				
		Q3				
	SPB	Q1		25		
		Q2		50		
		Q3		725		
	EPB	Q1	0	413	100	50
		Q2	0	650	150	50
		Q3	50	1275	150	50
	PRG	Q1	0	100	100	50
		Q2	0	300	225	50
		Q3	100	700	1362	150
		$\chi2$	3.450	148.841	0.165	0.2
		p	0.327	0.001	0.684	0.655
Sex	Male	Q1		50		
		Q2		150		
		Q3		600		
	Mare	Q1	0	100	100	50
		Q2	0	351	150	50
		Q3	50	750	375	100
		$\chi2$	0.364	7.942		
		p	0.546	0.005		

As drawing in Table 3, there were reached differences in the egg excretion of small strongyles regarding the breed and sex of the horses. The greatest numbers were observed in the English Pure Blood animals and in females, whereas no elimination was observed in Spanish Sport Horses.

No differences were obtained in the egg elimination of oxyurids and cestoda by considering the age, breed, or sex of the horses.

By means of Spearman's rank test, a statistical negative correlation between the age of the horses and the elimination of ascarids and strongyles eggs was proved ($r = -0.445$, $p = 0.001$ and $r = -0.167$, $p = 0.001$, resp.).

DISCUSSION

Worldwide, horses are exposed to helminth parasites from different groups resulting in significant morbidity and mortality [11]. The most common helminths of horses include the small and large strongyles, along with tapeworms, ascarids, pinworms, and the lungworms [12]. In the current study, we proved the existence of infection by ascarids, strongyles (small and large) and pinworms in horses from NW Spain, which agrees with data reported by Bucknell et al. [4] in Australia, Romaniuk et al. [13] in Polonia, and Pereira and Vianna [1] in Brazil, in horses housed under differing management schemes.

The main helminth parasites observed were strongyles, in agreement with previous investigations in areas with a similar weather [1, 14, 15]. Likewise, a low prevalence was obtained for tapeworms, although the low sensitivity of the fecal examination techniques in detecting cestode eggs could be the explanation to our results [16]. Meana et al. [17] pointed that the coprological methods have a lower likelihood of diagnosing cestode infection when horses have less than 100 tapeworms.

The lack of flukes and coccidia in the current study provides evidence to back up the rarity of infection by this class of parasite [1, 13].

To get more knowledge about the factors influencing infections by helminths in horses, the coprological data were examined by considering the age, breed, and sex of the animals. Only P. equorum and strongyles showed any age effect. The values of prevalence and elimination of P. equi-eggs were significantly the highest in horses less than 3 years old, which agrees with Mfitilodze and Hutchinson [18] and Bucknell et al. [4].

The percentage of infection by strongyles was significantly greater in the horses less than 10 years old. It has been proved that age does not influence the cyathostome burdens [19], and Klei and Chapman [20] reported that the naturally acquired immunity against small strongyles slowly develops with age, but remains incomplete. This could be the explanation to the finding of a negative correlation between the age and the infection by ascarids and strongyles.

The conditions of housing and management are usually related to the horse breed. This explains why the autochthonous Pura Raza Galega horses, maintained under extensive forest conditions and receiving an inadequate keeping, attained the highest prevalence of infection by ascarids and strongyles. In addition, no helminth parasites were observed in the fecal samples from Spanish Sport horses, and the Spanish Pure Blood ones were few parasitized. Several studies did not match the influence of the horse breed on the helminthosis [18, 21].

It has been shown that helminth infection is ubiquitous in horses with access to pasture. The absence of positive results in the Sport Spanish horses seems to be attributable to a reduced possibility for pasturing and thus to contact to the infective phases (larval 3rd stages for the gastrointestinal nematoda) or to intermediate hosts (oribatids in the case of tapeworms). Another possible explanation could be that these are economically valuable horses, maintained under appropriate hygienic conditions, and receiving periodical veterinary attention. Moreover, the observation of elevated prevalences for gastrointestinal worms in the English Pure Blood and in the Spanish Pure Blood equids was an unexpected result, because of their economic value and the conditions of housing and keeping, similar to the Sport Spanish horses.

Our results showed that sex had influence on the prevalence of ascarids and strongyles, being the females more infected than the males, in agreement with Fikru et al. [21].

This is the first study about the effect of several intrinsic factors on the helminth parasites affecting horses from NW Spain, so the lack of coprological surveys makes more difficult the discussion of the results obtained in the current investigation. It must be taken into account that the presence of seasonal dynamics of egg expulsion influences the results for the intensity of parasitization [6].

The development of coprological surveys provides a very interesting and indispensable tool for knowing the main helminth parasites infecting the horses. In the light of our results we consider that the infections caused by helminths, especially the strongyles, are significantly common in the region of study, so that greater importance should be given to this situation. The elevated prevalence in the English Pure Blood and autochthonous horses underlines the need for the application of appropriate measure to the control of helminth parasites. More information is needed to know the applied ways for the control of parasites in equids, in particular that related to chemoprophylaxis.

ACKNOWLEDGMENTS

This work was supported, in part, by a research grant from the Xunta de Galicia (XUGA, Spain) to I. Francisco and R. Francisco, and by the Projects XUGA PGIDT06RAG26102PR and 07MDS021261PR (Xunta de Galicia, Spain), and complies with the current laws for Animal Health Research in Spain. They are in debt to Mrs. B. Valcárcel for preparing and editing the manuscript.

REFERENCES

1. J. R. Pereira and S. S. S. Vianna, “Gastrointestinal parasitic worms in equines in the Paraíba Valley, State of São Paulo, Brazil,” Veterinary Parasitology, vol. 140, no. 3-4, pp. 289–295, 2006.
2. E. Osterman Lind, J. Höglund, B.-L. Ljungström, O. Nilsson, and A. Uggla, “A field survey on the distribution of strongyle infections of horses in Sweden and factors affecting faecal egg counts,” Equine Veterinary Journal, vol. 31, no. 1, pp. 68–72, 1999.
3. M. M. Larsen, S. Lendal, M. Chriél, S. N. Olsen, and H. Bjørn, “Risk factors for high endoparasitic burden and the efficiency of a single anthelmintic treatment of Danish horses,” Acta Veterinaria Scandinavica, vol. 43, no. 2, pp. 99–106, 2002.
4. D. G. Bucknell, R. B. Gasser, and I. Beveridge, “The prevalence and epidemiology of gastrointestinal parasites of horses in Victoria, Australia,” International Journal for Parasitology, vol. 25, no. 6, pp. 711–724, 1995.
5. E. T. Lyons, S. C. Tolliver, and S. S. Collins, “Prevalence of large endoparasites at necropsy in horses infected with Population B small strongyles in a herd established in Kentucky in 1966,” Parasitology Research, vol. 99, no. 2, pp. 114–118, 2006.
6. T. A. Kuzmina, Y. I. Kuzmin, and V. A. Kharchenko, “Field study on the survival, migration and overwintering of infective larvae of horse strongyles on pasture in central Ukraine,” Veterinary Parasitology, vol. 141, no. 3-4, pp. 264–272, 2006.

7. R. P. Herd, "Performing equine faecal egg counts," Veterinary Medicine, vol. 87, pp. 240–244, 1992.
8. MAFF, Manual of Veterinary Parasitological Laboratory Techniques, Ministry of Agriculture, Fisheries and Food, HMSO, London, UK, 1986.
9. E. Osterman, Prevalence and control of strongyle nematode infections of horses in Sweden, Doctoral thesis, Swedish University of Agricultural Sciences, Uppsala, Sweden, 2005.
10. J. R. Lichtenfels, "Helminths of domestic equids: illustrated keys to genera and species with emphasis on North American forms," Proceedings of the Helminthological Society of Washington, vol. 42, pp. 1–92, 1975.
11. J. E. Hodgkinson, "Molecular diagnosis and equine parasitology," Veterinary Parasitology, vol. 136, no. 2, pp. 109–116, 2006.
12. B. O›Meara and G. Mulcahy, "A survey of helminth control practices in equine establishments in Ireland,"Veterinary Parasitology, vol. 109, no. 1-2, pp. 101–110, 2002.
13. K. Romaniuk, K. Reszka, and E. Lasota, "Influence of animal breeding manner on the occurrence of internal parasites," Wiadomosci Parazytologiczne, vol. 50, no. 3, pp. 647–651, 2004.
14. S. Love, D. Murphy, and D. Mellor, "Pathogenicity of cyathostome infection," Veterinary Parasitology, vol. 85, no. 2-3, pp. 113–122, 1999.
15. E. T. Lyons, T. W. Swerczek, S. C. Tolliver, H. D. Bair, J. H. Drudge, and L. E. Ennis, "Prevalence of selected species of internal parasites in equids at necropsy in central Kentucky (1995–1999)," Veterinary Parasitology, vol. 92, no. 1, pp. 51–62, 2000.
16. C. J. Proudman and G. B. Edwards, "Validation of a centrifugation/flotation technique for the diagnosis of equine cestodiasis," Veterinary Record, vol. 131, no. 4, pp. 71–72, 1992.
17. A. Meana, M. Luzon, J. Corchero, and M. Gómez-Bautista, "Reliability of coprological diagnosis ofAnoplocephala perfoliata infection," Veterinary Parasitology, vol. 74, no. 1, pp. 79–83, 1998.
18. M. W. Mfitilodze and G. W. Hutchinson, "Prevalence and intensity of non-strongyle intestinal parasites of horses in northern Queensland," Australian Veterinary Journal, vol. 66, no. 1, pp. 23–26, 1989.
19. C. Collobert-Laugier, H. Hoste, C. Sevin, C. Chartier, and P. Dorchies, "Mast cell and eosinophil mucosal responses in the large intestine of horses naturally infected with cyathostomes," Veterinary Parasitology, vol. 107, no. 3, pp. 251–264, 2002.
20. T. R. Klei and M. R. Chapman, "Immunity in equine cyathostome infections," Veterinary Parasitology, vol. 85, no. 2-3, pp. 123–136, 1999.
21. R. Fikru, D. Reta, and M. Bizunesh, "Prevalence of equine gastrointestinal parasites in western high lands of Oromia, Ethiopia," Bulletin of the Animal Health Production in Africa, vol. 53, no. 3, pp. 161–166, 2005.

CHAPTER 18

PARASITE CONTROL PRACTICES ON SWEDISH HORSE FARMS

Eva Osterman Lind, Erik Rautalinko, Arvid Uggla, Peter J Waller, David A Morrison and Johan Höglund

BACKGROUND

The horse is host to a great number of gastrointestinal helminths, of which nematodes of the family Strongylidae, the roundworm *Parascaris equorum* and the cestode *Anoplocephala perfoliata* are the most important. These parasites are ubiquitous and have been recognised as significant causes of clinical disease in horses. A previous Swedish study has shown that 2–3 year-old horses on stud farms, particularly in the south of the country, often shed high numbers of strongyle eggs [1]. Although the occurrence of the most pathogenic species, *Strongylus vulgaris*, has decreased markedly during the past 3 decades, eggs of this nematode were still found in samples from 14% of the investigated farms [1]. Furthermore, studies of *A. perfoliata* have revealed a high prevalence of this parasite in horses of all ages [2].

The officially estimated number of horses in Sweden is 283,100 [3], of which the great majority are leisure and sports horses. Generally, the control of endoparasites of Swedish horses relies largely on anthelmintics, which are easy to administer and rarely cause negative clinical side effects. Unfortunately, excessive use of anthelmintic drugs has led to the development of resistance in populations of cyathostomins worldwide [4]. Moreover, cases of decreased susceptibility of *P. equorum* to macrocyclic lactones were reported recently from The Netherlands and Canada [5, 6]. In Sweden, benzimidazole resistance in cyathostomins was shown on 96% of the farms [7], and recently occurrence of pyrantel resistance has been recognised [8]. Despite its widespread use for 20 years there are still no reports of resistance to ivermectin in horse strongyles. Nevertheless, in parallel to the situation in e.g. sheep trichostrongylids, it is believed that resistance against macrocyclic lactones will appear also in equine parasites [9].

In view of emerging anthelmintic resistance it is important to develop more sustainable control strategies, which are adapted to different types of horse management. The aim of the present questionnaire was to obtain information in order to describe the current routines and practices used by Swedish horse owners for the control of endoparasites. No previous work of this type has been performed in Sweden.

METHODS

A questionnaire on management practices and parasite control routines was developed and tested on 60 horse owners in a pilot study prior to commencing the main study. Subsequently the form was slightly revised, and the final version comprised 26 questions, of which 3 were open-ended and the rest closed (Table 1).

Citation: Eva Osterman Lind, Erik Rautalinko, Arvid Uggla, Peter J Waller, David A Morrison and Johan Höglund, "Parasite control practices on Swedish horse farms," Acta Veterinaria Scandinavica200749:25. DOI: 10.1186/1751-0147-49-25.

Table 1: Summary of questions in the questionnaire

Question	***Reply options***
Type of establishment	
Type of horses[1]	Trotters; riding horses; cold-blooded trotters; ponies; working horses; Thoroughbreds; Icelandic
Type of establishment[1]	Stud; livery; trotting stable; riding school; small private farm
Total number of horses	
Number of individuals younger than 5 years	
Pasture management	
Access to grazing area	No access; pasture summertime; all-year-round paddocks with grass
Do you practice mixed or rotational grazing?	Yes; no
Grazing areas and procedures practiced[1]	Permanent pastures; fertilizers used; aftermath grazed; ploughing and re-seeding every 2nd–3rd year; rotation between clean plots; pasture clipping/harrowing; grazing areas are part of crop rotation system
Do you remove manure from the grazing areas?	No; at least once per week; at least once per month; at least once per year
Use of anthelmintic drugs	
Do you de-worm your horses?	Yes; no
Person responsible for de-worming	Horse owners; manager; staff; veterinarian; other
How is the dosage calculated?	By guessing the horse weight; by measuring the horse weight; by age; one tube of paste per animal
Which drug brands were used at different months for the last 12 months[2]?	
When did you de-worm horses <5 yrs for the last 12 months?[3]	
When did you de-worm horses >4 yrs for the last 12 months?[3]	
Do you de-worm regularly against tapeworm?	No/sporadically; yes with double dose of pyrantel; yes with praziquantel; do not know
Which of the following drugs have you used during the past 24 months[1]?	All anthelmintic drugs and brands registered for horse are shown to the responder
Which routines are practiced on your farm?[1]	De-worming of new horses; individual de-worming programmes; horses sharing pasture de-wormed together; horses of the same age de-wormed together; all horses on the farm de-wormed together
What time of the year do you think is the most important for de-worming?	Jan-March; April-June; July-Sept; Oct-Dec
Do you look for parasites in faeces after deworming?	Yes; no
Attitudes and encountering of parasite problems	
Have you seen bot flies/eggs for the last 2 years?	Yes; no
What is your attitude regarding anthelmintic usage? State the importance on a 1–5 scale.	Environmental aspects; cost; resistance; targeted de-worming; alternatives to anthelmintic drugs
Have you had a faecal sample analyzed from a healthy horse?	No; once; several times; regularly
For how many years have you been active with horses?	
Do you consider helminth infection as a problem in horses? State the magnitude of the problem on a 1–5 scale.	

Have you experienced problems caused by endoparasites?	Yes; no
How important are the following sources of information for you? State the importance on a 1–5 scale.	Information on the package of the drug; other horse owners; Apoteksbolaget (Swedish Pharmacy Chain); books; internet; veterinarian; horse magazines

[1] Possibility to choose more than one option

[2] Respondents were to combine anthelmintic trade names and months of the year in a chart

[3] The months were to be marked by the respondent

In order to include the main types of horse establishments in the study, names of respondents were obtained from the following lists:

- Individuals who had horses insured by Agria, the principal Swedish insurance company for horses;
- Riding clubs that were members of Svenska Ridsportförbundet (the Swedish Riding Association);
- Professional trainers with an A-licence from Svenska Travsportens Centralförbund (the Swedish Trotting Association);
- Members of the Svenska hingsthållarföreningen (Swedish Stallion Holders› Association);
- Stallion studs that were members of Avelsföreningen för Svenska Varmblodiga Hästen (the Swedish Warmblood Association).

From each of these lists, establishments were selected randomly using slips of paper or random numbers generated by the computer. The questionnaire was finally posted to 627 horse establishments (out of approximately 56 thousand) in 2003. To maximize the number of respondents, a book on horses was rewarded those who completed the questionnaire. In addition, reminder letters were posted to those who had not returned the questionnaire after 2 and 4 weeks.

Based on information from the completed questionnaires, respondents were classified into the following types of establishments:

- Stud farms – at least 10 horses; several foals bred every year;
- Livery yards – mainly horses older than 4 years; different horse owners;
- Trotting stables – often large establishments with a high proportion of young horses being trained; a great turnover of horses;
- Riding schools – usually horses older than 4 years; generally short grazing periods;
- Small private – establishments with a small number of horses; often one owner.

A few establishments were multipurpose stables. These were classified according to what seemed to be the principal type.

Data summaries and descriptive statistical analyses were calculated using Microsoft Excel X for Mac Service Release 1 (Microsoft Corporation). The frequency data were analyzed with log-likelihood contingency (for 4 variables) or goodness-of-fit (for 1 variable) tests with Williams correction for continuity (G-tests; [10]), using Microsoft Excel X for Mac Service Release 1 (Microsoft Corporation). The continuous data were analyzed by 2-factor orthogonal analyses of variance, using SYSTAT 9 for Windows (SPSS Inc, Chicago IL, USA). For all three analyses one factor was the type of establishment, with the other factor being either horse age, anthelmintic feature or information source. It all cases it is the interaction hypothesis that is of interest. In order to assess the effect of possible non-normality on the analyses, they were repeated using non-parametric 2-factor orthogonal Kruskal-Wallis tests [11]. For all three analyses the same qualitative result was obtained from both the parametric and non-parametric tests; and so only the parametric results are presented here (i.e. means and interaction F-values). All tests were considered to be statistically significant at $P < 0.05$.

RESULTS

Response

In total, replies were obtained from 447 (71%) of the establishments. However, 3 respondents were excluded because less than half of the questions had been answered (Table 2). The response rate was good in all types of farms (66–78% depending on type). For each question the amount of missing data varied from 0 to 12%. In all cases, our reported percentages are the percentage of those who responded to the question.

Table 2: Data on establishments that returned the questionnaire

	Stud farms	*Livery yards*	*Trotting stables*	*Riding schools*	*Small private*	*Total*
Number of respondents	51	44	112	117	120	444
%	12%	10%	25%	26%	27%	
Response rate	70%	72%	66%	78%	72%	71%
Mean number of horses (range)	53 (10–200)	15 (3–70)	31 (4–130)	35 (9–90)	6 (1–36)	26
Proportion <5 yrs (range)	50% (13–100)	21% (0–80)	68% (20–100)	4% (0–24)	22% (0–100)	31%

Pasture Management

Overall, 97% of the respondents (n = 429) stated that their horses had access to grazing areas. On all stud farms and small private farms horses had access to grazing areas, whereas 89% of the trotting stables, 98% of the livery yards and 99% of the riding schools kept horses on grazing areas.

Most establishments, particularly livery yards, stated that the pastures were permanent, i.e. used solely for horses for several consecutive years (Table 3). Pasture clipping, or chain harrowing, were the most common pasture hygiene procedures undertaken; 36% of the respondents clipped or harrowed their pastures. Twenty-six percent of the establishments carried out more than one of the pasture improvement procedures shown in Table 3. On stud farms a majority (74%) used more than one of these procedures.

Table 3: Percentage of respondents that carried out different pasture management procedures

Pasture procedures	*Stud farms*	*Livery yards*	*Trotting stables*	*Riding schools*	*Small private*	*Total* n = 429
Permanent pastures	61%	93%	83%	87%	83%	83%
Aftermath grazed	16%	12%	5%	9%	15%	11%
Ploughing and re-seeding	20%	5%	8%	4%	17%	11%
Rotation between clean plots	24%	7%	4%	12%	13%	11%
Pasture clipping/harrowing	76%	28%	35%	25%	33%	36%
Pastures part of crop rotation system	43%	7%	6%	3%	10%	11%

Forty-one percent of the respondents (n = 179) stated that they removed faeces from the grazing areas (Fig 1). Of those, 6% stated that they did it at least once per week, whereas 11% did it at least once per month and 24% once per year. In addition, only 10% (n = 47) practiced mixed or rotational grazing with other animal species, such as cattle or sheep. The proportion of respondents that did practice mixed or rotational grazing with other livestock species varied from 4% (trotting stables) to 18% (stud farms).

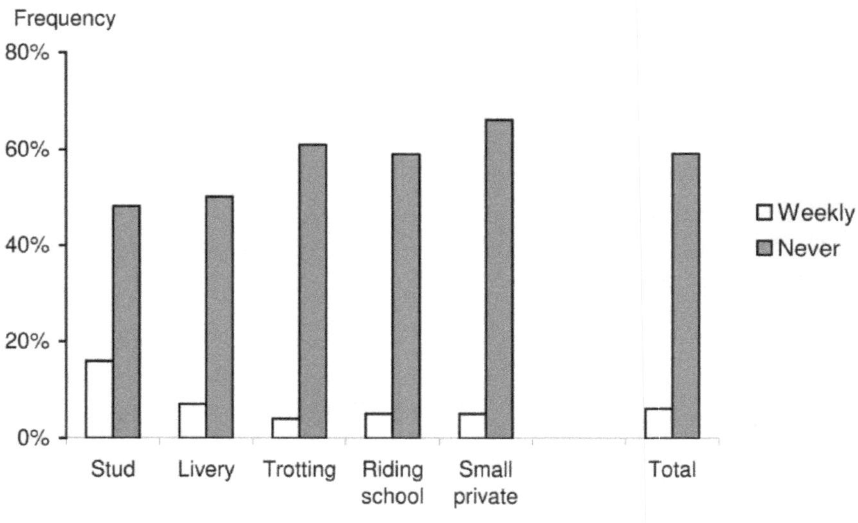

Figure 1: Percentage of respondents who removed manure weekly or never did it. Other options are not displayed in the figure.

Use of Anthelmintic Drugs

Virtually all respondents (99.5%, n = 442) stated that they de-wormed their horses. Only 8 respondents (2%) considered winter (Jan-March) as the most important time for de-worming. This was significantly ($G = 28.3$, $df = 3$, $P < 0.001$) fewer than for other times of the year (Fig 2).

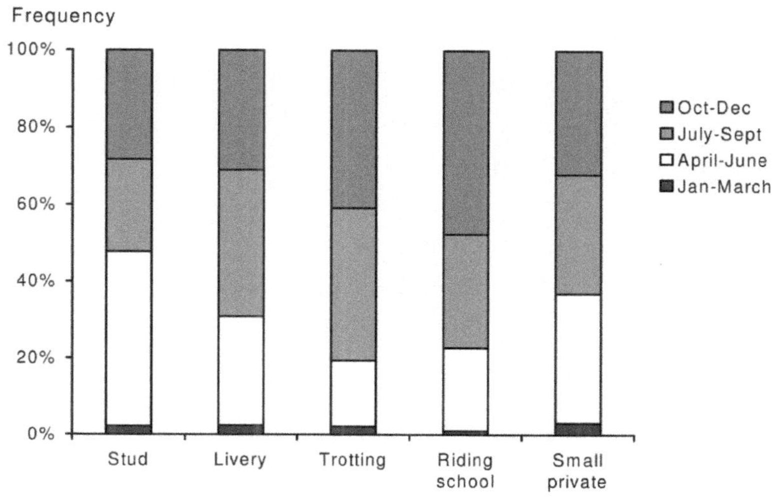

Figure 2: Times of the year considered to being the most important for de-worming (n = 387).

To calculate the dosage of anthelmintic, 13% out of 441 stated that they measured the horse's weight (girth tape or scale), 67% guessed the weight, and the remainder, particularly trotting stables, administered one tube of anthelmintic paste per animal. Eighty-two percent of 439 respondents stated that they de-wormed all horses on the farm at the same time and 38% de-wormed new horses on arrival at the farm. Nearly all (98%, n = 431) respondents stated that treatments were performed by either the horse owners or farm managers. Ten farms (2%), of which 6 were trotting stables, stated that anthelmintic treatments were carried out by a veterinarian. The number of anthelmintic treatments per year varied from 1–8 with an average of 3.2. Generally ($F = 13.10$, $df = 4$, $P < 0.001$), horses younger than 5 years were treated more frequently (3.5 times) than older horses (3.0 times). This was particularly evident for stud farms, where young horses were treated 4.4 times per year and older horses 3.3 times. Stud farms and trotting stables treated horses of all ages more frequently than did other types of establishments. In livery yards, riding schools and small private establishments, the adult horses were treated 2.6–2.8 times per year, and for livery yards and small private establishments there was no difference in treatment frequency between young and old horses.

Anthelmintic treatments were performed during all months of the year, but most respondents stated that they used anthelmintics less during the winter months (Jan-March; Fig 3). Those who de-wormed their horses in the winter were mainly respondents on stud farms and trotting stables. The percentages of establishments that de-wormed in May (55%) and September (42%) were significantly ($G = 284.9$, $df = 11$, $P < 0.001$) higher than during other times of the year.

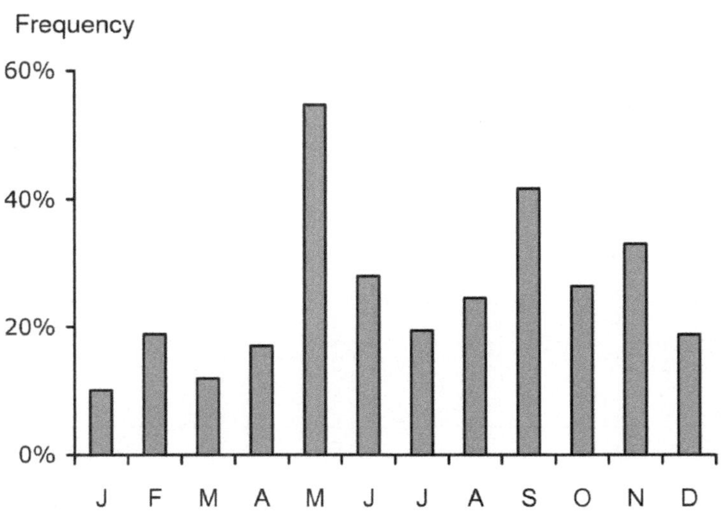

Figure 3: Frequency distribution of anthelmintic treatments performed during the previous 12 months. Note that numbers add up to more than 100 because the horses are dewormed more than once per year.

Ivermectin and pyrantel were the most commonly used drugs. The benzimidazoles were used in only 0–2% of the treatments (Fig 4). There was a significant (G = 127.8, df = 9, P < 0.001) seasonally related difference between the use of pyrantel and ivermectin drugs: pyrantel dominated in the spring and ivermectin in the autumn. Less than half of the respondents (41%, n = 180) had observed bot flies or their eggs during the previous 24 months.

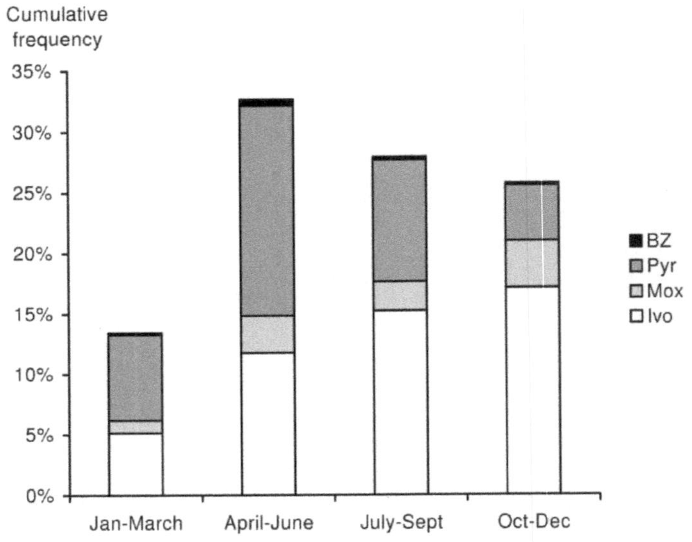

Figure 4: Usage of different anthelmintic drugs at various times of the year. BZ – benzimidazoles; Pyr – pyrantel; Mox – moxidectin; Ivo – ivermectin.

The majority of the respondents (65%, n = 272) had used 2 different classes of anthelmintic drugs (excluding praziquantel) during the previous 12 months; 9% (n = 38) had used 3 classes and the remaining had used one class. Furthermore, it was stated by 50% of the respondents that they de-wormed with pyrantel at 38 mg/kg bodyweight against tapeworms, whereas 1% used praziquantel. Most of the treatments against tapeworms were performed in May, although all months of the year were represented. Thirty-nine percent did not de-worm against tapeworm, and 10% did not know if they did.

Attitudes To and Encountering of Parasite Related Problems

Some features regarding attitude to anthelmintic treatment are presented in Table 4. Respondents from all types of farms considered anthelmintic resistance to be of great importance (mean 4.6 out of 5), whereas a demand for faecal analysis prior to de-worming was of low importance (mean 2.3). The cost of anthelmintic compounds was listed as most important for riding schools. Generally (F = 2.40, df = 16, P = 0.001), establishments with trotters considered that all features specified in Table 4 were of less importance than did other types of establishments.

Table 4: Mean scores regarding anthelmintic treatment related features, This was classified on a scale 1–5, where 1 was irrelevant and 5 very important

Classified features	*Stud farms*	*Livery yards*	*Trotting stables*	*Riding schools*	*Small private*	*Total (St.dev)* n = 429
Environmental aspects	3.1	3.3	2.8	3.3	3.2	3.1 (1.2)
Cost of drug	3.3	3.0	2.3	3.5	2.7	2.9 (1.3)
Anthelmintic resistance	4.7	4.5	4.3	4.7	4.6	4.6 (0.8)
Demand for faecal egg counts prior to de-worming	2.3	2.8	2.0	2.5	2.4	2.3 (1.0)
Alternatives to anthelmintics	3.5	3.3	2.9	3.4	3.5	3.3 (1.1)

Only 1% (n = 5) of the respondents sent faecal samples for parasitological analysis on a regular basis. Sixty-eight percent (n = 302) had never sent a sample and the remaining 31% (n = 135) had sent samples occasionally once or several times. The proportion of respondents that had sent samples several times was significantly (G = 64.2, df = 12, P < 0.001) higher among trotting stables than other types of establishments.

Seventy-two percent of the respondents had never experienced any problems that they could associate with helminth infections (Fig 5). Still, they scored the problem of helminth infections in horses as a mean of 2.5 on a 1–5 scale. Significantly (G = 39.0, df = 4, P < 0.001) higher proportions of respondents on stud farms and trotting stables stated that they had experienced problems with helminth infections than those on other types of farms.

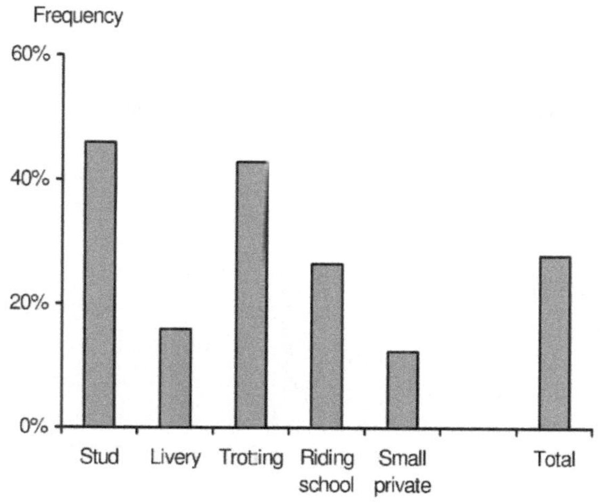

Figure 5: The proportion of respondents (n = 444) who had personal experience of helminth related problems in their horses.

In general, information regarding parasites and parasite control seemed to be of significance. All respondents considered the veterinarian to be the most important information source, whereas information gained from the internet and other horse owners were the least important (Table 5). With the exception of veterinarians, information sources were generally scored lower by trotting stables and stud farms than by other categories of respondents ($F = 3.06$, $df = 24$, $P < 0.001$).

Table 5: Mean scores regarding information on parasites and control, This was classified on a scale 1–5, where 1 was totally unimportant and 5 very important

Information source	*Stud farms*	*Livery yards*	*Trotting stables*	*Riding schools*	*Small private*	*Total (St. dev)* **n = 437**
The package of the drug	3.8	4.3	4.0	4.1	4.3	4.1 (1.0)
Other horse owners	2.7	3.2	2.5	2.8	3.2	2.9 (1.1)
Swedish Pharmacy Chain (Apoteksbolaget)	3.0	3.9	2.9	3.5	3.8	3.4 (1.3)
Books	3.5	3.9	3.1	3.6	3.6	3.5 (1.1)
Internet	2.5	3.4	2.3	2.9	2.9	2.7 (1.3)
Veterinarians	4.5	4.7	4.7	4.8	4.5	4.7 (0.7)
Horse magazines	4.2	3.9	3.4	4.1	3.7	3.8 (1.1)

DISCUSSION

The overall response rate was good for all types of farms. However, valid conclusions may be drawn only if the returned questionnaires are representative of all Swedish horse establishments. We consider this likely to be true. First, a representative range of establishments was targeted for the survey. Second, the response rate was high across all categories of establishments. Third, we attempted to independently verify the accuracy of our data. For example, anthelmintic treatments as described by the respondents to the survey were compared to statistics on the sales of anthelmintic drugs for horses, and they were found to be in agreement.

As 97% of the respondents stated that their horses had access to grazing areas, usually permanent pastures, it can be concluded that the conditions on Swedish horse farms are favorable for the transmission of pasture-borne endoparasites. In general, pasture hygiene was infrequently practiced. However, stud farms appeared to apply pasture hygiene practices to a greater extent than respondents on other types of farms, which suggests an awareness of contaminated pasture as the main source of infection for important endoparasites. Pasture clipping and/or chain harrowing obviously were the most commonly used procedures, especially on stud farms (76%). The main reason for clipping the pasture is to improve the re-growth of grass and to remove weeds. During the process of clipping, the faeces will disperse over the pasture, sometimes after it has been broken up by a cutter, which can be attached to the clipper. Chain harrowing is primarily performed to prevent high levels of infective larvae on pasture. As a consequence of pasture clipping or chain harrowing during hot and dry weather, the infective larvae will die from desiccation [12]. Still, only 6% of the respondents removed faeces at least once per week, which is considerably lower than has been reported from the UK, where 49% of the respondents stated that they collected faeces at least once per week [13]. Furthermore, 90% of the establishments in the present study did not practice mixed or rotational grazing with other livestock, although the benefit of such grazing management is often highlighted in parasite control recommendations. Thus, it appears that Swedish horse owners are less inclined, or have less possibility, to mix or rotate grazing with sheep or cattle than are horse owners in Denmark (18%), England (44%) or Ireland (71%) [14, 15, 16].

Practically all respondents de-wormed their horses, and only occasionally did a veterinarian perform these treatments. The exceptionally low use of benzimidazoles is in accordance with statistics from the Swedish Pharmacy Chain on the sales of anthelmintics for horses in Sweden. Ivermectin and pyrantel were the most frequently used drugs. Interestingly, late autumn was considered to be the most important time of the year for de-worming, although the frequency distribution of performed treatments showed that more farms had de-wormed in May (spring) than in any other month. The reason why the respondents regarded late autumn as the most important time for de-worming is most likely due to awareness of the bot fly, *Gasterophilus intestinalis*, which had been evident on 41% of the farms. Also, the increased use of macrocyclic lactones in late autumn indicates the concern among Swedish horse owners about *G. intestinalis*. In order to preserve the efficacy of anthelmintic drugs a number of recommendations have been developed, namely: (1) minimising the number of doses, (2) slow rotation between different drug classes, (3) correct dosing, (4) effective treatment of new individuals before introduction to the herd, and (5) regular monitoring for resistance [17]. Slow rotation of drug classes on an annual or biennial basis implies that *G. intestinalis* control is excluded in the years when macrocyclic lactones are not used. The same principle has to be applied to treatment with pyrantel against the tapeworm *Anoplocephala perfoliata*. However, administration of more than one drug class per year on 65% of the farms, and more than two classes on 9%, suggests that the recommendation of a slow rotation of drug classes has not been fully adopted in Sweden.

Compared to Ireland [15] and the UK [13], Swedish horse owners appear to de-worm less frequently. The most intensive anthelmintic control programmes were found on stud farms and trotting stables, i.e. establishments that typically accommodate a great number of young horses. However, it can be speculated that the treatment frequency for adult horses in Sweden is unnecessarily high. In a previous study of strongyle egg output in Swedish horses it was found that 59% of the animals older than 4 years excreted as few as 0–100 eggs per gram of faeces [1]. Moreover, in livery yards and small private establishments there was no difference in the number of treatments between young and adult horses, which either suggests overuse of anthelmintics in adult horses or the opposite in young horses.

The vast majority (82%) of respondents stated that all horses on their farm were treated at the same time. However, only 38% of the respondents treated new horses before introduction to the herd. In the future, treatment of new horses, preferably with macrocyclic lactones, obviously needs to be emphasised by veterinarians in order to avoid the introduction of resistant parasite strains.

In the control of endoparasites of livestock in general, increased attention is being paid to targeted selective anthelmintic treatments based on prior faecal egg count (FEC) monitoring [18]. For equines, studies have shown that targeted treatments may reduce the total number of treatments and thereby also the selection pressure for anthelmintic resistance [19, 20, 21]. Application of targeted treatments, as well as the recommendation to monitor regularly for anthelmintic resistance, require both the involvement of a veterinarian and laboratory analyses of faecal samples. In this study, only 1% of the respondents stated that they consign samples for FEC analysis on a regular basis, with the majority never sending faecal samples from healthy horses. Thus, it appears that Swedish horse owners perform FECs less frequently than do horse owners in Ireland, where 28% of the owners performed FECs at least once per year [15]. Reasons for a low frequency of FEC analysis could be: (1) in Sweden the analysis of a faecal sample is considerably more expensive than the dose of anthelmintic, (2) the cost of anthelmintics does not appear to be of decisive importance to the horse owners, and (3) lack of motivation, as it was generally considered that parasites are a minor problem, and 72% of the respondents had no personal experience of parasite related problems in their horses. Consequently, the respondents also considered that faecal sampling prior to de-worming was of minor importance. Methods alternative to anthelmintic treatment were considered as being of average importance. However, respondents on all types of farms considered anthelmintic resistance to be an important, or very important, issue. Altogether, these results indicate that Swedish horse owners are concerned about anthelmintic resistance but they lack the knowledge, or motivation, as how to delay its development.

Finally, it was evident in all categories of horse owners that veterinarians were the most important source of information regarding parasite control, whereas the internet still seems to be of minor importance. Hence, to increase horse owners' knowledge of endoparasites and parasite control, the most appropriate way would be to further educate veterinarians. This could be achieved by courses, leaflets and articles, but additionally a closer collaboration between parasitologists and veterinary practitioners would be beneficial for all parties concerned.

ACKNOWLEDGEMENTS

The study was supported financially by Agria Insurance Co, Stockholm, Sweden.

AUTHORS' CONTRIBUTIONS

EOL was responsible for the design of the study, performance of the pilot study, the distribution of the questionnaire and writing the draft of the manuscript. ER contributed in the design of the study and in the formulation of questions. AU, PJW and JH participated in the design of the study and helped to word the final version of the manuscript. DAM did most of the data analyses and the interpretation of these.

REFERENCES

1. Osterman Lind E, Höglund J, Ljungström BL, Nilsson O, Uggla A: A field survey on the distribution of strongyle infections of horses in Sweden and factors affecting faecal egg counts. Equine Veterinary Journal. 1999, 31: 68-72.
2. Nilsson O, Ljungström BL, Höglund J, Lundquist H, Uggla A: Anoplocephala perfoliata in horses in Sweden: prevalence, infection levels and intestinal lesions. Acta Veterinaria Scandinavica. 1995, 36: 319-328.

3. Swedish Board of Agriculture. [http://www.sjv.se/home/amnesomraden/statistics]

4. Kaplan RM: Anthelmintic resistance in nematodes of horses. Veterinary Reseach. 2002, 33: 491-507. 10.1051/vetres:2002035.

5. Boersema JH, Eysker M, Nas JWM: Apparent resistance of Parascaris equorum to macrocyclic lactones. The Veterinary Record. 2002, 150: 279-281.

6. Hearn FP, Peregrine AS: Identification of foals infected with Parascaris equorum apparently resistant to ivermectin. Journal of the American Veterinary Medical Association. 2003, 15 (223(4)): 482-485. 10.2460/javma.2003.223.482.

7. Nilsson O, Lindholm A, Christensson D: A field evaluation of anthelmintics in horses in Sweden. Veterinary Parasitology. 1989, 32: 163-171. 10.1016/0304-4017(89)90117-9.

8. Osterman Lind E, Kuzmina T, Uggla A, Waller PJ, Höglund J: A field study on the effect of some anthelmintics on cyathostomins of horses in Sweden. Veterinary Research Communications. 2007, 31: 53-65. 10.1007/s11259-006-3402-5.

9. Sangster NC: Pharmacology of anthelmintic resistance in cyathostomes: will it occur with the avermectin/milbemycins?. Veterinary Parasitology. 1999, 85: 189-204. 10.1016/S0304-4017(99)00099-0.

10. Sokal RR, Rohlf FJ: Biometry. 1981, San Francisco, W.H. Freeman

11. Zar JH: Biostatistical Analysis. 1984, Englewood Cliffs, Prentice-Hall, 2nd

12. Herd RP: Parasite hygiene: a nonchemical approach to equine endoparasite control. Modern Equine Practice. 1986, 36-38.

13. Lloyd S, Smith J, Connan RM, Hatcher MA, Hedges TR, Humphrey DJ, Jones AC: Parasite control methods used by horse owners: factors predisposing to the development of anthelmintic resistance in nematodes. Veterinary Record. 2000, 146: 487-492.

14. Pascoe RJ, Wilson TJ, Coles GC: Nematode control in eventer horses. The Veterinary Record. 1999, 145: 200-201.

15. O'Meara B, Mulcahy G: A survey of helminth control practices in equine establishments in Ireland. Veterinary parasitology. 2002, 109: 101-110. 10.1016/S0304-4017(02)00249-2.

16. Lendal S, Larsen MM, Bjørn H, Craven J, Chriél M, Olsen SN: A questionnaire survey on nematode control practices on horse farms in Denmark and the existence of risk factors for the development of anthelmintic resistance. Veterinary Parasitology. 1998, 78: 49-63. 10.1016/S0304-4017(98)00117-4.

17. Lloyd S, Soulsby EJL: Is anthelmintic resistance inevitable: back to basics?. Equine Veterinary Journal. 1998, 30: 280-283.

18. Hoste H, Chartier C, Lefrileux Y, Goudeau C, Broqua C, Pors I, Bergeaud JP, Dorchies P: Targeted application of anthelmintics to control trichostrongylosis in dairy goats: result from a 2-year survey in farms. Veterinary Parasitology. 2002, 110: 101-108. 10.1016/S0304-4017(02)00307-2.

19. Duncan JL, Love S: Preliminary observations on an alternative strategy for the control of horse strongyles. Equine vet J. 1991, 23: 226-228.

20. Krecek RC, Guthrie AJ, Van Nieuwenhuizen LC, Booth LM: A comparison between the effects of conventional and selective antiparasitic treatments on nematode parasites of horses from two management schemes. Journal of the South African Veterinary Association. 1994, 65: 97-100.

21. Döpfer D, Kerssens CM, Meijer YGM, Boersema JH, Eysker M: Shedding consistency of strongyle-type eggs in dutch boarding horses. Vet Parasitol. 2004, 124: 249-258. 10.1016/j.vetpar.2004.06.028.

SECTION V: PARASITES OF PIGS

CHAPTER 19

IMMUNOPROTEOMIC PROFILE OF TRICHINELLA SPIRALIS ADULT WORM PROTEINS RECOGNIZED BY EARLY INFECTION SERA

Jing Yang, Wei Pan, Ximeng Sun, Xi Zhao, Gu Yuan, Qing Sun, Jingjing Huang and Xinping Zhu

Keywords: *Trichinella spiralis,* Adult worm, Mass spectrometry, Immunoproteomics, Diagnosis

BACKGROUND

Trichinellosis, which is caused by infection with the nematode *Trichinella spiralis* remains an important food-borne parasitic zoonosis worldwide. It not only causes a public health hazard but also represents an economic problem in porcine animal production and food safety [1,2]. Human trichinellosis is primarily caused by ingesting the raw or undercooked meat of pigs and other animals containing *T. spiralis* larvae [3]. The disease affects as many as 11 million people and is regarded as a re-emerging disease [4]. From 2005 to 2009 in China, 15 outbreaks of human trichinellosis were reported, with 1387 cases and four deaths [5]. *T. spiralis* is a tissue-dwelling parasitic nematode, and its life cycle is completed in a single host, including all stages of the adult worm (Ad), newborn larvae (NBL) and muscle larvae (ML). After ingestion, muscle larvae are released from the capsules and develop into sexually mature adult worms in the intestine. Each female worm can produce 500-1000 NBL in a period of 5-10 days. Then, the NBL migrate through the lymphatic system and the general circulatory system. Subsequently, the parasites develop into infective muscle larvae encapsulated in the host skeletal muscles [6]. During all developmental stages, *T. spiralis* expresses many immunodominant antigens that elicit a protective immune response, as well as antigens useful for the serodiagnosis of trichinellosis [7,8].

Because trichinellosis manifests as nonspecific signs and symptoms, the clinical diagnosis of this disease is difficult [9]. Currently, the diagnosis of trichinellosis relies on detection of the larvae in a muscle biopsy or highly specific immunodiagnostic tests. The immunological tests current available use excretory-secretory products (ES) secreted by the living larvae as antigens to detect antibodies in the sera of infected individuals. However, testing is not widely available because of the limited availability of antigens produced by *T. spiralis* larvae. These tests are also not sensitive for the detection of the early stage of infection and may cross-react with other parasites [10,11]. Another weakness of serologic methods using ES products as antigens is the high rate of false negative results, even with a combination of ELISA and Western blot, which may increase the detection sensitivity [10,11]. Anti-helminthic drugs are more effective against the adult worms remaining in the intestine during early infection than the encapsulated muscle larvae. After the newborn larvae are released by the adult worm, the NBL migrate to the muscle tissue to be encapsulated that are more resistant to anthelmintic therapy and cause greater pathology; therefore, it is critical to identify and diagnose early infection for timely treatment [9,12]. The antigens from the early stage of infection, such as adult worms and newborn larvae, are immunogenic and induce immune responses in an infected host and may be used for early immunodiagnosis [7]. Although previous studies showed that some antigens derived from newborn larvae are recognized by *T. spiralis*-infected animal sera or have potential as vaccine antigens [13,14], these antigens have not shown satisfactory results for detecting early infections or vaccine development. Therefore, it is necessary to identify sensitive and specific novel antigens derived from adult worms or newborn larvae to detect early infection by *T. spiralis* to achieve better therapeutic effects.

Two-dimensional electrophoresis (2-DE), combined with mass spectrometry (MS) is an effective approach for

Citation: Jing Yang, Wei Pan, Ximeng Sun, Xi Zhao, Gu Yuan, Qing Sun, Jingjing Huang and Xinping Zhu, "Immunoproteomic profile of Trichinella spiralis adult worm proteins recognized by early infection sera," Parasites Vectors (2015) 8: 20. doi:10.1186/s13071-015-0641-8.

high resolution analysis of complex groups of proteins [15]. Combining these techniques with Western blot using a specific antibody allows us to identify antigens that induce host immune responses during infection and could therefore be used for immunodiagnosis and/or vaccine development. This immunoproteomics tool provides information on both the characteristics of immunogenic proteins and the serological response directed against parasites, such as *Schistosoma japonicum* [16], *Toxoplamsma gondii* [17], *Ascaris lumbricoides* [18] and *Taenia solium* [19]. In fact, several excretory-secretory (ES) proteins and surface proteins from *T. spiralis* muscle larvae were identified by using this immunoproteomic tool [20-22]. These results suggest that proteins, such as serine protease, p43 glycoprotein and 5′-nucleotidase, are potential diagnostic antigens and the targets for vaccines in host-parasite interactions. However, these antigens are derived from muscle larvae and may not be suitable for the early diagnosis of *Trichinella* infection.

In this study, to identify antigens recognized by the host immune system during early enteric infection, *T. spiralis* adult worm extracts were separated by 2-DE and recognized using sera from pigs and mice infected with *T. spiralis* for 7 days. The primary immunoreactive spots recognized using the early infection sera were characterized by MALDI-TOF/TOF-MS analyses in combination with bioinformatics. The antigens recognized by the sera during this early stage may be used to immunodiagnose the early infection by *T. spiralis*. The results of this study will facilitate the selection of antigens as reagents for early serological diagnosis and possibly vaccine development.

METHODS

Animals

Experimental animals (mice and pigs) were purchased from the Laboratory Animal Services Center of Capital Medical University (Beijing, China). Experimental procedures for *T. spiralis* infection were reviewed and approved by the Capital Medical University Animal Care and Use Committee and were consistent with the NIH Guide for the Care and Use of Laboratory Animals.

Maintenance and Collection of *T. spiralis* Worms and Protein Sample Preparation

The *T. spiralis* ISS 533 strain used in this study was maintained in female ICR mice in our laboratory, and *T. spiralis* muscle larvae were recovered from the muscles of infected mice with a standard pepsin/hydrochloric acid digestion method [23]. The adult worms were collected from the small intestine of experimentally infected Wistar rats at 4 days after experimental infection.

The collected adult worms were washed several times in PBS and then homogenized in lysis buffer containing 7 M urea, 2 M thiourea, 4% CHAPS, 65 mM Tris, 2% DTT, and 1% Bio-Lyte (pH3-10). The adult worm lysates were centrifuged at 20,000 × g at 4°C for 60 min and the supernatant was collected as adult extracts. The total protein concentration was determined using a 2D Quant kit (GE Healthcare, USA) and stored at -80°C until use for proteomic analysis.

Collection and Preparation of *T. spiralis* Infected Animal Sera

T. spiralis infected pig sera were collected from 4 pigs orally infected with 20,000 *T. spiralis* muscle larvae each for 7 days and pooled. The infected mouse sera were obtained from 10 BALB/c mice orally infected each with 500 *T. spiralis* muscle larvae for 7 days. Uninfected sera from normal pigs and mice were collected as negative controls.

Two-dimensional polyacrylamide gel electrophoresis (2-DE)

Approximately, 400 μg of *T. spiralis* adult extracts were used for each 2-DE analysis. The worm extracts with bromophenol blue were loaded into 17 cm pH 3-10 immobilized pH gradient (IPG) strips (Bio-Rad, USA) and separated by isoelectric focusing (IEF) using a Protean IEF Cell (Bio-Rad, USA). IEF was performed at 20°C with rehydration at 20°C for 12 h, followed by isoelectric focusing according to the manufacturer's instructions. After isoelectric focusing, the IEF strips were equilibrated for 15 min in a reducing buffer (6 M urea, 2% SDS, 0.375 M Tris-HCl pH 8.8, 20% glycerol, and 2% DTT), followed by 15 min in an alkylation buffer (6 M urea, 2% SDS, 0.375 M Tris-HCl, pH8.8, 20% glycerol, and 2.5% iodoacetamide). For the second dimension, the equilibrated IPG strips were placed on 12% SDS-PAGE and run at 15 mA/gel for 30 min. The gels were either stained with Coomassie Blue R-350 or transferred to a PVDF membrane for Western blot. Three gels were run for the adult worm extracts under the same conditions.

Western Blot Analysis

The separated protein spots from the 2-DE gels were transformed onto PVDF membranes (Millipore, USA) using a Trans-blot semi-dry Transfer Cell TM (Bio-RAD, USA) for 90 min at 18 V. The membranes were blocked with 5% skimmed milk in PBS, pH 7.4 for 2 h at room temperature and then incubated with either *T. spiralis* infected swine pooled sera or infected mouse sera diluted 1:1 00 in PBS, pH7.4, with 0.05% Tween 20 (PBST). After 3 washes in PBST, the membranes were incubated with the horseradish peroxidase-conjugated rabbit anti-swine IgG or goat anti-mouse IgG (Sigma, USA). Reproducibility of the immune recognition was verified by repeating the immunoblot at least three times. The sera collected from normal swine or mice were used as controls. The PDQuest™ 2-D Analysis Software (Bio-RAD, USA) was used for matching and analysis of the antigenic protein spots on the 2-D gels.

In-Gel Tryptic Digestion

Only those spots recognized by the infection sera from both the pigs and mice were selected for further study. Following the selection of spots of interest by matching with the immunoblot image, the protein spots on the Coomassie Blue-stained gels were carefully excised. The excised gel pieces were incubated with 100 mM NH_4HCO_3 and 30% CAN in the dark, washed with 100 mM NH_4HCO_3 and dried. Then, the gel species were further rehydrated in digestion buffer containing trypsin (Promega, USA) and incubated at 37°C overnight. The trypsin-digested peptides were subsequently extracted with 100 μl of

60% ACN/0.1% trifluoroacrtic acid (TFA) and prepared for MALDI-TOF/TOF-MS analysis.

Protein Identification using MALDI-TOF /TOF-MS Analysis

The resulting peptides from the above extraction were analyzed on an Applied Biosystem Sciex 4800 mass spectrometer (Applied Biosystems, USA). The MS spectra were recorded in reflector mode in a mass range from 800 to 4000. The peptide mass fingerprints (PMFS) were obtained. The peaks with the highest mass intensities were selected for MS/MS for protein identification. Each peptide assignment was also manually verified. The PMFS and MS/MS data were searched from the NCBI and SwissProt databases of the existing *T. spiralis* genome or ESTs using MASCOT version 2.2 (Matrix Science, LTD). Protein identification was considered accurate when the confidence scores >95% and the MASCOT score was >50. The identified proteins were categorized by their protein sequences according to the information obtained from the InterProsan software. The outputs were subjected to analysis by the GO categories using the Web Gene Ontology Annotation Plotting (WEGO, http://wego.genomics.org.cn/cgi-bin/wego/index.pl).

Expression and Immunological Test of Recombinant *Ts*14-3-3 (r*Ts*14-3-3)

DNA coding for the full length *Ts*14-3-3 was amplified from total cDNA reverse-transcribed from total *T. spiralis* adult RNA using primers designed according to *Ts*14-3-3 sequence (GenBank accession no. XM_003378886) (the forward primer: 5′-CGGGATCCATGACCGAAAAGGAAGACAT-3′ and the reverse primer: 5′-CGGAATTC CTGCCCAGCGGC TGTATCTT-3′). The amplified DNA products were cloned into the expression vector pET-28a (+) (Novagen, Germany) using BamHI and XhoI sites. The recombinant pET-28a (+)/*Ts*14-3-3 plasmids were transformed into the *E. coli* BL21. The recombinant protein (r*Ts*14-3-3) was induced with 1 mM IPTG and the expressed soluble recombinant *Ts*14-3-3 was purified using His-Bind Purification Kit (Novagen, USA).

Following SDS-PAGE, the r*Ts*14-3-3 was transferred onto nitrocellulose membrane. The membrane was incubated with the same *T. spiralis*-infected swine or mice sera used for identifying the immunogenic antigens described above. The recombinant *Ts*14-3-3 was used to immunize mouse to obtain antiserum in order to detect the expression of native *Ts*14-3-3 in adult worm and muscle larvae stages of *T. spiralis*.

RESULTS

2-DE Analysis of *T. spiralis* Adult Extracts

The somatic proteins of the *T. spiralis* adult extracts were separated on a 2-DE gel, and the protein spots were visualized following Coomassie R-350 staining (Figure 1A). Image analysis revealed more than 300 spots stained on the gel, the majority of which migrated between pH 4 and 10 over a broad range of molecular masses between 10-150 kDa.

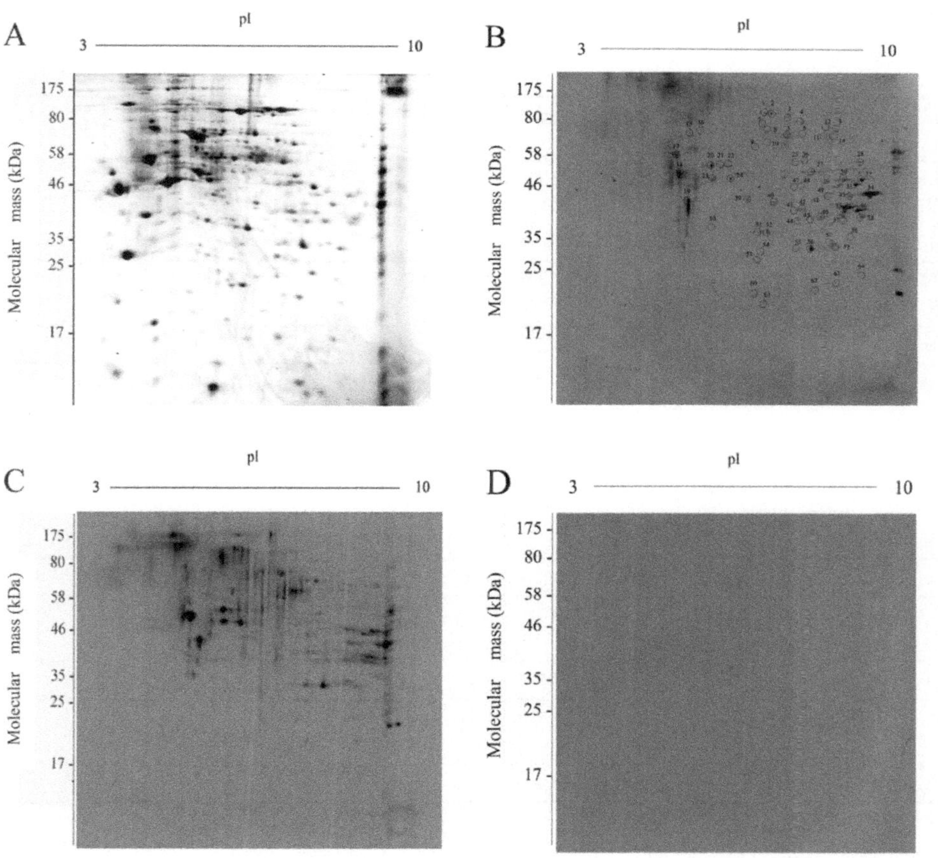

Figure 1: 2-DE and Western blot analysis of *T. spiralis* adult worm proteins. A. 2-DE gel of adult worm proteins separated in the first dimension in the pH range 3-10 and in second dimension on a 12% polyacrylamide gel. The 2-DE gel was stained with Coomassie Blue G-350. **B.** Western blot of adult worm proteins probed with pig infection sera at 7 days post infection. The protein spots selected for further analysis are numbered. **C.** Western blot of adult worm proteins probed with mouse infection sera at 7 days post infection. **D.** Western blot of adult worm proteins probed with normal swine sera.

Immunoreactive Antigens Recognized by Early Infected Swine and Mouse Sera

The PDQuest software allowed us to overlap shared spots between the 2 species, swine and mouse, based on the same MWs and isoelectric points. As shown in Figure 1B and Figure 1C, there were more than sixty protein spots recognized by sera from both swine and mice infected with *T. spiralis* for 7 days, with molecular weights ranging from 20 kDa to 180 kDa, and pI values from 3-10. Most of the recognized antigens were between 30 kDa to 150 kDa, with pI values between 4 and 9. The spots and their corresponding proteins on the gel were labeled individually with the same number. No proteins reacted to normal swine or mouse serum (Figure 1D).

Identification of Protein Spots by MALDI-TOF MS Analysis

The immunoblot and the Coomassie Blue stained gel were aligned and matched with the PDQuest™ 2-D Analysis Software. Sixty-four of the positive spots recognized by swine and mice sera infected with *T. spiralis* for 7 days were matched and located on the Coomassie blue stained gel, and then excised for in-gel tryptic digestion. The digested peptides were then subjected to MALDI-TOF/TOF-MS analysis. The proteins listed in the table are the highest ranked candidates that were unambiguously identified in the MASCOT search (Table 1) with molecular weights listed from high to low. A total of 55 immunoreactive proteins were identified by peptide mass fingerprinting. Nine spots selected for MS analysis did not generate any MS data. Several proteins, such as the intermediate filament protein, actin-5c, 14-3-3, inorganic pyrophosphatase, putative thioredoxin, and serine protease inhibitor were identified in several spots next to each other. Actin-5c was identified in spots 19, 20, 21, and 22. The 14-3-3 protein was found in spots 60 and 61. Putative thioredoxin was identified in spots 42, 51 and 52. Spots 56, 57 and 59 were the serine protease inhibitor kazal-type 4. As a consequence, a total of 40 distinct immunoreactive proteins were identified. Notably, several house-keeping genes were identified, such as actin and intermediate filament protein. Several proteins were involved in bioprocessing, metabolism and signaling pathways, such as cysteine proteases, inorganic pyrophosphatase protein-tyrosine phosphatase, heat shock protein and developmental-regulated GTP-binding protein.

Table 1: Identification of *T. spiralis* adult worm proteins recognized by pig and mouse infection sera at 7 DPI

Spot no.	Protein name	NCBI ID	pI	MW (kDa)	Protein score	Protein score C.I.%	Coverage (%)	No. matched peptides
1	intermediate filament protein ifa-1	gi|316973417	5.96	73.218	816	100	62	34
2	6-phosphofructokinase	gi|316973417	7.97	93.66	93	100	15	11
3	heat shock protein 70 (*Trichinella britovi*)	gi|2104672	5.77	71.86	33	99.5	18	11
4	MAP/microtubule affinity-regulating kinase 3	gi|316978564	9.25	78.23	115	100	18	11
5	chaperone protein DnaK	gi|316972817	5.43	73.47	494	100	36	22
6	32 kDa beta-galactoside-binding lectin (Galectin-1)	gi|316970057	9.04	55	85	100	17	7
7	F-box/WD repeat-containing protein sel-10	gi|316975364	6.29	67.25	67	100	19	9
8	HAD-superfamily hydrolase	gi|316976388	7.8	66.01	56	98.7	10	6
9	cysteine protease ATG4B	gi|316968242	5.79	47.54	68	100	20	6
10	developmentally-regulated GTP-binding protein 1	gi|316965924	8.97	48.51	52	99.6	20	7
11	dolichyl-diphosphooligosaccharide—protein glycosyltransferase subunitSTT3A	gi|316976331	8.85	62.448	62	97.996	25	11
12	HAD-superfamily hydrolase	gi|316976388	7.8	66.01	56	98.7	10	6
13	putative glutaredoxin-like protein	gi|316970937	6.21	91.79				13
14	MYND finger protein	gi|316977375	8.8	56.83	64	100	12	5
15	intermediate filament protein ifa-1	gi|316973417	5.96	73.21	478	99.9	51	31
16	acyl-protein thioesterase	gi|316970759	5.02	55.8	108	100	13	5

17	putative stress-induced-phosphoprotein 1	gi|316977783	6.01	58.16	93	100	22	9
18	7 transmembrane receptor	gi|316965614	5.82	41.87	89	100	38	14
19	Actin-5c	gi|316970244	5.3	42.21	280	100	36	10
20	Actin-5c	gi|316970244	5.3	42.21	422	100	34	9
21	Actin-5c	gi|316970244	5.3	42.21	133	100	17	5
22	Actin-5c	gi|316970244	5.3	42.21	133	100	17	5
23	inorganic pyrophosphatase	gi|316967781	5.76	41.796	96	100	12	4
24	inorganic pyrophosphatase	gi|316967781	5.76	41.796	96	100	12	4
25	No identified							
26	No identified							
27	adenosine deaminase	gi|47934208	5.93	39.787	61	97.4	13	4
28	putative LIM and SH3 domain protein	gi|316973491	9.47	33.96	63	98.7	33	9
29	hypothetical protein Tsp_11860	gi|316969203	8.09	39.25	65	98.2	25	8
30	hypothetical protein Tsp_11860	gi|316969203	8.09	39.25	68	97.8	25	8
31	ubiquitin-conjugating enzyme E2 1	gi|316968002	7.07	41.31	65	100	19	8
32	phosphomannomutase 2	gi|316975006	5.76	31.86	379	100	43	12
33	zinc metallo protein	gi|316965635	5.93	32.23	73	100	23	6
34	hypothetical protein Tsp_11358	gi|316966928	9.51	34.91	82	100	34	8
35	Tas retrotransposon peptidase A16 superfamily protein	gi|316959639	8.6	37.73	64	99.8	23	9
36	putative trypsin	gi|316978020	8.53	39.6	89	100	23	7
37	No identified							
38	protein-tyrosine phosphatase	gi|316967260	5.92	25.75	94	100	21	5
39	putative nudix hydrolase 6	gi|339244291	5.21	32.98	63	98.44	15	4
40	Actin-depolymerizing factor 2	gi|316972221	6.37	40.828	123	100	10	4
41	26S protease regulatory subunit 6B	gi|316968151	5.47	39	88	100	19	5
42	putative thioredoxin	gi|316967722	5.56	36.88	217	100	34	8
43	26S protease regulatory subunit 7	gi|316970971	5.67	49	97	100	22	9
44	vacuolar proton pump subunit E	gi|316974496	5.8	26.14	163	100	30	5
45	inositol monophosphatase	gi|316978221	5.65	23.35	185	100	38	5
46	No identified							
47	hypothetical protein Tsp_11860	gi|316969203	8.09	39.25			25	8
48	hypothetical protein Tsp_11860	gi|316969203	8.09	39.25			25	8
49	No identified							
50	No identified							
51	putative thioredoxin	gi|316967722	5.56	36.88	217	100	34	8
52	putative thioredoxin	gi|316967722	5.56	36.88	217	100	34	8
53	No identified							
54	tumor protein D52	gi|316971259	5.98	16.889	84	97.9	59	7
55	No identified							
56	serine protease inhibitor Kazal-type 4	gi|316969591	8.56	24.89	72	99.875	27	4
57	serine protease inhibitor Kazal-type 4	gi|316969591	8.56	24.89	72	99.875	27	4
58	No identified							
59	serine protease inhibitor Kazal-type 4	gi|316969591	8.56	24.89	72	99.875	27	4
60	14-3-3 protein	gi|257219670	4.83	28.29	74	99.855	24	6
61	14-3-3 protein	gi|257219670	4.83	28.29	74	99.855	24	6
62	tumor protein D52	gi|316971259	5.98	16.889	84	97.9	59	7

63	translation initiation factor eIF-5A	gi|316973471	5.17	12.32	113	100	57	4
64	tumor protein D52	gi|316971259	5.98	16.889	84	97.9	59	7

Distribution of the Identified Protein Spots

The molecular weight (MW) and isoelectric point (pI) of the identified proteins were analyzed (Figure 2A). The MW of 55 proteins was ranged from 12.32 to 93.66 kDa. Twenty-eight of 55 (50.9%) proteins ranged from 30 to 50 kDa. The pI was between 4.83 and 9.04, and 29 of 55 (52.7%) proteins were in the range of pI 5~6 (Figure 2B). The two-dimensional distribution of the 55 identified proteins is shown in Figure 2C.

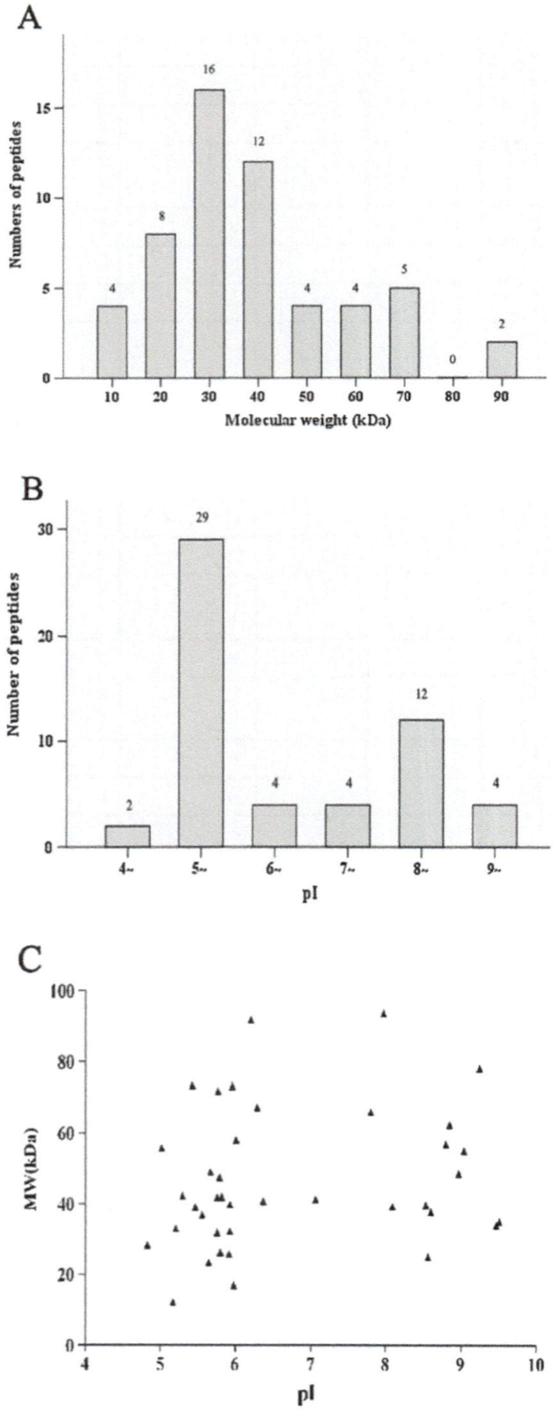

Figure 2: Distributions of *T. spiralis* adult worm proteins spots recognized by both pig and mouse anti-*T. spiralis*sera at 7 DPI. **(A)** Distributions of molecular weight (MW) for *T. spiralis* adult worm proteins recognized by both pig and mouse anti-*T. spiraliss* era at 7 DPI. **(B)** Distributions of isoelectric point (pI) for *T. spiralis* adult worm protein spots recognized by both pig and mouse anti-*T. spiralis* sera at 7 DPI. **(C)** The two-dimensional distribution of *T. spiralis* adult worm protein spots recognized by both pig and mouse anti-*T. spiralis* sera at 7 DPI.

Gene Ontology Analysis

To further understand the functions of these identified immunoreactive proteins, the InterPro database was searched based on the BLASTP results. A total of 40 proteins, not including the 15 repeated protein spots, were categorized by cellular component, molecular function, and biological process using WEGO. The primary molecular functions were catalytic activity (GO: 0003824) and binding (GO: 0005488). These proteins were classified into eight categories related to their biological process as follows: biological regulation, cellular component organization, cellular process, establishment localization, metabolic process, pigmentation, and response to stimulus. For the biological process function, a large proportion was metabolic process (GO: 0008152) and cellular process (GO: 0009987). These results are shown in Figure 3.

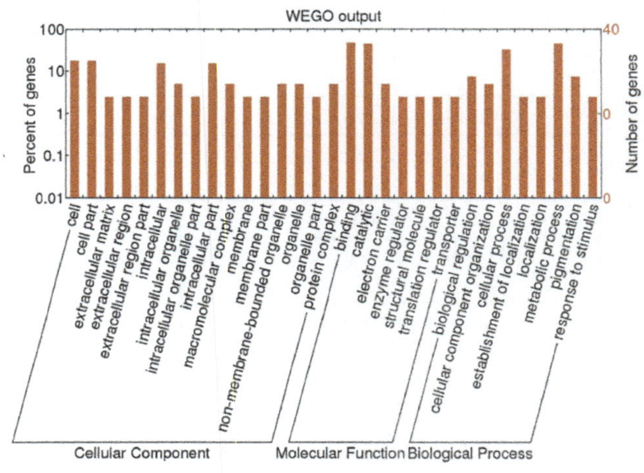

Figure 3: GO categories of *T. spiralis* immunoreactive adult worm proteins. The proteins were classified into cellular component, molecular function and biological process by WEGO according to their GO signatures.

Expression feasibility of r*Ts*14-3-3 and its Recognition by Infected Sera

To validate the potential of *Ts*14-3-3 as vaccine or diagnostic antigen, the *Ts*14-3-3 was successfully cloned and expressed in *E. coli* BL21 as soluble recombinant protein. As shown in Figure 4A, the recombinant protein (r*Ts*14-3-3) was highly induced in BL21 in soluble and insoluble fractions. The molecular mass of the r*Ts*14-3-3 (with the histidine tag) was approximately 30 kDa, which corresponded well to the predicted size of the gene product. The r*Ts*14-3-3 was easily purified with Ni-affinity chromatography. The purified r*Ts*14-3-3 was able to be strongly recognized by the same *T. spiralis*-

infected swine and mouse sera used for identifying the immunogenic antigens by immunoproteomic approach, but not by normal swine and mice sera (Figure 4B). The r*Ts*14-3-3 was recognized not only by the early infected swine sera (7 dpi) but also by the sera from swine infected with *T. spiralis* for up to 28 days (Figure 4C). The expression of native *Ts*14-3-3 was detected in both stages of *T. spiralis* by using mouse antisera against r*Ts*14-3-3 (Figure 4D).

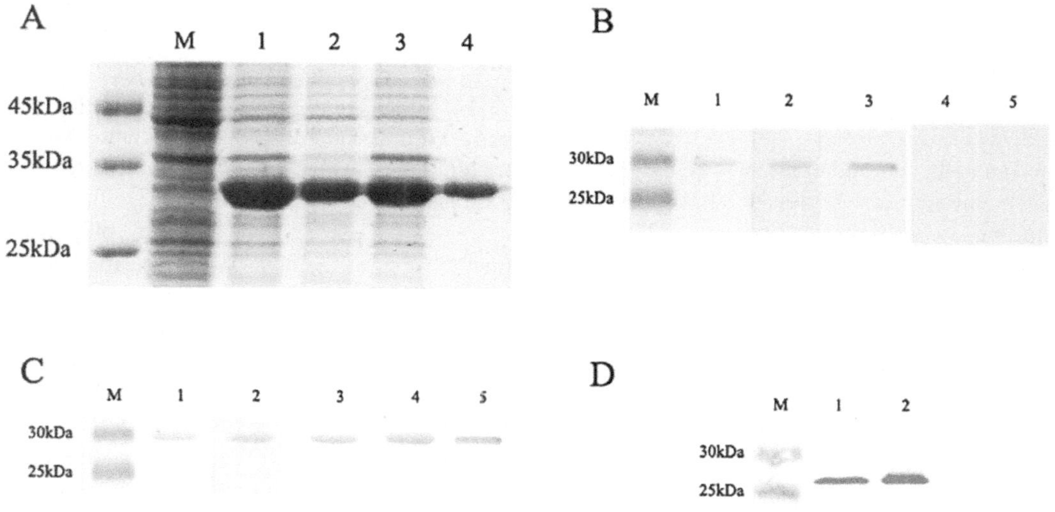

Figure 4: SDS-PAGE and Western blot analysis of r*Ts*14-3-3 expressed in *E. coli*BL21. (A) Bacterial lysates or purified recombinant protein were analyzed by SDS–PAGE and stained with Coomassie blue. Lane M, protein marker; lane 1, uninduced *E. coli* lysate; lane 2, IPTG-induced *E. coli* lysate; lane 3, insoluble fraction of induced *E. coli* lysate ; lane 4, soluble fraction of induced *E. coli* lysate ; lane 5, r*Ts*14-3-3 purified by Ni-affinity chromatography. **(B)** Western blot analysis of r*Ts*14-3-3. The r*Ts*14-3-3 was transferred on individual lane and recognized by *T. spiralis* infected swine sera at 7 dpi (lane 1); *T. spiralis* infected mouse sera at 7 dpi (lane 2) and anti-His monoclonal antibody (lane 4).**(C)**. The r*Ts*14-3-3 was recognized by sera of swine infected with *T. spiralis* for 7 days (lane 1); 14 days (lane 2); 21 days (lane 3) and 28 days (lane 4) or by anti-His antibody as control (lane 5). **D**. Western blot analysis of native *Ts*14-3-3 in adult extracts (lane 1) and in muscle larval extracts (lane 2) of *T. spiralis* by antibody against r*Ts*-14-3-3.

DISCUSSION

In recent years, trichinellosis has become an emerging and re-emerging parasitic diseases and the severity of trichinellosis in human ranges from subclinical to fatal [24]. Early diagnosis of the infection is critical for the timely and effective treatment of trichinellosis because anthelmintic drugs are much more effective against adult worms in the intestine than to the encapsulated larvae in the muscle [9,12]. Therefore, it is important to identify antigens recognized by the host immune system during the early infection stage. These immunodominant antigens can be developed as biomarkers for the early diagnosis of trichinellosis or even as vaccine candidates to better control this food-borne zoonotic disease.

Although a number of *Trichinella* antigens, such as TSL-1, serine protease and histidine-tailed metalloprotein, have been identified as immunodominant antigens recognized by the host immune system during natural infection [8,25,26], these antigens do not meet the requirements for the early diagnosis of infection. Some somatic antigens from adult *T. spiralis* worms were recognized by *Trichinella* early or late infection sera from pigs by immunoscreening the adult worm cDNA library [27]. Therefore, it is possible to identify and develop these immunodominant antigens from adult worm as immunological reagents for the early diagnosis of *Trichinella* infection because the adult stage only exists during the early stage of infection.

In this study, a novel immunoproteomics approach was used to identify potential immunogens for the early diagnosis of trichinellosis or to develop an effective vaccine. The soluble extracts from *T. spiralis* adult worms were separated by 2-DE and detected with early infection sera from swine or mice infected with *T. spiralis* for only 7 days. During this period of infection,*Trichinella* infective larvae develop only into adult worms in the intestine of the infected host; therefore, the antigens from the adult worms that elicit an early immune response in infected animals may be used as potential target antigens for early diagnosis and/or vaccines against trichinellosis.

More than 60 *T. spiralis* adult worm proteins were recognized by the pooled early infection sera from infected pigs and mice, and 55 of these proteins were identified by MALDI-TOF/TOF-MS. The MW of the identified antigens ranged from 12.3 kDa to 93.7 kDa, and the pI ranged from pH 5.0 and 9.5. The fifty-five identified antigens represent 40 different proteins. Several antigens had more than one spot with different pIs, such as intermediate filament protein, actin-5c, 14-3-3, inorganic pyrophosphatase, putative thioredoxin, and serine protease inhibitor. It is possible that these antigens have more than one isoform with different post-translation modifications or binding to different co-factors that change their pI or molecular weight. Remarkably, these proteins are involved in a wide range of biological functions, such as biological regulation, cellular process, metabolic process, and localization.

Among the potential immunogens in present study, several structural proteins, including cytoskeleton and muscle proteins, such as actin-5c was also identified. Studies indicated that actin is related to the invasion of worm into the intestinal epithelial cells, indicating this protein may be involved in the early survival of the parasites within the host [28]. Mice infected with*Echinostoma caproni*, an intestinal trematode, produce early immune responses to actin, suggesting that this protein is exposed early to the host and may be of importance in the establishment of parasitism [29].

Heat shock proteins (HSPs) are traditionally considered a highly immunogenic and conserved family of proteins. These proteins were identified as potential vaccine candidate antigens and may also function as immunological modulators of immune responses [30]. Of these, HSP70 is a major target of immune responses of the host to infections by helminths and protozoan parasites [31,32]. Previous studies indicated that SmHSP70 elicited an early humoral immune response and may be a good target for the immunodiagnosis of schistosomiasis [33]. HSP70 in*Echinostoma caproni* also induced a strong early immune response in mice [29]. Moreover, our previous study indicated that *Ts*-Hsp70 from adult *T. spiralis* is highly immunogenic and may be a good vaccine candidate [34,35]. In this study, *Ts*-HSP70 was recognized by early infection sera, indicating that this protein has potential for the early diagnosis of trichinellosis.

Another interesting protein recognized by early infected sera in this study is cysteine protease. This protease is a key molecule in host-parasite interactions, which has gained significant attention as a target for chemotherapy or immunoprophylaxis [36]. Vaccination with cysteine protease coding DNAs induced significant protection against several helminth and protozoan infections by reducing the parasite burden or fecal egg count and reducing egg viability [37]. In addition, many cysteine proteases can be used for the immunodiagnosis of parasitic diseases with good sensitivity and specificity [38,39]. Recognition of the cysteine protease by early *T. spiralis* infection sera in this study suggests that *T. spiralis* cysteine protease is not only a good target for vaccine but also a promising target for immunodiagnostic antigen.

Of the immunogens identified in the present study, the 14-3-3 protein is of particular interest. There were two protein spots that matched the 14-3-3 protein of *T. spirali*, which indicates that the 14-3-3 protein was a strong immunogenic antigen during the early infection. The 14-3-3 proteins, a series of abundant acidic proteins which belong to a family of conserved regulatory molecules, play key roles in several eukaryotic biochemical processes, such as signal transduction, transport, regulation, cell differentiation and cell survival, and have been identified in several helminth parasites [40,41]. Studies indicated that this protein could be used for routine immunodiagnosis and serological epidemiological surveys as well for helminthic diseases with high sensitivity and specificity [42,43]. In addition, for parasites, such as *S. mansoni* and *E. granulosus*, the 14-3-3 proteins can induce humoral and cellular immune responses and have been tested as potential vaccine targets [44,45]. Therefore, it intrigues our interest to evaluate *Ts*14-3-3 identified in this study as a reagent for the early serologic diagnosis for trichinellosis or even for the target of vaccine against *Trichnelle* infection. Primary expression assay demonstrated that *Ts*14-3-3 is feasible to be expressed as soluble recombinant protein in *E. coli* and the purified recombinant *Ts*14-3-3 from induced bacterial lysates was able to be recognized not only by the early *T. spiralis*-infected sera from swine and mice (7 dpi), but also by sera of swine infected for up to 28 days. In addition, this antigen exists in both adult and muscle larvae stages, indicating this *Ts*14-3-3 can be used not only for early diagnosis but also for detecting whole period of infection. These results further confirm that *Ts*14-3-3 is an immunodominant antigen recognized by *T. spiralis* infected sera and could be a good target for early immunodiagnosis of trichinellosis. The sensitivity and specificity of recombinant *Ts*14-3-3 as an antigen for serological diagnosis of *Trichinella* infection is under investigation by testing the defined sera from patients with trichinellosis compared with normal sera and sera from patients with other helminthiases.

In this study, we identified candidate antigens for early immunodiagnosis and vaccine development against trichinellosis using an immunoproteomics approach. The proteins identified in this study, specifically *Ts*14-3-3 protein, cysteine protease and HSP70, may play critical roles in the maintenance of the host-parasite relationship during the early stage of*Trichinella* infection, therefore are good targets for vaccine and early immunodiagnosis as well. Except for *Ts*14-3-3 that has been successfully expressed in *E. coli* as soluble recombinant protein that can be recognized by *Trichinella*-infected swine and mouse sera, other identified antigens are also being evaluated for their potential as immunodiagnostic or vaccine reagents using *in vitro* expression of the recombinant proteins, immunological test for defined infection sera and challenge study with *T. spiralis* infection animal model.

CONCLUSIONS

In this study, 2-DE and Western blot were used to characterize the diagnostic antigens or vaccine candidates from *T. spiralis* adult worm. A total of 64 proteins from the adult worm were recognized by early infection sera from pigs and mice infected with *T. spiralis* for 7 days. The proteins identified in this study, especially 14-3-3 protein, possess significant potential as early diagnostic reagents or vaccine candidates.

ACKNOWLEDGEMENTS

This study was supported by grants from the National Natural Science Foundation of China (81201313, 81171598), the Natural Science Fundation of Beijing (5122007), and the National Science and Technology Major Project (2012ZX10004220-012). We thank Yuwan Hao, Yaping Yang, Fengyun Wang and Jin Pan for their technical assistance.

AUTHORS' CONTRIBUTIONS

JY performed the experiments and drafted the manuscript. WP, XMS, XZ, YG, QS and JJH performed several experiments. XPZ designed the study and revised the manuscript. All authors read and approved the final manuscript.

REFERENCES

1. Dupouy-Camet J. Presidential address of ICT12 Conference: "Trichinella and trichinellosis–a never ending story". Vet Parasitol. 2009;159(3–4):194–6.
2. Chen MX, Ai L, Xu MJ, Chen SH, Zhang YN, Guo J, et al. Identification and characterization of microRNAs in *Trichinella spiralis* by comparison with Brugia malayi and *Caenorhabditis elegans*. Parasitol Res. 2011;109(3):553–8.
3. Pozio E. World distribution of *Trichinella spp.* infections in animals and humans. Vet Parasitol. 2007;149(1–2):3–21.

4. Wang ZQ, Cui J, Xu BL. The epidemiology of human trichinellosis in China during 2000-2003. Acta Trop. 2006;97(3):247–51.

5. Cui J, Wang ZQ, Xu BL. The epidemiology of human trichinellosis in China during 2004-2009. Acta Trop. 2011;118(1):1–5.

6. Kang SA, Cho MK, Park MK, Kim DH, Hong YC, Lee YS, et al. Alteration of helper T-cell related cytokine production in splenocytes during *Trichinella spiralis* infection. Vet Parasitol. 2012;186(3–4):319–27.

7. Zocevic A, Mace P, Vallee I, Blaga R, Liu M, Lacour SA, et al. Identification of *Trichinella spiralis* early antigens at the pre-adult and adult stages. Parasitology. 2011;138(4):463–71.

8. Yepez-Mulia L, Hernandez-Bello R, Arizmendi-Puga N, Fonseca-Linan R, Ortega-Pierres G. Contributions to the study of *Trichinella spiralis* TSL-1 antigens in host immunity. Parasite Immunol. 2007;29(12):661–70.

9. Dupouy-Camet J, Kociecka W, Bruschi F, Bolas-Fernandez F, Pozio E. Opinion on the diagnosis and treatment of human trichinellosis. Expert Opin Pharmacother. 2002;3(8):1117–30.

10. Gomez-Morales MA, Ludovisi A, Amati M, Cherchi S, Pezzotti P, Pozio E. Validation of an enzyme-linked immunosorbent assay for diagnosis of human trichinellosis. Clin Vaccine Immunol. 2008;15(11):1723–9.Central

11. Cuttell L, Gomez-Morales MA, Cookson B, Adams PJ, Reid SA, Vanderlinde PB, et al. Evaluation of ELISA coupled with western blot as a surveillance tool for *Trichinella*infection in wild boar (Sus scrofa). Vet Parasitol. 2014;199(3–4):179–90.

12. Nunez GG, Costantino SN, Venturiello SM. Detection of coproantibodies and faecal immune complexes in human trichinellosis. Parasitology. 2007;134(Pt 5):723–7.

13. Zarlenga DS, Boyd P, Lichtenfels JR, Hill D, Ray GH. Identification and characterisation of a cDNA sequence encoding a glutamic acid-rich protein specifically transcribed in*Trichinella spiralis* newborn larvae and recognised by infected swine serum. Int J Parasitol. 2002;32(11):1361–70.

14. Zhang Y, Wang Z, Li L, Cui J. Molecular characterization of *Trichinella spiralis*aminopeptidase and its potential as a novel vaccine candidate antigen against trichinellosis in BALB/c mice. Parasit Vectors. 2013;6:246.

15. Krah A, Jungblut PR. Immunoproteomics. Methods Mol Med. 2004;94:19–32.

16. Wang J, Zhao F, Yu CX, Xiao D, Song LJ, Yin XR, et al. Identification of proteins inducing short-lived antibody responses from excreted/secretory products of *Schistosoma japonicum* adult worms by immunoproteomic analysis. J Proteomics. 2013;87:53–67.

17. Sun XM, Ji YS, Elashram SA, Lu ZM, Liu XY, Suo X, et al. Identification of antigenic proteins of *Toxoplasma gondii* RH strain recognized by human immunoglobulin G using immunoproteomics. J Proteomics. 2012;77:423–32.

18. Acevedo N, Mohr J, Zakzuk J, Samonig M, Briza P, Erler A, et al. Proteomic and immunochemical characterization of glutathione transferase as a new allergen of the nematode *Ascaris lumbricoides*. PLoS One. 2013;8(11):e78353.

19. Santivanez SJ, Hernandez-Gonzalez A, Chile N, Oleaga A, Arana Y, Palma S, et al. Proteomic study of activated *Taenia solium* oncospheres. Mol Biochem Parasitol. 2010;171(1):32–9.

20. Bien J, Nareaho A, Varmanen P, Gozdzik K, Moskwa B, Cabaj W, et al. Comparative analysis of excretory-secretory antigens of *Trichinella spiralis* and *Trichinella britovi*muscle larvae by two-dimensional difference gel electrophoresis and immunoblotting. Proteome Sci. 2012;10(1):10.

21. Cui J, Liu RD, Wang L, Zhang X, Jiang P, Liu MY, et al. Proteomic analysis of surface proteins of *Trichinella spiralis* muscle larvae by two-dimensional gel electrophoresis and mass spectrometry. Parasit Vectors. 2013;6:355.

22. Wang L, Cui J, Hu DD, Liu RD, Wang ZQ. Identification of early diagnostic antigens from major excretory-secretory proteins of *Trichinella spiralis* muscle larvae using immunoproteomics. Parasit Vectors. 2014;7:40.

23. Gamble HR, Bessonov AS, Cuperlovic K, Gajadhar AA, van Knapen F, Noeckler K, et al. International Commission on Trichinellosis: recommendations on methods for the control of*Trichinella* in domestic and wild animals intended for human consumption. Vet Parasitol. 2000;93(3–4):393–408.

24. Frey CF, Schuppers ME, Nockler K, Marinculic A, Pozio E, Kihm U, et al. Validation of a western blot for the detection of anti-trichinella spp. Antibodies in domestic pigs. Parasitol Res. 2009;104(6):1269–77.

25. Wang B, Wang ZQ, Jin J, Ren HJ, Liu LN, Cui J. Cloning, expression and characterization of a *Trichinella spiralis* serine protease gene encoding a 35.5 kDa protein. Exp Parasitol. 2013;134(2):148–54.

26. Radoslavov G, Jordanova R, Teofanova D, Georgieva K, Hristov P, Salomone-Stagni M, et al. A novel secretory poly-cysteine and histidine-tailed metalloprotein (Ts-PCHTP) from*Trichinella spiralis* (Nematoda). PLoS One. 2010;5(10):e13343.

27. Liu P, Wu XP, Bai X, Wang XL, Yu L, Rosenthal B, et al. Screening of early antigen genes of adult-stage *Trichinella spiralis* using pig serum from different stages of early infection. Vet Parasitol. 2013;194(2–4):222–5.

28. Wang ZQ, Wang L, Cui J. Proteomic analysis of *Trichinella spiralis* proteins in intestinal epithelial cells after culture with their larvae by shotgun LC-MS/MS approach. J Proteomics. 2012;75(8):2375–83.

29. Sotillo J, Valero L, Sanchez DPM, Fried B, Esteban JG, Marcilla A, et al. Identification of antigenic proteins from *Echinostoma caproni* (Trematoda) recognized by mouse immunoglobulins M, A and G using an immunoproteomic approach. Parasite Immunol. 2008;30(5):271–9.

30. Colaco CA, Bailey CR, Walker KB, Keeble J. Heat shock proteins: stimulators of innate and acquired immunity. Biomed Res Int. 2013;2013:461230.

31. Kaur J, Kaur S. ELISA and western blotting for the detection of Hsp70 and Hsp83 antigens of *Leishmania donovani*. J Parasit Dis. 2013;37(1):68–73.

32. Liu F, Cui SJ, Hu W, Feng Z, Wang ZQ, Han ZG. Excretory/secretory proteome of the adult developmental stage of human blood fluke, Schistosoma japonicum. Mol Cell Proteomics. 2009;8(6):1236–51.

33. Kanamura HY, Hancock K, Rodrigues V, Damian RT. *Schistosoma mansoni* heat shock protein 70 elicits an early humoral immune response in *S. mansoni* infected baboons. Mem Inst Oswaldo Cruz. 2002;97(5):711–6.

34. Wang S, Zhu X, Yang Y, Yang J, Gu Y, Wei J, et al. Molecular cloning and characterization of heat shock protein 70 from *Trichinella spiralis*. Acta Trop. 2009;110(1):46–51.

35. Fang L, Sun L, Yang J, Gu Y, Zhan B, Huang J, et al. Heat shock protein 70 from*Trichinella spiralis* induces protective immunity in BALB/c mice by activating dendritic cells. Vaccine. 2014;32(35):4412–9.

36. Sajid M, McKerrow JH. Cysteine proteases of parasitic organisms. Mol Biochem Parasitol. 2002;120(1):1–21.

37. Jorgensen L, Buchmann K. Cysteine proteases as potential antigens in antiparasitic DNA vaccines. Vaccine. 2011;29(34):5575–83.

38. Pina R, Gutierrez AH, Gilman RH, Rueda D, Sifuentes C, Flores M, et al. A dot-ELISA using a partially purified cathepsin-L-like protein fraction from Taenia solium cysticerci, for the diagnosis of human neurocysticercosis. Ann Trop Med Parasitol. 2011;105(4):311–8.

39. Rabee I, Mahana NA, Badr AM. Immunodiagnosis of Egyptian human fasciolosis gigantica using Fas1 and Fas2 cysteine proteinase antigens. J Egypt Soc Parasitol. 2013;43(3):787–96.

40. Mrowiec T, Schwappach B. 14-3-3 proteins in membrane protein transport. Biol Chem. 2006;387(9):1227–36.

41. Obsil T, Obsilova V. Structural basis of 14-3-3 protein functions. Semin Cell Dev Biol. 2011;22(7):663–72.

42. Lee MR, Kim YJ, Kim DW, Yoo WG, Cho SH, Hwang KY, et al. The identification of antigenic proteins: 14-3-3 protein and propionyl-CoA carboxylase in *Clonorchis sinensis*. Mol Biochem Parasitol. 2012;182(1–2):1–6.

43. Luo QL, Qiao ZP, Zhou YD, Li XY, Zhong ZR, Yu YJ, et al. Application of signaling protein 14-3-3 and 26 kDa glutathione-S-transferase to serological diagnosis of *Schistosomiasis japonica*. Acta Trop. 2009;112(2):91–6.

44. Li ZJ, Wang YN, Wang Q, Zhao W. Echinococcus granulosus 14-3-3 protein: a potential vaccine candidate against challenge with *Echinococcus granulosus* in mice. Biomed Environ Sci. 2012;25(3):352–8.

45. Schechtman D, Tarrab-Hazdai R, Arnon R. The 14-3-3 protein as a vaccine candidate against schistosomiasis. Parasite Immunol. 2001;23(4):213–7.

CHAPTER 20

MOLECULAR EPIDEMIOLOGY OF ASCARIASIS: A GLOBAL PERSPECTIVE ON THE TRANSMISSION DYNAMICS OF ASCARIS IN PEOPLE AND PIGS

Martha Betson, Peter Nejsum, Richard P. Bendall, Rinki M. Deb and J. Russell Stothard

Keywords: *Ascaris*, giant roundworm, population genetics, soil-transmitted helminth, zoonosis, neglected tropical disease, microsatellite, barcode

Ascariasis is caused by infection with the giant roundworm *Ascaris lumbricoides*, with around 760 million cases worldwide [1]. Although infections are particularly common in developing countries where sanitation and hygiene is poor, ascariasis exhibits a cosmopolitan distribution, with cases also described in developed countries [2–4]. It was recently estimated that ascariasis contributes 1.31 million disability-adjusted life years to the global burden of disease [1, 5]. The closely related parasite *Ascaris suum* infects innumerable pigs across the globe and is especially common in organic and extensive farming systems [6, 7]. Infections in pigs are associated with production losses owing to reduced growth and low feed conversion efficiency, with livers unfit for human consumption [7].

Because adult *A. lumbricoides* and *A. suum* worms are morphologically indistinguishable, there has been much debate as to whether they represent the same or different species [8, 9]. In addition, the extent of natural cross-transmission of worms between pig and human hosts is unclear [10]. Experimental cross-infections have demonstrated that *A. suum* can infect humans and that *A. lumbricoides* can infect pigs, with host preference in the efficiency of infection establishment [10, 11]. Although no definitive molecular marker has been found that can clearly distinguish between so-called human worms and pig worms, a combination of markers has proven useful [11]. Molecular studies have demonstrated that human *Ascaris* infections in developed countries are predominantly of pig origin [2–4, 12], whereas in developing countries human-to-human transmission predominates [13–16]. However, in China, 14% of human worms were derived from pigs (i.e., were of zoonotic origin), indicating that cross-transmission in areas of endemicity may be more common than originally thought [17]. Hybrids between human and pig worms have been detected, indicating that mating can take place between *Ascaris* from the 2 host species [18].

Molecular markers have been used to investigate geographical differences in the population structure of *Ascaris* on a macroscale and microscale. Overall, the data support structuring of *Ascaris* populations between countries [13, 18–21]. However, results were more variable at a local scale [14, 19, 20, 22], which may reflect methodological differences and variations in transmission dynamics, migration, and farming practices. To date, sampling of *Ascaris* from Africa has not been extensive. Given that humans arose on this continent [23], it is plausible that there has been a long association between humans and the *Ascaris* parasite here.

In this study, we used mitochondrial and microsatellite markers to characterize a large collection of adult *Ascaris* worms acquired from human and pig hosts in areas where *A. lumbricoides* is considered endemic or nonendemic. The level of *Ascaris* cross-transmission between pig and human hosts was investigated, as was the geographical structuring of parasite populations. The results provide novel insights into the evolutionary origins of *Ascaris* in humans and pigs.

Citation: Martha Betson, Peter Nejsum, Richard P. Bendall, Rinki M. Deb, and J. Russell Stothard, "Molecular Epidemiology of Ascariasis: A Global Perspective on the Transmission Dynamics of Ascaris in People and Pigs," DOI: 10.1093/infdis/jiu193

MATERIALS AND METHODS

Ascaris Samples, Ethics Approval, and Informed Consent

The host and sampling location of the worms are summarized in Table 1. Many samples were collected during previous studies. Additional worms were obtained from humans in the United Kingdom, Kenya, and Bangladesh and from pigs in the United Kingdom, Denmark, and Tanzania. Ethics approval and informed consent were obtained for collection of worms from humans [13, 14, 19, 20, 24, 26]. Sixteen worms from humans had been submitted to the Clinical Microbiology Laboratory, Royal Cornwall Hospital, for routine identification.

Table 1. Characteristics of *Ascaris* Samples Included in This Study

Country, Location	**Host**	**Samples, No.**	***cox*1**	**MS**	**Reference**
United Kingdom					
Cornwall	Humans	15	14	11	[3], this study
Abattoir, Bedfordshire	Pigs	49	38	41	This study
Denmark					
Unspecified	Humans	2	2	2	This study
Unspecified	Pigs	31	27	31	This study
Uganda					
Mayengo, Kabale District	Humans	10	10	10	[24]
Nyamirima, Kabale	Humans	9	9	9	[24]
Katuna, Kabale	Humans	1	1	1	[24]
Kiniogo, Kabale	Humans	9	9	8	[24]
Nyakitokoli, Kabale	Humans	41	41	18	[24]
Habutobere, Kabale	Humans	37	37[a]	32[a]	[20]
Musezero, Kisoro District	Humans	62	61[a]	56[a]	[20]
Hamukaaka, Kabale	Humans	19	19[b]	9[b]	[19]
Kapchorwa, Kapchorwa District	Humans	2	2	0	Davies et al (unpublished data)
Katuna, Kabale	Pigs	23	23	21	[25]
Burambira-Katuna, Kabale	Pigs	6	6	5	[25]
Kamugangguzi, Kabale	Pigs	11	11	9	[25]
Rwakakobe, Kabale	Pigs	12	8	9	[25]
Mugyenyi Lane, Kabale	Pigs	7	7	6	[25]
Abattoir, Kampala	Pigs	55	52	6	This study
Zanzibar					
Kandwi	Humans	5	5[b]	4[b]	[19]
Kizimibani	Humans	8	8[b]	8[b]	[19]
Ghana	Humans	18	15[b]	16[b]	[19]
Tumbatu-Jongowe	Humans	29	29[b]	25[b]	[19]
Miscellaneous	Humans	2	2[b]	0	[19]
Tanzania					
Abattoir	Pigs	38	37	36	This study
Kenya					
Kwale	Humans	6	6	0	This study
Zambia					
Traveler (worm sampled in the United Kingdom)	Humans	1	1	0	This study
Bangladesh					
Unspecified	Humans	41	37	37	This study
Nepal					

Unspecified	Humans	5	5	0	[21]
Philippines					
Unspecified	Pigs	6	3	0	[13]
Guatemala					
Santa Cruz Naranjo and Chaimal, Santa Rosa Province	Humans	6	6	0	[14, 26]
Santa Cruz Naranjo, Santa Rosa	Pigs	6	5	0	[14, 26]
Total	Humans and pigs	572	536	410	...

Abbreviation: MS, microsatellite.

[a] *Cox*1 and microsatellite data published [20].

[b] *Cox*1 and microsatellite data published but only 5 microsatellite loci were analysed in the published study [19].

DNA Extraction

Genomic DNA was extracted from worm gonads or muscle tissue [4, 19], using the CTAB method [27], the Genomic DNA Isolation Kit for Tissue and Cells (nexttec, Hilgertshausen, Germany), or the DNeasy Blood and Tissue Kit (Qiagen, Manchester, United Kingdom).

*Cox*1 Sequencing and Microsatellite Amplification

A 450-bp fragment of the *Ascaris cox*1 gene was amplified using primers As-Co1F and As-Co1R [15], and the fragments were sequenced [19]. Eight microsatellite loci (ALAC07, ALAC09, ALGA48, ALTN04, ALGA31, ALGA15, ALAC32, and ALAC08) were individually amplified by polymerase chain reaction from a subset of samples (Table 1), and fragment sizes were determined, as published elsewhere [28].

Sequence Analysis

*cox*1 sequences were assembled and manually edited using Sequencher v4.8 (Gene Codes Corporation, Ann Arbor, MI). A 383-bp consensus sequence was obtained for each sample and aligned using MacClade v4.08 (Sinauer Associates, Sunderland, MA). Collapse v1.2 was used to identify samples with identical haplotypes. BLAST was used to search for exact sequence matches in GenBank and novel haplotypes were submitted to GenBank (accession numbers KF719094–151). A minimum-spanning parsimony network was constructed in TCS v2.1. jModeltest v2.1.3 was used to determine the best-fitting nucleotide substitution model [29], using a data set containing all unique haplotypes and a selection of previously identified haplotypes (CavHap1, CavHap3, CavHap5, and CavHap13–9) [12] obtained from GenBank. The resulting model (Hasegawa-Kishino-Yano, with gamma distributed rates) was used for construction of a maximum likelihood tree in MEGA v5.05, with branch support provided by bootstrapping (1000 replications). The same software was used to determine *p*-distances between clusters.

Microsatellite Analysis

Microsatellite allele sizes were determined using PeakScanner v1.0 (Applied Biosystems). PowerMarker v3.25 [30] was used to determine the number of alleles per locus (N_A), observed heterozygosity (H_O), and expected heterozygosity (H_E). Numbers of private alleles (N_P) and allelic richness (R_A) were calculated using FSTAT v2.9.3.2 [31]. To take into account potential relatedness of parasites from the same host individual, genetic differentiation between populations was analyzed using the hierarchical analysis of molecular variance procedure in Arlequin v3.5.1.2 [32]. Pairwise estimates of F_{ST} (a measure of genetic differentiation) between populations were generated, and permutation tests of genetic differentiation (101 000 permutations) were conducted. Genetic distances between parasite populations (Cavalli-Sforza and Edwards' chord distances) [33] were estimated in PowerMarker and visualized using a neighbor joining clustering algorithm with bootstrapping (1000 replications) to determine phenogram reliability. Consense (Phylip v3.65) was used to compute a consensus tree, which was visualized using DrawTree (Phylip v3.65). This was done for *Ascaris* populations from different host types, countries, villages, or individuals (in which the number of worms per village/host was ≥6).

Population structure was also inferred from the microsatellite data set using Bayesian analysis in STRUCTURE v2.3.4 [34, 35]. An admixture model assuming correlated allele frequencies was used (burn-in length, 50 000; run length, 100 000). Values of *K* from 1 to 14 were tested, and 20 independent runs were performed for each *K*. To determine the most likely true value of *K*, the mean Ln P(D) value (an estimate of posterior probability) was determined for each *K* and plotted against *K*. If there was no obvious peak in the plot, Δ*K* was calculated and plotted against *K* [36]. This analysis indicated that 2 was the most likely true value of *K*. To examine whether further substructuring existed, samples were assigned to one of 2 groups on the basis of a *Q* value of >0.5 in the STRUCTURE output. The simulation was run again for each group separately, testing values of *K* from 1 to 10, using a burn-in of 100 000 and a run length of 1 000 000 to improve stability between runs. The presence of cross-transmission and hybrids between pig and human worms was investigated using STRUCTURE, NewHybrids [37], and BAPS [38], as described elsewhere [17, 18].

RESULTS

*Cox*1 Haplotypes

We analyzed *cox*1 sequences from 319 *Ascaris* worms collected from humans and 217 worms collected from pigs (Table 1). A total of 75 different haplotypes were identified, 43 of which were novel. Table 2summarizes haplotype abundance by host and location. H1 was by far the most abundant haplotype, particularly in worms from humans. H3 was also common in human *Ascaris*. In contrast, H7, H28, H52, and H64 were abundant in pig worms, but of these only H64 was unique to *Ascaris* from pigs.

Table 2. *Cox*1 Haplotype Abundance, by Country and Host

Haplotype	UK		DK		UG		ZZ	TZ	KE	ZA	BA	NP	PH	GT	
	H	P	H	P	H	P	H	P	H	H	H	H	P	H	P
H1	…	…	…	…	134	4	29	…	1	…	23	…	…	…	…
H2	…	…	…	…	2	…	1	…	…	…	…	…	…	…	…
H3	…	…	…	…	23	…	12	…	…	…	…	…	…	1	…
H4	…	…	…	…	…	…	3	…	…	…	…	…	…	…	…
H5	…	…	…	…	…	…	2	…	…	…	…	…	…	…	…
H7	…	5	…	4	1	33	2	1	…	…	…	…	…	2	…
H8	…	…	…	…	…	…	2	…	…	…	1	…	…	…	…
H11	…	…	…	…	2	…	1	…	…	…	1	…	…	…	…
H21	…	…	…	…	2	…	…	…	…	…	…	…	…	…	…
H24	…	…	…	…	1	…	…	…	…	…	1	…	…	…	…
H28	8	8	1	19	1	16	…	28	…	…	…	…	2	…	3
H29	…	…	…	…	2	…	…	…	…	…	…	…	…	…	…
H32	…	…	…	…	…	3	…	2	…	…	1	2	…	2	…
H33	…	…	…	…	…	1	…	…	…	…	1	…	…	…	…
H47	…	…	…	…	2	…	…	…	…	…	…	…	…	…	…
H52	1	…	…	…	…	41	…	…	…	…	…	…	…	…	…
H57	…	…	…	…	…	3	…	…	…	…	…	…	…	…	…
H60	…	…	…	…	…	…	…	…	…	…	…	…	…	…	2
H64	…	22	…	1	…	2	…	3	…	…	…	…	…	…	…
H66	…	1	…	…	…	…	…	1	…	…	…	…	…	…	…
H74	2	…	…	…	…	…	…	…	…	…	…	…	…	…	…
H75	…	…	…	…	…	…	…	…	4	1	…	…	…	…	…
H77	…	…	…	…	1	…	…	…	1	…	…	…	…	…	…
Rare[a]	3	2	1	3	18	4	7	2	…	…	9	3	1	1	0
Total	14	38	2	27	189	107	59	37	6	1	37	5	3	6	5

Abbreviations: BA, Bangladesh; DK, Denmark; GT, Guatemala; H, humans; KE, Kenya; NP, Nepal; P, pigs; PH, Philippines; TZ, Tanzania; UG, Uganda; UK, United Kingdom; ZA, Zambia; ZZ, Zanzibar.

[a] Haplotypes that were only sampled once in this study.

In a minimum spanning parsimony network of all haplotypes, 3 main groups could be observed (Figure 1). Cluster C sequences differed by >8 base pairs from other haplotypes and so were not connected to the main network. There was no obvious segregation of haplotypes on the basis of geographical location. Clusters A and B contained haplotypes from both pig and human worms, but there was a tendency for haplotypes from human *Ascaris* to cluster around H1 and H3 and those from pig *Ascaris* to cluster around H7, H28, and H52. Cluster C only contained 1 sequence from a human worm (from the United Kingdom). A maximum likelihood tree was constructed on the basis of these haplotypes and included additional, recently published *Ascaris cox*1 sequences [12] (Supplementary Figure 1). The tree revealed the same 3 groupings of *Ascaris* sequences with strong bootstrap support for separation between the 3 groups. Mean *p*-distances were 2.8% between clusters A and B, 5.4% between clusters A and C, and 4.2% between clusters B and C. None of the sequences from other ascarids fell into these groups. Whereas clusters A and B contained sequences from *Ascaris* collected from both host species and all 4 continents, cluster C contained only sequences from Europe and Africa.

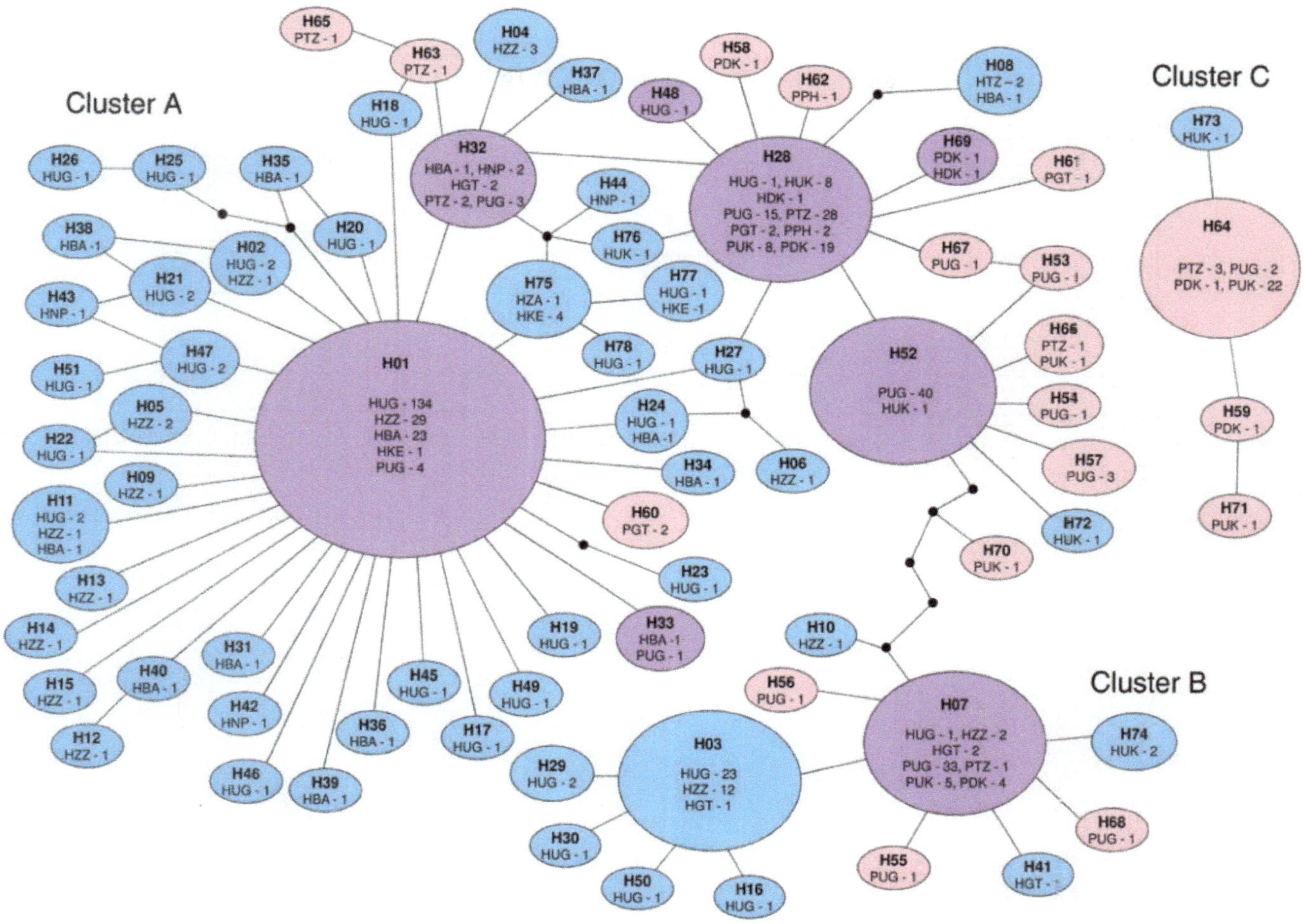

Figure 1. Minimum spanning TCS network of all *cox*1 haplotypes identified. A line indicates 1 base change. A black dot indicates a nonsampled or extinct haplotype. The size of the ovals is representative of the number of samples with a particular haplotype. Blue ovals represent haplotypes only found in worms from humans, pink ovals indicate haplotypes only found in worms from pigs, and purple ovals indicate haplotypes identified in worms from both hosts. The haplotype number is displayed in bold. The host type and geographical location are also indicated. Numbers indicate number of samples from each host type and location with the specific haplotype. The 3 clusters are labeled cluster A, cluster B, and cluster C. Abbreviations: BA, Bangladesh; DK, Denmark; GT, Guatemala; H, humans; KE, Kenya; NP, Nepal; P, pigs; PH, Philippines; TZ, Tanzania; UG, Uganda; UK, United Kingdom; ZA, Zambia; ZZ, Zanzibar.

Microsatellite Analysis

Microsatellite data were analyzed from 246 human and 164 pig worms (Table 1). Microsatellite allelic diversity stratified by locus, host species, and location is summarized in Supplementary Table 1. Mean allelic richness was somewhat higher in *Ascaris* from human hosts than those from pigs ($P = .062$; 15 000 permutations); this was more apparent when *Ascaris* from humans in the United Kingdom were classified as pig *Ascaris*($P = .041$). There was no difference in observed or expected heterozygosity between human and pig *Ascaris* (H_O, $P = .426$; H_E, $P = .200$).

Genetic flow between *Ascaris* populations from different hosts and locations was investigated through estimation of pairwise F_{ST} values and permutation tests of genetic differentiation (Table 3). There was evidence of genetic differentiation between nearly all *Ascaris* populations. However, differentiation between worms from sympatric pig and human hosts was higher than between populations from the same host in different geographical areas, except for human worms from United Kingdom. When genetic distances between *Ascaris* populations were visualized using a consensus neighbor-joining tree, populations from pig hosts clustered together and populations from humans grouped together, apart from United Kingdom human worms, which clustered with pig worms (Figure2*A*). Populations were then subdivided on the basis of village or individual host, and genetic distances were determined (Figure 2*B*). The same major division between worms from pig and human hosts was observed, with further clustering by location. *Ascaris* from humans in Uganda divided into 2 main clusters, one containing worms from Habutobere and Musezero and the other containing worms from other villages. The worms from Bangladesh grouped with those from Zanzibar. *Ascaris* worms from humans in the United Kingdom appeared most similar to worms from pigs in Tanzania and Denmark. *Ascaris* populations from different pig hosts in the United Kingdom were genetically differentiated.

Table 3. Pairwise Differentiation Between *Ascaris* Populations From Different Hosts and Countries, Based on Microsatellite Data

Host, Country	Host, Country							
	P, UK	H, UK	P, DK	H, UG	P, UG	H, ZZ	P, TZ	H, BA
P, UK	...	.153	.030	.001	.005	.025	.059	.004
H, UK	.037	...	.001	<.0001	.0002	.122	.009	<.0001
P, DK	.057	.029	...	<.0001	.0002	.012	<.0001	<.0001
H, UG	.065	.092	.101	...	<.0001	.013	<.0001	<.0001
P, UG	.056	.041	.050	.100	...	.004	<.0001	<.0001
H, ZZ	.056	.050	.070	.033	.068	...	.069	<.177
P, TZ	.064	.040	.071	.116	.051	.071	...	<.0001
H, BA	.065	.081	.100	.051	.092	.012	.106	...

Data below the diagonal denote pairwise F_{ST} (a measure of genetic differentiation) values based on hierarchical analysis, and data above the diagonal denote *P* values from the permutation test of genetic differentiation (10 100 permutations).

Abbreviations: BA, Bangladesh; DK, Denmark; H, humans; P, pigs; TZ, Tanzania; UG, Uganda; UK, United Kingdom; ZZ, Zanzibar.

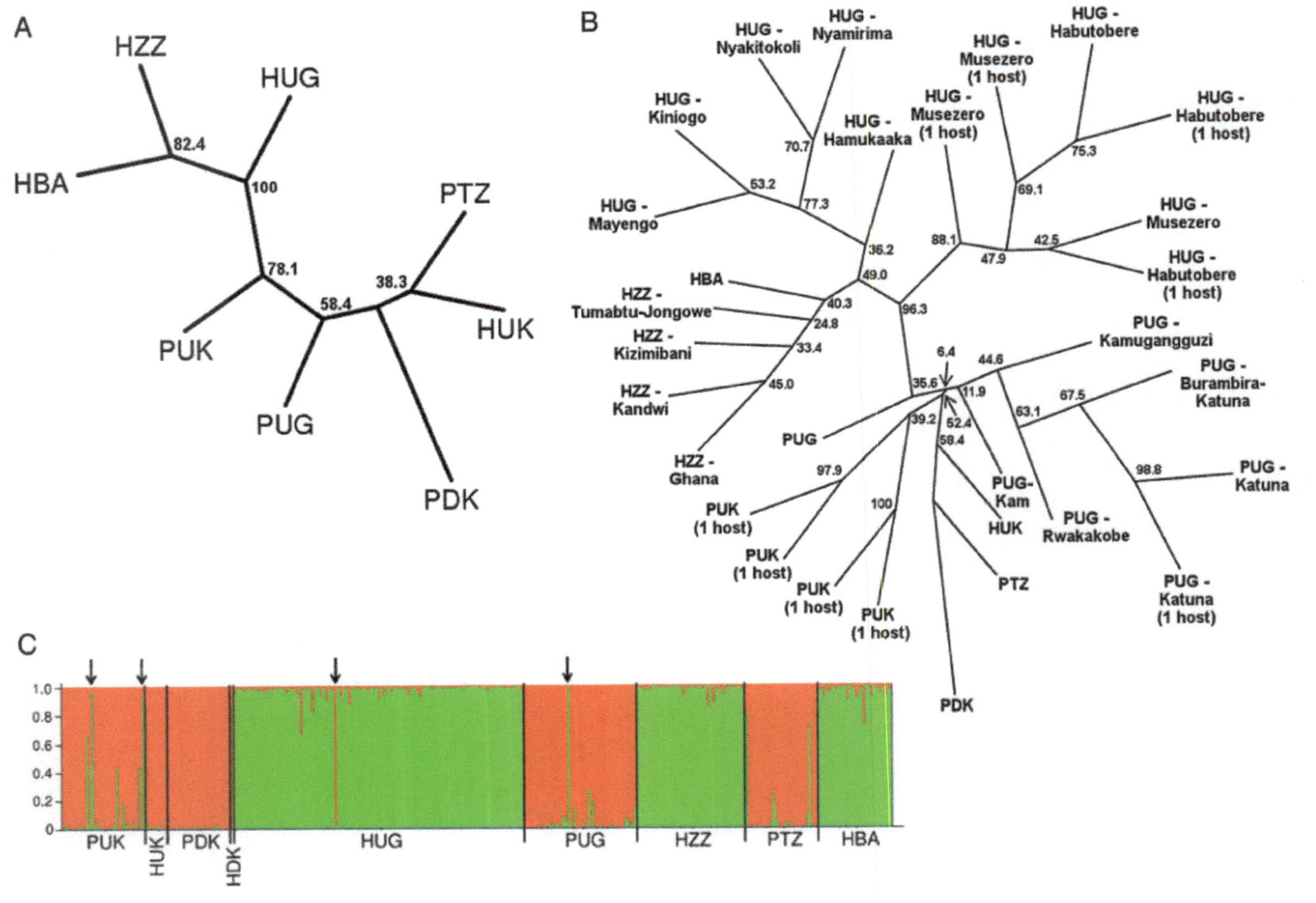

Figure 2. *A–B*, Cavalli-Sforza and Edwards' chord distances between *Ascaris* populations from different host types and locations represented in consensus neighbor joining trees based on 8 microsatellite markers. *A*, Populations stratified by host type and country. *B*, Populations stratified by host type and by country, by village, or by individual host, depending on the number of worms sampled for each location and host and whether information on individual hosts was available. Names of villages are provided in panel *B*, and if a population corresponds to worms from only 1 host, this is indicated in brackets. Bootstrap values are displayed and are based on 1001 replications. *C*, Assignment of *Ascaris* samples to clusters on the basis of STRUCTURE analysis. Output from a representative STRUCTURE run is presented. One cluster is indicated in red (mostly worms from pigs) and green (mostly worms from humans). Each narrow column corresponds to 1 sample. Examples of cross-transmission between human and pig hosts are indicated with black arrows. In addition, most worms from humans in the United Kingdom and Denmark appear to have originated from pigs. Abbreviations: BA, Bangladesh; DK, Denmark; GT, Guatemala; H, humans; KE, Kenya; NP, Nepal; P, pigs; PH, Philippines; TZ, Tanzania; UG, Uganda; UK, United Kingdom; ZA, Zambia; ZZ, Zanzibar.

Bayesian Analysis

Bayesian analysis of the microsatellite data, using STRUCTURE, was used to assign worms to clusters without prior knowledge of host type or sampling location. On the basis of posterior probabilities, the true value of*K* (ie, the number of clusters) was most likely 2. A bar plot from a representative STRUCTURE run is shown in Figure 2*C*. It was apparent that the 2 clusters corresponded to host type, apart from worms from humans in Europe, which mainly clustered with worms from pigs. To investigate further substructuring in the data set, worms were designated to one of 2 groups on the basis of the STRUCTURE output, and the simulation was run again for each group separately. Additional structure was evident, with a likely *K* of 4 for each group. The 4 clusters for human worms loosely corresponded to location (Table 4): Uganda (Musezero and Habutobere), Uganda (other villages), Zanzibar, and Bangladesh. However, clusters 3 and 4 both contained worms from Zanzibar and Bangladesh. For the group mainly consisting of pig worms (Table 4), the clusters also corresponded to geographical area: United Kingdom (cluster 1), Denmark (cluster 2), Uganda (cluster 3), and Tanzania (cluster 4). The human worms from Denmark and the United Kingdom shared genomes mainly with pig worms from Denmark (cluster 2), and the human worm from Uganda mainly with pig worms from Uganda (cluster 3).

Table 4. Proportions of Each *Ascaris* Population Originating Predominantly From Humans and Pigs That Were Assigned to Each of the 4 Clusters Identified in STRUCTURE

Population, Host and Country	Worms, No.	Cluster 1	Cluster 2	Cluster 3	Cluster 4
Human *Ascaris*					
P, UK	3	0.406	0.013	0.027	0.553
H, UK	1	0.178	0.005	0.006	0.811
H, DK	1	0.179	0.005	0.006	0.809
H, UG	142	0.568	0.326	0.047	0.059
P, UG	1	0.978	0.006	0.009	0.067
H, ZZ	53	0.017	0.113	0.741	0.129
P, TZ	2	0.110	0.035	0.065	0.790
H, BA	37	0.044	0.051	0.267	0.638
Pig *Ascaris*					
H, UG	1	0.021	0.073	0.559	0.347
P, UG	55	0.034	0.145	0.751	0.071
P, TZ	34	0.012	0.361	0.016	0.611
P, UK	38	0.708	0.160	0.035	0.096
H, UK	10	0.045	0.707	0.060	0.188
P, DK	31	0.038	0.843	0.083	0.037
H, DK	1	0.008	0.844	0.094	0.055

Data are proportion of worm genomes, unless otherwise indicated.

Abbreviations: BA, Bangladesh; DK, Denmark; H, humans; P, pigs; TZ, Tanzania; UG, Uganda; UK, United Kingdom; ZZ, Zanzibar.

To investigate whether there were any cases of cross-transmission and hybridization between worms from human hosts and worms of pig origin, simulations using BAPS, NewHybrids, and STRUCTURE were conducted (Table 5). Hybrids were identified by STRUCTURE but not by BAPS or NewHybrids, suggesting that these represented false positives. All programs identified 12 worms from humans in the United Kingdom and Denmark and 1 worm from humans in Uganda as belonging to the pig cluster. In addition, 2 *Ascaris* from pigs in the United Kingdom and 1 worm from Uganda were assigned to the human cluster. These worms likely represent examples of cross-transmission between humans and pigs (Supplementary Table 2).

Table 5. Summary of STRUCTURE, BAPS, and NewHybrids Analyses

Host, Country, Program	Population 1	Population 2	Hybrid	NC	Total
Human *Ascaris*					
United Kingdom and Denmark					
STRUCTURE	0	11	2	0	13
BAPS	0	13	0	0	13
NewHybrids	2	11	0	0	13

Uganda					
STRUCTURE	140	1	2	0	143
BAPS	142	1	0	0	143
NewHybrids	140	3	0	0	143
Zanzibar					
STRUCTURE	54	0	0	0	53
BAPS	54	0	0	0	53
NewHybrids	53	1	0	0	53
Bangladesh					
STRUCTURE	37	0	0	0	37
BAPS	37	0	0	0	37
NewHybrids	36	0	0	1	37
Pig *Ascaris*					
United Kingdom					
STRUCTURE	2	34	5	0	41
BAPS	4	37	0	0	41
NewHybrids	5	35	0	1	41
Denmark					
STRUCTURE	0	31	0	0	31
BAPS	0	31	0	0	31
NewHybrids	0	31	0	0	31
Uganda					
STRUCTURE	1	52	3	0	56
BAPS	1	55	0	0	56
NewHybrids	1	54	0	1	56
Tanzania					
STRUCTURE	0	33	3	0	36
BAPS	2	34	0	0	36
NewHybrids	2	34	0	0	36

Data are no. of worms.

Abbreviation: NC, not classified.

DISCUSSION

Here, we describe the first large-scale molecular analysis of human and pig *Ascaris* from different locations across the globe using mitochondrial and microsatellite markers including better sampling of African isolates. We found strong genetic differentiation between *Ascaris* originating from human and pig hosts. However, there was also evidence of cross-transmission of *Ascaris* between pigs and humans, with practically all European human *Ascaris* infections originating from pigs and sporadic zoonotic and anthroponotic transmission in areas of endemicity.

The *cox*1 haplotypes identified add to the growing database of *Ascaris cox*1 sequences from human and pig hosts [12, 15, 19, 20, 39, 40]. They fell into 3 groups, which correspond to clusters A–C, identified previously [12, 40]. The *p*-distances between cluster C and clusters B and A were surprisingly high but still lower than the 10% that is normally seen for*cox*1 sequences between different helminth species [41]. In addition, it should be noted that the existence of 3 taxonomic clusters was not supported by the microsatellite data, highlighting the complex nature of mitochondrial inheritance and the pitfalls associated with using a single marker for molecular epidemiological studies [42]. The extremely frequent sampling of H1 and its central position in cluster A suggest that this may be an ancestral haplotype, originating in Africa, that has subsequently diverged and spread. Moreover, we did not find a strict segregation between *cox*1 haplotypes from worms of human or pig origin. Nevertheless, there were constellations of *Ascaris* haplotypes originating predominantly from 1 host species, suggesting that there are local barriers to the exchange of genetic material between pig and human*Ascaris* and adaptations to particular host species. Interestingly, haplotypes from human *Ascaris* in the United Kingdom and Denmark cluster practically exclusively with pig worms, indicating a zoonotic origin for these infections.

Using different approaches for analysis of microsatellite data, we observed genetic differentiation between human and pig *Ascaris* in developing countries. These results are in accordance with findings from a number of published studies [4, 13, 16–18, 43]. In contrast, *Ascaris* from humans in Europe clustered with pig worms rather than human worms from other areas, providing further evidence that *Ascaris* infection is a zoonosis in developed countries [2–4, 12]. Using Bayesian analysis, there were no worms of pig origin found in humans from Zanzibar or Bangladesh, which is unsurprising given that both are Muslim countries where pig farming is uncommon. In Uganda, where around 18% of households keep pigs [44], 1 of 143 human worms (0.7%) was of pig origin and 1 of 56 pig worms (1.8%) was of human origin. In China, 13.9% of worms (n = 137) in humans were zoonotic and 0.8% of worms in pigs (n = 121) were anthroponotic [17]. The differences in level of zoonotic transmission between the 2 countries likely represent variations in farming practices, feces disposal, and human-pig contact. Intriguingly, there were 2 worms in pigs from the United Kingdom that clustered with human worms, although one had a pig-like *cox*1 haplotype (H64). These *Ascaris* parasites came from an organic abattoir in Bedfordshire, but the location of the farm(s) where the pigs were reared is not known. It is possible that a human *Ascaris* transmission cycle exists in pigs, an extremely surprising result which warrants further investigation. No examples of hybridization between pig and human worms were found in any location. In contrast, 7.8% of worms in China (n = 258) and 4% in Guatemala (n = 24) were identified as hybrids using 23 microsatellite markers, indicating the potential for exchange of genetic material between pig and human *Ascaris* populations [17, 18]. The fact that we did not find evidence of hybridization might reflect variations in transmission dynamics of *Ascaris* worms in different locations. Alternatively, the 8 markers we used may not provide sufficient resolution to identify hybrids.

As anticipated [4, 13, 18, 20], we found significant genetic differentiation between *Ascaris* populations from different countries. Additional structuring of parasite populations at the village or individual host level was also apparent, particularly in Uganda where the largest sample of worms originated. This may be related to the well-documented overdispersed distribution and clustering of *Ascaris* infections at household level [22, 45]. Genetic substructuring at the individual host level has also been observed in Guatemala and Denmark [4, 14]. The 4 clusters predicted by Bayesian analysis for human worms mainly corresponded to country, although the Ugandan worms also clustered by village. Interestingly, whereas cluster 4 contained mainly worms from Bangladesh, worms from Zanzibar were also found here. Similarly, Zanzibari and some Bangladeshi worms were assigned to cluster 3. This may reflect the long history of and ongoing traffic between Zanzibar and the Indian subcontinent.

Because of greater sampling, our study provides a better picture of the genetic diversity of *Ascaris* in Africa. Since the evolution of early hominids is thought to have taken place here [23], it is possible that there has been a long-standing association between humans and ascarids on this continent and that humans migrating from Africa facilitated the spread of a proto-*Ascaris*. The oldest ascarid eggs discovered so far were found in France [46]. However, Africa is poorly represented in the archeological record and further historical phylogeographical studies are required to determine where *Ascaris* originated. It is clear that, ascariasis has been intimately intertwined with humans for thousands of years, as recently demonstrated by infections discovered within the body of King Richard III [47].

The older evolutionary origin of *Ascaris* in human and pig hosts is contested. It is unclear whether *A. lumbricoides* and *A. suum* are separate species derived from a common ancestor, multiple host colonization events took place after geographical subdivision of host populations [18], or *A. lumbricoides* and *A. suum* are really a single species with regional variants [8]. This discussion depends on a consistent definition of "species." Defining species as "groups of actually or potentially interbreeding natural populations which are reproductively isolated from other such groups" [48], we suggest that *A. lumbricoides* and *A. suum* are 2 separate species, since there are high levels of genetic differentiation between pigs and human worms in sympatric areas. Although hybrids between pig-derived and human-derived worms have been identified, these are rare and likely to have reduced fitness, otherwise population structuring between the hosts would not be observed [11]. Regarding host switching, our results are less conclusive. Like Anderson et al but in contrast to Criscione et al, we find that, in broad terms, differentiation between worms was based primarily on host affiliation, with further differentiation based on geographical location [13]. This could indicate a single historical host switch of *Ascaris* populations infecting pigs or humans. However, the mitochondrial data and the fact that no single diagnostic marker has been identified to distinguish between *A. lumbricoides* and *A. suum* favor an alternative model of multiple host switches over time, with subsequent merging of worm populations in the 2 hosts [18]. This explanation may be more consistent with the history of pig domestication across Eurasia [49].

The current mainstay of control programs against ascariasis in humans is preventive chemotherapy, involving periodic treatment of preschool and school-aged children in *Ascaris*-endemic communities with anthelmintic drugs, and there are real prospects for local elimination of disease by treatment scale-up [50]. In areas where it is common for households to keep pigs and/or where pig manure is used as a fertilizer, however, the progress toward elimination may be hampered if there is significant cross-over of transmission. Thus, with forthcoming scale up of preventive chemotherapy, it may be that sources of zoonotic transmission will become ever more important, and, if so, they should be taken into account by mathematical models currently being developed to explore the stability and dynamics of end points of control.

In conclusion, our results provide novel insights into the transmission dynamics and speciation of *Ascaris* from humans and pigs. Although *A. lumbricoides* and *A. suum* appear to be 2 separate species over most of their range, the process of speciation is not so far advanced that they are entirely host specific or unable to exchange genetic information, and cross-transmission between pig and human hosts takes place across the globe. The level of cross-transmission is likely to depend on local farming and hygiene practices. However, it is possible that we underestimated the zoonotic potential of *A. suum,* as we only analyzed adult worms (i.e., *Ascaris* that completed hepato-tracheal migration and established in the intestine). It is probable that *A. suum* commonly undergoes visceral larvae migration in humans, but because of host preferences most larvae are expelled on return to the intestine. Zoonotic and anthroponotic transmission could lead to greater morbidity because hosts are less well-adapted to the parasite. In addition, potential exchange of genetic information between

A. lumbricoides and *A. suum* could allow the spread of drug-resistance and virulence genes between parasite populations in different hosts, although it is also possible that if humans are treated but pigs are not, the untreated parasite population will act as refugia, diluting the alleles linked to resistance.

ACKNOWLEDGMENTS

We thank everyone who donated *Ascaris* samples or DNA for this study, including Helena Ngowi (Sokoine University of Agriculture, Tanzania), Ida-Hella Poulsen and Sofie Nissen (University of Copenhagen, Denmark), Jaap Boes (Danish Cattle Federation, Denmark), Harriet Namwanje (Ministry of Health, Uganda), Rashidul Haque (International Center for Diarrheal Diseases Research, Bangladesh), and Tim J. C. Anderson and Sarah Williams-Blangero (Southwest Foundation for Biomedical Research, Texas); and Rebecca Kane, for laboratory assistance.

REFERENCES

1. Pullan RL, Brooker S. Ascaris lumbricoides and ascariasis: estimating numbers infected and burden of disease. In: Holland C, ed. Ascaris the neglected parasite. London: Academic Press, 2013:343–62.
2. Anderson TJC. Ascaris infections in humans from North America: molecular evidence for cross-infection. Parasitology 1995; 110:215–9.
3. Bendall RP, Barlow M, Betson M, Stothard JR, Nejsum P. Zoonotic ascariasis, United Kingdom. Emerg Infect Dis 2011; 17:1964–6.
4. Nejsum P, Parker ED, Frydenberg J, et al. Ascariasis is a zoonosis in Denmark. J Clin Microb 2005; 43:1142–8.
5. Murray CJ, Vos T, Lozano R, et al. Disability-adjusted life years (DALYs) for 291 diseases and injuries in 21 regions, 1990–2010: a systematic analysis for the Global Burden of Disease Study 2010. Lancet 2012; 380:2197–223.
6. Roepstorff A, Mejer H, Nejsum P, Thamsborg SM. Helminth parasites in pigs: new challenges in pig production and current research highlights. Vet Parasitol 2011; 180:72–81.
7. Thamsborg SM, Nejsum P, Mejer H. Impact of Ascaris suum in livestock. In: Holland C, ed. Ascaris the neglected parasite. London: Academic Press, 2013.
8. Leles D, Gardner SL, Reinhard K, Iniguez A, Araujo A. Are Ascaris lumbricoides and Ascaris suum a single species? Parasit Vectors 2012; 5:42.
9. Peng W, Criscione CD. Ascariasis in people and pigs: New inferences from DNA analysis of worm populations. Infect Genet Evol 2012; 12:227–35.
10. Nejsum P, Betson M, Bendall RP, Thamsborg SM, Stothard JR. Assessing the zoonotic potential of Ascaris suum and Trichuris suis: looking to the future from an analysis of the past. J Helminthol 2012; 86:148–55.
11. Betson M, Nejsum P, Stothard JR. From the twig tips to the deeper branches: new insights into evolutionary history and phylogeography of Ascaris. In: Holland C, ed. Ascaris the neglected parasite. London: Academic Press, 2013.
12. Cavallero S, Snabel V, Pacella F, Perrone V, D'Amelio S. Phylogeographical studies of Ascaris spp. based on ribosomal and mitochondrial DNA sequences. PLoS Negl Trop Dis 2013; 7:e2170.
13. Anderson TJC, Jaenike J. Host specificity, evolutionary relationships and macrogeographic differentiation among Ascaris populations from humans and pigs. Parasitology 1997; 115:325–42.
14. Anderson TJC, Romero-Abal ME, Jaenike J. Mitochondrial DNA and Ascaris microepidemiology: the composition of parasite populations from individual hosts, families and villages. Parasitology 1995; 110:221–9.
15. Peng WD, Yuan K, Hu M, Zhou XM, Gasser RB. Mutation scanningcoupled analysis of haplotypic variability in mitochondrial DNA regions reveals low gene flow between human and porcine Ascaris in endemic regions of China. Electrophoresis 2005; 26:4317–26.
16. Peng WD, Yuan K, Zhou XM, Hu M, El Osta YGA, Gasser RB. Molecular epidemiological investigation of Ascaris genotypes in China based on single-strand conformation polymorphism analysis of ribosomal DNA. Electrophoresis 2003; 24:2308–15.
17. Zhou C, Li M, Yuan K, Deng S, Peng W. Pig Ascaris: an important source of human ascariasis in China. Infect Genet Evol 2012; 12:1172–7.
18. Criscione CD, Anderson JD, Sudimack D, et al. Disentangling hybridization and host colonization in parasitic roundworms of humans and pigs. Proc Biol Sci 2007; 274:2669–77.
19. Betson M, Halstead FD, Nejsum P, et al. A molecular epidemiological investigation of Ascaris on Unguja, Zanzibar using isoenyzme analysis, DNA barcoding and microsatellite DNA profiling. Trans R Soc Trop Med Hyg 2011; 105:370–9.
20. Betson M, Nejsum P, Llewellyn-Hughes J, et al. Genetic diversity of Ascaris in southwestern Uganda. Trans R Soc Trop Med Hyg 2012; 106:75–83.
21. Nejsum P, Frydenberg J, Roepstorff A, Parker ED. Population structure in Ascaris suum (Nematoda) among domestic swine in Denmark as measured by whole genome DNA fingerprinting. Hereditas 2005; 142:7–14.
22. Criscione CD, Anderson JD, Sudimack D, et al. Landscape genetics reveals focal transmission of a human macroparasite. PLoS Negl Trop Dis 2010; 4:e665.
23. Willoughy PR. The evolution of modern humans in Africa: A comprehensive guide. Langham, MD: AltaMira Press, 2007.
24. Olsen A, Namwanje H, Nejsum P, Roepstorff A, Thamsborg SM. Albendazole and mebendazole have low efficacy against Trichuris trichiura in school-age children in Kabale District, Uganda. Trans R Soc Trop Med Hyg 2009; 103:443–6.
25. Nissen S, Poulsen IH, Nejsum P, et al. Prevalence of gastrointestinal nematodes in growing pigs in Kabale District in Uganda. Trop Anim Health Prod 2011; 43:567–72.

26. Anderson TJC, Romero-Abal ME, Jaenike J. Genetic structure and epidemiology of Ascaris populations: patterns of host affiliation in Guatemala. Parasitology 1993; 107:319–34.

27. Standley CJ, Kabatereine NB, Lange CN, Lwambo NJ, Stothard JR. Molecular epidemiology and phylogeography of Schistosoma mansoni around Lake Victoria. Parasitology 2010; 137:1937–49.

28. Criscione CD, Anderson JD, Raby K, et al. Microsatellite markers for the human nematode parasite Ascaris lumbricoides: Development and assessment of utility. J Parasitol 2007; 93:704–8.

29. Posada D. jModelTest: phylogenetic model averaging. Mol Biol Evol 2008; 25:1253–6. 30. Liu K, Muse SV. PowerMarker: an integrated analysis environment for genetic marker analysis. Bioinformatics 2005; 21:2128–9.

30. Goudet J. FSTAT (Version 1.2): A computer program to calculate F-statistics. J Heredity 1995; 86:485–6.

31. Excoffier L, Lischer HE. Arlequin suite ver 3.5: a new series of programs to perform population genetics analyses under Linux and Windows. Mol Ecol Resour 2010; 10:564–7.

32. Cavalli-Sforza LL, Edwards AW. Phylogenetic analysis. Models and estimation procedures. Am J Hum Genet 1967; 19:233–57.

33. Falush D, Stephens M, Pritchard JK. Inference of population structure using multilocus genotype data: linked loci and correlated allele frequencies. Genetics 2003; 164:1567–87.

34. Pritchard JK, Stephens M, Donnelly P. Inference of population structure using multilocus genotype data. Genetics 2000; 155:945–59.

35. Evanno G, Regnaut S, Goudet J. Detecting the number of clusters of individuals using the software STRUCTURE: a simulation study. Mol Ecol 2005; 14:2611–20.

36. Anderson EC, Thompson EA. A model-based method for identifying species hybrids using multilocus genetic data. Genetics 2002; 160: 1217–29.

37. Corander J, Marttinen P. Bayesian identification of admixture events using multilocus molecular markers. Mol Ecol 2006; 15:2833–43.

38. Iniguez AM, Leles D, Jaeger LH, Carvalho-Costa FA, Araujo A. Genetic characterisation and molecular epidemiology of Ascaris spp. from humans and pigs in Brazil. Trans R Soc Trop Med Hyg 2012; 106:604–12.

39. Snabel V, Taira K, Cavallero S, D'Amelio S, Rudohradska P, Saitoh Y. Genetic structure of Ascaris roundworm in Japan and patterns of its geographical variation. Jpn J Infect Dis 2012; 65:179–83.

40. Blouin MS. Molecular prospecting for cryptic species of nematodes: mitochondrial DNA versus internal transcribed spacer. Int J Parasitol 2002; 32:527–31.

41. Anderson TJC. The dangers of using single locus markers in parasite epidemiology: Ascaris as a case study. Trends Parasitol 2001; 17:183–8.

42. Peng W, Zhou X, Cui X, et al. Transmission and natural regulation of infection with Ascaris lumbricoides in a rural community in China. J Parasitol 1998; 84:252–8.

43. Statistical Abstract 2011. Entebbe: Ugandan Ministry of Agriculture Animal Industries and Fisheries. http://www.agriculture.go.ug/userfiles/ Statistical%20Abstract%20 2011.pdf.

44. Walker M, Hall A, Basanez MG. Individual predisposition, household clustering and risk factors for human infection with Ascaris lumbricoides: new epidemiological insights. PLoS Negl Trop Dis 2011; 5:e1047.

45. Loreille O, Bouchet F. Evolution of ascariasis in humans and pigs: a multi-disciplinary approach. Mem Inst Oswaldo Cruz 2003; 98:39–46.

46. Mitchell PD, Yeh HY, Appleby J, Buckley R. The intestinal parasites of King Richard III. Lancet 2013; 382:888.

47. Mayr E. Systematics and the origin of species. New York: Columbia University Press, 1942:120.

48. Larson G, Dobney K, Albarella U, et al. Worldwide phylogeography of wild boar reveals multiple centers of pig domestication. Science 2005; 307:1618–21.

49. WHO. Eliminating soil-transmitted helminthiasis as a public health problem in children: progress report 2001–2010 and strategic plan 2011–2020. Geneva: World Health Organization, 2012.

CHAPTER 21

EFFICACY AND SAFETY OF ANTHELMINTICS TESTED AGAINST TAENIA SOLIUM CYSTICERCOSIS IN PIGS

Ernatus Martin Mkupasi, Chummy Sikalizyo Sikasunge, Helena Aminiel Ngowi, Maria Vang Johansen

INTRODUCTION

Making safe and evidence-based recommendations for porcine cysticercosis treatment requires adequate information on the efficacy and safety of the anthelmintics to be used [1]. It has been reported that the policy of confiscating cysticercosis-infected pig carcasses from official slaughter houses without compensation only drives farmers to illegal slaughter and consumption or sale, increasing the possibility of infecting more people [2]. Effective treatment of infected pigs will increase the value of pork and access to formal marketing systems, which will be strong incentives for farmers to treat their pigs and increase compliance with other control activities such as health education, sanitation, and human treatment. However, in order to improve the economic value of pork, its appearance should be clean and similar to noninfected meat [3].

Efforts to treat *T. solium* cysticercosis in pigs started in late 70s after promising results from human neurocysticercosis treatment with praziquantel. Since then, seven anthelmintics have been evaluated in treatment of porcine cysticercosis employing naturally infected pigs [4]. The seven anthelmintics comprise five benzimidazoles (BZ), praziquantel, and nitazoxanide. The BZ represents a class of broad-spectrum anthelmintics, which have the great merit of being available in a wide variety of formulations and routes of administration [5]. Since their introduction in the early 60s, they have had a major impact on safe and effective management of helminths in both humans and animals [6], [7]. Praziquantel, on the other hand, is a prazinoisoquinoline derivative, and is highly effective against a broad range of trematodes and cestodes [8]. Nitazoxanide is a nitrothiazolyl-salicylamide derivative, the prodrug which is metabolised to form tizoxanide, the main active metabolite [9]. This work focuses on evaluating the efficacy and safety of flubendazole, fenbendazole, albendazole, albendazole sulphoxide, oxfendazole, praziquantel, and nitazoxanide anthelmintics, which have been tested for treatment of porcine cysticercosis.

A literature search was performed using the databases CAB, Web of Science, Medline, Agricola, and Agris, provided by the University of Copenhagen Library. Porcine cysticercosis treatment information published in English through August 2012 was evaluated. A total of twelve publications about porcine cysticercosis chemotherapy were obtained and summarised in this review. As no formal guidelines exist for assessing drug efficacy against porcine cysticercosis, the studies vary significantly regarding setup, number of pigs included, methodology, and ways of assessing and reporting the outcome [10]. For each study, we have included information about the dependent and independent variables, methodology, and duration of the study. The summary of the drugs' efficacy and safety are presented in the Table 1 and Table 2, respectively.

Citation: Mkupasi EM, Sikasunge CS, Ngowi HA, Johansen MV (2013) Efficacy and Safety of Anthelmintics Tested against Taenia solium Cysticercosis in Pigs. PLoS Negl Trop Dis 7(7): e2200. doi:10.1371/journal.pntd.0002200.

Table 1. Efficacy of different anthelmintics tested against porcine cysticercosis

Reference	Anthelmintic	Dose (mg/kg)	Treated pigs	Control pigs	TE (wks)	KR	Effect on MC	Effect on BC
12	FLU	5.5–40	15	11	1–4	0–100	Variable	Variable
14	FBZ	5–45	16	2	3–5	NR	Good	Variable
17	ABZ	30 & 50	12	5	10–12	89–99	Good	Variable
20	ABZSO	15	4	3	12	59–100	Variable	Variable
23	PZQ	50	4	4	10–12	0–10	No effect	No effect
23	PZQ+OFZ	30+50	4	"	10–12	100	Good	Good
23	OFZ	30	4	"	10–12	100	Good	Good
24	OFZ	10	6	6	10	88–96	Good	Low
24	OFZ	20	6	"	10	100	Good	Good
24	OFZ	30	5	"	10	100	Good	Good
25	OFZ	30	16	4	1–12	80–100	Good	Variable
26	OFZ	30	20	40	32	100	Good	NE
27	OFZ	30	20	20	1–26	82–100	Good	Low
32	PZQ	50	11	2	1–65	20–75	Variable	Variable
33	PZQ	25	6	6	5	55–100	Variable	Variable
33	PZQ	50	6	"	5	78–100	Good	Variable
33	PZQ	100	6	"	5	18–100	Variable	Variable
34	NZX	150	6	6	10	0	No effect	No effect

KR - Killing rate, TE - Time evaluated, MC - Muscular cysts, BC - Brain cysts, NE - Not evaluated, NR - Not reported, wks - weeks.

doi:10.1371/journal.pntd.0002200.t001

Table 2. Reported adverse effects after anthelmintics treatment of porcine cysticercosis

Reference	Anthelmintic	Dose (mg/kg)	Treatment duration	Adverse effects
12	FLU	5.5–40	10 consecutive days	Reduced appetite
14	FBZ	5–45	7 or 14 consecutive days	Slightly reduced appetite
17	ABZ	30	3 consecutive days	Lethargy and anorexia
17	ABZ	50	Single-dose treatment	Prostration, anorexia, lethargia, and death
20	ABZSO	15	8 consecutive days	Ulcers developed in 2 pigs at injection site
23	PZQ	50	Single dose	No side effect reported
23	PZQ+OFZ	30+50	Single dose	No side effect reported
23	OFZ	30	Single dose	No side effect reported
24	OFZ	10 20 & 30	Single dose	No side effect observed
25	OFZ	30	Single dose	No side effect observed
26	OFZ	30	Single dose	Not reported
27	OFZ	30	Single dose	Not reported
32	PZQ	50	>15 days	Not reported
33	PZQ	25, 50 & 100	Single day	Not reported
34	NZX	150	7 consecutive days	No side effect observed

doi:10.1371/journal.pntd.0002200.t002

Flubendazole (FLU)

Flubendazole has both antinematodal and anticestodal activities [11]. The drug is registered for use in pigs for control of helminth infections other than *T. solium* cysticercosis with doses between 1.6–4 mg/kg [5]. Early efforts to control porcine cysticercosis evaluated the effect of FLU in two treatment trials. In the first experiment conducted in Mexico [12], the efficacy of FLU on *T. solium* metacestodes was determined using 17 naturally infected pigs. Nine pigs were allocated into two groups of five and four pigs and treated with individual doses ranging from 5.5–6.4 mg/kg and 8.3–28.5 mg/kg, respectively. The drug was administered orally mixed in feed twice a day for ten consecutive days, while eight pigs were left untreated (Table 1).

The efficacy of the drug was evaluated 25 days after treatment by morphological changes, viability test, and histological assessment of the metacestodes in the treated pigs as compared to the control. In treated pigs, the metacestodes showed degenerative changes, being smaller, dry, and yellowish in color. The doses between 5.5–6.4 mg/kg showed low efficacy, as these had 82–98% of the metacestodes viable, while doses between 8.3–28.5 mg/kg had only 0–8% metacestodes viable, as compared to control pigs in which 60–100% metacestodes were viable. The study did not differentiate the effect of the treatment according to the location of metacestodes either in muscles or in brain tissues (Table 1).

In the second experiment [12], nine naturally infected pigs

were divided into treatment and control groups comprising six and three pigs, respectively. The treated pigs were administered FLU mixed in feed in a dosage of 40 mg/kg daily for ten consecutive days. One pig died from an undetermined cause on day seven and was evaluated for the effect of treatment. Two pigs were sacrificed on days 12 and 14, respectively and the remaining three pigs on day 25. Three percent of muscular metacestodes were viable in the pig evaluated on day seven; the remainder had no viable metacestodes with exception of one pig evaluated on day 14, which had almost 100% viable muscular metacestodes. However, the pig was reported to have been reluctant to eat the medicated feed. The viability of brain metacestodes was found to be 28% in the pig evaluated on day seven and 98% in the pig evaluated on day 14. In the control group, the viability was about 98 and 88% for muscular and brain metacestodes, respectively (Table 1).

Histopathological examination further revealed destruction of metacestodes, which appeared swollen, edematous with acute inflammatory reaction seven days after treatment. At day 25, the metacestodes were completely destroyed with tissue necrosis. No adverse effects were reported at the dosage used apart from one pig from the second study, which died on day seven of treatment (Table 2). Doses between 8.3–40 mg/kg were found to be effective against metacestodes in muscles, but were less effective for brain metacestodes. The repeated treatment required makes it uneconomical and impractical for porcine cysticercosis control under field conditions in endemic areas.

Fenbendazole (FBZ)

Fenbendazole has a broad spectrum of activity against gastrointestinal and respiratory helminths in domestic animals. It is registered for use in pigs at a dose of 5 mg/kg [13]. The efficacy of FBZ in treatment of porcine cysticercosis was evaluated in Korea [14], using 18 naturally infected pigs. The pigs were allocated into nine groups of two pigs each; eight groups were treated with a pig feed formulation of the drug and one group served as an untreated control. The first treated group was administered 45 mg/kg and the second group 20 mg/kg FBZ for 14 consecutive days. The third and fourth groups were both given 25 mg/kg and the fifth and sixth groups received 15 mg/kg also for 14 consecutive days. The remaining two groups were treated with 5 mg/kg per day for seven consecutive days.

The efficacy of the drug was assessed by sacrificing the pigs at days 20–39 after last treatment, and the metacestode morphological changes were evaluated grossly and by use of scanning and transmission electron microscopes. The study showed that FBZ was effective at all doses and regimens used (Table 1). The metacestodes in muscle were more affected than in the brain; they were deflated and shrunk and appeared as small rice grains in size and shape. However, the effect on the brain metacestodes varied as the cysts appeared to be in the process of disintegration. Generally FBZ was found to be safe; the only reported side effect was the slight decrease in appetite during the treatment in some treated pigs, but eventually they gained weight as compared to the controls (Table 2). Based on the treatment of four pigs, it was concluded that FBZ at 5 mg/kg for seven consecutive days was effective in treatment of porcine cysticercosis. However, the prolonged treatment duration required limits its use in control of porcine cysticercosis in endemic areas.

Albendazole (ABZ)

Albendazole, another BZ anthelmintic, is oxidized to albendazole sulphoxide, the systematically active metabolite, and then further oxidized to albendazole sulphone, which is inactive [15]. It is a broad-spectrum anthelmintic that is effective against nematode, trematode, and cestode infections in sheep and cattle at a dose between 5–10 mg/kg [6], [15]. It has been reported to have better efficacy in treatment of human neurocysticercosis than praziquantel [16]. It is not registered for use in pigs.

An evaluation of the efficacy of ABZ in single- and multiple-dose regimens in treatment of porcine cysticercosis in naturally infected pigs was conducted [17]. Seventeen pigs were allocated into two treatment groups of six pigs each and a control group of five pigs. The first treatment group was administered with ABZ in a single dose of 50 mg/kg, the second group with 30 mg/kg every day for three days given orally mixed in feed, and the third control group was left untreated (Table 1).

The efficacy was assessed 10–12 weeks after treatment; the pigs were sacrificed and the effect of the treatment evaluated by metacestodes count and viability test. The three-day regimen of 30 mg/kg was effective, killing all metacestodes in muscles but not the brain metacestodes. In this group, the pigs developed adverse effects such as lethargy and anorexia (Table 2). In the group treated with a single dose of 50 mg/kg, the drug was less effective compared to 30 mg/kg for three days, leaving 11.4% and 6.7% viable metacestodes in muscular and brain tissues, respectively (Table 1). In addition, the pigs developed marked adverse effects such as severe prostration, complete anorexia, and lethargy, and one pig died on the third day after treatment (Table 2). In both groups, the calcified metacestodes were still visible in meat 10–12 weeks after treatment. The authors concluded, based on the 12 treated pigs, that although the three-day administration of albendazole was highly effective, the side effects observed and the multiple doses limit its applicability in the field. Additionally, the prolonged use of the drug in humans [18] and in dogs and cats [19] is reported to induce bone marrow toxicosis, which may lead to lethal pancytopenia.

Albendazole sulphoxide (ABZSO)

Albendazole sulphoxide is available for use in ruminants for control of intestinal nematodes and some trematodes and cestodes at doses between 5–7.5 mg/kg [6]. It is not registered for use in pigs. The efficacy of ABZSO against porcine cysticercosis was evaluated in Mexico [20]. Seven naturally infected pigs (four sows and two boars) with age ranging between 6–12 months were divided into two groups of four and three pigs for treatment and control, respectively. The treatment group received a dosage of 15 mg/kg ABZSO by subcutaneous injection for eight consecutive days, and the control group was given a 0.9% saline solution (Table 1).

The efficacy of ABZSO was reported to be 100% in the muscle metacestodes when evaluated 12 weeks after treatment. The metacestodes were examined macroscopically for vesicular or micro-calcified cysts and by viability test. The metacestodes were reported to be degenerated but were still visible 12 weeks post treatment. ABZSO was ineffective against brain metacestodes as it left 41.1% of the metacestodes viable. In the control group, 91.5% of muscular and 75.8% of brain metacestodes were viable. Histopathological evaluation of muscle tissues indicated complete destruction of the metacestode with necrosis. The treatment was reported to be well tolerated; however, two pigs developed ulcers at injection sites. Based on the treatment of four pigs, it was concluded that 15 mg/kg ABZSO was 100% effective for muscle cysts treatment but less effective for brain cysts. However, the required multiple treatments and low efficacy to the brain cysts limits its use in control of porcine cysticercosis.

Oxfendazole (OFZ)

Oxfendazole has broad-spectrum activity against inhibited larval stages of gastrointestinal roundworms, tapeworms, and lungworms in many animal species at doses between 4.5–10 mg/kg [21]. Unlike other BZ compounds, OFZ is absorbed more readily from the gastrointestinal tract. OFZ is metabolically interconvertable to FBZ, and then extensively metabolised to fenbendazole sulphoxide, an active metabolite, then oxidized to the inactive fenbendazole sulphone. This is responsible for prolonged systemic bioavailability of the drug, accounting for the reported high efficacy against porcine cysticercosis. Following oral administration at 30 mg/kg in pigs, it rapidly absorbed, reaching very high plasma levels and systemic exposure after two hours, and persisted in plasma up to 96 hours post treatment. The elimination half-life is about 7.5 hours in sheep. The dose is well tolerated in all tested pigs [21],[22]. However, the drug is not registered for use in pigs.

Studies have been conducted to evaluate OFZ's efficacy, safety, killing time, and cyst clearance rates in pigs naturally infected with porcine cysticercosis (Table 1). In the first study conducted in Peru [23], sixteen adult pigs naturally infected with *T. solium* cysticercosis were divided into four groups that were randomly allocated to PZQ, PZQ plus OFZ, and OFZ treatment groups and a control group, respectively. The pigs were kept at a veterinary facility, free from infection transmission throughout the study period. The drugs were mixed in feed and administered orally. In the groups treated with OFZ alone or the PZQ plus OFZ combination, the drugs were found to be 100% effective as no metacestodes evaginated from either muscle or brain tissue 10–12 weeks after treatment, as compared to controls where nearly 100% viable metacestodes were found (Table 1). Praziquantel at 50 mg/kg alone was not effective as nearly 100% of metacestodes were viable in both muscle and brain tissue, similar to the control group [23]. The dosage regime was safe as no side effect were noted during the observation period.

In another study [24], 24 adult pigs naturally infected with cysticercosis were allocated into four groups and treated with 10, 20, and 30 mg/kg OFZ mixed with feed or left untreated, respectively. The pigs were kept at the veterinary facility, free from any risk of the transmission of cysticercosis, for the whole study period. The pigs were sacrificed eight to ten weeks post treatment for metacestodes evaluation. Up to 25 metacestodes from selected muscles, heart, and brain were excised and tested for viability by evagination. Doses of 10 and 20 mg/kg were not effective as 4–12% of metacestodes were still viable in both muscle and brain tissues, but 30 mg/kg OFZ showed high efficacy as no metacestodes were viable in either muscle or brain tissue. More than 75% of the cysts in the control group were viable irrespective of the anatomical location (Table 1).

The time taken for OFZ to kill the cysticerci was evaluated using 20 adult pigs naturally infected with cysticercosis, where 16 pigs were treated with 30 mg/kg OFZ and four were left untreated[25]. The cysticercosis-infected pigs were brought to and reared at an infection-free veterinary facility for the duration of the study. The OFZ-treated pigs were sacrificed at weeks one, four, and 12 after treatment, where all control pigs were sacrificed at week 12. The viability of metacestodes was assessed by evagination test. It was observed that the metacestode viability was significantly reduced one week following OFZ treatment, but at week four some viable metacestodes were still observed. At week twelve, all metacestodes had disappeared leaving only minuscule scars except in one animal that had viable brain metacestodes. In the controls, the average metacestode viability was 66% and 58% from muscle and brain tissue, respectively.

Protection against reinfection after OFZ treatment was evaluated using 20 adult pigs naturally infected with cysticercosis [26]. The pigs were drenched with 30 mg/kg OFZ and kept in the disease-free facility in the veterinary faculty for eight weeks. After that period, each treated pig was matched with two naïve pigs similar in age and sex, obtained from disease-free farms, and exposed in a high-risk environment for the infection. Three months later, the pigs in both groups were dissected to evaluate their infection status. New infections were detected in 15 of the 32 controls (42%) by serology and by the presence of metacestodes in 12 pigs (37%), whereas no viable metacestodes were detected in the muscles of the previously treated pigs. From this study, the OFZ was demonstrated to have an added advantage: that following treatment, infected pigs were protected against reinfection for at least three months [26].

The efficacy, killing time, and cyst clearance rate in *T. solium*–infected pigs treated with OFZ was evaluated in Zambia using 40 (22 males and 18 females) infected pigs [27]. The pigs were kept in a disease-free facility at veterinary school premises. They were divided into treated and control groups; the treated group received 30 mg/kg OFZ given orally mixed in feed. The pigs were sacrificed at one, four, eight, and 26 weeks after treatment. In pigs killed at one week, both live and dead metacestodes were recovered with mean (± S.D.) of 18±17% and 92±5% in treated and control groups, respectively. However, one striking finding at one week post treatment was that in treated pigs all metacestodes in the heart were dead. At four and eight weeks after treatment, all muscle metacestodes were calcified, but brain metacestodes were viable. At 26 weeks post treatment, in four out of five carcasses the metacestodes had completely disappeared with normal meat appearance, but one carcass had visible calcified metacestodes in the muscles. The brain metacestodes were still viable with mean (± S.D.) of 36±49% and 91±8% in treated and control groups, respectively. From this study, it was concluded that OFZ at 30 mg/kg body weight killed all muscular metacestodes as early as four weeks after treatment, but brain metacestodes were not significantly affected. It was demonstrated that complete clearance of metacestodes occurred between 8–26 weeks or more. The authors hypothesized that the clearance of the dead metacestodes from the muscle tissue depends on the intensity of the infection at the time of treatment [27]. In three treatment trials [23]–[25], the dose of 30 mg/kg OFZ was reported to be safe in infected pigs (Table 2).

An intervention field treatment trial using OFZ in mass chemotherapy of pigs in endemic villages in Peru in combination with taeniasis chemotherapy in humans using PZQ as a control program has been reported with promising results [28]. A single dose of 5 mg of PZQ was given to eliminate intestinal taeniasis in humans, and two rounds of OFZ (30 mg/kg) were administered to all pigs. There was a decrease of prevalence of the condition at the end of the intervention period. The impact of the intervention was low and did not attain the goal of elimination of transmission due to less than 100% coverage in both human and pig populations.

In another study, a randomized controlled trial was conducted to evaluate the effectiveness of OFZ treatment for control of porcine cysticercosis in endemic villages of Mozambique [29]. A substantial benefit of treating pigs with OFZ using the single oral dose of 30 mg/kg was clearly demonstrated, since the prevalence and incidence in groups of treated pigs was significantly lower compared to the group of untreated pigs [29]. The results from the two intervention studies showed that OFZ treatment was effective to control porcine cysticercosis; however, it needs to be integrated with other control approaches.

In all studies, 30 mg/kg OFZ was 100% effective in treating muscle cysticerci with variable efficacies in the brain cysticerci. The reason for the reported low efficacy against the brain cysticerci is not clear; genetic variation of the cysticerci or differences in location of the cysticerci within the brain tissues may have influenced the effectiveness of OFZ treatment. However, in most endemic areas pork goes uninspected, but the pig brain is not commonly eaten raw; thus, it is not likely that cysts that survive only in the brain will be ingested and perpetuate the cycle. The withdrawal period has been recently reported to be 17 days, making it safe for pre-slaughter treatment of infected pigs [22]. The use of OFZ in pregnant sows at 13.5 mg/kg has been reported to be safe [30]; however, the 30 mg/kg dose recommended for *T. solium* cysticercosis treatment needs to be further evaluated. The safety of the dose to the piglets should also be evaluated. In spite of the mentioned limitations, the drug is safe, inexpensive, and easily administered in suspension preparation, making it a good candidate to be promoted for use in endemic areas.

Although OFZ worked significantly better than the other BZ, it is not ideal, as studies have shown variable effects on brain metacestodes. More research is needed to fully assess the efficacy and effectiveness of OFZ against *T. solium* cysticercosis and other pig parasitoses before it can be recommended for use as a regular anthelmintic in endemic areas. The drug needs to be registered for use in pigs and made available in cysticercosis endemic areas.

Praziquantel (PZQ)

Praziquantel is effective against a wide range of trematodes and cestodes in dogs and cats at a dose of 5 mg/kg, being generally less effective against nematodes [8], [31]. It is not registered for use in pigs. The use of PZQ for control of porcine cysticercosis at different doses has been evaluated (Table 1). In the first experiment, the effect of PZQ treatment was evaluated using 13 naturally infected adult pigs, divided into two groups of 11 and two pigs [32]. The first group was treated with PZQ at 50 mg/kg per day, divided into three portions mixed in feed for a period of 15 days. The second group of two pigs was the infected control, left untreated and monitored for 13 months. Nine noninfected pigs were used as noninfected treated controls.

The efficacy of the treatment was monitored through CT scans and histopathogical and viability evaluations of the metacestodes. Results of the CT scans indicated both morphological and size change following treatment. Metacestodes became irregular, smaller, and less clearly defined after treatment. Although the decrease in number of metacestodes was observed in both brain and muscle tissues from the first day after treatment, some metacestodes were still visible on day 47 after the last treatment. For morphological and viability evaluation, samples were taken from the masseters of two pigs at days 1 and 8 after the first treatment and then from pigs killed on 2, 5, 7, 10, 15, 25, 28, 32, 57, 63, and 65 days after the last dose of PZQ. The two untreated pigs were necropsied after 13 months. Macroscopic evaluations of muscles showed sequential changes in metacestodes. At first, the vesicular fluid became turbid with white capsule of varying thickness. In more advanced stages, either the tissue cavities where the parasite lodged contained yellowish, caseous materials, or the parasites looked like small rice grains. From day 57 onward, muscle parasites could not be identified, only small scars suggesting their previous presence.

The results of the viability study indicated that only the pig evaluated on day one during treatment had 8/10 (80%) viable muscle metacestodes, while in those evaluated on the following days all muscle metacestodes were dead. Viable brain metacestodes were found in two treated pigs; one on day 15 (1/6) and the other on day 25 (2/8). Histopathologically, the metacestodes in muscles showed severe degenerative changes. In the brain, the results were variable as many metacestodes were intact, surrounded with limited inflammatory infiltrate. It was concluded that the drug damaged the metacestodes in muscles, as demonstrated by morphological change and inhibition of evagination afterward, and that the inflammatory reaction killed and eliminated the metacestodes.

In efforts to overcome the limitations of multiple doses of 50 mg/kg PZQ [32], a one-day PZQ treatment at three different doses of 25, 50, and 100 mg/kg against muscular and brain metacestodes was evaluated in Mexico [33]. Twenty-four naturally infected pigs divided into four groups of six animals each were employed. Three groups were administered with a total dose of 25, 50, and 100 mg/kg, respectively, given in three portions in the morning, afternoon, and evening mixed in feed. The fourth group was left untreated. The effect of the treatment was assessed through morphological, histological, and viability evaluations.

Thirty-four days post treatment, all pigs were sacrificed and cysts were evaluated. Macroscopic examination revealed viable cysts in all six untreated pigs, as compared to 4/6 in those treated with 25 mg/kg and 3/6 in the groups treated with 50 or 100 mg/kg. Metacestodes were degenerated, appearing as small rice grain in most pigs from the treated groups. Following viability evaluation in the group treated with 25 mg/kg, viable cysts were observed in 4/5 pigs with viability ranging between 5–45% and 15–30% for muscle and brain metacestodes, respectively. In the 50 mg/kg treated group, viable cysts were observed in 3/6 pigs with viability of 18–22% and 5–22% for muscle and brain metacestodes, respectively. In the 100 mg/kg treated group, a viability of 20–72% and 10–22% for muscle and brain mesacestodes was observed, respectively, in 3/6 pigs. While in the control group, the viability ranged between 68–100% and 70–100% in muscle and brain cysts, respectively (Table 1).

Most metacestodes in the muscles and brain of all treated pigs exhibited a histological picture of dying or dead parasites except in two pigs that were similar to the control group. The study showed that the treatment had some effect on the metacestodes, and that the effect correlated positively with increasing dose as evaluated by viability and histological statuses of the metacestodes at 34 days post treatment. A single dose of 50 mg/kg PZQ reduced the number of metacestodes but did not affect the viability of the remaining metacestodes. This study did not demonstrate the time taken to clear cysts from the meat as the pigs were evaluated one month after treatment.

Though good efficacy has been demonstrated using 50 mg/kg PZQ for 15 days in treatment of porcine cysticercosis [32], the long duration of treatment will be costly and impractical for the control of porcine cysticercosis in endemic areas. The safety of the treatment regimens for the infected pigs was not reported.

Nitazoxanide (NZX)

A recent study was conducted in Peru using naturally infected pigs to explore the efficacy of combined therapy (ABZ plus PZQ) versus ABZ, PZQ, OFZ, or NZX alone at the dose of 15, 75, 30, and 150 mg/kg, respectively [34]. Fifty-four infected pigs were used, randomly allocated into nine groups with six pigs each. All drugs were administered orally, mixed with feed. The pigs were kept at the School of Veterinary Medicine facilities for ten weeks and then euthanized and subjected to necropsy study to determine the efficacy of the treatment.

Results showed that a combination of ABZ and PZQ, ABZ alone, and OFZ alone were effective antiparasitic drugs for treatment of cysticercosis, and the combined schemes had the best antiparasitic effect in the brain with a statistically significant reduction in viable brain cysts. Nitazoxanide at 150 mg/kg for seven consecutive days was not effective as it left many surviving cysts similar to control pigs, suggesting minimal or no cysticidal effect [34].

CONCLUSION

The evaluated studies varied greatly in design and sample size, methodology was insufficiently described, and almost all studies reported different ways of assessing viability, a key dependent variable for evaluating efficacy. Time points for assessing efficacy, killing, or cyst clearance rates vary between the studies, making comparison between them difficult. Most publications inadequately recorded adverse drug reactions [35]. Due to difficulties in attaining an artificial infection pig model under laboratory conditions, recruiting homogenous groups as much as possible is suggested. Young infected pigs between 3–6 months of age are suggested to avoid the effect of natural involution of the parasite rather than the effect of the drug evaluated. The pigs should be randomized according to age, sex, and level of infection based on either number of tongue cysts and/or level of cysticercal antigens. Also, each group should not have less than six animals [10]. Based on the observations from the studies conducted and reviewed here, the cysts killing time and clearance rate should be evaluated at four and 12 weeks, respectively. Apart from ABZSO, all tested drugs were applied orally mixed in feed, which might be practical, but since BZ have generally poor absorption after oral administration, alternative routes of administration might be more appropriate when testing efficacy against a muscle and brain parasite.

Although highly diverse in setup and methodologies, so far OFZ has proven to be the most promising drug since a single dose of 30 mg/kg has been shown to have high efficacy against muscle metacestodes and is safe, but is less effective for brain metacestodes. This warrants further systematic assessment using alternative formulations and routes of administration. However, no standardised guidelines are in place for assessing the efficacy of anthelmintics against porcine cysticercosis, unlike most other pig helminths [10], and are urgently needed. In conclusion, although the WHO now recommends anthelmintic treatment of pigs as a way to control and eliminate *T. solium* cysticercosis, we still lack the tool to do so. Proper assessment of efficacy, effectiveness, registration of the drug in a suitable pig formulation, and availability of the drug in the endemic areas will be the way forward.

REFERENCES

1. WHO (2009) Position paper on Taenia solium taeniasis/cysticercosis. World Health Organization expert meeting on food-borne trematode infections and taeniasis/cysticercosis. Vientiane, Lao People's Democratic Republic 59.
2. Cysticercosis Working Group in Peru (1993) The marketing of cysticercotic pigs in the Sierra of Peru. Bull World Health Organ 71: 223–228.
3. Gonzalez AE, Garcia HH, Gilman RH, Tsang VCW (2003) Cysticercosis Working Group in Peru (2003) Control of Taenia solium. Acta Trop 87: 103–109. doi: 10.1016/s0001-706x(03)00025-1
4. Gonzalez AE, Wilkins PP, Lopez T (2002) Porcine cysticercosis. In: Singh G, Prabhakar S, editors. Taenia solium cysticercosis: from basic to clinical science. Wallingford: CABI Publishing. pp 145–156.
5. Ramanpreet W, Hedaitullah MD, Naaz SF, Iqbal K, Lam HS (2011) Benzimidazole derivatives – an overview. International Journal of Research in Pharmacy and Chemistry 1: 2231–2781.
6. Campbell WC (1990) Benzimidazoles: veterinary uses. Parasitol Today 6: 130–133. doi: 10.1016/0169-4758(90)90231-r
7. Dubey AK, Sanya PK (2010) Benzimidazoles in a wormy world. Vet J 5 ISSN 0973-6980.
8. Watson MBS (2009) Praziquantel. Journal of Exotic Pet Medicine 18: 229–231. doi: 10.1053/j.jepm.2009.06.005
9. Anderson VR, Curran MP (2007) Nitaxoxanide: a review

of its use in the treatment of gastrointestinal infections. Drugs 67: 1947–1967. doi: 10.2165/00003495-200767130-00015

10. Hennessy D (2006) World association for the advancement of veterinary parasitology (WAAVP): second edition of guidelines for evaluating the efficacy of anthelmintics in swine. Vet Parasitol 141: 138–149. doi: 10.1016/j.vetpar.2006.04.038
11. Krizova V, Nobilis M, Pruskova L, Chladek J, Szotakova B, et al. (2009) Pharmacokinetics of flubendazole and its metabolites in lambs and adult sheep (Ovis aries). J Vet Pharmacol Ther 32: 606–612. doi: 10.1111/j.1365-2885.2009.01082.x
12. Tellez-Giron E, Ramos MC, Montante M (1981) Effect of flubendazole on Cysticercus cellulosae in pigs. Am J Trop Med Hyg 30: 135–138.
13. Heggem BBS (2008) Fenbendazole. Journal of Exotic Pet Medicine 17: 308–310. doi: 10.1053/j.jepm.2008.07.009
14. Cho K, Araki T, Takaichi S, Segawa T, Shiina T, et al.. (1982) Fenbendazole in cysticercosis cellulosae. In: Necoechea RR, Pijoan C, Casariin A, Guzman M, editors. Proceedings of the International Pig Veterinary Society Congress: 26th–31st July 1982; Mexico. p 179.
15. Venkatesan P (1998) Albendazole. J Antimicrob Chemother 41: 145–147. doi: 10.1093/jac/41.2.145
16. Matthaiou DK, Panos G, Adamidi ES, Falagas ME (2008) Albendazole versus praziquantel in the treatment of neurocysticercosis: a meta-analysis of comparative trials. PLoS Negl Trop Dis 2: e194 doi:10.1371/journal.pntd.0000194.
17. Gonzalez AE, Garcia HH, Gilman RH, Lopez MT, Gavidia C, et al. (1995) Treatment of porcine cysticercosis with albendazole. Am J Trop Med Hyg 53: 571–574.
18. Opatrny L, Prichard R, Snell L, Maclean JD (2005) Death related to albendazole-induced pancytopenia: case report and review. Am J Trop Med Hyg 72: 291–294.
19. Stokol T, Randolph JF, Nachbar S, Rodi C, Barr SC (1997) Development of bone marrow toxicosis after albendazole administration in a dog and cat. J Am Vet Med Assoc 210: 1753–1756.
20. Peniche-Cardena A, Dominguez-Alpizar JL, Sima-Alvarez R, Argaez-Rodriguez F, Fraser A, et al. (2002) Chemotherapy of porcine cysticercosis with albendazole sulphoxide. Vet Parasitol 108: 63–73. doi: 10.1016/s0304-4017(02)00177-2
21. Marriner S, Bogan JA (1981) Pharmacokinetics of oxfendazole in sheep. Am J Vet Res 42: 1143–1145. doi: 10.1007/bf02228633
22. Moreno L, Lopez-Urbina MT, Faras C, Domingue G, Donadeu M, et al. (2012) A high oxfendazole dose to control porcine cysticercosis: pharmacokinetics and tissue residue profiles. Food Chem Toxicol 50: 3819–3825. doi: 10.1016/j.fct.2012.07.023
23. Gonzalez AE, Garcia HH, Gilman RH, Gavidia CM, Tsang VCW, et al. (1996) Effective, single-dose treatment of porcine cysticercosis with oxfendazole. Am J Trop Med Hyg 54: 391–394. doi: 10.1136/vr.141.16.420
24. Gonzalez AE, Falcon N, Gavidia C, Garcia HH, Tsang VCW, et al. (1997) Treatment of porcine cysticercosis with oxfendazole: a dose-response trial. Vet Rec 141: 420–422. doi: 10.1136/vr.141.16.420
25. Gonzalez AE, Falcon N, Gavidia C, Garcia HH, Tsang VCW, et al. (1998) Time-response curve of oxfendazole in the treatment of swine cysticercosis. Am J Trop Med Hyg 59: 832–836.
26. Gonzalez AE, Gavidia C, Falcon N, Bernal T, Verastegui M, et al. (2001) Protection of pigs with cysticercosis from further infections after treatment with oxfendazole. Am J Trop Med Hyg 65: 15–18
27. Sikasunge CS, Johansen MV, Willingham AL III, Leifsson PS, Phiri IK (2008) Taenia solium porcine cysticercosis: viability of cysticerci and persistency of antibodies and cysticercal antigens after treatment with oxfendazole. Vet Parasitol 158: 57–66. doi: 10.1016/j.vetpar.2008.08.014
28. Garcia HH, Gonzalez AE, Gilman RH, Moulton LH, Verastegui M, et al. (2006) Combined human and porcine mass chemotherapy for the control of T. solium. Am J Trop Med Hyg 74: 850–855.
29. Pondja A, Neves L, Mlangwa J, Afonso S, Fafetine J, et al. (2012) Use of oxfendazole to control porcine cysticercosis in a high-endemic area of Mozambique. PLoS Negl Trop Dis 6: e1651 doi:10.1371/journal.pntd.0001651.
30. Morgan DW (1982) Toxicity study of oxfendazole in pregnant sows. Vet Rec 111: 161–163. doi: 10.1136/vr.111.8.161
31. Ali BH (2006) A short review of some pharmacological, therapeutic and toxicological properties of praziquantel in man and animals. Pakistan Journal of Pharmacological Science 19: 170–175.
32. Flisser A, Gonzalez D, Shkurovich M, Madrazo I, Correa D, et al. (1990) Praziquantel treatment of porcine brain and muscle Taenia solium cysticercosis. 1. Radiological, physiological and histopathological studies. Parasitol Res 76: 263–269. doi: 10.1007/bf00930823
33. Torres A, Plancarte A, Villalobos ANM, Aluja ASd, Navarro R, et al. (1992) Praziquantel treatment of porcine brain and muscle Taenia solium cysticercosis. 3. Effect of 1-day treatment. Parasitol Res 78: 161–164. doi: 10.1007/bf00931659
34. Gonzalez EA, Bustos JA, Jimenez JA, Rodriguez ML, Ramirez MG, et al. (2012) Efficacy of diverse antiparasitic treatments for cysticercosis in the pig model. Am J Trop Med Hyg 87: 292–296. doi: 10.4269/ajtmh.2012.11-0371
35. Edwards IR, Aronson JK (2000) Adverse drug reactions: definitions, diagnosis, and management. Lancet 356: 1255–1259. doi: 10.1016/s0140-6736(00)02799-9

CHAPTER 22

PREVALENCE OF GASTROINTESTINAL PARASITES AND CRYPTOSPORIDIUM SPECIES IN EXTENSIVELY MANAGED PIGS IN MEKELLE AND URBAN AREAS OF SOUTHERN ZONE OF TIGRAY REGION, NORTHERN ETHIOPIA

Zewdneh Tomass, Ekwal Imam, Tsegabirhan Kifleyohannes, Yohannes Tekle and Kidane Weldu

Keywords: Ascaris spp., Cryptosporidium spp., Ethiopia, extensive pig management, gastrointestinal parasites, Mekelle, Tigray Region

INTRODUCTION

Infection of pigs with gastrointestinal (GIT) parasites is widely reported from all corners of the world and shown to be influenced by the type of pig management practiced [1]. Extensive production of pigs for commercial purpose is widely practiced in developing countries of Africa. Availability of cost free feed (household or municipal garbage) and possibilities for the animals to get better nutrition through scavenging initiate pig growers of developing countries to prefer extensive management. In this regard 70-95% of pig raising sectors of developing countries practice extensive husbandry [2].

Poor environmental hygiene coupled with extensive managements is reported as risk factors of infection of pigs with GIT parasites [1]. Gastrointestinal helminths including *Oesophagastomum dentatum*, *Trichuris suis*, *Ascaris suum*, *Oesophagastomum quadrispinulatum*, *Trichostrongylus axei*, *Strongyloides ransomi*, *Hyostrongylus rubidus* and *Physocephalus sexalutus* have been identified in pigs raised under extensive production in Kenya, Ghana and Burkina Faso [3-5]. Semi-extensively managed pigs are reported to harbor *Taenia solium,* in Nigeria [6]. Pigs rose under semi-intensive and extensive husbandry were found to be infected with *Ascaris suum* and *Oesopha-gostomum* spp. in Holeta, Ethiopia [7]. In addition to helminths, extensively managed pigs are also reported to harbor intestinal protozoans including *Cryptosporidium* spp., *Giardia lambelia*, *Balantidium coli* and *Eimeria* spp. in developing countries [8]. Among other intestinal protozoans *Cryptosporidium* has been given much attention because of its occurrence in various domestic and wild animals and and its potential for causing emerging cryptosporidiosis [9].

Phylum Apicomplexa and family Cryptospordiidae that causes severe diarrhea, anorexia and weight loss, especially in immunocompromised animals and humans (mainly children bellow five years of age and HIV/ AIDS patients). Cryptosporidiosis is caused by several genotypes and phenotypically diverse *Cryptosporidium* species and has been emerging over the past decade. [9].

At present more than 22 *Cryptosporidium* species have been identified [9] however, over 60 genotypes remain undefined [10]. Recent genetic characterization studies revealed that pigs are infected with genetically distinct and host-adapted form of *Cryptosporidium*, *Cryptosporidium* "pig"genotype [11]. However, pigs can also be infected with the zoonotic

Citation: Tomass Z, Imam E, Kifleyohannes T, Tekle Y, Weldu K. Prevalence of gastrointestinal parasites and Cryptosporidium species in extensively managed pigs in Mekelle and urban areas of southern zone of Tigray region, Northern Ethiopia. Vet World. 2013; 6(7): 433-439. doi:10.5455/vetworld.2013.433-439.

Cryptosporidium parvum, "cattle" genotype, indicating their potential as reservoirs of zoonotic infection to humans [11]. So far Haileyesus [12], reported prevalence of *Cryptosporidium parvum* and *C. hominis* in extensively managed cattle and HIV/AIDS patients in Ethiopia. However, there is lack of data regarding the prevalence of *Cryptosporidium* spp. in extensively managed pigs in Ethiopia. Hence, it is crucial to determine the prevalence of *Cryptosporidium* species in pigs before classifying them as one of the reservoirs for zoonotic cryptosporidiosis in Ethiopia.

Pig infected with GIT parasites had poor feed conversion rate and delays in achievement of market weight. Some of the GIT parasites of pigs result in condemnation of organs or entire carcasses causing economic losses in pork industry [13]. In addition, pigs infected with GIT parasites may act as source of zoonoses through contaminating the environment with infective stages of intestinal parasites present in their excreta [11]. The epidemiology of pig born GIT parasites may further be complicated when some of the parasites of pigs infect man and vice versa. *Ascaris* spp. is typical example [14].

In Ethiopia the population of pigs has shown slight increment since 1980. However, pig raising is at its infancy in the country with a total population of about 1900 [15]. Recently small scale pig husbandry is being practiced in urban areas of Ethiopia, however, the management is mainly extensive whereby pigs are allowed to scavenge on household wastes at backyards and municipal garbage dumping sites at peri-urban areas [7]. Such extensive pig husbandry coupled with poor environmental hygiene and pigs' voracious feeding behavior may render infection of the animals with helminth and GIT parasites in Ethiopia. Nevertheless, few studies have been done on prevalence of GIT parasites in extensively managed pigs in Ethiopia in general and Tigray Region in particular [7]. Therefore, this study was initiated to investigate prevalence of GIT parasites in extensively managed pigs and associated environmental health risks in Mekelle and urban areas of southern zone of Tigray Region, Ethiopia.

MATERIALS AND METHODS

Study Areas

This study was carried out in Mekelle and Southern Zones of Tigray Region, Ethiopia (Fig-1). Mekelle is the capital city of Tigray Region located 780 km north of Addis Ababa, the capital city of Ethiopia. Its geographic location is 13° 32' N and 39° 33' E. It has an average altitude of 2200 m.a.s.l with a mean minimum and mean maximum monthly temperatures of 8.7 and 26.8 respectively. Mekelle receives an average 600 mm of rainfall annually and more than 70% of it falls between July and August, followed by long dry season (October to May) [16]. Mekelle has an estimated total human population of 215,546 [17]. Urban agriculture is a common practice in Mekelle [18]. The livestock management system practiced in Mekelle includes extensive, intensive and semi-intensive [19]. Pigs are recently introduced into Mekelle and raised by few households under extensive management.

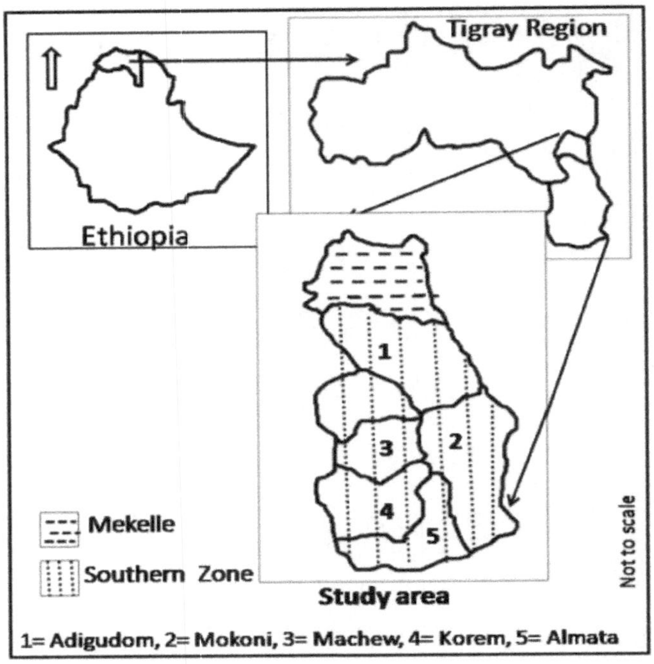

Figure 1: Map of the study area

Southern zone of Tigray Region is located in northern Ethiopia (longitude 39° 5'-39° 8' and latitude 12° 3'- 13° 7' (Fig-1). Here agriculture involves mixed crop and livestock farming. The climate is characterized by bimodal rainfall. About 70–80% of the rain falls in the Kiremt season (June–September) [20]. The mean minimum and maximum temperature ranges from 8° C to 30° C, with small annual variations. This zone is composed of 11 districts (Weredas). According to the 2007 census, the total urban and rural human population of the zone is estimated to be 1,004,558 [17]. This zone includes major urban areas of Alamata, Mekoni, Korem, Maychew and Adigudom. Recently the number of households engaged in extensive pig husbandry are increasing in urban areas of southern zone of Tigray region.

Animals Studied

This study was conducted during June - September 2012. Seven hundred fourteen extensively managed pigs (336 males and 378 females) owned by a total of 38 households in Mekelle and urban areas of southern zone of Tigray Region were included in the study. On the basis of the pig owning household head's declaration, the animals were categorized into three age groups of < 5 months old, 5-12 month old and > 12 months old. Distribution of the pigs with respect to sex and age is given in Table-1.

Table 1. Distribution of sample pigs (n=714) with respect to sex and age in Mekelle and urban areas of Southern Zone of Tigray Region, Ethiopia

Sex	Age category of pigs			Total
	< 5 months	5-12 month	>12 months	
Male	177	143	16	336
Female	163	154	61	378
Total	340	297	77	714

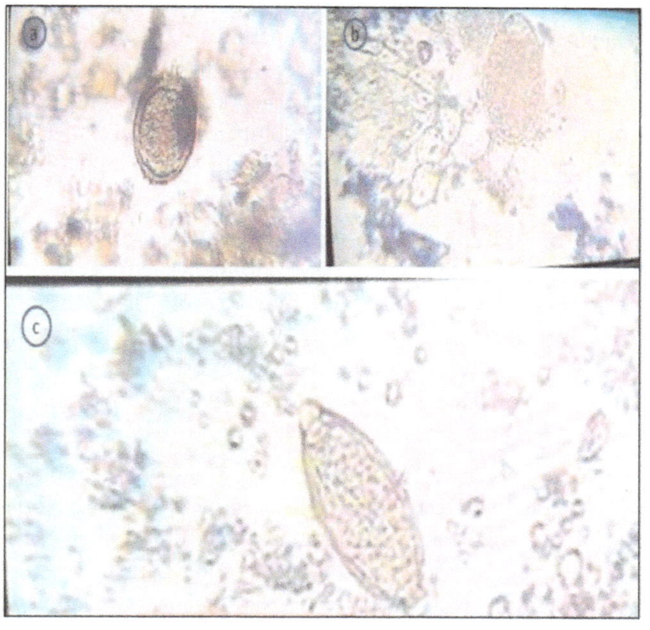

Figure 2: Eggs of gastrointestinal helminths isolated from extensively managed pigs in Mekelle and urban areas of Southern Zone of Tigray Region, Ethiopia; *Ascaris suum* (a), *Fasciola hepatica* (b) and *Trichuris suis* (c)

Collection of Fecal and Environmental Samples

Fecal samples were collected directly from the rectum of pigs with strict sanitation in the morning, when households release the animals from their pens. About 5 gram of the collected fecal sample was put in screw cap bottles containing 10% formalin. Soil samples were collected from backyards of pig pens using clean zipped plastic bags. Fecal and soil samples were transported to the Parasitology Laboratory, Department of Biology, Mekelle University (Ethiopia) on same day and stored at -20 °C until processed and examined for eggs and oocysts of gastrointestinal helminths and protozoans, respectively.

PROCESSING AND EXAMINATION FECAL AND SOIL SAMPLES

Zinc Sulphate Flotation

Three grams of fecal samples were mixed with 50 ml of 0.4g/ml Zinc Sulphate (flotation fluid) using mortar and pistil. Similarly soil samples were also mixed with 50 ml of 0.4g/ml Zinc Sulphate. The resulting fecal or soil suspension was poured through a tea strainer into a beaker. Then suspension was poured from the beaker into a test tube leaving a convex meniscus at the top. A cover slip was then carefully placed on top of the test tube and the test tube was let to stand for 20 minutes and after that cover slip was carefully lifted from the tube together with a drop of fluid adhering to it and immediately placed on a glass slide for microscopic examination [21]. These procedures were used to recover eggs intestinal helminths and oocysts of *Eimeria* spp.

Table 2. Demographic information and pig husbandry conditions practiced by households in Mekelle and Southern Zone of Tigray Region, Ethiopia

Variables	No. (%) pig owning per households
Sex	
Male	38(100)
Female	0(0)
Pig raising as an occupation	
Par time	16(42.11)
Full time	22(57.89)
Purpose of pig raising	
For market	38(100)
For food/other purpose	0(0)
Tap water supply for the household	
Yes	32(84.21)
No	6(15.79)
Toilet for the household	
Yes	32(84.21)
No	6(15.79)
Damping site for pig slurry	
Municipal garbage container	12(31.58)
Nearby garden/farm	19(50)
Municipal wastewater canal	7(18.42)
Floor condition of pig pen	
Cemented/cobbled with stone	6(15.79)
None cemented /non stone cobbled	32(84.21)

Sedimentation

In case of using NaCl as a flotation solution, the flotation technique was supplemented with sedimentation to recover eggs of intestinal helminths such as *Fasciola hepatica* which do not float well in sodium chloride solution. For this purpose, 3 g of fecal or soil samples was put in a conical flask and mixed with 30 ml of water; the mixture was then sieved through a tea strainer into a beaker and transferred into a centrifuge tube for centrifuging at 1500 rotation per minute for 3 minutes. The supernatant was then discarded and sediment was mixed with 1% of methylene blue and examined under the microscope using 40objective lens [22].

Modified Ziehl–Neelsen Technique

A total of 276 randomly selected pig fecal samples from Mekelle and urban areas of southern zone of Tigray Region were examined for *Cryptosporidium* oocyts by the modified Ziehl – Neelsen technique [21]. Thin fecal smear was prepared from each of the fecal samples, air-dried, fixed with absolute methanol and stained with a carbol-fuchsin (primary stain) for 30 minutes. The smear was then washed with tap water and decolorized with 1% acid-alcohol (1ml HCl and 99ml of 96% ethanol) for 2 minutes; washed again with tap water and counterstained with 1% methylene blue for another 2 minutes, then rinsed again in tap water and air-dried. The smear slides were then examined under a microscope at 1000x magnification for detection of *Cryptosporidium* oocysts.

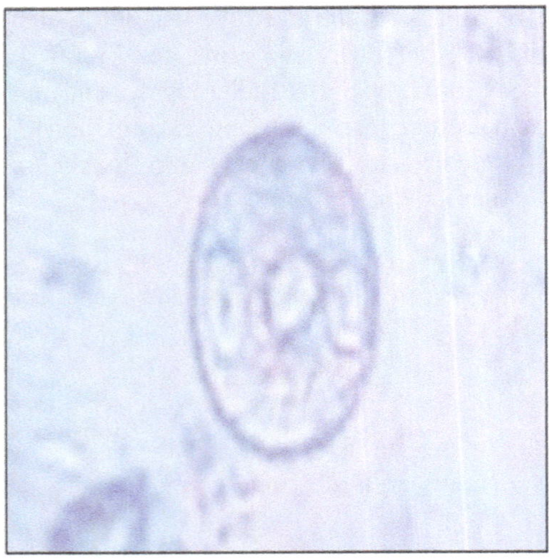

Figure 3: Oocyst of *Eimeria* species isolated from extensively managed pigs in Mekelle and urban areas of Southern Zone of Tigray Region, Ethiopia

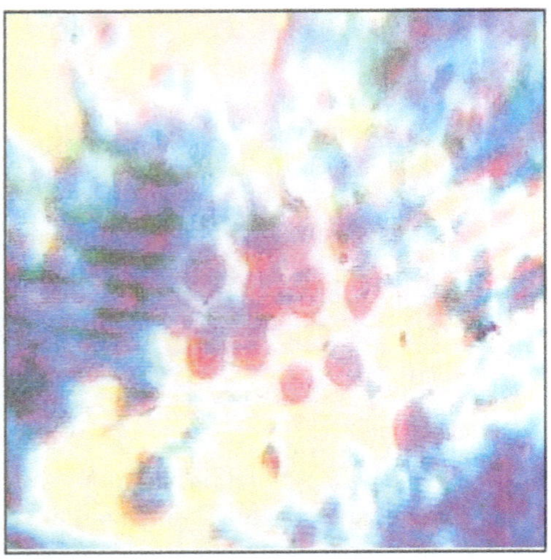

Figure4: Oocysts of *Cryptosporidium* species detected from extensively managed pigs in Mekelle and urban areas of Southern Zone of Tigray Region, Ethiopia.

Survey for Demographic Information and Pig Husbandry Conditions

A close ended interview questionnaire containing variables including characteristics of pig owning households and demographic information was first prepared in English and then translated into the local language of Tigriyna, to collect data on pig owning households. Interviews were administered to a total of 38 household heads encountered during the study. Observational check list containing variables such as presence of toilet and tap water supply for the household, site for dumping of pig slurry and floor condition of pig pens was prepared to collect data on pig husbandry condition at household level.

Statistical Analysis

Descriptive statistics was used to summarize data on prevalence of gastrointestinal parasites in pigs and contamination of soil by helminth eggs in Mekelle and urban areas of southern zone of Tigray Region, Ethiopia. Chi-square test using SPSS10 [23] software was conducted to see if there is any difference between prevalence of gastrointestinal parasites with respect to age and sex of the pigs as well as among different study sites.

RESULTS

A total of 38 male household heads with ages ranging from 15-69 years were identified engaged in extensive pig management in Mekelle and urban areas of southern zone of Tigray Region. Pig husbandry was a fulltime occupation for about 22 (58%) of the households. Fifty percent of the pig owning house-holds dump slurry of the animals in the nearby agricultural farms as manure (Table-2). The mean number of family size and pigs owned by households were found to be 4.05+0.379 and 20.82+2.89, respectively.

Out of 714 coprological samples of pigs examined, 195 (27.3%) were positive for at least one of the gastrointestinal parasites in Mekelle and southern zones of Tigray Region (Table-3). During microscopic examination 169 (94.94%), 05 (2.81%) and 01 (0.56%) pigs were found to be positive for eggs of *Ascaris suum, Fasciola* and *Trichuris suis* respectively (Figure 2).

On the other hand, 3 (1.69%) pigs were found to be positive for oocysts of *Eimeria* spp. (Figure 3, Table 4). About 26% of the parasitized pigs were infected with *A. suum* either as a single or multiple infections with other parasite species. However, there is no statistically significant association in the prevalence of intestinal parasites in pigs between Mekelle zone and southern zone of Tigray Region (÷^{2}[df 1] = 0.320; *P=0.572*). There is also no association in the prevalence of parasites between male and female pigs in the study areas (÷^{2}[df 1] = 1.921; *P=0.166*). On contrary, there is significant association between different age categories and prevalence of parasites, where majority of infection occurring in pigs with ages ranging from 5-12 months (÷^{2}[df 2] = 8.376; *P=0.015*).

Moreover, Out of 276 fecal samples examined for oocytss of *Cryptosporidium* spp. (Figure4), 20 (7.2%) were found to be positive. Regarding parasitological contamination of the environment in the study areas, soil samples collected from backyards of pig pens were found to be contaminated with eggs of *Ascaris* spp. (Table-5).

DISCUSSION

In this study it was possible to recover eggs and oocysts of gastrointestinal helminths and protozoans, respectively. Twenty seven percent of the pigs were infected with one or more gastrointestinal parasite species. *Ascaris suum* was the most common helminth in all age categories of pigs examined in the present study. This is in agreement with similar studies in extensively managed pigs [24, 25]. On the contrary, Tiwari et al. [26] reported no evidence of *A. suum* infection in pigs in Grenada, West Indies. Though, *A.* suum is naturally a parasite of pigs, but it can also infect human [14]. The potential of *A. suum* to infect human might be due to the fact that it shares similar protein molecules with *Ascaris lumbricoides* for which man is the natural host [27, 28]. Therefore, it is not surprising to say extensively managed pigs in the present study areas may act as potential reservoir hosts of human ascariasis.

Table 3. Prevalence of intestinal parasites in pigs in Mekelle and Southern Zone of Tigray Region, Ethiopia (2012)

Study Areas	No. of pigs sampled	Single infection*	Mixed infection@	Total No. of Positive
Mekelle	310	A 83, F 1, E 1	4 (A & E)	89
Urban areas of southern zone of Tigrey region				
Adigudom	35	A 8	1(A & F), 1(A & E), 1(A & T)	11
Maychew	190	A 38, F 3, E 1	1(A & F), 1(A & E)	42
Alamata	139	A 30, F 1, T 1, E 2	6(A & F), 3 (A & E)	42
Korem	20	A 7	1 (A & T)	8
Mekoni	20	A 3	0	3
Total	714			195 (27.3%)

A= *Ascaris suum*, F= *Fasciola hepatica*, E= *Eimeria* spp., T= *Trichuris suis*; *Single infection means, infection of pigs with any one of the parasites; #For example, in 3rd column it means 83 pigs were infected with *Ascaris suum* (A), 01 with *Fasciola hepatica* (F) and 01 with *Eimeria* spp. (E) and similarly for other rows in the same columns. @Multiple infections mean, pigs infected with more than one parasite.

Table 4. Prevalence of gastrointestinal parasites in different age groups of pigs in Mekelle and urban areas of Southern Zone of Tigray Region, Ethiopia*

Age groups	*A. suum*		*F. hepatica*		*Eimeria* spp.		*T. suis*	
	No	%	No	%	No	%	No	%
<5 months (n=340)	71	20.9	6	1.8	6	1.8	0	0
5-12 months (n=297)	96	32.3	6	2.0	6	2.0	1	0.3
> 12 months (n=77)	18	23.4	1	1.3	0	0.0	1	1.3
All age groups (n=714)	185	25.9	13	1.8	12	1.7	2	0.3

* Both single and multiple infections were considered to calculate the prevalence

Table 5. Contamination of soil by eggs of *Asacris* spp. at backyards of pig pens in the study areas.

Study areas	No. of soil samples examined	Prevalence of *Ascaris* spp.No.(%)
Mekelle Zone	8	6(75)
Urban Areas of Southern Zone of Tigray Region		
Adigudom	2	02(100)
Maychew	10	06 (60)
Korem	1	01(100)
Mekoni	1	0 (0)
Alamata	3	3(100)

The prevalence of the second nematode parasite, *Trichuris suis,* was very low in different age groups of pigs examined. This low prevalence agrees with the findings of earlier studies in Africa and West Indies [26, 29, 30]. This supports the speculations that *T. suis* eggs are highly susceptible to environmental factors. The prevalence of *Fasciola hepatica* was low (2.81%) in this study. On the contrary, Apt et al. [31] reported higher prevalence *F hepatica* in pigs of the Chilean provinces.

Factors such as presence of reservoir hosts, presence of snail intermediate hosts and ability of *F. hepatica* to colonise and adapt new hosts contribute for its spread in livestock in an area [32]. The transmission ecology of our present study areas are not far away from fulfilling the aforementioned epidemiological determinants of fasciolosis in livestock. Mekelle and urban areas of southern zone of Tigray Region are centers of livestock marketing, so that farmers from surrounding rural areas bring livestock to the urban markets. Therefore, such livestock migration from rural villages to markets in the urban areas may contribute for the introduction of gastrointestinal parasites including *F hepatica* to the urban areas. In addition, there is huge cattle transport to Mekelle from different districts of the region for the Abregele meat factory. Irrigated urban and pre-urban crop production practice through ditching urban wastewater may render suitable habitats for snail intermediate hosts of *F hepatica* in the present study areas. From our personal observation, pigs in the study areas browse grasses along the irrigation water ditches which may expose them to infection with the metacercaria of *F hepatica* [33]. This may also contributes for contamination of the ditched water with eggs or oocyts of gastro-intestinal parasites contained in pig feces.

The prevalence of *Eimeria* spp. in this study was much lower than a similar survey in Ethiopia [7] and Zimbabwe [34], respectively. This difference in prevalence of *Eimeria* spp. may be attributed to the underlining difference in epidemiology of *Eimeria* spp. in the areas and methods used to recover oocysts from fecal samples.

In the present study, out of 276 pigs examined 20 (7.2%) were positive for *Cryptosporidium* spp. This result is consistent with the findings of Morgan et al. [11]. However, the modern Merifluor *Cryptosporidium* immunofluorescence assay revealed higher positivity of *Cryptosporidium* spp. in 217 intensively managed pigs in Lusaka, Zambia [35]. Nevertheless previous study by Haileyesus [12] showed prevalence of *Cryptosporidium parvum* and *C. hominis* in extensively managed cattle and HIV/AIDS patients, respectively in Ethiopia.

There is no statistically significant difference in the prevalence of gastrointestinal parasites (*Ascaris suum,*

Trichuris suis, Fasciola hepatica and *Eimeria* spp.) in Mekelle and urban areas of southern zone of Tigray Region ($\div^2$[df 1] = 0.320; *P=0.572*). This may be due to the reason that pigs of both of the study areas are under similar risk factors of infection with gastro-intestinal parasites. During our field survey it was observed that pigs were scavenging on household and municipal garbage in both Mekelle and urban areas of southern zone of Tigray Region. Even in few sites of the study areas it was recorded that children were defecating outside to their home and pigs were allowed to feed on children's fecal material. Consumption of human fecal material by pigs may complicate the epidemiology of gastrointestinal parasites such as *Ascaris suum* and *Cryptosporidium* spp. that can infect both pigs and man [10].

There was also no statistically significant difference in the prevalence rate of gastrointestinal parasites between male and female pigs ($\div^2$[df 1] = 1.921; *P=0.166*). This result is consistent with the finding of previous study in Holeta, Ethiopia [7]. However, Tamboura et al. [4] reported higher prevalence of gastrointestinal nematodes in female pigs than in males in Burkina Faso. The reason for equal exposure of both sexes of pigs to GIT parasites in the present and previous study [7] in Ethiopia may be due to voracious feeding of both sexes on household and municipal garbage in the study areas.

A significant association was recorded between chances of gastrointestinal parasites infections and different age categories of pigs. It was observed that majority of infection occurring in pigs with ages ranging from 5-12 months ($\div^2$[df 2] = 8.376; *P=0.015*). On the contrary, Abdu and Gashaw [7] reported statistically insignificant difference in infection rate of gastrointestinal parasites in pigs of different age groups in Holeta, Ethiopia. However, Obonyo et al. [36] reported high prevalence of gastrointestinal infections in finishers than in adults in Kenya. The lower prevalence of gastrointestinal parasites in the youngest (<5 months) and in the oldest (>12 month) age groups might be because, the youngest pigs are lactating and hence partially scavenging on garbage for feed, whereas, most of the oldest pigs were either pregnant females (sows) or males kept for breeding (boars) and therefore were given special attention by the owners in terms of additional feed to reduce their scavenging dependency on garbage which is considered to be one of the risk factors for infection with gastrointestinal parasites.

Eggs of *Ascaris* spp. were recorded in soil samples collected from backyards of pig pens in the study areas. The reason for the occurrence of eggs of *Ascaris* spp. in soil may be due to its resistance to environmental factors [37]. Speciation of *Ascaris* isolates of soil was not possible as eggs of *Ascaris suum* are morpholo-gically identical to eggs of the human parasite, *Asacris lumbricoides*. This implies the source of *Ascaris* egg contamination of soil could be either *Ascaris suum* or *Asacris lumbricoides*, which was due to poorly managed pig slurry and outside defecation practices of humans.

CONCLUSION AND RECOMMENDATION

Gastrointestinal parasites (*Ascaris suum, Trichuris suis, Fasciola hepatica, Eimeria* spp.) and *Cryptospo-ridium* spp. have been investigated from extensively managed pigs in Mekelle and southern zone of Tigray Region, Ethiopia. *A. suum* was most prevalent either as a single or multiple infections with other parasites in pigs examined. The possibilities of *Ascaris* spp. of pigs to infect man and vice versa coupled with unhygienic environmental condition may complicate the epidemiology and control of ascariasis in the study areas. In the present study extensively managed pigs are also reported to harbor *Fasciola hepatica* and *Cryptosporidium* spp. suggesting the potentials of pigs as reservoirs hosts of the parasites. Further investigations are recommended for molecular characterization of *Ascaris* and *Cryptosporidium* isolates of pigs to clearly determine the species of the parasites responsible for swine ascariasis and cryptosporidiosis, respectively in the study areas.

AUTHORS' CONTRIBUTION

ZT was the project leader and designer of the study in addition to drafting and revising the manuscript. EI was responsible for statistical analysis of data, preparation of study area map and edition of the Manuscript. TK was in charge of sample collection and examination. YT was responsible for sample processing. KW rendered overall assistance during sample collection, processing and examination. All authors read and approved the final manuscript.

ACKNOWLEDGEMENTS

The authors would like to acknowledge the Department of Biology and College of Veterinary Medicine, Mekelle University, for laboratory facilities. This study received financial support from the MU-UMB, Mekelle University. We would like to thank the representatives of veterinary health centers for their unreserved assistance in facilitating the field work. Furthermore, we would like to extend our gratitude to the pig owning households for participation in the study.

REFERENCES

1. Nansen P and Roepstorff A. (1999) Parasitic helminths of the pig: factors influencing transmission and infection levels, International Journal of Parasitology, 29: 877–891.
2. http://dx.doi.org/10.1016/S0020-7519(99)00048-X
3. Lekule F.P. and Kyvsgaard N.C. (2003) Improving pig husbandry in tropical resource-poor communities and its potential to reduce risk of porcine cysticercosis, Acta Tropica, 87: 111-117. http://dx.doi.org/10.1016/S0001-706X(03)00026-3
4. Nganga C.J., Karanja D.N. and Mutune M.N. (2008) The prevalence of gastrointestinal helminth infection in pigs in Kenya, Tropical Animal Health and Production, 40: 331-334. http://dx.doi.org/10.1007/s11250-007-9112-3
5. Tamboura H.H., Banga-Mboko H., Maes D., Youssao I., Traore A., Bayala B. and Dembele M.A. (2006) Prevalence of common gastrointestinal nematode parasites in scavenging pigs of different ages and sexes in eastern centre province, Burkina Faso, Onderstepoort Journal of Veterinary Research, 73: 53-60. http://dx.doi.org/10.4102/ojvr.v73i1.169
6. Permin A,Yelifari L, Bloch P, Steenhard N, Hansen N.P. and Nansen P. (1999) Parasites in cross-bred pigs in the Upper East region of Ghana, Veterinary Parasitology, 87: 63-71. http://dx.doi.org/10.1016/S0304-4017(99)00159-

4

7. Gweba M, Faleke O.O., Junaidu A.U., Fabiyi J.P. and Fajinmi A.O. (2010) Some risk factors for Taenia Solium cystycercosis in semi-intensively raised pigs in Zuru, Nigeria, Veterinaria Italiana, 46: 57-67.

8. Abdu S. and Gashaw A. (2010) Production system dynamism and parasitic interaction of swine in and around Holetta, Ethiopia, Ethiopian Veterinary Journal, 14: 71-81.

9. Uysal H. K., Boral O., Metiner K and Ilgaz A. (2009) Investigation of Intestinal Parasites in Pig Feces That Are also Human Pathogens, Türkiye Parazitoloji Dergisi, 33: 218-221.

10. Ramirez N. E., Ward L. A. and Sreevatsan S. (2004) A review of the biology and epidemiology of cryptosporidiosis in humans and animals, Microbes and Infection, 6: 773-785. 10. Fayer R. (2010) Taxonomy and species delimitation in Cryptosporidium.Experimental, Parasitology, 124: 90-97.

11. Morgan U. M., Buddle R, Armson A and Thompson R. C. A. (1999) Molecular and biological characterisation of Cryptosporidium in pigs, Australian Veterinary Journal, 77: 44-47. http://dx.doi.org/10.1111/j.1751-0813.1999.tb12428.x

12. Haileyesus A. (2010) The prevalence of intestinal parasites and molecular characterisation of Cryptoporidium species in Ethiopia. Ph.D. Thesis, Addis Ababa University, Ethiopia. Pp.117.

13. Hale O. M. and Stewart T. B. (1998) Losses to Internal Parasites in Swine Production, Journal of Animal Sciences, 66: 1548-1554.

14. Arizono, N., Yoshimura, Y., Tohzaka, N., Yamada, M., Tegoshi, T., Onishi, K. and Uchikawa, R. (2010) Ascariasis in Japan: Is pig-derived Ascaris infecting humans, Japanese Journal of infectious diseases, 63: 447-448.

15. CSA. (2004) Central Statistical Authority. National Statistics Abstract, Addis Ababab, Ethiopia.

16. Kibrom G. (2005) Investigation into engineering properties of Mekele soils with an emphasis on expansive soils, M.Sc. thesis, Addis Abeba University, Addis Ababa, Ethiopia.

17. CSA. (2008) Central Statistical Authority. National Statistics Abstract, Addis Ababab, Ethiopia.

18. Ashebir D., Pasquini M. and Bihon W. (2007) Urban agriculture in Mekelle, Tigray state, Ethiopia: Principal characteristics, opportunities and constraints for further research and development, Cities, 24: 218-228. http://dx.doi.org/10.1016/j.cities.2007.01.008

19. MZAO. (2011) Mekelle Zonal Agricultural Office. Mekelle, Ethiopia.

20. Araya A. and Stroosnijder L. (2011) Assessing drought risk and irrigation need in northern Ethiopia, Agricultural and forest meteorology, 151: 425-436. http //dx.doi.org/10.1016/j.agrformet.2010.11.014

21. WHO (1991) Basic laboratory methods in medical parasitology. World Health Organization, Geneva.

22. Bayou K. (2005) Standard veterinary laboratory diagnostic manual. Volume III. Ministry of Agriculture and Rural Development, Animal Health Department. Addis Ababa, Ethiopia.

23. SPSS-10. (1988) SPSS-X user's guide. 3rd ed. Chicago (IL): SPSS Inc.

24. Salifu D.A., Manga T.B. and Onyali, I.O. (1990) A survey of gastrointestinal parasites in pigs of the Plateau and Rivers States, Nigeria, Revue d'Elevage et de Médecine Vétérinaire des Pays Tropicaux, 43(2):193-196.

25. Nsoso S.J., Mosala K.P., Ndebele R.T. and Ramabu S.S.(2000) The prevalence of internal and external parasites in pigs of different ages and sexes in Southeast District, Botswana, Onderstepoort Journal of Veterinary Research, 67: 217-220.

26. Tiwari K. P., Chikweto A, Belot G, Vanpee G, Deallie C, Stratton G and Sharma R.N. (2009) Prevalence of intestinal parasites in pigs in Grenada, West Indies, West Indian Veterinary Journal, 9 (1): 22-27.

27. Alba J. E., Comia M.N., Oyong G. and Claveria F. (2009). Ascaris lumbricoides and Ascaris suum: A comparison of electrophoretic banding patterns of protein extracts from the reproductive organs and body wall, Veterinarski arhiv, 79: 281-291.

28. Leles D, Gardner S. L., Reinhard K, I-iguez A and Araujo A. (2012) Are Ascaris lumbricoides and Ascaris suum a single species, Parasit Vectors, 5: 42. http://dx.doi.org/10.1186/1756-3305-5-42

29. Esrony K., Kambarage D. M., Mtambo M. M., Muhairwa A. P. and Kusiluka L.J. (1997) Helminthosis in local and cross-bred pigs in the Morogoro region of Tanzania, Preventive Veterinary Medicine, 32:41–46. http://dx.doi.org/10.1016/S0167-5877(97)00011-1

30. Marufu M.C., Chanayiwa P, Chimonyo M and Bhebhe E. (2008) Prevalence of gastrointestinal nemtodes in Mukota pigs in a communal area of Zimbabwe, African Journal of Agricultural Research, 3(2): 91-95.

31. Apt W., Aguilera X, Vega F, Alcaíno H, Zulantay I, Apt P, González V, Retamal C, Rodríguez J and Sandoval J. (1993). Prevalence of fascioliasis in humans, horses, pigs, and wild rabbits in 3 Chilean provinces, Biol Oficina Sanit Panam, 115: 405-414.

32. Mas-Coma S., Bargues M.D. and Valero M.A. (2005) Fascioliasis and other plant-borne trematode zoonoses, International Journal of Parasitology, 35: 1255–1278. http://dx.doi.org/10.1016/j.ijpara.2005.07.010

33. PHAO. (2011) Fasciola hepatica: Pathogen safety data sheet - infectious substances. Public Health Agency of Canada. 19 Aug 2011.

34. Chhabra R. C. and Mafukidze R.T. (1992) Prevalence of coccidia in pigs in Zimbabwe, Veterinary Parasitology, 41: 1-5. http://dx.doi.org/10.1016/0304-4017(92)90002-Q

35. Siwila, J. and Mwape, K. E. (2012) Prevalence of Cryptosporidium spp. and Giardia duodenalis in pigs in Lusaka, Zambia, Onderstepoort Journal of Veterinary Research, 79(1): 1-5, Art. #404, http:// dx.doi.org/10.4102/ojvr. v79i1. 404.

36. Obonyo F. O., Maingi N., Githigia S. M. and Ng'ang'a C. J. (2012) Prevalence, intensity and spectrum of

helminths of free range pigs in Homabay District, Kenya. Livestock Research for Rural Development. Volume 24, Article #48. http://www.lrrd.org/lrrd24/3/obon24048.htm, Retrieved, 27-10-2012.

37. Lewis-Jones R and Winkler M. (1991) Sludge parasites and other pathogens. Ellis Horwood Limited, Chichester, England.

SECTION VI: PARASITES OF DOGS AND CATS

CHAPTER 23

PREVALENCE OF HELMINTHS IN DOGS AND OWNERS' AWARENESS OF ZOONOTIC DISEASES IN MAMPONG, ASHANTI, GHANA

Papa Kofi Amissah-Reynolds, Isaac Monney, Lucy Mawusi Adowah and Samuel Opoku Agyemang

INTRODUCTION

Dogs live in close association with humans, providing them with companionship and security, among others [1]. However, these companion animals can as well transmit diseases to humans who have close contact with them [2, 3]. Infections could be transmitted to humans through contact with animal hair [4, 5], food and water contaminated with dog excreta or secretions, and/or consumption of dog meat [6]. According to the literature, dogs can host well-known zoonotic parasites, including Toxocara canis, Diphyllobothrium latum, Ancylostomaspp., Uncinaria stenocephala [7], and Echinococcus granulosus [8]. The presence of these parasites in dogs causes different clinical symptoms depending on the parasite species and density [9].

There are numerous reports on canine intestinal parasites worldwide. Some studies reported prevalence of between 4 and 40% [7, 10–12]. Others reported higher prevalence of over 60% [9, 13–16]. The varying prevalence reported could be due to differences in status of dog sampled, geographical location, and the diagnostic techniques used [17, 18]. Gastrointestinal parasites are more common in dogs in developing countries [19]. High prevalence and heavy infections are often reported in such countries. This is attributed to the fact that dogs in these regions are rarely treated for parasitic diseases and policies on pet ownership are usually lacking [15] or poorly enforced, thereby providing fertile grounds for zoonotic transmission of parasites.

In Ghana, very little attention has been given to parasites in dogs and only two studies have been conducted in this regard. Studies conducted by Anteson and Corkish [20] and Johnson et al. [21] identified a total of 9 species of intestinal helminths in dogs in Ghana. Anteson and Corkish highlighted the ineffectiveness of antihelminthics, while asserting the possible transmission of zoonotic parasites to children [20]. Johnson et al. [21] identified housing styles, sources of dogs, and purpose of keeping dogs as significant factors associated with infection. Data from these studies were however not population-based as they focused only on owned dogs, but not stray or unowned dogs.

To the best of our knowledge, there has been no survey on intestinal helminths in dogs in Mampong, Ashanti. Current epidemiological data is therefore needed for establishing effective control measures in animal and public health. We report for the first time the prevalence and types of helminths in dogs, deworming practices, and knowledge of pet owners on zoonotic parasites in the area.

Citation: Papa Kofi Amissah-Reynolds, Isaac Monney, Lucy Mawusi Adowah, and Samuel Opoku Agyemang, "Prevalence of Helminths in Dogs and Owners' Awareness of Zoonotic Diseases in Mampong, Ashanti, Ghana,"Journal of Parasitology Research, vol. 2016, Article ID 1715924, 6 pages, 2016. doi:10.1155/2016/1715924.

EXPERIMENTAL SECTION

Study Area and Study Design

Mampong, Ashanti, is the capital of the Mampong Municipal Assembly in the Ashanti region of Ghana. Geographically, it is located on latitude 7°05′42″N and longitude 1°24′49″W, approximately 60 km northeast of the regional capital, Kumasi. It has an estimated population of 40,000 people, accounting for approximately half of the population of the entire municipality. The town lies within a wet semiequatorial forest zone and has scenic undulating land forms which range from scarps and hills to low lying tropical areas. Farming activities are predominant in the township owing to the fertile soil.

The study area was divided into three sites according to the planning of settlements. Site 1 is a poorly planned settlement with dispersed housing system and poor environmental conditions. Site 2 and Site 3 have better community setup in terms of housing and environmental conditions compared to Site 1.

Dogs were classified into three age groups as puppies (0–6 months), young dogs (>6 months to 12 months), and adults (>12 months) as described by Bone, 1988 (cited in [9]). They were further categorized into stray, semidomestic, and domestic based on a modified description from the one used by Perera et al. [19]. Domestic dogs were the ones with owners, kept under strict confinement, who do not mingle with stray or semidomestic dogs and may or may not be dewormed and/or vaccinated against rabies and other diseases. The semidomestic dogs were the ones who had owners, who mingle with stray dogs and may or may not be dewormed and/or vaccinated against rabies and other diseases. Stray dogs were the free-ranging ones that did not have owners, fed off the streets, and had no deworming and vaccination against rabies and other diseases.

Random house-to-house screening of dogs of all age groups, sexes, housing styles, and functions was conducted between March and July 2015. Stool samples of one hundred and fifty-four (154) dogs were collected in sterile containers labelled with identification data. After collection, samples were taken to the Laboratory of Veterinary Service, Kumasi, and kept frozen until use. With the informed consent of dog owners, a structured questionnaire was also used to assess the dog management practices and owners' awareness of zoonotic canine parasites.

Laboratory Procedure

Stool samples of dogs were analyzed for eggs of parasites using saturated sodium chloride solution as a floatation medium. Samples were observed under the light microscope at 10x objective. The parasites were classified according to their species based on existing keys and descriptions [22]. The results were analyzed using SPSS version 17 to determine frequencies and percentages. Test for associations was conducted with the Chi-square (χ^2) test at 5% significance level.

Assessment of Pet Management Practices and Awareness of Zoonotic Diseases

Questionnaires were administered to 100 dog owners who consented to be interviewed. The questionnaires were divided into two distinct sections to capture information on reasons for keeping dog(s), number of dogs kept, knowledge of zoonosis, and pet management practices including deworming frequency, housing and feeding mode, and veterinary care.

RESULTS AND DISCUSSION

Results

Out of the 154 dog excrement samples examined, approximately 53% were infected with at least one parasite. Overall, 13 parasite species were found in the dog excrement, with the top four parasites being Toxocara canis(18.8%), Ancylostoma sp. (16.9%), Troglotrema salmincola (7.8%), and Diphyllobothrium latum (7.1%) (Figure1). Nematodes were more common than cestodes in the study dogs.

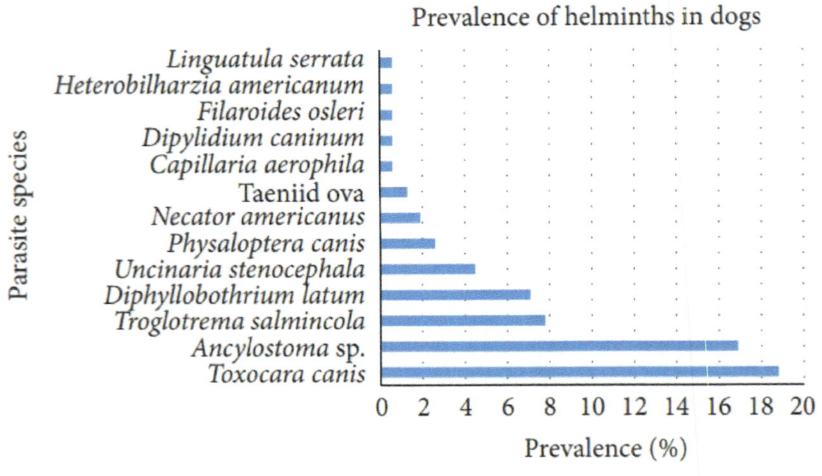

Figure 1: Distribution of helminths found in dog excrement (n = 154).

The prevalence pattern by age of the four most predominant parasites is presented in Figure 2. Only two fish parasites, namely, Troglotrema salmincola and Diphyllobothrium latum, showed an association with age. While the former showed decreasing prevalence with age of dogs, the latter showed a reverse trend.

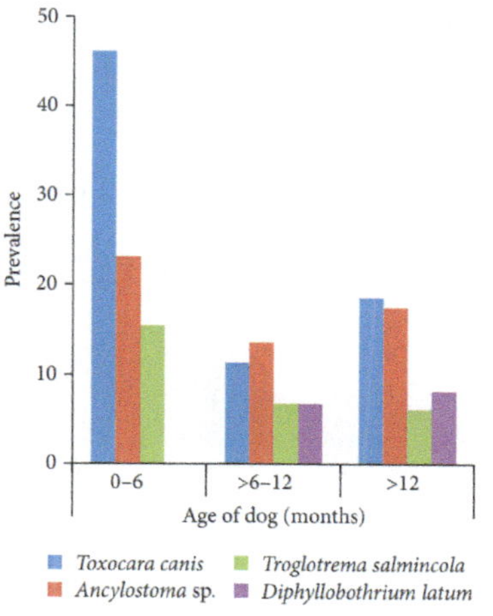

Figure 2: Prevalence pattern of parasites by age.

The prevalence of helminths in dogs in relation to age and sex is shown in Table 1. Among the three age groups, the highest prevalence (86.7%) was recorded in puppies, followed by adult dogs (52.0%) and young dogs (41.5%). Male dogs recorded slightly higher prevalence (55.1%) than female dogs (48.2%), though the difference was not statistically significant ($p > 0.05$). Eleven (11) species of parasites were recovered from male dogs compared to six (6) from the females.

Table 1: Prevalence of helminths in dogs in relation to age and sex ($N = 154$)

Variable	Number examined	Number infected	Infection rate (%)	*p* value
Age (months)				
0–6	15	13	86.7	
>6–12	41	17	41.5	$p = 0.011$; $\chi^2 = 9.034$
>12	98	51	52.0	
Sex				
Male	98	54	55.1	
Female	56	27	48.2	$p = 0.410$; $\chi^2 = 0.678$
Total	**154**	**81**	**52.6**	

The frequency of single and mixed infections is presented in Figure 3. Single infections were more common (42.2%) than multiple infections (10.4%). The percentage of dogs harboring mixed infections of two and three parasites was 7.8% and 2.6%, respectively. Interestingly, 13 male dogs (13.2%) harbored multiple parasites compared to 3 female dogs (5.4%). No female dog harbored more than two parasites. Multiple infections were recorded in dogs sampled from Site 1 and Site 2 only.

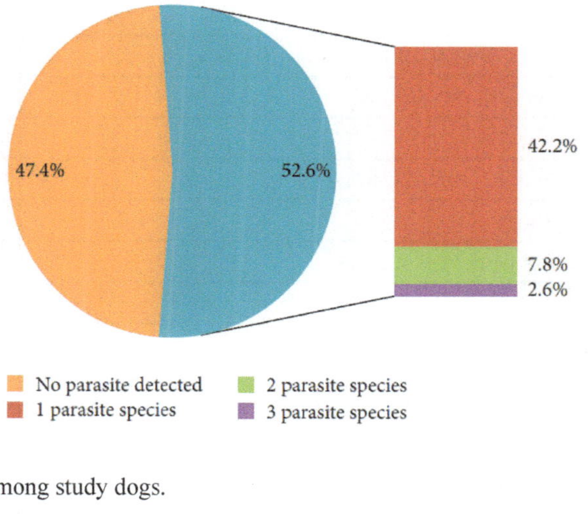

Figure 3: Pattern of parasitic infection among study dogs.

The prevalence of helminths in relation to the functions of the 145 owned dogs sampled is presented in Table 2. Though dogs who were kept for companionship recorded higher prevalence (69.2%) than dogs used for hunting (66.7%) and security (44.0%), the difference was not statistically significant (). Approximately 70% of the owned dogs sampled were kept for security.

Table 2: Prevalence of helminths in relation to dog function

Function of dog	Number of dogs examined	Number of dogs infected	Infection rate (%)	*p* value
Companionship	39	27	69.2	
Hunting	6	4	66.7	$p = 0.59$; $\chi^2 = 5.650$
Security	100	44	44.0	
Total	**145**	**75**	**51.7**	

Table 3 shows the prevalence of helminths in dogs in relation to their housing styles. Stray dogs recorded the highest prevalence (66.7%), followed by domestic (61.1%) and semidomestic dogs (50.4%), respectively. Nearly 90% of the dogs sampled were allowed to roam about in the community.

Table 3: Prevalence of helminths in relation to mode of housing

Mode of housing	Number of dogs examined	Number of dogs infected	Infection rate (%)	*p* value
Domestic	18	11	61.1	
Stray	9	6	66.7	$p = 0.476$; $\chi^2 = 1.485$
Semidomestic	127	64	50.4	
Total	**154**	**81**	**52.6**	

A statistically significant association ($p = 0.02$; $\chi^2 = 12.323$) was found between location and helminthic infections in dogs. The relation between location and prevalence of helminths is shown in Table 4.

Table 4: Prevalence of helminths based on location of dog

Location	Number of dogs examined	Number of dogs infected	Infection rate (%)	*p* value
Site 1	48	30	62.5	
Site 2	50	32	64.0	$p = 0.02$; $\chi^2 = 12.323$
Site 3	56	19	33.9	
Total	**154**	**81**	**52.6**	

None of the 100 dog owners interviewed fed their dogs with standard dog feed and close to three-quarters (73%) fed their dogs off the bare floor (Table 5). Awareness of rabies disease in dogs was comparable (62%) to that of helminth infestation in dogs (60%) among the dog owners. Most dog owners (93%) allowed their dogs to defecate anywhere without any restriction and close to 9 out of 10 dog owners had never taken their dogs to a veterinary clinic although there is one present in the town. Regular deworming of dogs is an uncommon practice among dog owners; close to half of the dog owners had never dewormed their dogs and a significant proportion (76%) had no knowledge of the transmission of zoonotic diseases to humans. About a third of dog owners (32%) kept their dogs in kennels and close to half of them (46%) cleaned the kennels once a month. The median number of dogs kept per owner was 2 (range 1–15).

Table 5: Dog management practices and awareness of zoonotic parasites (N = 100)

Type of feed given to dog	
Dog feed	0%
Raw meat products and household leftovers	100%
How do you feed your dog?	
In a bowl	13%
In a bowl and/or on the floor	14%
On the floor	73%
Awareness of rabies in dogs	
Yes	62%
No	38%
Awareness of helminthic infections in dogs	
Yes	60%
No	40%
Where do(es) your dog(s) usually defecate?	
Within the house	7%
Within and/or outside the house (anywhere)	93%

Have you ever taken your dog(s) to a veterinary clinic?	
Yes	12%
No	88%
Frequency of deworming dog(s)	
Once every 3 months	16%
Once every 6 months	13%
Once a year	25%
Never	46%
Awareness of risk of zoonotic transmission of parasites	
Yes	24%
No	76%
Do you keep your dogs in kennels?	
Yes	32%
No	68%
How often do you clean the kennels?	
Daily	22%
Weekly	32%
Monthly	46%

*n = 32

Discussion

The present study reports for the first time on helminth parasites in dogs in Mampong, Ashanti, Ghana. The two previous studies on dogs in Ghana were done on owned dogs in a different location [20, 21]. All the parasites reported in this study have been previously documented in dogs elsewhere, but with regional variation in prevalence and parasite species.

In the present study, we recorded lower overall prevalence compared to previous data in Africa [9, 13, 15, 16]. The use of single faecal floatation in the present study may have underestimated the prevalence, as a combination of methods has been reported to increase the chances of recovering more parasites [19]. Also, ecological and epidemiological differences, as well as the faecal floatation methods used [11], may account for the variations in distribution and prevalence of parasites. Single infections were more common than multiple infections and this agrees with the findings of Ugbomoiko et al. [15] and Kimura et al. [12]. In contrast, other studies [9, 16, 19] reported higher frequencies of multiple parasites compared to single parasites.

Data from the present study is consistent with previous works in Ghana and other parts of Africa which have reported Toxocara canis, Ancylostoma sp., Dipylidium caninum, and Taeniidae as some of the helminths parasitizing dogs [9, 13, 15, 16, 21]. Trichuris vulpis, Strongyloides sp., and Spirocerca lupi were absent in the present study though these parasites have also been previously reported. The absence of Spirocerca lupi eggs in our study may be due to the use of sodium chloride as a floatation medium [9].

Our present results agree with Ugbomoiko et al. [15] and Kimura et al. [12], who reported Toxocara canis as the most common helminth in dogs. Toxocara canis is a soil-transmitted helminth; thus, habits like feeding off floors and sleeping on bare grounds in the study dogs could account for this observation. Though the prevalence pattern of Toxocara canis was not age-dependent, the highest prevalence of this nematode was found in puppies. The older dogs may have developed specific immunity to Toxocara canis through frequent exposure at an early age. We also found two fish parasites, Diphyllobothrium latum and Troglotrema salmincola, in the dogs sampled. Our results also showed that the prevalence pattern for the fish parasites was age-dependent; Troglotrema salmincola decreased with age, whereas Diphyllobothrium latum showed a reverse trend. The age-dependent prevalence pattern of fish parasites may be due to the role of immune responses in dogs. This role is however unclear and needs to be elucidated. These parasites have only been previously reported in dogs which feed on raw/fresh fish products. Considering that nearly all the dogs sampled fed on raw fish products or viscera, we predict that this prevalence pattern observed is largely due to the feeding habit of the dog rather than the age.

We recorded lower prevalence of Dipylidium caninum (0.6%) than has been previously reported elsewhere in Africa. Studies by Anteson and Corkish [20] and Zewdu et al. [9] recorded significantly higher prevalence ofDipylidium caninum by postmortem compared to coproscopy. Zewdu et al. [9] further indicated that necropsy provides more detailed information than coproscopy. However, we could not perform necropsy in the present study because the dogs could not be killed for such purposes.

Taeniid tapeworms are morphologically indistinguishable. Therefore, molecular analysis is needed to differentiate species of Taeniidae. Echinococcus granulosus is one of the Taeniid species found in dogs, which is also of zoonotic importance. However, the use of coproscopy in the present study did not allow us to detect the species of Taeniidae present.

Age, sex, location, and management practices (including housing styles and deworming practices) are some risk factors that predispose dogs to parasitism. Knowledge of risk factors of infection is vital in the development of effective control programs. Identification of risk factors is however a complex process, particularly in developing countries, given the high numbers of stray dogs with poor or no documented histories. In the present study, age of dog and location were identified as significant risk factors associated with parasitism. Perhaps, the low immunity of puppies compared to the older dogs accounts for the significantly higher prevalence of infection in the former. Though sex was not a significant risk factor, male dogs harbored more parasites species and more multiple infections compared to females. This could be attributed to the greater propensity for male dogs to roam about compared to females.

Ten (10) out of the 13 parasite species encountered were zoonotic, excluding Physaloptera canis, Filaroides osleri, and Heterobilharzia americanum. In addition, majority of the dogs were not regularly dewormed. Deworming of dogs did not appear to be associated with the reasons for keeping the dogs. For some dog owners, deworming was mostly done once a year by veterinary officers during community visits to vaccinate the pets against rabies. In areas where there are strict regulations on pet husbandry practices, dogs are generally given better care. These dogs are more regularly dewormed, mostly kept confined, or always accompanied outside and are not likely to defecate indiscriminately into the environment. These practices have the potential to limit the transfer of zoonotic agents. In comparison with these best practices, veterinary care for dogs in the study area was very poor. Except for yearly vaccination of dogs against rabies by veterinarians, awareness creation on zoonosis and proper pet management practices was virtually nonexistent. With most dogs harboring zoonotic parasites, having close bonds with dog owners who irregularly deworm their pets, and defecating indiscriminately, public health is threatened as a result of easy transfer of zoonotic parasites into the environment.

Compared to the most recent report on canine helminths in Ghana, we observed a number of similarities. The prevalence rate of 52.6% reported in our study is comparable with the 62.6% prevalence rate reported by Johnson et al. [21] in Accra, Ghana. The highest prevalence of Toxocara canis reported in both studies was found in puppies. Again, more than half of the dogs sampled in the two studies were kept for security and with a similar proportion being allowed to roam about in the communities. Most dog owners kept multiple dogs at home (median: 2 and 3, resp.), but pet management practices were poor. Both studies identified zoonotic canine parasites and reported low awareness of dog owners on risk of zoonotic transmission of parasites. Based on these findings, we predict that data from other parts of the country could show a similar trend and this could have serious implications for animal and public health, with dogs playing active roles in zoonotic transmission.

CONCLUSIONS

The study shows that more than half (approximately 53%) of the study dogs (N = 154) were infected with helminthic parasites, mostly nematodes. The top four parasites were Toxocara canis (18.8%), Ancylostoma sp. (16.9%), Troglotrema salmincola (7.8%), and Diphyllobothrium latum (7.1%). Age of dogs ($p = 0.011$; $\chi 2 = 9.034$) and location ($p = 0.02$; $\chi 2 = 12.323$) were significant risk factors of helminth parasitism, while mode of housing, function, and gender of dogs were not. Only close to a quarter (24%) of dog owners had knowledge of transmission of zoonotic diseases to humans and about half (46%) have never dewormed their dogs although most of them (73%) fed their dogs directly off the ground. Dogs in the area are potential agents of zoonotic transmission given direct excretion of helminth-infested excreta into the environment, cohabitation with owners, and poor pet management practices. The indiscriminate excretion of dogs in the environment is a blot on the landscape and poses a potential pollution source for adjoining surface water resources. The lack of awareness on the transmission of zoonotic diseases from dogs to humans and lack of proper veterinary care for the dogs are a serious public health risk. Dog owners need to be educated and veterinary services should be offered on door-to-door basis instead of the conventional centralized mode.

Given the species diversity of parasites in dogs in the region, we recommend the use of broad spectrum antihelminthics in the treatment of helminthiasis. The study needs to be replicated in other parts of the country to give a holistic impression of the spatial variation of helminth infection among dogs across the country.

AUTHORS' CONTRIBUTION

All the authors conceived and designed the experiments; Papa Kofi Amissah-Reynolds, Lucy Mawusi Adowah, and Samuel Opoku Agyemang performed the experiments; Papa Kofi Amissah-Reynolds and Isaac Monney analysed the data; all the authors contributed reagents/materials/analysis tools; Papa Kofi Amissah-Reynolds and Isaac Monney wrote the paper. Isaac Monney, Lucy Mawusi Adowah, and Samuel Opoku Agyemang contributed equally to this work.

ACKNOWLEDGMENTS

The authors acknowledge the contributions of the following staff of the Laboratory Service, Veterinary Directorate, Kumasi: Dr. Mabel Abudu, Ms. Belinda Sunu, Mrs. Irene, K. Afutu, and Mrs. Ernestina Antwi.

REFERENCES

1. M. Paul, L. King, and E. P. Carlin, "Zoonoses of people and their pets: a US perspective on significant pet-associated parasitic diseases," Trends in Parasitology, vol. 26, no. 4, pp. 153–154, 2010.
2. M. R. Lappin, "Pet ownership by immunocompromised people. Bayer Zoonosis Symposium," North American Veterinary Conference, vol. 24, no. 5, pp. 16–25, 2002.
3. N. Itoh, K. Kanai, Y. Hori, F. Hoshi, and S. Higuchi, "Prevalence of Giardia intestinalis and other zoonotic intestinal parasites in private household dogs of the Hachinohe area in Aomori prefecture, Japan in 1997, 2002 and 2007," Journal of Veterinary Science, vol. 10, no. 4, pp. 305–308, 2009.
4. W. F. El-Tras, H. R. Holt, and A. A. Tayel, "Risk of Toxocara canis eggs in stray and domestic dog hair in Egypt," Veterinary Parasitology, vol. 178, no. 3-4, pp. 319–323, 2011.
5. S. Öge, H. Öge, B. Gönenç, G. Özbakiş, and C. Yildiz, "Presence of Toxocara eggs on the hair of dogs and cats," Ankara Üniversitesi Veteriner Fakültesi Dergisi, vol. 60, pp. 171–176, 2013.

6. J. Cui and Z. Q. Wang, "Outbreaks of human trichinellosis caused by consumption of dog meat in China," Parasite, vol. 8, no. 2, supplement, pp. S74–S77, 2001. ·
7. D. Joffe, D. Van Niekerk, F. Gagne, J. Gilleard, S. Kutz, and R. Lobingier, "The prevalence of intestinal parasites in dogs and cats in Calgary, Alberta," Canadian Veterinary Journal, vol. 52, no. 12, pp. 1323–1328, 2011.
8. J. Abdi, K. Asadolahi, M. H. Maleki, and A. A. Hafez, "Prevalence of helminthes infection of stray dogs in Ilam province," Journal of Paramedical Sciences, vol. 4, no. 2, pp. 47–50, 2013.
9. E. Zewdu, Y. Semahegn, and B. Mekibib, "Prevalence of helminth parasites of dogs and owners awareness about zoonotic parasites in Ambo town, central Ethiopia," Ethiopian Veterinary Journal, vol. 14, no. 2, pp. 17–30, 2010.
10. M. C. Gaunt and A. P. Carr, "A survey of intestinal parasites in dogs from Saskatoon, Saskatchewan,"Canadian Veterinary Journal, vol. 52, no. 5, pp. 497–500, 2011.
11. M. Mirazaei and M. Fooladi, "The prevalence of intestinal helminths in owned dogs in Kerman city, Iran," Scientia Parasitologica, vol. 13, no. 1, pp. 51–54, 2012.
12. A. Kimura, Y. Morishima, S. Nagahama et al., "A coprological survey of intestinal helminthes in stray dogs captured in Osaka prefecture, Japan," Journal of Veterinary Medical Science, vol. 75, no. 10, pp. 1409–1411, 2013.
13. B. M. Anene, T. O. Nnaji, and A. B. Chime, "Intestinal parasitic infections of dogs in the Nsukka area of Enugu State, Nigeria," Preventive Veterinary Medicine, vol. 27, no. 1-2, pp. 89–94, 1996.
14. F. J. Martínez-Moreno, S. Hernández, E. López-Cobos, C. Becerra, I. Acosta, and A. Martínez-Moreno, "Estimation of canine intestinal parasites in Córdoba (Spain) and their risk to public health," Veterinary Parasitology, vol. 143, no. 1, pp. 7–13, 2007.
15. U. S. Ugbomoiko, L. Ariza, and J. Heukelbach, "Parasites of importance for human health in Nigerian dogs: high prevalence and limited knowledge of pet owners," BMC Veterinary Research, vol. 4, article 49, 2008.
16. E. T. Kutdang, D. N. Bukbuk, and J. A. A. Ajayi, "The prevalence of intestinal helminths of dogs (Canis familaris) in Jos, Plateau State, Nigeria," Researcher, vol. 2, no. 8, pp. 51–56, 2010.
17. I. D. Robertson, P. J. Irwin, A. J. Lymbery, and R. C. A. Thompson, "The role of companion animals in the emergence of parasitic zoonoses," International Journal for Parasitology, vol. 30, no. 12-13, pp. 1369–1377, 2000.
18. T. C. G. Oliveira-Sequeira, A. F. T. Amarante, T. B. Ferrari, and L. C. Nunes, "Prevalence of intestinal parasites in dogs from São Paulo State, Brazil," Veterinary Parasitology, vol. 103, no. 1-2, pp. 19–27, 2002.
19. P. K. Perera, R. P. V. J. Rajapakse, and R. S. Rajakaruna, "Gastrointestinal parasites of dogs in Hantana area in the Kandy District," Journal of the National Science Foundation of Sri Lanka, vol. 41, no. 2, pp. 81–91, 2013.
20. R. K. Anteson and J. D. Corkish, "An investigation of helminth parasites in well-cared for dogs in Accra,"Ghana Medical Journal, vol. 14, no. 3, pp. 193–195, 1975.
21. S. A. M. Johnson, D. W. Gakuya, P. G. Mbuthia, J. D. Mande, and N. Maingi, "Prevalence of gastrointestinal helminths and management practices for dogs in the Greater Accra region of Ghana."Heliyon, vol. 1, Article ID e00023, 2015.
22. E. J. L. Soulsby, Helminths, Arthropods and Protozoa of Domesticated Animals, Bailliere Tindall, London, UK, 7th edition, 1986.

CHAPTER 24 MOLECULAR DETECTION AND CHARACTERIZATION OF TICK-BORNE PATHOGENS IN DOGS AND TICKS FROM NIGERIA

Joshua Kamani, Gad Baneth, Kosta Y. Mumcuoglu, Ndadilnasiya E. Waziri, Osnat Eyal, Yifat Guthmann, Shimon Harrus

INTRODUCTION

Several tick-borne bacteria and parasites are important pathogens of humans and animals[1]. Being haematophagous, ticks are capable of transmitting disease agents such as viruses, bacteria and protozoa. Historically, they have been considered second only to mosquitoes in their ability to transmit disease agents [2]. Ticks attach to their hosts, facilitating transmission of infectious agents to the host and their spread to different geographical regions via traveling pets or other means of transportation [3]. Globalization and increased international trade, urbanization, climate change and increased travel and mobility of pets have resulted in rapid extension of the zoogeographical range for many tick species [1]. In areas where canine vector-borne diseases are endemic, dogs can be simultaneously or sequentially infected with more than one vector-borne agent [3], [4]. Because blood sucking vectors contain infected host blood and pathogens, they are reliable indicators for the existence of pathogens in a specific area [5]. Therefore, it is recommended to periodically screen animals and vectors for pathogen carriage.

Several molecular surveys have evaluated the existence of multiple vector borne pathogens in specific regions including, Europe [4], Middle East [6], Asia [7] and Africa [8]. Epidemiological surveillance of disease occurrence and prevalence is required to map local risk, to acquaint physicians and veterinarians with the prevalence of pathogens and emergence of new infectious agents and forecast possible vector-borne infection outbreaks. This can be achieved by the use of molecular diagnostic techniques, data analysis and mathematical models as well as veterinary clinical surveillance.

In Nigeria, the diagnosis of vector-borne pathogens (VBPs) is usually based on the microscopic detection of pathogens in peripheral blood smears, sometimes serology is employed and rarely molecular methods are used. Microscopic diagnosis may lack sensitivity and is time consuming while serology usually indicates exposure rather than active infection, and might mislead due to serological cross reactions with other closely related organisms. Conversely, molecular detection is more sensitive and specific. As data on canine vector-borne infections in Nigeria is scarce [9], [10], this study aimed at broadening the knowledge on these canine pathogens and their ectoparasites. The objective of this study was to molecularly detect and, characterize various vector-borne pathogens in dogs and ticks in four states of Nigeria.

Citation: Kamani J, Baneth G, Mumcuoglu KY, Waziri NE, Eyal O, Guthmann Y, et al. (2013) Molecular Detection and Characterization of Tick-borne Pathogens in Dogs and Ticks from Nigeria. PLoS Negl Trop Dis 7(3): e2108. doi:10.1371/journal.pntd.0002108.

MATERIALS AND METHODS

Study Area

The study was conducted in the 4 Nigerian states; Plateau (9°10′N9°45′E), Kaduna (10°20′N7°45′E), Kwara (8°30′N 5°00′E) and Rivers (4°45′N 6°50′E) (Figure 1).

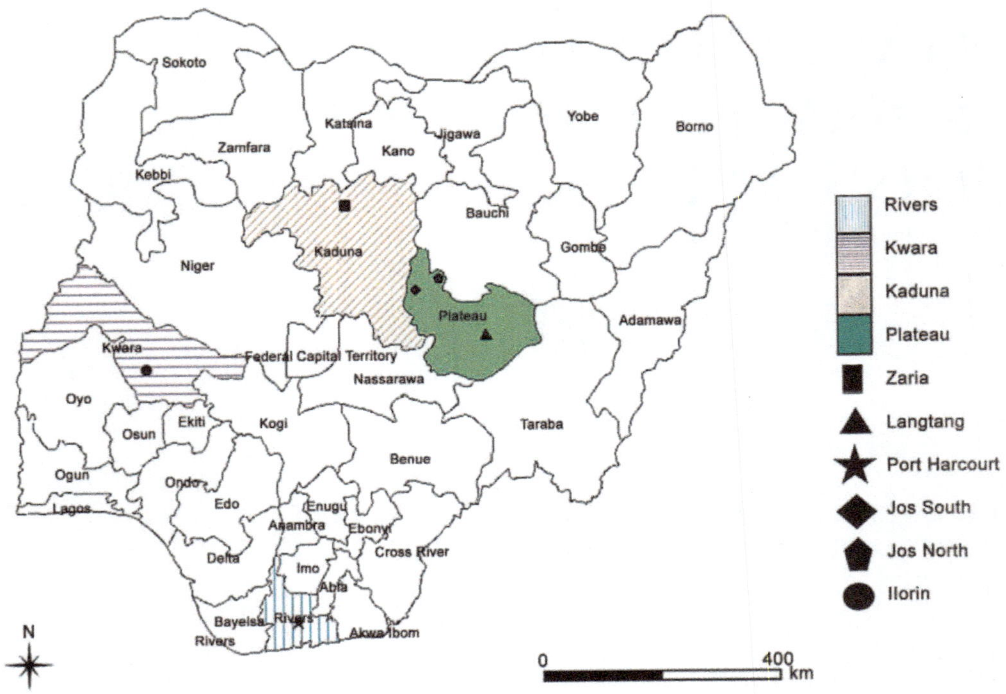

Figure 1. Map of Nigeria, West Africa showing states (shaded) where samples were collected. Legends describe the location of veterinary clinics and hospitals where samples were collected.

Ethics statement

The study protocol was read and approved by The National Veterinary Research Institute Vom, Nigeria Ethical Committee on Animal Use and Care. Animals were treated in a humane manner and in accordance with authorizations and guidelines for Ethical Conduct in the Care and Use of Nonhuman Animals in Research of the American Psychological Association (APA) for use by scientists working with nonhuman animals (American Psychological Association Committee on Animal Research and Ethics in 2010).

Sampling of Dogs

One hundred and eighty one dogs from 4 states of Nigeria presented to private or government veterinary hospitals between August and December 2011 were selected. The selection criteria included dogs infested with ticks or manifesting clinical signs of tick borne diseases, such as anemia, weakness, pyrexia, anorexia and haemoglobinuria. Demographic data, signalment (age, sex, and breed) and clinical signs were recorded for each dog. Five ml of blood were collected from the cephalic or jugular vein into sterile EDTA tubes, and kept at 4°C until arrival at the laboratory.

Sampling of Ticks

Ticks were collected from dogs infested at the time of presentation into test tubes containing absolute ethanol and transported to the laboratory. Thereafter, samples were preserved at −20°C and transported in a cool box to Israel for identification and DNA analysis. A total of 258 ticks were collected from 42 domestic dogs. After identification, ticks from each dog were grouped according to their species. One to three ticks from each dog were pooled for analysis. Seventy six tick pools were processed for DNA extraction. Most of the ticks selected were partially or fully engorged adult females, nymphs and larvae.

DNA Extraction

Blood samples

DNA was extracted from EDTA-anticogulated blood using the Illustra blood genomic Prep Mini Spin kit (GE Healthcare UK Limited) according to the manufacturer's instructions. DNA concentrations were determined by measuring the absorbance at 260 nm (A_{260}) with a NanoVue Spectrophotometer (GE Healthcare, UK Limited).

Ticks

Ticks were minced using a sterile scalpel blade before homogenization in sterile Eppendorf tubes containing 50 µl phosphate buffered saline (PBS). Total DNA was extracted from each tick pool using the Illustra tissue and cell genomic Prep Mini Spin kit (GE Healthcare UK Limited), adjusted in 100 µl of TE buffer and stored at −20°C until further use.

Real Time PCR for detection of Ehrlichia and Anaplasma spp

A 97 base pair segment of the 16S ribosomal RNA (16S rRNA) gene of *Ehrlichia canis* and*Anaplasma platys* was targeted using primers 16S-F and 16S-R as previously described [5]. DNA from *E. canis* 611 tissue culture was obtained from The Koret School of Veterinary Medicine, The Hebrew University of Jerusalem, Rehovot Israel and was used as a positive control. DNA from blood of a specific pathogen free (SPF) dog was used as a negative control. The negative and non-template controls (NTC) as well as the positive control were included in each reaction in duplicates. Non template control reactions were done using the same procedures and reagents described above but without DNA added to the PCR reaction to rule out PCR contaminations.

Real Time PCR for detection of Rickettsia spp

Initial detection of *Rickettsia* sp. was performed by screening all DNA samples for the presence of a 133-bp citrate synthase gene (*gltA*) fragment using primers rico173F and rico173R as previously described [11]. Positive samples from this reaction were further analyzed for the presence of a 178–189-bp fragment of the outer membrane protein A gene (*ompA*), using primers 107F and 299R as previously described [12]. DNA extracted from cultured *R. conorii israelensis* was used as a positive control, and two negative control samples containing all the ingredients of the reaction except DNA were used for all trials.

Conventional PCR assays for Babesia and Hepatozoon spp

A 408 base-pair fragment of the 18S ribosomal RNA (*18S rRNA*) gene of *Babesia* spp. was targeted using primers PIRO-A and PIRO-B as previously described [13]. For the detection of *Hepatozoon* spp., the forward primer HEP-F and the reverse primer HEP-R were used as previously reported targeting a 666 bp fragment of the *18S rRNA* gene [14], [15].

Positive controls of naturally infected dogs with *Babesia vogeli* (Bab 36799) and*Hepatozoon canis* (HEP 7423), as well as negative DNA controls from colony-bred dogs negative by PCR for vector-borne pathogens were run with each corresponding PCR reaction. Non-template control (NTC) reactions were done using the same procedures and reagents described above but without DNA added to the PCR reaction to rule out contaminations. PCR was performed using Syntezza PCR-Ready High Specificity (Syntezza Bioscience, Israel). Amplification was performed using a programmable conventional thermocycler (Biometra, Goettingen, Germany).

PCR products were electrophoresed on 1.5% agarose gels stained with ethidium bromide and checked under UV light for the size of amplified fragments by comparison to a 50 bp DNA molecular weight marker.

Sequencing

DNA amplicons from positive samples were purified (EXOSAP-IT, USB, Cleveland, Ohio, USA) and sequenced using forward primers at the Center for Genomics Technologies, Hebrew University of Jerusalem, Israel. DNA sequences obtained were evaluated with Chromas Lite software version 2.01(Technelysium pty Ltd) and compared for similarity to sequences deposited in GenBank, using the BLAST program hosted by NCBI, National Institutes of Health, Bethesda, MD USA http://www.ncbi.nlm.nih.gov/BLAST. Selected sequences were deposited in GenBank.

Statistics

Data generated in the study were analyzed by a χ^2 test using the Statistix 8 software. Association of pathogen DNA between dogs and ticks was computed using the Medcal statistical software [16]. P values <0.05 were considered significant.

RESULTS

Pathogen DNA in dog blood

A total of 181 dogs were examined during this study, 66 (36.5%) being males and 102 (56.4%) were females. No information on sex was available for 13 (7.2%) of the samples analyzed (Table 1). The age ranges of the study population were 0–6 months, 32%; 7–12 months, 30.9%; 13–24 months, 19.9%; 25–36 months, 3.9%; >36 months, 5%, while no information on age was available for 15 (8.3%) dogs. Seventy eight (43.1%) of the dogs studied belonged to a local (Nigerian) breed, 61 (33.7%) belonged to pure foreign breeds, 27 (14.9%) were of cross- breeds while no information on breed was available for 15 (8.3%) dogs. The majority of the sampled dogs were from Plateau State (150; 82.9%), followed by Rivers State (17; 9.4%), Kaduna State (11; 6.1%) and Kwara State (3; 1.7%).

Table 1. Distribution of vector-borne pathogens among dog population studied.

Variables	No. (%) examined	No. (%) positive for								Total
		E. canis	*A. platys*	*B. rossi*	*B. vogeli*	*Theileria* sp.	*H. canis*	*Rickettsia* spp.		
								gltA	*OmpA*	
Sex										
Male	66 (36.5)	4 (6.1)	5 (7.6)	3 (4.5)	0 (0)	0 (0)	27 (40.9)	5 (7.6)	1 (1.5)	44 (24.3)
Female	102 (56.4)	11 (10.8)	7 (6.9)	9 (8.8)	0 (0)	1 (0.9)	38 (37.3)	9 (8.8)	0 (0)	75 (41.4)
DNA	13 (7.2)	8 (61.5)	0 (0)	0 (0)	1 (1.7)	0 (0)	10 (76.9)	2 (15.3)	0 (0)	21 (11.6)
Age group (months)										
0–6	58 (32.0)	7 (12.1)	3 (5.2)	5 (8.6)	0 (0)	0 (0)	21 (36.2)	6 (10.3)	0 (0)	42 (22.7)
7–12	56 (30.9)	7 (12.5)	4 (7.1)	4 (7.1)	0 (0)	0 (0)	24 (42.9)	2 (3.6)	0 (0)	41 (22.1)
13–24	36 (19.9)	2 (5.6)	5 (13.9)	1 (2.8)	0 (0)	0 (0)	15 (41.7)	5 (13.9)	1 (2.8)	28 (15.5)
25–36	7 (3.9)	0 (0)	0 (0)	1 (14.3)	0 (0)	1 (14.3)	1 (14.3)	0 (0.0)	0 (0)	3 (1.7)
>36	9 (5.0)	0 (0)	0 (0)	0 (0)	0 (0)	0 (0)	2 (22.2)	1 (11.1)	0 (0)	3 (1.7)
DNA	15 (8.3)	7 (46.7)	0 (0)	1 (6.7)	1 (6.7)	0 (0)	12 (80.0)	2 (13.3)	0 (0)	23 (12.7)
Breed										
Local	78 (43.1)	7 (9.0)	5 (6.4)	5 (5.1)	0 (0)	0 (0)	35 (44.9)	9 (11.5)	1 (1.3)	61 (33.1)
Exotic	61 (33.7)	6 (9.8)	6 (9.8)	6 (9.8)	0 (0)	1 (1.6)	16 (26.2)	4 (6.6)	0 (0)	39 (215)
Cross	27 (14.9)	3 (11.1)	1 (3.7)	1 (7.4)	0 (0)	0 (0)	12 (44.4)	1 (3.7)	0 (0)	18 (9.9)
DNA	15 (8.3)	7 (46.7)	0 (0)	0 (0)	1 (6.7)	0 (0)	12 (80.0)	2 (13.3)	0 (0)	22 (12.2)
Sampling Area										
Rivers state	17 (9.4)	2 (11.8)	2 (11.8)	2 (11.8)	0 (0)	0 (0)	2 (11.8)	0 (0)	0 (0)	8 (4.4)
Kwara state	3 (1.7)	0 (0)	1 (33.3)	0 (0)	0 (0)	0 (0)	0 (0)	0 (0)	0 (0)	1 (0.6)
Kaduna state	11 (6.1)	7 (63.3)	0 (0)	0 (0)	1 (9.1)	0 (0)	9 (81.8)	2 (18.2)	0 (0)	19 (10.5)
Plateau State										
a. Jos North	41 (22.7)	7 (17.1)	4 (9.8)	6 (14.6)	0 (0)	0 (0)	11 (26.8)	2 (4.9)	0 (0)	30 (16.0)
b. Jos South	84 (46.4)	6 (7.1)	4 (4.8)	4 (4.8)	0 (0)	1 (1.2)	30 (35.7)	10 (11.9)	1 (1.2)	55 (30.4)
c. Lantang North	25 (13.8)	1 (4.0)	1 (4.0)	0 (0)	0 (0)	0 (0)	23 (92.0)	2 (8.0)	0 (0)	27 (14.9)
Total	**181 (100)**	**23 (12.7)**	**12 (6.6)**	**12 (6.6)**	**1 (0.6)**	**1 (0.6)**	**75 (41.4)**	**16 (8.8)**	**1 (0.6)**	**140 (77.3)**

DNA = Data not available; *E. canis* = *Ehrlichia canis*; *A. platys* = *Anaplasma platys*; *B. rossi* = *Babesia rossi*; *B. vogeli* = *Babesia vogeli*; *H. canis* = *Hepatozoon canis*.
doi:10.1371/journal.pntd.0002108.t001

Overall estimate of infection with VBPs was 77.3% (140/181) in sampled dogs. Single infections occurred in 73(40.3%) dogs while co- infection with more than one pathogen occurred in 67 (37%) of the dogs examined. Co- infections with *H. canis* were most prevalent (14.4%) followed by *E. canis* and *Rickettsia* spp. (6.6%) each (Table 2). Single infections occurred mostly in dogs within the age range of 9–12 months. Co-infections were mostly detected in dogs between 2–12 months of age.

Table 2. Number of dogs infected with single or multiple vector- borne pathogens.

Nature of infection	Pathogen species detected in dogs							
	E. canis	*A. platys*	*B. rossi*	*B. vogeli*	*Theileria* sp.	*H. canis*	*Rickettsia* sp.	Total (%)
Single infection	10	6	6	0	1	46	4	73 (40.3)
Co infection with								
E. canis	-	0	1	0	0	10	1	12 (6.6)
A. platys	0	-	1	0	0	5	2	8 (4.4)
B. rossi	1	1	-	0	0	4	1	7 (3.9)
B. vogeli	1	0	0	-	0	1	-	2 (1.1)
Theileria sp.	0	0	0	0	0	0	0	0(0)
H. canis	10	4	3	1	0	-	8	26 (14.4)
Rickettsia sp.	1	1	1	0	0	9	-	12 (6.6)
Total	**23**	**12**	**12**	**1**	**1**	**75**	**16**	**140 (77)**

E. canis = *Ehrlichia canis*; *A. platys* = *Anaplasma platys*; *B. rossi* = *Babesia rossi*; *B. vogeli* = *Babesia vogeli*; *H. canis* = *Hepatozoon canis*.
doi:10.1371/journal.pntd.0002108.t002

Hepatozoon canis was the most frequently detected pathogen in dogs (41.4%), followed by *E. canis*, *Rickettsia* spp., *Babesia rossi* and *A. platys* (12.7%, 8.8%, 6.6% and 6.6% respectively). *Babesia vogeli*, *Theileria* sp. and *R. conorii israelensis* were detected in one dog each (Table 1). There was no significant difference (p>0.05) in prevalence of these pathogens between the various groups of dogs studied (Table 1). Sequences of pathogens derived from dog's blood in this study were deposited in GenBank under the following accession numbers; *H. canis* (JQ976620–JQ976629); *B. rossi* (JQ976603–JQ976616); *B. vogeli* (JQ976617); *Theileria* sp. (JQ976619); *E. canis* (JQ976630–JQ976641) and *A. platys* (JQ976642–JQ976653).

Pathogen DNA in ticks

A total of 258 ticks (128 adults, 124 nymphs and 6 larvae) partially or fully engorged belonging to two genera *Rhipicephalus* and *Haemaphysalis*, removed from 42 dogs were examined for various VBPs. *Ehrlichia canis*, *H. canis* and *Rickettsia* spp. DNA were detected in *R. sanguineus*, *R. turanicus* and *H. leachi* ticks. NA of various VBPs was detected in all the different tick species examined in this study. A total of 76 tick pools were tested out of which 18 (23.7%), 16(21.1%), 8(10.5%) and 4(5.3%) were positive for the DNA of *E. canis*, *H. canis*, *Rickettsia* spp. and *Candidatus* N. mikurensis respectively, while *A. platys* and *R. conorii israelensis* DNA were detected in one tick pool each (Table 3). Sequences from ticks were assigned the following accession numbers: *H. canis* (JX027010–JX027020),*Candidatus* N. mikurensis (JX027021–JX027024), *E. canis* (JQ976654–JQ976665), *A. platys* (JQ976666) and *R. conorii israelensis* (JX259321 and JX259322).

Table 3. Comparison of DNA sequence similarities between pathogens detected in dogs and ticks in this study and GenBank deposited sequences.

Pathogen sequences from dog blood		Pathogen sequences from ticks	
Pathogen genotype (No. positive)-Accession No.	**First Genbank Match Accession No. (% sequence similarity)**	**Pathogen genotype (No. positive)- Accession No.**	**First GenBank Match Accession No. (% sequence similarity)**
***Babesia* spp.**			
B. rossi (1) –JQ976615	*Babesia rossi* -AB303074.1 (100)	-	-
B. rossi (9) - JQ976603	*Babesia rossi* -AB303074.1 (99)	-	-
B. rossi (2) –JQ976612	*Babesia rossi* -AB303074.1 (98)	-	-
B. vogeli (1) -JQ976617	Uncultured *Babesia* clone seqBCV79-JN717134.1 (99)	-	-
***Theileria* sp.**			
Theileria sp (1)-JQ976622	*Theileria ovis* -GU726904.1 (98)	-	-
***Ehrlichia* spp.**			
E. canis (17) - JQ976631	Uncultured *Ehrlichia* sp. clone -JQ260861 (100)	*E. canis* (15) - JQ976654	Uncultured *Ehrlichia* spp -JQ260861 (100)
E. canis (2)- JQ976630	Uncultured *Ehrlichia* sp. clone-JQ260861 (99)	*E. canis* (2) –JQ976659	*E. chaffensis*-JQ085940.1 (99)
E. canis (3) - JQ976639	Uncultured *Ehrlichia* sp. clone-JQ260861 (97)		
		***Candidatus* Neoehrlichia mikurensis**	
		C. N mikurensis (4) - JX027021	*C.N. mikurensis*- JQ359051 (100)
***Anaplasma* spp.**			
A. platys (8) - JQ976650	*Anaplasma platys* isolate A.pl -JQ 396431(100)	*A. platys* (1) - JQ976666	*Anaplasma platys* -JQ396431 (99)
A. platys (1) –JQ976643	*Anaplasma platys* isolate A.pl-JQ 396431 (99)		
A.platys (1) - JQ976648	*Anaplasma platys* isolate A.pl-JQ 396431 (97)		
Anaplasma sp (1)-JQ976642	uncultured Anaplasmataceae bacterium-JN581373.1 (99)		
Hepatozoon canis			
H. canis (6) –JQ976617	*Hepatozoon canis* -DQ 111754 (99)	*H. canis* (2)-JX027013	*Hepatozoon canis* -DQ111754 (100)
H. canis (3) JQ976626	*Hepatozoon canis* -EU289222 (99)	*H. canis* (5)-JX027011	*Hepatozoon canis* -DQ111754 (99)
H. canis (1)-JQ976629	*Hepatozoon canis* -JF 459994 (99)	*H. canis* (3) - JX027010	*Hepatozoon canis*-GU376457 (99)
***Rickettsia* spp.**			
Rickettsia sp (*gltA*) (16) JX259323	Uncultured *Rickettsia* sp JQ664729 (100)	*Rickettsia* sp (*gltA*) (6) JX259324	Uncultured *Rickettsia* sp JQ664729 (100)
R. c. israelensis (1) JX259321	*R. c. israelensis* (EU122392 (100)	*R. c. israelensis* (1) JX259322	*R. c. israelensis* EU122392 (100)

E. canis = *Ehrlichia canis*; *A. platys* = *Anaplasma platys*; *B. rossi* = *Babesia rossi*; *B. vogeli* = *Babesia vogeli*; *H. canis* = *Hepatozoon canis*; *E. chaffeensis* = *Ehrlichia chaffeensis*; C. N mikurensis = *Candidatus* N. mikurensis; *R. c. israelensis* = *Rickettsia. conorii israelensis*.

doi:10.1371/journal.pntd.0002108.t003

Comparison between the Presence of Pathogen DNA in Blood and Ticks from the Same Dog

Pathogen DNA as single or multiple infections were detected in 26/76 (34.2%) tick pools removed from dogs with tick infestation at the time of clinical presentation and sampling. Blood and ticks from 7 dogs (nos. 1, 8, 33, 34, 37, 38 and 39) were free from DNA of the various VBPs tested for in this study. DNA of pathogens was detected in ticks removed from 7 other dogs (nos. 3, 4, 12, 18, 25, 31 and 36) but none was detected in the blood of their dog host. Conversely, DNA of various pathogens was detected in 7 dogs (nos. 5,7,13, 16, 28, 29 and 49), but no pathogen DNA was detected in ticks removed from them. Ticks collected from 4 dog (nos. 2, 15, 22 and 23) as well as the dogs from which they were removed were both positive for *E. canis* DNA. Similarly, DNA of *H. canis* was detected in 3 dogs (nos. 20, 21 and 24) and ticks removed from each of them. However, DNA of *H. canis*only was detected in 3 dogs (nos. 11, 35 and 42) but DNA of both *H. canis* and *E. canis* was detected in ticks removed from them. Different pathogen's DNA was detected in 10 dogs (nos. 6, 9, 10 14, 17, 19, 26, 27, 35 and 40) as compared to the ticks removed from them. Nine (11.8%) of the tick pools were co-infected by two or more pathogens. There was a significant association between *H. canis* DNA in dogs and ticks removed from them (Relative risk=2.69; 95% Confidence Interval=1.2–

5.8; Z=2.51; p=0.012). However, there was no significant association between the detection of pathogen DNA in dogs blood and ticks removed from them for *E. canis*, (RR=1.56; 95% CI=0.44–5.45; Z=0.69; p=0.49), *A. platys*(RR=0.59; 95% CI=0.025–14.3; Z=0.32; p=0.75) or *B. rossi* (RR=0.07; 95% CI=0.004–1.13; Z=1.88; p=0.061). *Babesia* spp. and *Theileria* spp. DNA were not detected in any of the tick pools tested.

Identity of Pathogen Sequences Amplified from Dogs and Ticks

Babesia rossi and *B. vogeli* sequences from this study had 98–100% and 99% similarities, respectively, with the first matched BLAST result from GenBank (Table 3), while *Theileria* sp. had 98% sequence similarity with *Theileria ovis*. *Ehrlichia canis* sequences from blood of dogs and ticks in this study had 97–100% and 100% similarities, respectively, with the first matched BLAST result from GenBank. Two sequences had 99% similarity with *Ehrlichia chaffeensis* as the first GenBank match from BLAST. However, attempts to validate the identity of this species by PCR for secretory genes (*SodB/ VirB 3*, *VirB 4*, and *VirB 9*) did not yield confirmatory results. Four sequences from ticks had 100% sequence identity to*Candidatus* N. mikurensis. *Anaplasma platys* sequences from dogs and ticks had 97–100% and 99% sequences similarities, respectively, with the first matched BLAST result from GenBank. Similarly, *H. canis* sequences from dogs and ticks had 99% and 99–100% similarities, respectively, with *H. canis* sequences deposited in GenBank (Table 3).

The rickettsial *gltA* gene fragment was detected in 16 of 181 (8.8%) dog blood samples and in 8 of 76 (10.5%) tick pools examined. Rickettsial *ompA* DNA was found in one (0.6%) blood and one tick sample. Both sequences were identical and were 100% similar to *ompA*fragment from *R. conorii israelensis*. All the sequences detected in this study from dogs and the ticks removed from each of them were highly identical to each other (99–100%) for all the pathogens identified (Table 3).

DISCUSSION

Ticks and other haematophagous arthropods play a major role in the epidemiology of diseases of humans and animals globally. Their distribution and abundance determines the epidemiology of vector borne infections. The results of this study provide molecular evidence for the presence of *E. canis, H. canis, A. platys, B. rossi, B. vogeli, Theileria* sp., closely related to *T. ovis*, *Candidatus* N. mikurensis and *R. conorii israelensis* in dogs and ticks from Nigeria. DNA of at least one vector borne pathogen was detected in 77% of the dogs and 45% of the tick pools examined.

This is the first report documenting the identification of *Candidatus* N. mikurensis, *R. conorii israeliensis*, *A. platys* and *Theileria* sp. in dogs and ticks from Nigeria. In fact, it is the first detection of the zoonotic pathogen, *Candidatus* N. mikurensis, in Africa. *Candidatus* N. mikurensis is an emerging pathogen first described in 2004 affecting humans and animals with varying clinical manifestation [17]. This pathogen was reported in several hosts including *Ixodes* spp. ticks, *Rattus norvegicus*, humans and dogs from Japan, Switzerland and Germany [17]–[19]. Although *Ixodes* ticks of medical and veterinary importance are not found in Nigeria, *R. norvegicus* are common and serve as small mammal hosts to multi- host ticks during their life cycle. As engorged ticks were screened in this study, it is possible that *R. sanguineus* ticks acquired *Candidatus* N. mikurensis from infected *R. norvegicus* or dogs. Due to the fact that this agent is a potential threat to humans, physicians should consider this pathogen in their differential diagnosis list in complicated unexplained fever of unknown etiology cases in Nigeria.

Rickettsia gltA DNA was detected in 8.8% and 10.5% of dogs and ticks respectively in this study. These estimates are almost similar to the 7.8% previously reported [9] but lower than the 20.6% infection rate reported for *R. africae* in ticks collected from cattle and vegetation in Nigeria [10]. Another report of prevalence of 0.4% *R. conorii* and 94–100% *R. africae* in*Rhipicephalus evertsi* was made in Guinea and Liberia, West Africa [20]. In the present study, 8.8% of blood samples and 10.5% of tick pools were positive for the rickettsial *gltA* but only one blood sample (0.6%) and one *R. sanguineus* tick pool (1.3%) were found positive for the rickettsial *ompA* gene, and their sequences were 100% identical to *R. conorii israelensis*. This is the first report indicating the presence of the agent of Mediterranean Spotted Fever in Nigeria. Rickettsiae with *ompA* gene are considered to be pathogenic, while those who exclude this gene are probably non-pathogenic endosymbionts [21].*Rickettsia africae*, the etiologic agent of African tick fever in humans has been detected in ticks from Nigeria [9], [10] and other West African countries [20] but not in our study. It is possible *R. sanguineus*, *R. turanicus* and *H. leachi* found on dogs in this study are not competent vectors for this organism [20].

The detection of *A. platys* infection in Nigeria is also reported for the first time in this study. The estimate of 6.6% infection rate in dogs in this study is higher than the 4% reported for dogs in Italy [22], but lower than 16% reported in Venezuela [23]. *Anaplasma platys* is a thrombocytotropic bacteria of dogs that causes canine infectious cyclic thrombocytopaenia characterized by clinical abnormalities such as fever, anorexia, petechial haemorrhages, and uveitis [24].

Theileria sp. with 98% sequence similarity to *T. ovis* from a sheep in Iran [25] was detected in one dog in this study (Table 3). *Theileria* spp. have been reported in dogs from South Africa [26] and Spain [27]. The *Theileria* sp. in this study appears to be molecularly different from the previously described species.

The high estimate of *H. canis* (41.4%) and *E. canis* (12.7%) infections reported in dog blood in this study are higher than the 22% and 5%, respectively reported earlier in Zaria-Nigeria using microscopic examination of blood smears [28]. However, the estimate of 6.6% for *B. rossi* in this study is lower than previous reports of 10.2% [29] and 11.0% [30], and higher than 2.0% for dogs in Nigeria [28], but close to the 9.0% reported in Sudan [8]. Similarly, the estimate of 41.4% *H. canis* infection in this study is higher than the 20.3% previously reported in dogs from Nigeria, but almost similar to the 42.3% reported in Sudan [8]. The higher estimate of *H. canis* DNA in this study can be attributed to the sensitivity of the techniques used, enabling the detection of *E. canis* and *H. canis* at low bacterial and parasite loads. *Babesia canis* and *B.*

gibsoni were not detected in any of the samples tested. This finding is in agreement with earlier molecular surveys in dogs from Nigeria [30]and can be attributed to the absence of their tick vectors in Nigeria. Although a case of *B. rossi* and *B. canis* co-infection in a local Nigerian dog that never left the country has been reported [31], the source of that infection could not be elucidated.

One recent study in Nigeria did not detect *Ehrlichia* spp. in *R. sanguineus* ticks [9], while another study reported a prevalence of 5.7% *Ehrlichia* spp. in ticks collected from cattle [10]which is much lower than the 23.7% detected in this study. The difference in prevalence may be attributed to variation in techniques used and source of samples.

Dogs are competent reservoir- hosts of several zoonotic pathogens and are infested by many blood-feeding arthropods. The role of ticks as vectors of these pathogens can be asserted considering the high sequence similarities (99–100%) between the pathogens detected from the host and those detected in ticks removed from them (Table 3). Of the 18 tick pools positive for *E. canis*, and 16 positive for *H. canis*, 22% and 38% of the pools were from *E. canis* and *H. canis* positive hosts, respectively. There was a significant association between the detection of *H. canis* DNA in dogs and ticks removed from the same dog, but no association was found for *E. canis*, *A. platys* or *B. rossi*. As all ticks were removed from dogs while they were attached and most of them were partially or fully engorged, it is impossible to ascertain whether the ticks were fed with infected blood or if they served as vectors and transmitted the pathogen to their present host. Considering the fact that the tick species included in this study have multi- host life cycle, they could have acquired infection during feeding on a previous infected host and transmitted the infection during their next feeding.

Dog breeding is a lucrative business in Nigeria, where dogs are used for trade and security. Dogs also serve as a food source and their meat is considered as a delicacy among some ethnic groups in Nigeria. These can expose humans directly or indirectly to zoonotic agents during handling of dogs and ticks carrying pathogens, or during processing and consumption of their meat. Further investigation is required to elucidate the role of ticks and the effect of these pathogens in causing diseases in humans in Nigeria.

In conclusion, this study has confirmed that several vector borne pathogens of humans and animals are highly prevalent in Nigeria and West Africa where the incidence of tick-borne infections appears to be underestimated. Physicians and veterinarians should be aware of the existence of these pathogens in Nigeria and should include them in the differential diagnoses for clinical illnesses with compatible clinical signs. Screening targeted groups for VBPs as well as humans with fever of unknown origin or undiagnosed cases for infection with *R. conorii israelensis* and *Candidatus* N. mikurensis is recommended.

ACKNOWLEDGMENTS

The authors thank Abidoye Ebenezer (Ahmadu Bello University, Zaria), Ibitoye Timothy (IbitsonVet, Port Harcourt) and Oyewusi Joshua Adeoye (University of Agriculture, Abeokuta) for technical assistance during the collection of samples and Dr. Dmitry Apanaskevich for the identification of *Haemaphysalis leachi* tick. The technical assistance of Dr Nir Rudoler, Koret School of Veterinary Medicine, Israel is highly acknowledged.

AUTHOR CONTRIBUTIONS

Identified ticks: KYM. Conceived and designed the experiments: JK GB SH. Performed the experiments: OE YG JK. Analyzed the data: JK NEW. Contributed reagents/materials/analysis tools: GB SH. Wrote the paper: JK GB KYM SH.

REFERENCES

1. Shaw SE, Michael JD, Richard JB, Breitschwerdt EB (2001) Tick-borne infectious diseases of dogs. Trends Parasitol 17: 74–80. doi: 10. 1016/s1471-4922(00)01856-0
2. Hillyard PD (1996) Diseases carried by ticks in NW Europe: their medical and veterinary importance. In: Barnes, RSK, Coles, JH, eds. Ticks of North-West Europe. ynopses of the British Fauna (New Series). FSC Publications, 22–23
3. Otranto D, Dantas-Torres F, Breitschwerdt EB (2009) Managing canine vector borne diseases of zoonotic concern: part one. Trends Parasitol 25: 157–163. doi: 10. 1016/j. pt. 2009. 01. 003
4. Cardoso L, Yisaschar-Mekuzas Y, Rodrigues FT, Costa Á, Machado J, et al. (2010) Canine babesiosis in northern Portugal and molecular characterization of vector-borne co-infections. Parasite and Vectors 3: 27. doi: 10. 1186/1756-3305-3-27
5. Roux V, Raoult D (1999) Body lice as tools for diagnosis and surveillance of reemerging diseases. J. Clin. Microbiol 37: 596–599.
6. Peleg O, Baneth G, Eyal O, Inbar J, Harrus S (2010) Multiplex real-time qPCR for the detection of *Ehrlichia canis* and *Babesia canis vogeli*. Vet Parasitol 173: 292–299. doi: 10. 1016/j. vetpar. 2010. 06. 039
7. Suksawat J, Xuejie Y, Hancock SI, Hegarty BC, Nilumhang P (2001) Serologic and molecular evidence of co infection with multiple vector borne pathogens in dogs from Thailand. J Vet Int Med 15: 453–462. doi: 10. 1111/j. 1939-1676. 2001. tb01574. x
8. Oyamada M, Bernard D, Mickae B, Jacques D, Bruno B, et al. (2005) Detection of*Babesia canis rossi*, *B. canis vogeli*, and *Hepatozoon canis* in dogs in a village of Eastern Sudan by using a screening PCR and sequencing methodologies. Clin Diagn Lab Immunol 1343–1346. doi: 10. 1128/cdli. 12. 11. 1343-1346. 2005
9. Ogo NI, de Mera IG, Galindo RC, Okubanjo OO, Inuwa HM, et al. (2012) Molecular identification of tick-borne pathogens in Nigerian ticks. Vet Parasitol 187: 572–577. doi: 10. 1016/j. vetpar. 2012. 01. 029
10. Reye AL, Arinola OG, Hübschen JM, Muller CP (2012) Pathogen prevalence in ticks collected from the vegetation and livestock in Nigeria. Appl Environ Microbiol 78: 2562–2568. doi: 10. 1128/aem. 06686-11
11. Harrus S, Perlman-Avrahami A, Mumcuoglu KY, Morick D, Baneth G (2011) Molecular detection

of *Rickettsia massiliae*, *Rickettsia sibirica mongolitimonae* and*Rickettsia conorii israelensis* in ticks from Israel. Clin Microbiol Infect 17: 176–180. doi: 10. 1111/j. 1469-0691. 2010. 03224. x

12. Kidd L, Maggi R, Diniz PPVP, Hegarty B, Tucker M, et al. (2008) Evaluation of conventional and real-time PCR assays for detection and differentiation of Spotted Fever Group Rickettsia in dog blood. Vet Microbiol 129: 294–303. doi: 10. 1016/j. vetmic. 2007. 11. 035
13. Olmeda AS, Armstrong PM, Rosenthal BM, Valladares B, del Castillo A, et al. (1997) A subtropical case of human babesiosis. Acta Trop 229–234. doi: 10. 1016/s0001-706x(97)00045-4
14. Inokuma H, Okuda M, Ohno K, Shimoda K, Onishi T (2002) Analysis of the 18SrRNA gene sequence of a *Hepatozoon* detected in two Japanese dogs. Vet Parasitol 106: 265–271. doi: 10. 1016/s0304-4017(02)00065-1
15. Rubini AS, Paduan KS, Cavalcante GG, Ribolla PE, O'Dwyer LH (2005) Molecular identification and characterization of canine *Hepatozoon* species from Brazil. Parasitol Res 97: 91–93. doi: 10. 1007/s00436-005-1383-x
16. Medcalc Version 9. 6. 4. 0 (2008) Available: http://www. medcalc. be. accessed on 13thMay, 2010.
17. Kawahara M, Rikihisa Y, Isogai E, Takahashi M, Misumi H, et al. (2004) Ultrastructure and phylogenetic analysis of '*Candidatus* Neoehrlichia mikurensis' in the family Anaplasmataceae, isolated from wild rats and found in *Ixodes ovatus* ticks. Int J Syst Evol Microbiol 54 (Pt 5) 1837–1843. doi: 10. 1099/ijs. 0. 63260-0
18. Elena L, Luce B, Christèle D, Lise G (2012) Infections and coinfections of questing*Ixodes ricinus* ticks by emerging zoonotic pathogens in Western Switzerland. Appl Environ Microbiol 78: 4606. doi: 10. 1128/aem. 07961-11
19. Diniz PPVP, Schulz BS, Hartmann K, Breitschwerdt EB (2011) "*Candidatus*Neoehrlichia mikurensis" infection in a dog from Germany. J Clin Microbiol 2059–2062. doi: 10. 1128/jcm. 02327-10
20. Mediannikov O, Diatta G, Fenollar F, Sokhna C, Trape J-F, et al. (2010) Tick-Borne Rickettsioses, Neglected Emerging Diseases in Rural Senegal. PLoS Negl Trop Dis 4: e821 doi:10. 1371/journal. pntd. 0000821.
21. Foongladda S, Inthawong D, Kositanont U, Gaywee J (2011) *Rickettsia*, *Ehrlichia*,*Anaplasma*, and *Bartonella* in Ticks and Fleas from Dogs and Cats in Bangkok. Vector-Borne Zoon Dis 11: 1336–1341. doi: 10. 1089/vbz. 2010. 0174
22. de la Fuente J, Alessandra T, Victoria N Silviane N, Angelina A, et al. (2006) Molecular characterization of *Anaplasma platys* strains from dogs in Sicily, Italy. Vet Res 2: 24.
23. Huang H, Ahmet U, Miriam JP, Nelson GO, Yasuko R (2005) Prevalence and Molecular Analysis of *Anaplasma platys* in Dogs in Lara, Venezuela. Braz J Microbiol 36: 211–216. doi: 10. 1590/s1517-83822005000300002
24. Ulutas B, Bayramli G, Karagenc T (2007) First case of *Anaplasma* (*Ehrlichia*) *platys*infection in a dog in Turkey. Turk J Vet Anim Sci 31 (4) 279–282.
25. Zaeemi M, Haddadzadeh H, Khazraiinia P, Kazemi B, Bandehpour M (2011) Identification of different *Theileria* species (*Theileria lestoquardi*, *Theileria ovis*, and*Theileria annulata*) in naturally infected sheep using nested PCR-RFLP. Parasitol Res 108: 837–843. doi: 10. 1007/s00436-010-2119-0
26. Matjila PT, Leisewitz AL, Oosthuizen MC, Jongejan F, Penzhorn BL (2008c) Detection of a *Theileria* species in dogs in South Africa. Vet Parasitol 157: 34–40. doi: 10. 1016/j. vetpar. 2008. 06. 025
27. Dixit P, Alok K, Dixit J, Varshney P (2010) Evidence of new pathogenic *Theileria*species in dogs. J Parasit Dis 34: 29–32. doi: 10. 1007/s12639-010-0009-0
28. Ezekoli CD, Ogunkoya AB, Abdullahi R, Tekedek LB, Sannusi A, et al. (1983) Clinical and epidemiological studies on canine hepatozoonosis in Zaria, Nigeria. J Small Anim Pract 24: 455–460. doi: 10. 1111/j. 1748-5827. 1983. tb00385. x
29. Amuta EU, Atu BO, Houmsou RS, Ayashar JG (2010) *Rhipicephalus sanguineus*infestation and *Babesia canis* infection among domestic dogs in Makurdi, Benue State-Nigeria. Intl J Acadc Res 2/3: 170–172.
30. Sasaki M, Olutayo O, Morito T, Kaisaku O, Aya M, et al. (2007) Molecular survey of*Babesia canis* in dogs in Nigeria. J Vet Med Sci 69: 1191–1193. doi: 10. 1292/jvms. 69. 1191
31. Kamani J, Sannusi A, Dogo AG, Tanko TJ, Egwu OK, et al. (2010) *Babesia canis* and*Babesia rossi* co-infection in an untraveled Nigerian dog. Vet Parasitol 173: 334–335. doi: 10. 1016/j. vetpar. 2010. 06. 040

CHAPTER 25

SEROPOSITIVITY RATES FOR AGENTS OF CANINE VECTOR-BORNE DISEASES IN SPAIN: A MULTICENTRE STUDY

Guadalupe Miró, Ana Montoya, Xavier Roura, Rosa Gálvez and Angel Sainz

Keywords: Leishmaniosis Heartworm Ehrlichiosis Anaplasmosis Lyme disease Dog

BACKGROUND

The term canine vector-borne diseases (CVBD) includes a wide variety of diseases of infectious or parasitic aetiology whose agents are transmitted by ectoparasites such as ticks, fleas, lice, mosquitoes and sand flies [1]. Controlling these infectious agents is important because some are responsible for serious diseases in humans (e.g. *Anaplasma phagocytophilum, Bartonella* spp., *Borrelia burgdorferi, Leishmania infantum, Thelazia callipaeda*, etc.) [2]. However, their control can be extremely complex since they show a wide geographical distribution, and clinical signs in infected dogs can vary significantly [3, 4].

In addition, there is evidence to suggest that changing factors linked to climate and the environment could determine the expansion of the current geographical distribution ranges of these diseases and their arthropod vectors [5, 6, 7, 8, 9]. The transport of infected dogs from endemic areas has also been attributed an important role in the spread of CVBD to the north of Europe [10, 11]. Owing to an increase in this transport due to new habits such as travelling with dogs or adopting animals from other countries, the epidemiological status of these diseases in Europe, and especially across the Iberian Peninsula including Portugal, has changed considerably [12, 13, 14].

Citation: Miró et al.: Seropositivity rates for agents of canine vector-borne diseases in Spain: a multicentre study. Parasites & Vectors 2013 6:117.

CVBD may show no specific clinical signs or clinical-pathological abnormalities, or alternatively may present a varied clinical picture making the diagnosis of a CVBD extremely complex. Animals with subclinical infection have been described to show an increased risk of disease transmission [15, 16].

Anaplasma platys and *A. phagocytophilum* (An) are the aetiological agents of anaplasmosis, which affects a wide range of vertebrate hosts (rodents, dogs, humans). *A. phagocytophilum* is transmitted by ticks of the genus *Ixodes* and *A. platys* by the tick *Rhipicephalus sanguineus*. Both pathogens infect dogs in which the clinical picture ranges from subclinical disease to acute illness [17]. *A. phagocytophilum* can also infect humans causing febrile syndrome [18]. The reported seroprevalence of *Anaplasma* spp. in Spain has ranged from 5 to 19% for Galicia, Catalonia, Balearic Islands and Castilla-León [19, 20, 21].

Lyme disease is an infectious disease caused by spirochetes belonging to the *Borrelia burgdorferi* (Bb) *sensu lato* complex, transmitted by ticks of the genus *Ixodes*. Lyme disease shows a worldwide distribution, although its incidence is increasing in North America and Europe because of its association with this vector [22, 23, 24]. Bb affects a wide range of hosts, mainly humans and dogs. In humans, Lyme disease can produce chronic weakness with nonspecific clinical signs (fever, muscle and joint pain). Though few dogs show clinical signs, most are subclinical reservoirs [25, 26] and can be used as sentinels for this infection. In Spain, dogs seropositive for *B. burgdorferi* have been detected in Galicia (6.3%) [20], Mallorca (1.3%) [19] and Castilla -León (2.1 to 21%) [27, 28, 29].

Ehrlichia canis (Ec), an intracellular Gram-negative bacterium that infects monocytes, is the causative agent of canine monocytic ehrlichiosis, and is transmitted by the tick *Rhipicephalus sanguineus*[30]. The disease is characterized by three stages of varying severity. The acute stage produces clinical signs such as apathy, depression, anorexia, dyspnoea, fever, lymphadenopathy, splenomegaly, petechiae and echymotic haemorrhage in the skin and the mucous membranes, epistaxis, and vomiting. Laboratory abnormalities are usually thrombocytopenia, leucopenia and mild to moderate normocytic, normochromic and non-regenerative anaemia. The second stage is subclinical with clinical-pathological abnormalities such as thrombocytopenia, anaemia or hyperproteinemia. The third or chronic stage is characterized by a very complex clinical picture: haemorrhage, weakness, apathy, sustained weight loss, fever, lymphadenopathy, splenomegaly and peripheral oedema in the hind limbs and scrotum and a wide variety of clinical-pathological abnormalities [31, 32]. In Spain, the seroprevalence of Ec in dogs ranges from 3.1 to 19%, with cited rates of 3.1-6.5% for Galicia, Madrid and Zaragoza [20, 33, 34] and higher rates for Mediterranean regions (Catalonia, Valencia, Baleares) [19, 35, 36] and Castilla-León (12-20%) [35].

Dirofilaria immitis (Di) is a filarial worm transmitted by mosquitoes (Culicidae) to carnivores and other hosts. Since the vector is not very host specific, many mammals can become infected including humans [37]. *D. immitis* is a cosmopolitan parasite, mainly found in southern European countries including Spain, where it is endemic in the regions Valencia, Balearic Islands, Andalucia, Aragon and the Canary Islands with prevalences of 6.3-67.02% [38, 39, 40, 41, 42]. Lower prevalences have been reported for other regions, although recently cases have been detected in two northern provinces: La Rioja (12%) and La Coruña (4.2%) [43, 44]. *D. immitis,*also known as heartworm, mainly affects dogs but has also been detected in cats [45]. In dogs, the course of disease is chronic due to changes in the pulmonary arteries and lung parenchyma [46]. In humans, the parasite cannot complete its whole life cycle, yet produces a serious infection in which parasitic granulomas can be observed in the lung parenchyma [47].

Canine leishmaniosis (CanL), a zoonotic disease endemic in southern Europe caused by the protozoan*Leishmania infantum* (Li), is transmitted to humans and animals by blood-sucking phlebotomine sand flies [48,49]. Until recently, CanL was considered to be limited to the Mediterranean basin, with an estimated seroprevalence in Spain ranging from 3% in the north [50] to 34.6% for Malaga province on the south coast [51]. Northern Spain was considered a non-endemic area but CanL and its sand fly vectors have been detected in the northeast and northwest where the disease was previously unknown [50, 52, 53, 54]. At our latitude, dogs are considered the main reservoir for human infection [55, 56]. Clinical CanL shows a wide spectrum of clinical signs and severity because of the many pathogenic mechanisms involved and the particular immune response produced in the host [57]. The main clinical signs of CanL are one or more of the following: weight loss, lethargy, muscular atrophy, anaemia, lymphadenomegaly, splenomegaly, epistaxis, diarrhoea, renal disorders, ocular lesions, polyarthritis, onycogryphosis and skin lesions [58, 59, 60]. In endemic areas, a high proportion of clinically healthy dogs are able to transmit the infection causing a serious public health problem [61]. In Europe, human infection with *L. infantum* is observed mainly in children and immunocompromised adults, but a recent outbreak (2010) in southwest Madrid (Spain) indicates the epidemiology of this disease is complex and subject to constant change [62, 63].

Information emerging from Spain on some of these vector borne diseases has been limited. Most studies have addressed canine leishmaniosis in the Mediterranean basin and a few reports have dealt with ehrlichiosis, dirofilariosis, *Borrelia* and *Anaplasma* infection in specific areas of the country.

The present study was designed to establish seropositivity rates and epidemiological associations for these five CVBD by determining antibodies against *Anaplasma* spp. (An), *Borrelia burgdorferi* (Bb), *Ehrlichia canis*(Ec), and *Leishmania infantum* (Li) and the *Dirofilaria immitis* (Di) antigen in dogs from different Spanish regions.

METHODS

Bioclimatic Characteristics of the Study Area

The survey was carried out in seven different eco-epidemiological regions of Spain. The Iberian Peninsula shows two main regions of flora and vegetation, the Mediterranean and Eurosiberian regions. This last region covers the north of Spain where climate and vegetation are typically oceanic, with warm summers and cool winters and rainfall evenly distributed all year round. The rest of the peninsula falls within the Mediterranean region. Here, summers are dry and hot, and most rainfall occurs in autumn and spring. Moreover, coastal areas show a milder, more humid climate, and mountain ranges have a shielding effect from an oceanic influence determining a climate of extremely cold winters and very hot summers.

Veterinary Clinics and Dogs

The study was carried out in accordance with the International Guiding Principles for Biomedical Research Involving Animals, issued by the Council for the International Organizations of Medical Sciences. The owners of the dogs enrolled were previously informed about the study protocol.

The dogs examined were 1100 owned dogs attending 57 veterinary clinics in central (187 dogs; 7 clinics), eastern (90 dogs; 5 clinics), southern (75 dogs; 5 clinics), southeastern (105 dogs; 5 clinics), northern (15 dogs; 1 clinic), northeastern (465 dogs; 22 clinics) and northwestern (163 dogs; 11 clinics) Spain (see Figure 1).

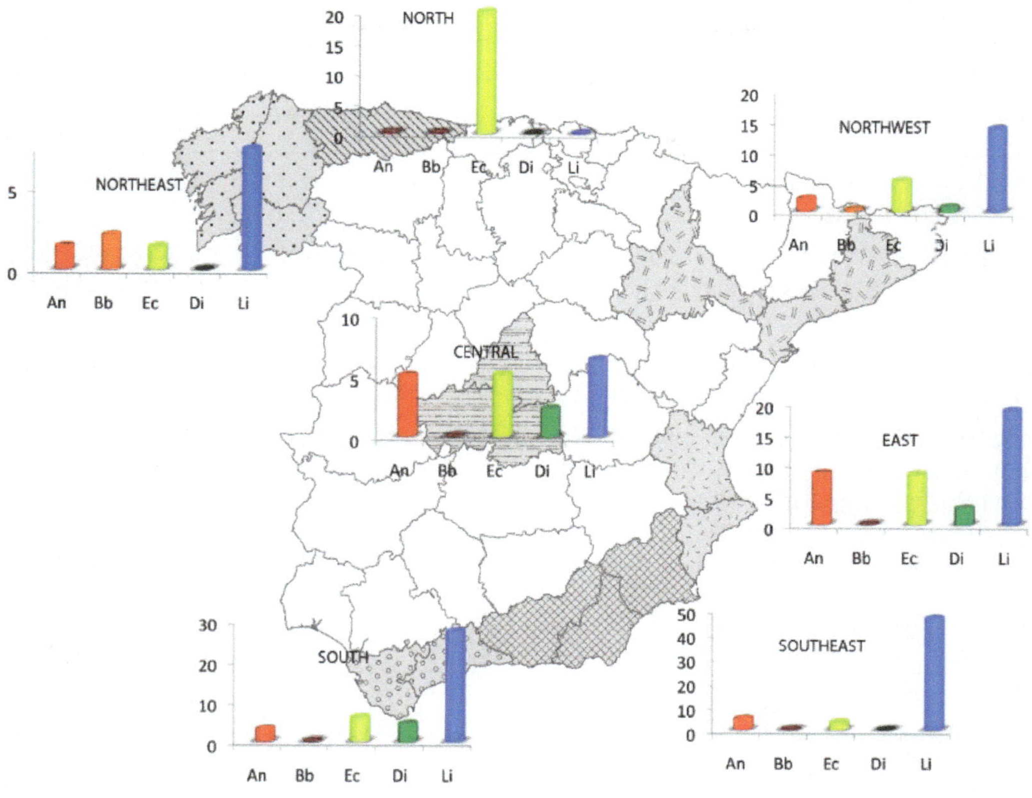

Figure 1: CVBD seropositivity recorded for seven Spanish geographical regions.

Dogs were subjected to the same protocol to compile a brief clinical record based on a questionnaire and physical examination. Blood samples were collected from all dogs. The data collected were correlated with age, sex, abode (indoors, outdoors or mixed), and the presence of clinical signs compatible with any CVBD. The dogs were 6 months to 18 years of age; 593 were male (489 entire, 104 neutered) and 507 female (405 entire, 102 neutered).

Serologic Testing

Anti-An, -Bb, and -Ec antibodies and the Di antigen were determined using the 4DX SNAP® Test (IDEXX Laboratories) and anti-*L. infantum* (Li) antibodies using the *Leishmania* SNAP® Test (IDEXX Laboratories) in blood and/or serum samples.

Statistical Analysis

Seropositivity rates were compared according to age, sex, abode and the presence of clinical signs. Associations between CVBD-agent seropositivity and the remaining variables were assessed using the chi-squared test. All statistical tests were performed using SPSS 19.0 software (SPSS Inc., Chicago, IL, USA). Significance was set at $p \leq 0.05$.

RESULTS

Overall seropositivity rates for the five CVBD agents were: Li (15.7%), Ec (5%), An (3.1%), Di (1.25%) and Bb (0.4%). Rates obtained by geographic region are shown in Table 1. Seropositivity to the Bb antibody and Di antigen was similar in the seven regions. Seropositivity to An was significantly higher (8.3%) in the east than the remaining regions (0-5%), the rate for Ec was significantly higher in the north (20%) and that for Li was significantly higher in the south (46.6%) and southeast (27.4%). In the north of Spain, no dog tested was Li seropositive (Table 1).

Table 1: Seropositivity for the CVBD studied by geographical region

Geographic region		CVBD				
	Positive/Total (%)					
	An	Bb	Ec	Di	Li	
Central	(n=187)	9/180 (5)	0/176 (0)	9/176 (5.1)	4/176 (2.3)	10/157 (6.4)
Northeast	(n=465)	9/451 (2)	1/451 (0.2)	23/451 (5.1)	3/451 (0.7)	60/434 (13.8)
East	(n=90)	6/72 (8.3) *	0/73 (0)	6/73 (8.2)	2/73 (2.7)	13/69 (18.8)
Southeast	(n=105)	2/45 (4.4)	0/30 (0)	1/33 (3)	0/31 (0)	41/88 (46.6) **
South	(n=75)	2/68 (2.9)	0/68 (0)	4/68 (5.9)	3/68 (4.4)	20/73 (27.4) **

Northwest	(n=163)	2/143 (1.4)	3/143 (2.1)	2/143 (1.4)	0/142 (0)	12/159 (7.5)
North	(n=15)	0/15 (0)	0/15 (0)	3/15 (20) *	0/15 (0)	0/15 (0) **
Total	**(n=1100)**	30/976 (3.1)	4/956 (0.4)	48/959 (5)	12/957 (1.25)	156/995 (15.7)
p value		*p=0.04*	*p=0.07*	*p=0.04*	*p=0.06*	*p<0.001*

* $p<0.05$; **$p<0.001$. Abbreviations: An, *Anaplasma phagocytophilum/Anaplasma platys*; Bb, *Borrelia burgdorferi*; Ec,*Ehrlichia canis*; Di, *Dirofilaria immitis*; Li, *Leishmania infantum*.

No associations were observed between sex and any CVBD ($p \geq 0.05$). Seropositivity towards Ec (40%) and Bb (6.7%) was higher in dogs under one year of age compared to adults ($p<0.05$), while no differences in the rates recorded for An, Di or Li were detected between the two age groups.

Seropositivity to An and Li was significantly higher for dogs that lived outdoors compared to indoors. No link was detected between the seropositivity rate observed for Bb, Ec and Di, and place of abode.

When stratified by the presence or absence of clinical signs, percentages of An, Bb, Ec, Di and Li seropositive dogs were 2.1%, 0%, 1.7%, 0.5% and 4.2% for the subset of dogs with no clinical signs (n=556), and 3.8%, 0.6%, 7.5%, 1.8% and 25.9% for those with clinical signs compatible with CVBD respectively (n=507) (Table 2). The main clinical signs described by the veterinarians were: apathy, anorexia, anaemia, lymphadenomegaly, digestive disorders, skin lesions characterized by alopecia, seborrhoeic dermatitis, erythema, scaling and hyperkeratosis, as well as ulcerative lesions, and onychogryposis.

Table 2: Seropositivity for CVBD according to the epidemiological variables analyzed

Epidemiological variable		**CVBD**				
	Positive/Total (%)					
	An	**Bb**	**Ec**	**Di**	**Li**	
Age (years)	<1	2/17 (11.8)	1/15 (6.7)**	6/15 (40)**	0/15 (0)	0/14 (0)
	1-3	12/369 (3.2)	1/361 (0.3)	7/362 (1.9)	2/361 (0.5)	60/370 (16.2)
	3-7	7/269 (2.6)	0/261 (0)	12/261 (4.6)	2/262 (0.8)	50/270 (18.5)
	>7	7/307 (2.3)	2/305 (0.6)	23/307 (7.5)	6/305 (2)	44/327 (13.5)
	Unknown	2/14 (14.3)	0/14 (0)	0/14 (0)	2/14 (14.3)	2/14 (14.3)
	p value	*p=0.14*	*p=0.001*	*p<0.001*	*p=0.3*	*p=0.14*
Sex	Male	21/531 (4)	3/526 (0.6)	23/528 (4.4)	9/527 (1.7)	94/546 (17.2)
	Female	9/445 (2)	1/430 (0.2)	25/431 (5.8)	3/430 (0.7)	62/449 (13.8)
	p value	*p=0.08*	*p=0.16*	*p=0.4*	*p=0.14*	*p=0.16*
Clinical signs	Asymptomatic	9/433 (2.1)	0/416 (0)	7/417 (1.7)	2/416 (0.5)	19/449 (4.2)
	Symptomatic	19/506 (3.8)	3/503 (0.6)	38/505 (7.5)**	9/504 (1.8)	133/513 (25.9)**
	Unknown	2/37 (5.4)	1/37 (2.7)	3/37 (8.1)	1/37 (2.7)	4/33 (12.1)
	p value	*p=0.13*	*p=0.11*	*p<0.001*	*p=0.07*	*p<0.001*
Place of abode	Indoor	6/360 (1.7)	0/346 (0)	14/346 (4)	2/346 (0.6)	26/354 (7.3)
	Outdoor	18/357 (5)*	1/355 (0.3)	22/355 (6.2)	5/355 (1.4)	86/362 (23.8)**
	Mixed	5/256 (2)	3/252 (1.2)	12/255 (4.7)	5/253 (2)	43/276 (15.6)
	Unknown	1/3 (5.2)	0/3 (0)	0/3 (0)	0/3 (0)	1/3 (5.2)
	p value	*p=0.01*	*p=0.07*	*p=0.23*	*p=0.28*	*p<0.001*

* $p<0.05$; **$p<0.001$. Abbreviations: An, *Anaplasma phagocytophilum/Anaplasma platys*; Bb, *Borrelia burgdorferi*; Ec,*Ehrlichia canis*; Di, *Dirofilaria immitis*; Li, *Leishmania infantum*.

In addition, seropositivity rates for Li and Ec were correlated with the presence of clinical signs in the dogs examined. No correlation was detected, however, between seropositivity for Bb, An and Di and the presence of clinical signs.

DISCUSSION

This study is the most complete survey of CVBD-agent seropositivity conducted in Spain. Most prior studies have been limited to a single region [21]. Overall, 37.1% of the dogs were seropositive for at least one of the five CVBD agents examined. The highest seropositivity rate detected was that of Li (15.7%) and the lowest Bb (0.4%), the seropositivity rate for each of these CVBD pathogens varying according to the geographic region. Despite differences detected in seropositivity to each CVBD-agent among each of the seven regions, the travel history of each dog was not included in the questionnaire, such that we cannot rule out the possibility that dogs were infected outside their home region [14].

The present study examines several epidemiological variables to assess possible associations with CVBD-agent seropositivity. No link was detected between sex and each CVBD ($p \geq 0.05$) although seropositivity rates for Ec (40%)

and Bb (6.7%) were higher in dogs under one year of age compared with adults ($p<0.05$). These data suggest a need for further studies designed to determine the effects of age on CVBD-agent seropositivity since we only examined 17 young dogs.

No significant correlation was detected in our study between the presence of clinical signs in a dog and its positivity for Bb, An or Di. In contrast, Li or Ec positivity was correlated with the presence of clinical signs in the dogs examined ($p<0.05$). This finding is consistent with reports indicating that clinical signs are commonly observed in dogs infected with *L. infantum* and *E. canis*[14, 16, 64, 65].

CVBD have been correlated with the presence of vectors such that prevalences should be higher in dogs living outdoors due to their greater cumulative exposure to the agents these vectors transmit. However, we detected no association between positivity for Bb, Ec and Di and place of abode, though dogs living outside showed a higher rate of An and Li. Seropositivity towards An was significantly higher in dogs living outdoors, in agreement with data obtained in dog shelters in northwest (45.3%) and central (19%) Spain [20, 21]. It would be interesting to collect information on whether the dogs were protected with an ectoparasiticidal agent since some of these insecticides are able to prevent CVBD [66, 67, 68, 69, 70]. Macrocyclic lactones have also been found to be effective against canine heartworm [46].

In Europe, *A. phagocytophilum* is transmitted by the tick *Ixodes ricinus*, whose distribution range is limited to areas of high humidity and cold temperatures, while *A. platys* could be transmitted by *Rhipicephalus sanguineus,* widely distributed across the Iberian Peninsula. Our results revealed a high seropositivity for this agent in eastern (8.3%) and central (5%) Spain, and a lower seropositivity in the north (0-2%). In prior studies conducted on dogs attending veterinary clinics in the northwest and east of Spain, similar rates of 5% and 11.5%, respectively, have been reported [19, 20]. Despite the good sensitivity and specificity of the test used to detect antibodies against *Anaplasma* (99.1% and 100%, respectively), serological cross-reactivity between *A. phagocytophilum* and *A. platys* has been described in experimentally infected dogs [71]. Thus, PCR is needed to identify the *Anaplasma* species. Our results could therefore indicate exposure to the *Anaplasma* genus with no information provided at the species level. So far, *A. phagocytophilum* has not been isolated in Spanish dogs. It is likely that the antibodies detected in this study were anti-*A. platys* antibodies since we noted a higher seropositivity to An in areas where the presence of *R. sanguineus* is common. It is also true that *I. ricinus* is the common vector of *B. burgdorferi* and *A. phagocytophilum*, yet we found no An/Bb co-infections. However, dogs from some regions could be infected with *A. phagocytophilum* since this agent has been isolated from *Ixodes* ticks [72, 73] and has also been detected in sheep, goats, cows, deer, birds [73, 74, 75] and even human beings [76, 77].

Antibodies against Bb were only detected in four dogs, three in the northwest (2.1%) and one in the northeast (0.2%). The Snap 4DX kit only detects these antibodies during active infection [78] such that this could explain the low seroprevalence recorded. Other serological studies in which the Snap 3DX or 4DX methods were used have provided similar results [19, 21]. Our data indicate significantly higher seropositivity for Bb in the younger dogs (<1 year), though this finding requires confirmation since our study only included 17 young dogs.

The bacterium Ec is transmitted by *R. sanguineus*. This tick is the most common tick found in dogs which explains the wide distribution of the disease [79]. *R. sanguineus* has been detected across Spain though we observed a significantly higher seropositivity to Ec in the north, where 6 out of 15 dogs were seropositive, while the overall prevalence of Ec was 5%. The low number of dogs surveyed precludes reliable estimates of the real prevalence of this disease. However, the higher seropositivity rate detected in the north could reflect the fact that *E. canis* infection is not limited to dogs, and that other wild canids (wolves, foxes, coyotes) may serve as reservoirs of infection [80]. Effectively, in northern Spain (Asturias), wild canids could live in close contact with domestic canids. There is also evidence that the prevalence of Ec is higher in rural areas or among stray dogs [20] than in urban areas [81]. Other authors have reported a similar Ec seroprevalence for different areas of the country in household dogs (3.13- 16.7%) [19, 20] along with a higher seroprevalence (54.7%) in stray dogs from the northwest of Spain [20].

D. immitis antigen was detected in 1.25% of the dogs examined here. Higher rates were recorded for central (2.3%) and eastern (2.7%) regions of the country while Di antigen was not detected in dogs from the north and northwest. It is known that climate and environmental factors determine the geographical distribution of its vector (Culicidae), allowing it to complete its life cycle and consequently the life cycle of Di [42, 82]. In Spain, similar surveys have identified Di in large areas of the country, often in irrigated zones [42]. A high prevalence of Di has been reported in the Canary Islands (19.2-67.02%)[38, 40, 41, 83], Mediterranean coast (6.3-39%)[84] and southern regions (8.5-36.7%) [38, 39]. At present, while in certain areas (e.g. Gran Canaria) prevalence is decreasing probably due to preventive measures [41, 42], in other areas where Di was considered non-endemic (La Rioja and La Coruña), the first cases of canine dirofilariosis have been detected [43, 44, 85]. A possible explanation for the lower prevalences detected here is that the ELISA test can give rise to false negatives in dogs with low heartworm burdens or in blood samples from dogs infected only by male worms [86]. Besides, these types of study are difficult to compare due to differences in the diagnostic techniques used (PCR, agglutination test, ELISA, etc.), the size and origin of samples, and the study season.

As expected, seropositivity towards *L. infantum* was the highest of all the CVBD-agents analyzed (15.7%). Li antibodies were detected in all the geographic regions except the north, and higher rates were recorded for the south (27.4%) and southeast (46.6%). Our Li seropositivity map is similar to those emerging from other Spanish surveys [65, 87, 88]. Other studies conducted in Spain [50, 89] have detected a higher seroprevalence in some northern areas. Such differences between studies could be attributable to the different population analyzed, the sampling season and the diagnostic technique used.

Among the dogs testing seropositive for Li, 85.2% (133/156) showed clinical signs of leishmaniosis in the physical exam performed by the veterinarians (Table 2).

This can be explained by the fact that CanL is well known to Spanish practitioners despite the wide variety of clinical signs this disease can show [53, 90]. In addition, Li seropositivity was significantly higher in the subset of dogs that lived outdoors compared to those living at home or even both indoors and outdoors. The explanation for this could lie in the increased exposure of dogs that spend more time outdoors to phlebotomines [65, 88, 91]. Arthropod vector distribution and density cause differences in the regional distribution of CVBD-agent seropositivity. To understand the potential role of the vector, knowledge of its environmental requirements is fundamental. There is indeed a need for research targeted at the prevention, diagnosis, treatment and prevention of CBVD. Information on the prevalence and geographical distribution of these infections is essential for planning control measures and their surveillance thereafter. This preliminary overview of the current situation in Spain requires further work to complete the prevalence map of agents causing CBVD in this country.

CONCLUSION

The findings of this study reveal that dogs in Spain are at risk of acquiring any of the five CVBD examined (leishmaniosis, heartworm, ehrlichiosis, anaplasmosis and Lyme disease). They also indicate that veterinarians across Spain need to include these diseases in their differential diagnosis and recommend the use of repellents along with prophylactic measures to prevent disease transmission by arthropod vectors. In addition, greater involvement on the part of public health authorities is needed given that some of the CVBD detected can be transmitted to humans.

DECLARATIONS

Acknowledgements

This study was funded by Bayer HealthCare (Animal Health) and IDEXX (Spain). Publication of the CVBD8 series of articles was sponsored by Bayer Animal Health GmbH. The authors are indebted to the veterinarians participating in this study.

Competing interests

The authors declare that they have no competing interests.

Authors' contributions

GM, AS and XR designed the survey, GM drafted the first version of the manuscript and finalized the manuscript. AM performed the statistical analysis of data, constructed the tables, drafted the first version of the manuscript and finalized the manuscript. RG prepared the figures and reviewed and finalized the manuscript. All authors read and approved the final version of the manuscript.

REFERENCES

1. Otranto D, Dantas-Torres F, Breitschwerdt EB: Managing canine vector-borne diseases of zoonotic concern: part one. Trends Parasitol. 2009, 25 (4): 157-163. 10.1016/j.pt.2009.01.003.
2. Otranto D, Dantas-Torres F, Brianti E, Traversa D, Petri 263 D, Genchi C, Capelli G: Vector-borne helminths of dogs and humans in Europe. Parasit Vectors. 2013, 6 (1): 16-10.1186/1756-3305-6-16.
3. Otranto D, Dantas-Torres F, Breitschwerdt EB: Managing canine vector-borne diseases of zoonotic concern: part two. Trends Parasitol. 2009, 25 (5): 228-235. 10.1016/j.pt.2009.02.005.
4. Day MJ: The immunopathology of canine vector-borne diseases. Parasit Vectors. 2011, 4: 48-10.1186/1756-3305-4-48.
5. Randolph SE: Perspectives on climate change impacts on infectious diseases. Ecology. 2009, 90 (4): 927-931. 10.1890/08-0506.1.
6. Rogers DJ, Randolph SE: Climate change and vector-borne diseases. Adv Parasitol. 2006, 62: 345-381.
7. Semenza JC, Menne B: Climate change and infectious diseases in Europe. Lancet Infect Dis. 2009, 9 (6): 365-375. 10.1016/S1473-3099(09)70104-5.
8. Jaenson TG, Jaenson DG, Eisen L, Petersson E, Lindgren E: Changes in the geographical distribution and abundance of the tick Ixodes ricinus during the past 30 years in Sweden. Parasit Vectors. 2012, 5: 8-10.1186/1756-3305-5-8.
9. Medlock JM, Hansford KM, Bormane A, Derdakova M, Estrada-Peña A, George JC, Golovljova I, Jaenson TG, Jensen JK, Jensen PM: Driving forces for changes in geographical distribution of Ixodes ricinus ticks in Europe. Parasit Vectors. 2013, 6: 1-10.1186/1756-3305-6-1.
10. Menn B, Lorentz S, Naucke TJ: Imported and travelling dogs as carriers of canine vector-borne pathogens in Germany. Parasit Vectors. 2010, 3: 34-10.1186/1756-3305-3-34.
11. Impact of pet travel on animal and public health. Vet Rec. 2008, 162 (14): 429-430.
12. Tabar MD, Francino O, Altet L, Sánchez A, Ferrer L, Roura X: PCR survey of vectorborne pathogens in dogs living in and around Barcelona, an area endemic for leishmaniasis. Vet Rec. 2009, 164 (4): 112-116. 10.1136/vr.164.4.112.
13. Beugnet F, Marié JL: Emerging arthropod-borne diseases of companion animals in Europe. Vet Parasitol. 2009, 163 (4): 298-305. 10.1016/j.vetpar.2009.03.028.
14. Cardoso L, Mendão C, Madeira de Carvalho L: Prevalence of Dirofilaria immitis, Ehrlichia canis, Borrelia burgdorferi sensu lato, Anaplasma spp. and Leishmania infantum in apparently healthy and CVBD-suspect dogs in Portugal--a national serological stud. Parasit Vectors. 2012, 5: 62-10.1186/1756-3305-5-62.
15. Baneth G, Bourdeau P, Bourdoiseau G, Bowman D, Breitschwerdt E, Capelli G, Cardoso L, Dantas-Torres F, Day M, Dedet JP: Vector-borne diseases–constant challenge for practicing veterinarians: recommendations from the CVBD World Forum. Parasit Vectors. 2012, 5: 55-10.1186/1756-3305-5-55.
16. Sainz A: Ehrlichiosis/Anaplasmosis. Enfermedades Vectoriales del Perro y el Gato. 2012, Madrid: Acalanthis Comunicación y Estrategias SLU, 203-226.

17. Foglia Manzillo V, Cappiello S, Oliva G: Tick-transmitted diseases in dogs: clinicopathological findings. Parassitologia. 2006, 48 (1–2): 135-136.

18. Jin H, Wei F, Liu Q, Qian J: Epidemiology and control of human granulocytic anaplasmosis: a systematic review. Vector Borne Zoonotic Dis. 2012, 12 (4): 269-274. 10.1089/vbz.2011.0753.

19. Solano-Gallego L, Llull J, Osso M, Hegarty B, Breitschwerdt E: A serological study of exposure to arthropod-borne pathogens in dogs from northeastern Spain. Vet Res. 2006, 37 (2): 231-244. 10.1051/vetres:2005054.

20. Amusategui I, Tesouro MA, Kakoma I, Sainz A: Serological reactivity to Ehrlichia canis, Anaplasma phagocytophilum, Neorickettsia risticii, Borrelia burgdorferi and Rickettsia conorii in dogs from northwestern Spain. Vector Borne Zoonotic Dis. 2008, 8 (6): 797-803. 10.1089/vbz.2007.0277.

21. Couto CG, Lorentzen L, Beall MJ, Shields J, Bertolone N, Couto JI, Couto KM, Nash S, Slack J, Kvitko H: Serological study of selected vector-borne diseases in shelter dogs in central Spain using point-of-care assays. Vector Borne Zoonotic Dis. 2010, 10 (9): 885-888. 10.1089/vbz.2009.0063.

22. EUCALB (European Union Concert Action On Lyme Borreliosis).http://www.eucalb.com/,

23. Greene CE, Straubinger RK: Borreliosis. Enfermedades Infecciosas del Perro y el Gato. Volume 1. Edited by: Greene C. 2008, Intermedica editorial, 464-484. 3

24. Sprong H, Hofhuis A, Gassner F, Takken W, Jacobs F, van Vliet AJ, van Ballegooijen M, van der Giessen J, Takumi K: Circumstantial evidence for an increase in the total number and activity of borrelia-infected ixodes ricinus in the Netherlands. Parasit Vectors. 2012, 5: 294-10.1186/1756-3305-5-294.

25. Hovius KE, Stark LA, Bleumink-Pluym NM, van de Pol I, Verbeek-de Kruif N, Rijpkema SG, Schouls LM, Houwers DJ: Presence and distribution of Borrelia burgdorferi sensu lato species in internal organs and skin of naturally infected symptomatic and asymptomatic dogs, as detected by polymerase chain reaction. Vet Q. 1999, 21 (2): 54-58. 10.1080/01652176.1999.9694992.

26. Speck S, Reiner B, Streich WJ, Reusch C, Wittenbrink MM: Canine borreliosis: a laboratory diagnostic trial. Vet Microbiol. 2007, 120 (1–2): 132-141.

27. Delgado S, Cármenes P: Seroepidemiological survey for Borrelia burgdorferi (Lyme disease) in dogs from northwestern of Spain. Eur J Epidemiol. 1995, 11 (3): 321-324. 10.1007/BF01719437.

28. Rojo Vázquez J: [Seroprevalence of the infections caused by Borrelia Burgdorferi and Rickettsia Conorii in humans and dogs in primary health care of San Andreas del Rabanedo (León, Spain)]. Rev Esp Salud Publica. 1997, 71 (2): 173-180. 10.1590/S1135-57271997000200008.

29. Merino FJ, Serrano JL, Saz JV, Nebreda T, Gegundez M, Beltran M: Epidemiological characteristics of dogs with Lyme borreliosis in the province of Soria (Spain). Eur J Epidemiol. 2000, 16 (2): 97-100. 10.1023/A:1007690807637.

30. Stich RW, Schaefer JJ, Bremer WG, Needham GR, Jittapalapong S: Host surveys, ixodid tick biology and transmission scenarios as related to the tick-borne pathogen. Ehrlichia canis. Vet Parasitol. 2008, 158 (4): 256-273. 10.1016/j.vetpar.2008.09.013.

31. Skotarczak B: Canine ehrlichiosis. Ann Agric Environ Med. 2003, 10 (2): 137-141.

32. McClure JC, Crothers ML, Schaefer JJ, Stanley PD, Needham GR, Ewing SA, Stich RW: Efficacy of a doxycycline treatment regimen initiated during three different phases of experimental ehrlichiosis. Antimicrob Agents Chemother. 2010, 54 (12): 5012-5020. 10.1128/AAC.01622-09.

33. Sainz A, Amusategui I, Tesouro MA: Canine ehrlichiosis in the Comunidad de Madrid in central Spain. Ann N Y Acad Sci. 1998, 849: 438-440. 10.1111/j.1749-6632.1998.tb11091.x.

34. Ciudad MJ, Cuevas M, Elvira A, López M, Pérez M: Estudio de seroprevalencia frente a *Ehrlichia canis* en la ciudad de Zaragoza. Consulta de Difusión Veterinaria. 2004, 12 (113): 67-69.

35. Sainz A, Delgado S, Amusategui I, Tesouro MA, Cármenes P: Seroprevalence of canine ehrlichiosis in Castilla-León (North-West Spain). Prev Med Vet. 1996, 29: 1-7. 10.1016/S0167-5877(95)01060-4.

36. González JM, Puig V, Collado E, Simeón S: Seroprevalencia de la ehrlichiosis canina en la provincia de Valencia. Consulta de Difusión Veterinaria. 2000, 76: 67-71.

37. Simón F, Morchón R, González-Miguel J, Marcos-Atxutegi C, Siles-Lucas M: What is new about animal and human dirofilariosis?. Trends Parasitol. 2009, 25 (9): 404-409. 10.1016/j.pt.2009.06.003.

38. Guerrero J, Rojo F, Ródenas A: Estudio de la incidencia de la enfermedad del gusano del corazón en la población canina española. Med Vet. 1989, 6: 217-220.

39. Ortega-Mora LM, Gómez-Bautista M, Rojo-Vázquez F, Rodenas A, Guerrero J: Survey of the prevalence of canine filariasis in Spain. Prev Vet Med. 1991, 11: 63-68. 10.1016/S0167-5877(05)80045-5.

40. Montoya JA, Morales M, Ferrer O, Molina JM, Corbera JA: The prevalence of Dirofilaria immitis in Gran Canaria, Canary Islands, Spain (1994–1996). Vet Parasitol. 1998, 75 (2–3): 221-226.

41. Montoya-Alonso JA, Carretón E, Corbera JA, Juste MC, Mellado I, Morchón R, Simón F: Current prevalence of Dirofilaria immitis in dogs, cats and humans from the island of Gran Canaria. Spain. Vet Parasitol. 2011, 176 (4): 291-294. 10.1016/j.vetpar.2011.01.011.

42. Morchón R, Carretón E, González-Miguel J, Mellado-Hernández I: Heartworm Disease (Dirofilaria immitis) and Their Vectors in Europe - New Distribution Trends. Front Physiol. 2012, 3: 196-

43. Morchón R, Moya I, González-Miguel J, Montoya MN, Simón F: Zoonotic Dirofilaria immitis infections in a province of Northern Spain. Epidemiol Infect. 2010, 138 (3): 380-383. 10.1017/S0950268809990434.

44. Simón F, Morchón R, González J: Dirofilariosis canina

en La Coruña. Argos. 2009, 106: 10-12.

45. Bowman D, Hendrix C, Lindsay D, Barr S: Dirofilaria immitis. Feline Clinical Parasitology. Edited by: Bowman D, Hendrix C, Lindsay D, Barr S. 2002, Iowa: Iowa State University Press, 331-334.

46. Bowman DD, Atkins CE: Heartworm biology, treatment, and control. Vet Clin North Am Small Anim Pract. 2009, 39 (6): 1127-1158. 10.1016/j.cvsm.2009.06.003. vii

47. Simón F, López-Belmonte J, Marcos-Atxutegi C, Morchón R, Martín-Pacho JR: What is happening outside North America regarding human dirofilariasis?. Vet Parasitol. 2005, 133 (2–3): 181-189.

48. Molyneux D, Killick-Hendrick R: The leishmaniasis in Biology and Medicine. Edited by: Killick-Kendrick WPaR. 1987, London: Academic, 121-176.

49. Killick-Kendrick R: Phlebotomine vectors of the leishmaniases: a review. Med Vet Entomol. 1990, 4 (1): 1-24. 10.1111/j.1365-2915.1990.tb00255.x.

50. Miró G, Checa R, Montoya A, Hernández L, Dado D, Gálvez R: Current situation of Leishmania infantum infection in shelter dogs in northern Spain. Parasit Vectors. 2012, 5: 60-10.1186/1756-3305-5-60.

51. Morillas F, Sanchez Rabasco F, Ocaña J, Martin-Sanchez J, Ocaña-Wihelmi J, Acedo C, Sanchiz-Marin MC: Leishmaniosis in the focus of the Axarquía region, Malaga province, southern Spain: a survey of the human, dog, and vector. Parasitol Res. 1996, 82 (6): 569-570. 10.1007/s004360050164.

52. Ballart C, Barón S, Alcover MM, Portús M, Gállego M: Distribution of phlebotomine sand flies (Diptera: Psychodidae) in Andorra: first finding of P. perniciosus and wide distribution of P. ariasi. Acta Trop. 2012, 122 (1): 155-159. 10.1016/j.actatropica.2011.11.011.

53. Ballart C, Alcover MM, Picado A, Nieto J, Castillejo S, Portús M, Gállego M: First survey on canine leishmaniasis in a non classical area of the disease in Spain (Lleida, Catalonia) based on a veterinary questionnaire and a cross-sectional study. Prev Vet Med. 2013, 109 (1-2): 116-127. 10.1016/j.prevetmed.2012.09.003.

54. Amusategui I, Sainz A, Aguirre E, Tesouro MA: Seroprevalence of Leishmania infantum in northwestern Spain, an area traditionally considered free of leishmaniasis. Ann N Y Acad Sci. 2004, 1026: 154-157. 10.1196/annals.1307.022.

55. Solano-Gallego L, Koutinas A, Miró G, Cardoso L, Pennisi MG, Ferrer L, Bourdeau P, Oliva G, Baneth G: Directions for the diagnosis, clinical staging, treatment and prevention of canine leishmaniosis. Vet Parasitol. 2009, 165 (1–2): 1-18.

56. Alvar J, Cañavate C, Molina R, Moreno J, Nieto J: Canine leishmaniasis. Adv Parasitol. 2004, 57: 1-88.

57. Baneth G, Koutinas AF, Solano-Gallego L, Bourdeau P, Ferrer L: Canine leishmaniosis - new concepts and insights on an expanding zoonosis: part one. Trends Parasitol. 2008, 24 (7): 324-330. 10.1016/j.pt.2008.04.001.

58. Solano-Gallego L, Miro G, Koutinas A, Cardoso L, Pennisi MG, Ferrer L, Bourdeau P, Oliva G, Baneth G: LeishVet guidelines for the practical management of canine leishmaniosis. Parasit Vectors. 2011, 4 (1): 86-10.1186/1756-3305-4-86.

59. Miró G, Cardoso L, Pennisi MG, Oliva G, Baneth G: Canine leishmaniosis–new concepts and insights on an expanding zoonosis: part two. Trends Parasitol. 2008, 24 (8): 371-377. 10.1016/j.pt.2008.05.003.

60. Baneth G, Aroch I: Canine leishmaniasis: a diagnostic and clinical challenge. Vet J. 2008, 175 (1): 14-15. 10.1016/j.tvjl.2006.11.011.

61. Molina R, Amela C, Nieto J, San-Andrés M, González F, Castillo JA, Lucientes J, Alvar J: Infectivity of dogs naturally infected with *Leishmania infantum* to colonized *Phlebotomus perniciosus*. Trans R Soc Trop Med Hyg. 1994, 88 (4): 491-493. 10.1016/0035-9203(94)90446-4.

62. Molina R, Jiménez MI, Cruz I, Iriso A, Martín-Martín I, Sevillano O, Melero S, Bernal J: The hare (Lepus granatensis) as potential sylvatic reservoir of Leishmania infantum in Spain. Vet Parasitol. 2012, 190 (1–2): 268-271.

63. Aguado M, Espinosa P, Romero-Maté A, Tardío JC, Córdoba S, Borbujo J: Outbreak of Cutaneous Leishmaniasis in Fuenlabrada. 2013, Madrid: Actas Dermosifiliogr

64. Miró G, Solano-Gallego L: Enfermedades Vectoriales del Perro y el Gato. 2012, Madrid: Acalanthis Comunicación y Estrategias, SLU

65. Gálvez R, Miró G, Descalzo MA, Nieto J, Dado D, Martín O, Cubero E, Molina R: Emerging trends in the seroprevalence of canine leishmaniasis in the Madrid region (central Spain). Vet Parasitol. 2010, 169 (3–4): 327-334.

66. Otranto D, Paradies P, Lia RP, Latrofa MS, Testini G, Cantacessi C, Mencke N, Galli G, Capelli G, Stanneck D: Efficacy of a combination of 10% imidacloprid/50% permethrin for the prevention of leishmaniasis in kennelled dogs in an endemic area. Vet Parasitol. 2007, 144 (3–4): 270-278.

67. Otranto D, Paradies P, Testini G, Latrofa MS, Weigl S, Cantacessi C, Mencke N, de Caprariis D, Parisi A, Capelli G: Application of 10% imidacloprid/50% permethrin to prevent Ehrlichia canis exposure in dogs under natural conditions. Vet Parasitol. 2008, 153 (3–4): 320-328.

68. Otranto D, de Caprariis D, Lia RP, Tarallo V, Lorusso V, Testini G, Dantas-Torres F, Latrofa S, Diniz PP, Mencke N: Prevention of endemic canine vector-borne diseases using imidacloprid 10% and permethrin 50% in young dogs: a longitudinal field study. Vet Parasitol. 2010, 172 (3–4): 323-332.

69. McCall JW, Baker CF, Mather TN, Chester ST, McCall SD, Irwin JP, Young SL, Cramer LG, Pollmeier MG: The ability of a topical novel combination of fipronil, amitraz and (S)-methoprene to protect dogs from Borrelia burgdorferi and Anaplasma phagocytophilum infections transmitted by Ixodes scapularis. Vet Parasitol. 2011, 179 (4): 335-342. 10.1016/j.vetpar.2011.03.046.

70. Stanneck D, Ebbinghaus-Kintscher U, Schoenhense E, Kruedewagen EM, Turberg A, Leisewitz A, Jiritschka W, Krieger KJ: The synergistic action of imidacloprid

and flumethrin and their release kinetics from collars applied for ectoparasite control in dogs and cats. Parasit Vectors. 2012, 5: 73-10.1186/1756-3305-5-73.

71. Chandrashekar R, Mainville CA, Beall MJ, O'Connor T, Eberts MD, Alleman AR, Gaunt SD, Breitschwerdt EB: Performance of a commercially available in-clinic ELISA for the detection of antibodies against Anaplasma phagocytophilum, Ehrlichia canis, and Borrelia burgdorferi and Dirofilaria immitis antigen in dogs. Am J Vet Res. 2010, 71 (12): 1443-1450. 10.2460/ajvr.71.12.1443.

72. Oporto B, Gil H, Barral M, Hurtado A, Juste RA, Garcia-Perez AL: A survey on Anaplasma phagocytophila in wild small mammals and roe deer (Capreolus capreolus) in Northern Spain. Ann N Y Acad Sci. 2003, 990: 98-102. 10.1111/j.1749-6632.2003.tb07344.x.

73. Portillo A, Pérez-Martínez L, Santibáñez S, Santibáñez P, Palomar AM, Oteo JA: Anaplasma spp. in wild mammals and Ixodes ricinus from the north of Spain. Vector Borne Zoonotic Dis. 2011, 11 (1): 3-8. 10.1089/vbz.2009.0214.

74. Barandika JF, Hurtado A, García-Esteban C, Gil H, Escudero R, Barral M, Jado I, Juste RA, Anda P, García-Pérez AL: Tick-borne zoonotic bacteria in wild and domestic small mammals in northern Spain. Appl Environ Microbiol. 2007, 73 (19): 6166-6171. 10.1128/AEM.00590-07.

75. Garcia-Perez AL, Barandika J, Oporto B, Povedano I, Juste RA: Anaplasma phagocytophila as an abortifacient agent in sheep farms from northern Spain. Ann N Y Acad Sci. 2003, 990: 429-432. 10.1111/j.1749-6632.2003.tb07406.x.

76. García JC, Núñez MJ, Castro B, Fraile FJ, López A, Mella MC, Blanco A, Sieira C, Loureiro E, Portillo A: Human anaplasmosis: the first Spanish case confirmed by PCR. Ann N Y Acad Sci. 2006, 1078: 545-547. 10.1196/annals.1374.106.

77. Oteo JA, Gil H, Barral M, Pérez A, Jimenez S, Blanco JR, Martinez De Artola V, García-Pérez A, Juste RA: Presence of granulocytic ehrlichia in ticks and serological evidence of human infection in La Rioja, Spain. Epidemiol Infect. 2001, 127 (2): 353-358.

78. Liang FT, Steere AC, Marques AR, Johnson BJ, Miller JN, Philipp MT: Sensitive and specific serodiagnosis of Lyme disease by enzyme-linked immunosorbent assay with a peptide based on an immunodominant conserved region of Borrelia burgdorferi vlsE. J Clin Microbiol. 1999, 37 (12): 3990-3996.

79. Nicholson WL, Allen KE, McQuiston JH, Breitschwerdt EB, Little SE: The increasing recognition of rickettsial pathogens in dogs and people. Trends Parasitol. 2010, 26 (4): 205-212. 10.1016/j.pt.2010.01.007.

80. Fishman Z, Gonen L, Harrus S, Strauss-Ayali D, King R, Baneth G: A serosurvey of Hepatozoon canis and Ehrlichia canis antibodies in wild red foxes (Vulpes vulpes) from Israel. Vet Parasitol. 2004, 119 (1): 21-26. 10.1016/j.vetpar.2003.08.012.

81. Sainz A, Delgado S, Amusategui I, Tesouro MA, Cármenes P: Seroprevalence of canine erhlichiosis in Castilla-León (north-west Spain). Vet Med. 1996, 29: 1-7.

82. Pou Barreto MC, Melero Alcibar R, Gálvez R, Guerrero I, Morchón García R, Carretón E, González Martín C, Del Castillo Remiro A, Molina R, Valladares B: Environmental factors influencing on mosquito distribution in Canary Islands (Spain). International Workshop of Dirofilaria. 2011, Spain: Las Palmas de Gran Canaria, 48-49.

83. Sosa N, Montoya J, Juste M: Situación epidemiológica actual de la dirofilariosis canina en la isla de Gran Canaria. I Congreso Universitario de Ciencias Veterinarias y Afines. 2002, Madrid

84. Rodes D: Últimos datos epidemiológicos sobre filariosis canina. Argos. 2006, 79: 52-

85. Mañas S, Ferrer D, Castellà J, Maria López-Martín J: Cardiopulmonary helminth parasites of red foxes (Vulpes vulpes) in Catalonia, northeastern Spain. Vet J. 2005, 169 (1): 118-120. 10.1016/j.tvjl.2003.12.011.

86. Atkins CE: Comparison of results of three commercial heartworm antigen test kits in dogs with low heartworm burdens. J Am Vet Med Assoc. 2003, 222 (9): 1221-1223. 10.2460/javma.2003.222.1221.

87. Fisa R, Gállego M, Castillejo S, Aisa MJ, Serra T, Riera C, Carrió J, Gállego J, Portús M: Epidemiology of canine leishmaniosis in Catalonia (Spain) the example of the Priorat focus. Vet Parasitol. 1999, 83 (2): 87-97. 10.1016/S0304-4017(99)00074-6.

88. Martín-Sánchez J, Morales-Yuste M, Acedo-Sánchez C, Barón S, Díaz V, Morillas-Márquez F: Canine leishmaniasis in southeastern Spain. Emerg Infect Dis. 2009, 15 (5): 795-798. 10.3201/eid1505.080969.

89. Amusátegui I, Sainz A, Aguirre E, Tesouro MA: Seroprevalence of *Leishmania infantum* in northwestern Spain, an area traditionally considered free of leishmaniasis. Ann N Y Acad Sci. 2004, 1026: 154-157. 10.1196/annals.1307.022.

90. Gálvez R, Miró G, Descalzo MA, Molina R: Questionnaire-based survey on the clinical management of canine leishmaniosis in the Madrid region (central Spain). Prev Vet Med. 2011, 102 (1): 59-65. 10.1016/j.prevetmed.2011.07.002.

91. Zaffaroni E, Rubaudo L, Lanfranchi P, Mignone W: Epidemiological patterns of canine leishmaniasis [correction of leishmaniosis] in Western Liguria (Italy). Vet Parasitol. 1999, 81 (1): 11-19. 10.1016/S0304-4017(98)00237-4.

CHAPTER 26

METHODS OF CONTROL OF THE LEISHMANIA INFANTUM DOG RESERVOIR: STATE OF THE ART

Michele Podaliri Vulpiani, Luigi Iannetti, Daniela Paganico, Filomena Iannino, and Nicola Ferri

INTRODUCTION

Leishmania infantum is a protozoa, obligatory intracellular parasite of mammalian macrophages. This parasite is transmitted by phlebotomine sandflies causing severe vector-born visceral infectious diseases: zoonotic visceral leishmaniosis (ZVL) in human and canine leishmaniosis (CanL) in dogs. Infected dogs, both owned and not, can be an important threat to public health, because L. infantum has the domestic dog as principal reservoir. To date, ZVL is endemic to large areas of Europe, Asia, and Africa, particularly in the countries of the Mediterranean Basin [1, 2]. In Latin America ZVL is linked to L. chagasi, now considered as a synonymous ofL. infantum and therefore included in the same species [3–5].

During the past years, the importance of ZVL public health concerns has increased, considering the increase in risk factors associated with environmental changes, human migration, and, mostly, the presence of Leishmania infantum-infected dogs in previous nonendemic areas. In fact, the emergence of cases of ZVL in new territories is usually preceded by an increase in the prevalence of CanL. An effective control of CanL is therefore crucial for the prevention of ZVL in humans: in particular, vector control through the employment of repellent drugs seems to be an efficient tool for the reduction of seroprevalence [5–9]. Culling of infected dogs is also used in some areas, but animal welfare concerns could arise from this issue, and its real usefulness is debated: epidemiological studies reported evidences of the inefficacy of ZVL control programs that provide for the elimination of infected dogs [10–12]. Treatment of infected dogs reduces or eliminates clinical signs, but it is not usually parasitological curative [13] and treated dogs could still be capable of transmitting the parasite [14]. Recently, a canine vaccine has been licensed in some countries and has been proved to be an efficient preventive tool in order to diminish both the number of human and canine cases [1, 12]. However, the use of this vaccine is still debated in many countries, considering its possible effect on the serological condition of healthy vaccinated individuals and, therefore, on the efficacy of serological control campaigns [15, 16].

Here, after a wide description of ZVL and CanL clinical and epidemiological aspects in humans and dogs, we consider what is the state of the art about CanL control methods, particularly regarding their efficacy and feasibility for large scale-control plans.

LEISHMANIA INFANTUM IN HUMANS: ZOONOTIC VISCERAL LEISHMANIASIS (ZVL)

Human leishmaniosis is a parasitic disease caused by intracellular protozoan of the genus Leishmania. These parasites infect many mammalian species, and the transmission from one species to another happens through arthropods

Citation: Michele Podaliri Vulpiani, Luigi Iannetti, Daniela Paganico, Filomena Iannino, and Nicola Ferri, "Methods of Control of the Leishmania infantum Dog Reservoir: State of the Art," Veterinary Medicine International, vol. 2011, Article ID 215964, 13 pages, 2011. doi:10.4061/2011/215964.

vectors, mostly phlebotomine sandflies. Among 15 species of Leishmania, 13 have a zoonotic nature and cause severe diseases transmitted from mammalian reservoirs to humans. There are two main forms of zoonotic leishmaniosis: the zoonotic visceral leishmaniosis (ZVL) and the zoonotic cutaneous leishmaniosis (ZCL).

ZCL is less severe, usually not fatal and self-healing, but responsible for a large number of cases, mostly in Latin America and Middle East [17]. It is caused by many different species of the genus Leishmania, including dermotropic L. infantum, but it is mostly due to L. major and other species hosted by rodents and many tropical wild animals (armadillos, sloths, and procavias). Clinical forms of ZCL in humans usually consist of localized noduloulcerative lesions; rarely these forms evolve to more severe and diffuse cutaneous leishmaniosis, with multiple nodules over large areas of skins.

ZVL is much more severe than ZCL, and it is caused by the viscerotropic L. infantum. Viscerotropic parasites addressed to the genus Leishmania have been classified into four species, precisely, L. donovani, L. archibaldi, L. infantum, and L. chagasi. The last one is now considered a New World synonymous of L. infantum [4]. In fact,L. infantum is thought to have been imported into the Americas by the dogs of European settlers during the colonization [18]. In humans, all these parasites cause visceral leishmaniosis, an acute, life-threatening disease during which the agents multiply in the macrophages of the reticuloendothelial system, resulting in generalized symptoms like fever, splenomegaly, and pancytopenia. L. donovani and L. archibaldi cause anthroponotic visceral leishmaniosis (AVL) that is only transmitted from human to human via sandfly bites and affects people of all ages while ZVL from L. infantum affects mainly young children and is transmitted from dogs. The only domestic and primary reservoir of this zoonotic disease is the dog [19], in which L. infantum causes the canine leishmaniosis (CanL). ZVL is a disease re-emerging in the whole Mediterranean Basin [19]: about 200 cases are yearly reported in Italy, usually in the same areas where CanL is endemic [20]. Worldwide reports show that sixty-six Old World and twenty-two New World countries are endemic for human leishmaniosis. The estimate yearly incidence of ZVL is 500,000 cases [21, 22]. About 90% of ZVL occur in rural and suburban areas of five countries (Bangladesh, India, Nepal, Sudan, and Brazil); however, this non uniform distribution is due to the evidence that official data are probably underestimated, because it was obtained through incomplete, passive case detection [17]. The clinic evolution of ZVL can greatly vary according to the immune status of the patient: in fact, it usually has a chronic course, but in people with reduced immune response (e.g., HIV-affected people) fulminant disease has been described [23]. In the classic, chronic evolution, early symptoms include abdominal pain, weight loss, weakness, and typically remittent febrile episodes, with two spikes per day. Later, lymphnodes swelling and liver and/or spleen enlargement may occur. Typically, there is hypergammaglobulinemia with circulating immune complexes and nephritis. Patients in the final stages of the disease show thrombocytopenia, bleeding, haematuria, and consequent anemia. Death may occur following hemorrhage and complications due to reduction of the immune response.

CANINE LEISMANIASIS (CANL): EPIDEMIOLOGY, PATHOGENESIS, AND CLINICAL SIGNS

Canine leishmaniosis (CanL) is a chronic visceral-cutaneous syndrome, which clinical signs could noticeably change from a patient to another: it may be manifested as a subclinical infection, often self-limiting [24] or can be a nonself-limiting and severe illness [25]. The transmission of L. infantum from domestic dogs to humans by the bite of previously infected sandflies was first demonstrated in 1930 [26, 27]. Since then, many studies confirmed the role of the domestic dog as the main reservoir of ZVL [17]. In fact, dogs have a high prevalence of both infection and infectiousness, have long-lasting infections, and are common in the peridomestic environment where usually the transmission to human occurs [5]. During the past years the scientific interest in CanL has grown considering the progressive increasing of the global incidence of ZVL and its occurrence in areas previously not involved, possibly as a consequence of global climate changes [17, 28]. Moreover, it is possible that the zoonotic potential of CanL has been enhanced, considering the more and more abundant presence of immunocompromised humans, particularly in developing countries [29–32]. However, even if dogs are recognized as the most important peridomestic reservoir of L. infantum infection to humans, only one study has shown that the owner of an infected dog could be at risk of transmission of the infection from his pet [33]. In fact, the presence of an infected dog in a household does not seem to increase the risk of infection for the members of the family in endemic areas [25], as the infected sandfly can transmit L. infantum in a range of 2.5 km [34]. Pathogenesis of CanL is common to others forms of leishmaniosis. In fact, all protozoan of the genus Leishmania are parasites that need two hosts to complete its life cycle: a phlebotomine sandfly vector and a mammal. The arthropod harbors the flagellated extracellular promastigote while the nonflagellated, intracellular amastigote develops in the mammal. The metacyclic promastigote (e.g., the final promastigote form) is transmitted to a new mammal host, that can belong to the same species of the previous extraphlebotomine host, or to another receptive species. The transmission occurs when an infected female sandfly feed on the mammal, inoculating promastigotes via the proboscis. Male sandflies are not effective vectors as they are not hematophagous [35]. In dogs, the subsequent course of infection is linked to the host immune response and to the degree of persistence and multiplication of the parasite [36]. As it has already been shown in humans [37], the presence or absence of T-cell response is important for the developing of clinical signs: analyses of circulating lymphocites in symptomatic dogs have shown low levels of $CD4^+$ and $CD8^+$ T-cells and a decrease in $CD21^+$ B-cells and $CD14^+$ monocytes, and changes related to bone marrow parasite density [38]. The absence of an adequate T-cell response leads to insufficient control of the parasite and consequent appearance of clinical signs, high Leishmania-specific antibody levels, and high parasite burdens in skin, bone marrow, spleen, liver, and lymphnodes [14, 39]. Asymptomatic dogs, in which Leishmania infection is manifested as a subclinical, self-limiting disease, are characterized by the presence of protective immunity that is $CD4^+$ T-cells-mediated [11, 40, 41]. On the contrary, symptomatic dogs are characterized by disease susceptibility associated to the production of a marked humoral non-protective immune response and a reduced cell-mediated immunity [36, 42]. Therefore, CanL can range from a mild dermatitis associated with specific cellular immunity and low humoral response to a severe disease characterized by immune complex deposition due to a massive humoral, non-protective response and renal damage consequent to the frequent development of glomerulonephritis and tubulointerstitial nephritis [43, 44].

Clinical signs of CanL show after a period of incubation from two to eight months [45], and up to fifteen months [46]. One author reported the development of clinical signs in dogs living in a nonendemic country after 5–7 years they had visited an endemic area [47]. Clinical signs vary widely from a patient to another due to the diversity of immune responses and the variety of organs affected, resulting in several clinical findings [36,42, 48]. Any organ could be potentially involved; however, some signs are more frequent than others. The main groups of clinical signs of CanL are described below.

Cutaneous Lesions

Cutaneous lesions are the most common clinical manifestations of CanL, they are reported in more than 50% of cases [36], even 90% according to several authors [36, 47], and an extensive range of dermatological entities have been described and classified in groups (reported percentages are from a study of Ferrer on 43 dogs): (1) alopecia and peeling (nonpruritic exfoliative dermatitis) generalized or localized over face, ears, and limbs (60%); (2) ulcerative dermatitis with ulcers in the skin of the limbs and joints (23%); (3) focal or multifocal nodular dermatitis (11%); (4) pustular dermatitis and general exanthema (6%). Papular dermatitis has also been described [44] and therefore considered as the fifth group of main dermatological entities associated to CanL [25]. Other less frequent cutaneous manifestations are depigmentation, digital, and nasal hyperkeratosis, while pyodermitis by Staphylococcus spp. is a frequent complication [25, 49]. Onychogryphosis has been reported as present in 75% of cases in a study by Semiao-Santos et al. [50]. Perionyxis and onychorrhexis have also been reported [47, 50].

Lymphadenopathy and Splenomegaly

Lymphadenopathy (increasing of size and consistency of lymph nodes) is a very common clinical sign, usually appearing relatively early during the course of the disease. The presence of this clinical sign has been reported in the 93.5% of cases [36, 50]. The general increase of limph nodes size facilitate palpating of superficial ones, in particular, popliteal, prescapular, and submaxillar [36]. Considerable splenomegaly have also been described [25, 47].

Ocular Manifestations

Ocular manifestations are quite frequent during CanL, being reported from 16 to 80% of cases [25]. The most frequent eye lesions are conjunctivitis, with mucous to mucopurulent conjunctivitis reported in 18.5% of cases [50]. These are characterized by a yellowish secretion that adhere to the lacrimal margins while the mucosa is usually pale, due to anemia [36]. Similarly, blepharitis (exfoliative, ulcerative, or nodular), anterior uveitis and keratoconjunctivitis have also been reported [51]. Keratoconjunctivitis can also progress to ulceration and blindness [52]. Uncommon are ocular consequences of systemic hypertension (e.g., retinal detachment), reported in 5.7% of hypertensive dogs with CanL [25, 53].

Renal Disease

Renal disease may be the only clinical manifestation of CanL [25]. Glomerulonephritis and tubulointerstitial nephritis due to the deposition of immune complex are the most common pathological findings in leishmaniotic dogs that develop chronic renal failure [43], which is the principal cause of death in CanL [25,36]. However, renal disease associated to this pathology does not always reach these severe developments: membranoproliferative glomerulonephritis is usually associated with chronic renal failure while dogs without clinical evidence of renal disease more frequently reveal mesangioproliferative lesions [54].

Other Clinical Signs

CanL is a systemic disease that could involve many organs, so a variety of other clinical signs are possible, often making difficult differential diagnosis to other diseases. Weight loss, locomotor abnormalities, apathy and anorexia are still quite frequent, being reported in 15–30% of cases; less frequent are polydypsia, poliphagia, polyuria, epistaxis, vomiting, and diarrhea [36, 50]. In particular, cachexia and muscular atrophy are common findings in dogs at the final stages of the disease, when locomotor abnormalities are also frequent. These could be associated to arthritis, osteomyelitis, and arthrosynovitis in uncommon clinical forms of leishmaniosis [47,55]. Other uncommon clinical forms include neurological disease and polymyositis [56], as well as various autoimmune and cardiovascular disorders (pericarditis, vasculitis) [25].

CANINE LEISMANIASIS (CANL): LABORATORY DIAGNOSIS

Accurate and early diagnosis of CanL is crucial to identify infectious dogs and organize control strategies. In order to diagnosis CanL, clinical, anatomopathological, and laboratory findings should be evaluated together. However, control programs are usually based mostly on mass screening, therefore laboratory techniques will be primarily taken into consideration: a large part of the CanL reservoir is composed by infected clinically healthy dogs. As concerns clinical signs and anatomopathological findings in CanL patients, also useful for the diagnosis in infected dogs with clinically evident disease, we recommend to refer to the previous chapter.

Different methods of laboratory diagnosis are currently available, and they can be divided between (1) parasite isolation (direct and indirect) and (2) immunodiagnostic techniques for the detection of cellular and humoral responses [36]. The detection of the parasite is the main conclusive diagnosis and it is usually carried out directly through the demonstration of amastigotes in smears or after culture of samples (aspirates) obtained from cutaneous lesions, bone marrow, lymphnodes, and spleen [25]. The most important indirect method of detection of the parasite is the polymerase chain reaction (PCR), characterized by high sensitivity and specificity. It can be carried out from samples of blood, skin, lymphnodes, conjunctiva, and bone marrow [36]. Obtaining blood could be the most simple and noninvasive procedure in order to perform PCR, but the parasite load is often lower than in other tissues. Therefore, the application of parasite detection techniques is often difficult when a high number of animals have to be sampled for screening purposes. In this cases, immunodiagnostic techniques are of great utility, in order to detect anti-Leishmania circulating antibodies (mainly IgG): immunofluorescent antibody test (IFAT), enzyme linked immunosorbent assay (ELISA), and direct agglutination test (DAT) are the most used methods. To date the IFAT test, the most specific and sensitive among the serological techniques mentioned above, is reasonably considered the "gold standard" for mass screening of dogs [57, 58]. In fact, infectiousness is positively associated with high antiparasite antibody response and low $CD4^+$ T-cell count [11, 40, 41], therefore high antibody levels are considered conclusive of a diagnosis of CanL [25, 38]. However, false-positive results due to serological cross-reactivity with other pathogens (e.g., Trypanosoma cruzi) have been described [59] and low sensitivity in detecting asymptomatic dogs has also been reported [60]. The cutoff titre to distinguish positive and negative results ranges from 1 : 40 to 1 : 160 according to different laboratories [61].

LEISHMANIA INFANTUM VECTORS: SANDFLY AND NON-SANDFLY TRANSMISSION ROUTES

Leishmania infantum is transmitted from the canine reservoir to other dogs or humans via sandflies bites. There is an exclusive association between sandfly species and Leishmania species due to specific enzyme and ligands present in the gut of these insects: only specific Leishmania spp. are allowed to attach to gut's wall and replicate without being excreted [62]. Therefore, the transmission of each Leishmania species occurs only in that areas where the specific vectors species are present. In particular, female sandflies of the genus Phlebotomus (Europe, Asia, and Africa) and Lutzomya (Latin America) are the vectors of L. infantum [19, 34, 35]. In the countries of the Mediterranean Basin the most important vector species is Phlebotomus perniciosus [63–65]. Other proven sandfly vectors present in the Mediterranean Basin and in the Middle East are P. ariasi, P. neglectus, P. perfiliewi,P. langeroni, and P. tobbi [5, 19, 35]. In northern Africa also P. sergenti and P. arabicus have been reported as proven vectors of L. infantum [25]. These arthropods are present both in tropical and temperate areas, but in the last ones they are usually active only during warm months, from spring to autumn, at temperatures between 15° and 28°C [25, 35]. The importance of sandfly transmission routes in the epidemiology of ZVL and CanL is demonstrated by the spatial and temporal overlapping of clinical cases and the presence of incriminated vector species [5]. For example, new cases of autochthonous ZVL in humans have been reported in areas of Northern Italy previously considered free [20], in consequence to new CanL outbreaks [66–68] and the proven northerly expansion of two specific vector species P. perniciosus and P. neglectus [28]. This situation has been attributed, just as new northward cases of CanL, to climate changes [17]. A recent European Union-funded project "Climate Change and Adaptation Strategies for Human Health in Europe" (cCASHh) concluded that so far there are no evidences that sandfly distributions in Europe have altered after recent climate changes, but it also stated that a considerable potential for climate-driven changes could be in Leishmaniosis distribution in the future [69, 70]. Moreover, the EDEN project (Emerging Diseases in a Changing European Environment) has highlighted the potential of leishmaniosis to expand to new territories with its vector as environments change, and various researches carried out in the framework of this project have come to the conclusion that significant changes have occurred in the geographic distribution of CanL and VZL cases and of flebotomine vectors, involving areas previously considered as nonendemic [71–74].

Non-sandfly transmission routes should be also considered. In fact, symptomatic CanL is characterized by widespread dissemination not only in blood but also in other body fluids, like semen or saliva, therefore biting [5], blood transfusions [75], and used needles [76, 77] have been suggested to be non-sandfly transmission routes, as well as sexual contact [78], congenital transmission [79, 80] and mechanical dog-to-dog transmission via ticks [81]. However, non-sandfly transmission seems to play only a marginal role in the epidemiology of leishmaniosis [25].

LEISHMANIA INFANTUM DOG RESERVOIR: METHODS OF CONTROL

The primary objective of the control of CanL is to reduce the cases of ZVL in humans through the reduction of the prevalence in dogs. Different methods of control are available for the control of the L. infantum canine reservoir. Control methods could be divided into two different groups: (1) methods aimed at infectious dogs (direct control methods) and (2) methods aimed at vectors (indirect control methods). As concern the first group, a big issue is to identify what dogs should be subjected to control methods. Infectious dogs should be recognized, and this is not an easy work. According to the guidelines by Solano-Gallego et al. [25], dogs in CanL endemic regions could be divided into sick (animals with clinical leishmaniosis) and healthy. Moreover, healthy dogs encompasses both noninfected and infected clinically healthy animals. Only part of infected clinically healthy dogs could develop disease (potentially "presymptomatic" dogs): in fact, there are CanL-infected dogs that could be considered "resistant" to clinical leishmaniosis that will never develop clinical signs. There is a debate about the degree of infectiousness of infected clinically healthy and infected sick dogs, also linked to the usefulness or not of therapeutic treatment on dogs for the control of ZVL in humans. Moreover, it is debated if only sick dogs are worth subjecting to direct control methods (e.g., clinical treatment or culling) in order to limit the transmission of L. infantum. In fact, infectiousness would increase with clinical severity, but the infectiousness of infected clinically healthy dogs would also be sufficiently high that direct control needs to be targeted to all serologically positive dogs [5]. However, according to a longitudinal study by Courtenay et al. [11], dogs infected but "resistant" to clinical leishmaniosis would contribute very little to transmission. So, direct control methods targeted to infectious dogs (presymptomatic and symptomatic dogs) could be effective if a reliable test were available. Although of undoubted utility in mass screening, IFAT is not a sensitive and specific test to detect infectiousness, neither are skin biopsies, in fact, studies comparing infectiousness and parasite loads in the skin or lymphnodes have not shown the presence of a correlation [82]. The use of quantitative PCR for the assessment of skin parasite load could be more informative [5], but to date the detection of anti-Leishmania circulating antibodies with a serological titre ≥ 1 : 160 is the preferred screening method to identify dogs with a very high chance to be infectious and, therefore, worth to be subjected to direct control methods [19]. It is obvious that all dogs (infectious and noninfectious) should be subjected to indirect control methods. Hereinafter, direct and indirect control methods are described, including their efficacy, advantages, and disadvantages.

Direct Control Methods

Culling

The removal of infectious, serologically positive dogs through euthanasia could seem the most obvious direct control method of the Leishmania infantum reservoir. In fact, this is a debated issue, as different studies tried to demonstrate the efficacy of this tool, without reaching definitive evidences [83, 84]. The new sensitivity of a large part of population, particularly in most developed countries, considers this kind of approach ethically unacceptable [7, 85]. For this reason, more and more countries are choosing to follow only no-kill strategies for the control of free-roaming dogs and, therefore, for the control of the canine reservoir of ZVL. However, the main evidence against the dog culling approach to control leishmaniosis is the failure of large programs of systematic elimination of seropositive dogs carried on during past years that did not result in any reduction in the number of human cases [86]. A high proportion of dogs should be euthanized to achieve effective reduction in disease transmission [87], and this is often a too ambitious objective, mostly in undeveloped countries with limited economic resources. Moreover, the diagnosis of infectious dogs can be very difficult: sometimes serological diagnosis produces false negatives and often there is a long interval before the effective elimination of infectious dogs [88]. Finally, the removal of dogs only subjected to serological diagnosis can have counterproductive effects: infected dogs, when removed, would be replaced by susceptible dog that could become infectious in a short time [11].

Treatment

Treatment of symptomatic or asymptomatic dogs with high levels of anti-Leishmania circulating antibodies is the only way to reduce the infectiousness of these subjects in countries where culling is not allowed. Infectious dogs should always be treated, not only for ethical reasons, but also for public health reasons. In fact, there is a correlation between infectiousness of dogs and parasite burden: the reduction of parasite loads after treatment would reduce the possibility of transmission of Leishmania infantum to vectors and, therefore, to other dogs or humans [89, 90]. Response to treatment vary from a patient to another and according to the protocol used, but particularly for the first choice drugs it is normally quick: in few days weight increases, cutaneous lesions reduce, blood parameters return to normality, and there is general improvement of the dog's condition [36].

To date, there are different protocols of treatment for leishmaniosis in dogs, using drugs from different categories. The "classic" and still considered "first choice" treatment is based on the use of pentavalent antimonial compounds. In particular, meglumine antimoniate (Glucantime), is the most used commercial formulation, usually combined with allopurinol, according to several different protocols. Considering the possibility of significant side effects, many different protocols have been suggested, varying considerably regarding the dosage, dose interval, and duration of treatment. Possible adverse effects may be arthralgias, myalgias, gastrointestinal problems, alterations in hepatic function and nephrotoxicity [36]. The last one is the most severe effect, and occurs mostly in dogs with reduced glomerular filtration rate [25]. The preferred route for the administration of antimonial compounds is subcutaneous [25]. Intramuscular or intravenous administration has also been suggested [36], even though they could be cause of muscular fibrosis, abscess formation [13], and thrombophlebitis [47]. Allopurinol is always administered orally. Allopurinol has synergic effect in CanL therapy, therefore it is used in many different protocols. It is an inhibitor of xanthine oxidase, that results in the inhibition of the synthesis of parasite proteins [91]. It has scarce side effects (xanthine urolithiasis) and therefore can be used for long periods [92, 93]. The protocol based on the combined use of antimonials and allopurinol considered as "first line treatment" by the guidelines from Solano-Gallego et al. [25] and Oliva et al. [94] is: meglumine antimoniate (MA) 75–100 mg/kg/SID S.C. for 4–8 weeks + allopurinol (A) 10 mg/kg/BID P.O. for six months or more [95–98]. Another effective protocol based on the use of the same drugs is: MA 50–75 mg/kg/BID S.C. for 1-2 months + A 10–20 mg/kg/die P.O. for 1–8 months [19, 99]. During treatment clinicopathological parameters should be monitored, including complete CBC, biochemical profile, serum protein electrophoresis, and urinalysis, after the first month of analysis and then at least every 3-4 months [25]. In order to limit side effects, modulation of doses according to kidney and liver functions has also been used [9]: MA 75 mg/kg/BID S.C. + A 20 mg/kg/SID P.O. were used in dogs with GOT, GPT, BUN and creatinine inside normal range; MA 50 mg/kg/SID S.C. and A 20 mg/kg/SID P.O. were used in dogs with liver or renal failure. In the same study, the moment of stopping antimonial treatment was decided on the basis of results from serum protein electrophoresis, enduring the treatment until the albumin/globulin was ≥0.80.

The second choice "classic" treatment for the therapy of CanL is amphotericin B: it is a very powerful anti-Leishmania drug [100], but it is preferably administered by slow intravenous infusion [25, 101], although also subcutaneous administration has been suggested [102]. The speed of intravenous infusion is closely related to the occurrence of side effects like trembling, fever, nausea, and vomiting [103]. Another important disadvantage of amphotericin B is its severe nephrotoxicity, resulting in decreasing of the rate of glomerular filtration with consequent increasing in levels of serum creatinine and urea nitrogen [36]. The recommended protocol foresees the administration of doses from 0.1 to 1 mg/kg/SID or twice per week (lower doses when administration is daily) I.V. for two months [101, 102]. The development of formulations of amphotericin B in lipid carriers has been performed to diminish toxicity [104], but these products have high costs. Moreover, these are the first line drugs for the therapy of human leishmaniosis, so their use in dogs is not recommended to avoid drug parasite resistance [25]. Experimentally, liposomal amphotericin B has been used in dogs at the dose of 3 mg/kg/SID I.V. for five consecutive days, intravenously: results were good, but clinical signs usually reappeared after 4–6 months [105].

Recently, miltefosine has been successfully used in association with allopurinol for the treatment of CanL [6,106]. It is an antineoplastic agent that has proved to be efficient against Leishmania [107], now registered for the use in dogs as Milteforan. The main advantages of this drug are the oral administration and the low toxicity, even if some gastrointestinal side effects (vomiting, diarrhea) have been reported, mostly at high doses, so that administration with food is recommended [108, 109]. Another possible side effect could be the early development of drug resistance due to the long half-life of this agent [110]. The protocol successfully used [6] foresees the administration of miltefosine 2 mg/kg/SID P.O. for four weeks and allopurinol 10 mg/kg/BID P.O. for six months.

Vaccine and Immunotherapy

The use of an anti-Leishmania dog vaccine could be the most practical and efficient tool for the control and, possibly, the eradication of the disease in endemic areas [3, 87]. In the last years, many studies have been carried on several immunoprophylactic vaccine candidates, in order to find an efficient tool able to directly prevent leishmanian infections [111–117]. To date, only two vaccines have been licensed, both in Brazil, precisely the Leishmune (Fort Dodge Animal Health) and the Leish-Tec (Hertape Calier Saùde Animal). The second one consists of adenovirus expressing a Leishmania donovani A2 antigen, but only partial results on field trials testing its efficacy have been published so far [14, 118, 119]. Leishmune vaccine has already shown its efficacy in various field studies [15, 113, 120, 121]. It is a FML-saponin vaccine that protect 98% of vaccinated dogs [15], blocking the transmission of the disease to sandfly vectors. This tool acts on a crucial moment of the life cycle of Leishmania infantum, with important epidemiological effects: in fact, it was demonstrated that vaccinated dogs do not present the parasite in blood, skin and lymph nodes [120], not exposing the parasite to sandflies. In some areas of Brazil, the anti-Leishmania vaccination of healthy dogs has been used as a preventive tool systematically used in association to regular culling of serologically positive dogs, with encouraging effects: from 2004 to 2006 the vaccination of 5.7% of the healthy dogs led to a decrease of 25% of cases of CanL in dogs and of 61% of cases of ZVL in humans [12]. Anti-Leishmania vaccination is debated because of the possible effects on the serological response of vaccinated, healthy dogs: after vaccination they could present seroconversion, therefore being indistinguishable from infectious dogs [15, 16]. So, serological control campaigns, employing either ELISA or IFAT serological screening tests, would be no more useful, because more than 70% of vaccinated dogs would result positive [12, 16]. Recently, it has been reported that the use of a specific anti-Leishmania ELISA test, suggested by the Brazilian Ministry of Health, would be able to detect only 1.3% of positivity among uninfected vaccinees [12], therefore not interfering with regular serological control campaigns.

The anti-Leishmania vaccine has also demonstrated its efficacy as immunotherapic agent, used alone or in association with allopurinol and amphotericin B (chemoimmunotherapy) for the treatment of symptomatic dogs [1]. For these purposes, a vaccine formulation, different from the one registered for prophylactic purposes, was used, with positive effects both considering immunotherapy (reduction of symptomatic cases from 100% to 38%) and chemoimmunotherapy (reduction of symptomatic cases from 100% to 12%). In particular, the combination chemotherapy-vaccine (chemoimmunotherapy) resulted very effective in eliminating also latent infections, given that 80% of patients showed PCR negative lymphnodes after eight months of treatment, versus only 33% of patients treated with immunotherapy alone.

Indirect Control Methods

Repellent Tools

During the last decade, a number of studies have been carried out demonstrating the efficacy of topical insecticides treatment of dogs exposed to sandfly bites in order to control the canine reservoir of Leishmania infantum [5, 6, 25]. It is now widely accepted that the prevention of sandfly bites on dogs is efficient in reducing not only the incidence of CanL [7, 122], but also the risk of human infections [33, 123]. There are three different types of topical preventive tools, namely, collars, spot-on and spray formulations, all based on synthetic pyrethroids at various concentrations: permethrin 50%-imidacloprid 10% (spot-on), permethrin 65% (spot-on), permethrin 1.9%-pyriproxyfen 0.02% (spray), and deltamethrin 4% (collar). These tools are efficient through two actions. (1) antifeeding effect: the presence of the insecticide on the skin has a strong repellent effect, so the sandfly has only a fleeting contact with the dog, that is sufficient to disorientate and irritate the insect, resulting in absence or reduction of the blood feeding; (2) insecticide effect: usually the sandfly, even if disorientated and incapable of feeding, remains on the skin for quite long time, absorbing a dose sufficient to achieve toxic effects [35, 124]. Therefore, these topical insecticides not only manage to prevent sandfly bites and, consequently, L. infantum transmission, but also can reduce the number of infectious phlebotomus by direct elimination of them. Deltamethrin-impregnated collars have antifeeding and lethality effects for six months [6], while spot-on and spray formulations have shorter effects, so they have to be applied at least once a month [7]. On the contrary, because of the slow release of the insecticide, collars achieve full protective activity only 1 week after application while spot-on formulations need 24–48 hours, and sprays are immediately active [123]. Collars have demonstrated to have a protective effect from 72% to more than 90% according to different studies [6, 36, 122]; moreover, they have shown to have a mortality effect ranging from 30% to 67% [36]. Spot-on formulations have demonstrated to be more effective, with a protection rate ranging from 88.9% to 97.7% and even to 100%, according to the intervals between one application and another (once or twice a month) [7,124, 125]. On the contrary, the insecticide effect of spot-on formulations seems to not differ very much from the one attributed to collars, ranging from 23% to 67% [123]. The only available spray formulation has shown a repellent efficacy of 71.4% but an insecticide effect just of 7.2%, after 21 days [126, 127].

Field studies have been performed for collars and spot-on formulations, in order to evaluate the impact of mass use on the incidence of leishmaniosis, reporting reductions from 50% to 53% in tropical or subtropical countries [128, 129] and from 86% (collars) to over 90% (spot-on) in temperate countries [7, 9, 122, 130]. Moreover, in an Iranian study based on the application of deltamethrin impregnated collars a reduction of 43% of the odds of seroconversion in children was reported [33], highlighting the indirect effects of these tools on human visceral leishmaniosis. These are important achievements, but even more important results could be obtained in the future through these tools. In fact, so far these control methods have been used only in reduced and controlled areas: the application of topical insecticides in wider areas, involving entire communities and a consistent percentage of the dog population (free-roaming and not) could have a greater effect on the incidence of both CanL and ZVL.

Environmental Control

The efficacy of environmental insecticides in order to control the sandfly population is debated, considering high costs, difficulties in application, pollution concerns, and the possibility of resistances. There is a great variety of species of vectors, and in some cases the presence of resistance was reported, in particular forPhlebotomus papatasi (resistance to DDT, permethrin, and lambdachyalothrin) and Phlebotomus argentipes(permethrin and deltamethrin) [131]. However, other studies have reported that sandfly control by insecticides should be a very effective control method: the increase of sandfly mortality reduces the number of vectors, directly influencing the disease transmission [87]. Synthetic pyrethroids are at present the most used anti-sandfly insecticides, even if their short-lived residual activity compared to DDT could be a limitation and a reason of the low efficacy sometimes reported [132]. The effectiveness of control campaigns based on insecticide spraying for the reduction of ZVL cases was reported in Italy [133], India, Greece, Israel [36] and in China [84]. In particular, the efficacy of insecticide spraying was reported to be more evident in the intra- or peridomiciliary environment, rather than reduce the overall sandfly population [134], as this kind of control is effective on adult insects only, because it is not known were immature forms live [133]. Moreover, spraying in areas like forests, burrows, caves, and other places where sandfly larvae and pupae are suspected to live is technically very difficult [36], and could have effects on other insects species, with consequent environmental damages. It has been suggested to concentrate spraying in the peridomiciliary environment to the inside walls of houses, doors, windows, kennels, hen houses, and drains [36] in order to maximize its effect against indoor-biting vectors. Recently, the use of insecticide-treated nets has been suggested as a preventive tool for ZVL in humans [135, 136]. The reduction of microhabitats favorable to sandflies has also been reported as a step to be taken in order to achieve effective prevention [25]. However, the use of repellent tools on dogs remains the most effective antivectorial method to control the L. infantum canine reservoir, and the use of environmental control in association to spot-on formulation should be particularly efficient in areas with large and concentrate dog populations (i.e., dog shelters).

Contemporary Use of Direct and Indirect Methods

A number of studies have shown the efficacy of single control methods of the Leishmania infantum dog reservoir, inducing the ministry, health organizations, and groups of scientists to suggest the contemporary use of different tools, particularly preventive and therapeutic tools, in order to enhance their effects [19, 35, 36,133]. However, these guidelines reported the absence of field studies or mathematically predictive studies on the effect of this "holistic" approach on the prevalence and the incidence of leishmaniosis [19]. It has been hypothesized that reinfection in endemic areas is likely [25], due to the persisting action of sandflies also on subjects treated with therapeutic protocols [137]. Recently, a field study of the authors [9] reported long term effects (4-year period) of therapeutic treatment associated with the application of spot-on preventive tools. The retrospective study was carried on in a dog shelter sited in an endemic area in Central Italy, reporting a significant, progressive reduction of prevalence and incidence of serologic reactivity to L. infantum with a very low rate of relapses (only 8% after 4 years in a pool of 67 subjects that were already seropositive at the beginning of the study). A total of 656 dogs sheltered in a municipal dog kennel were included in the study. Antimonial treatment was administered to animals assigned to one of the following three classes: (1) serological titre $\geq 1:160$, (2) serological titre $= 1:80$, albumins/globulins ratio $< 0{,}80$, and (3) serological titre $= 1:80$ titre, albumins/globulins ratio $\geq 0{,}80$, and presence of clinical signs of CanL. The therapeutic protocol was based on the administration of meglumine antimoniate and allopurinol. Doses were individually adjusted according to kidney and liver functions (meglumine antimoniate 75 mg/kg/BID + allopurinol 20 mg/kg/SID in dogs with normal functions, meglumine antimoniate 50 mg/kg/SID + allopurinol 20 mg/kg/SID in dog with kidney or liver failure). Antimonial treatment endured until the serum protein electrophoresis gave an albumins/globulins ratio ≥ 0.80; however, it was never longer than 12 months or shorter than 2 months. Allopurinol administration continued until complete serum protein electrophoresis normalization. Since the second year of the study a spot-on preventive treatment was applied once a month to all dogs that were in the shelter, using imidacloprid 10%-permethrin 50% (Advantix; Bayer; Germany) at a dose of 1 mL/10 kg. A progressive reduction of prevalence and incidence of seroreactivity to L. infantum was observed. In particular, during the four-year period seroprevalence was lowered from 10.8% to 4% ($\chi2 = 22.02$; $P = 0.000$, significant); while incidence was reduced from 8.92% to 1.63% ($\chi2 = 52.226$; $P = 0.000$, significant Figure 1). It should be highlighted that the introduction of the association of preventive and curative treatment was followed by a significant reduction in prevalence from the second to the third year of study (reduction of prevalence from 10.63 to 6.41; $\chi2 = 6.90$; $P = 0.009$), which contrasts with what had been observed from the first to the second year, probably as a consequence of the absence of preventive treatment (reduction of prevalence from 10.79 to 10.63; $\chi2 = 0.08$; $P = 0.928$, not significant). The very low rate of relapses could be considered as the key of this success. In fact, previous studies using antimonial treatment without preventing tools had reported seroreversion rates of 32% [138], 74.3% [99], 39.6% [139], and 86% [140]; these are values much more higher than the 8% reported in the research above described [9]. However, more studies are needed in order to confirm the role of preventive tools in reducing the rate of relapses and reinfections in endemic areas.

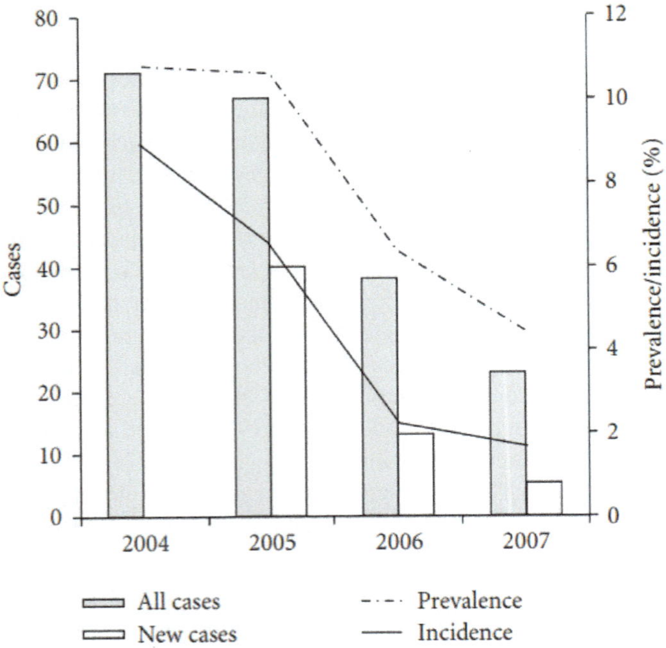

Figure 1: Evolution of prevalence and incidence of serological reactivity versus Leishmania infantum in two dog shelters during a 4-year period of contemporary use of direct (treatment with meglumine antimoniate and allopurinol) and indirect (spot-on repellent formulation imidacloprid 10%-permethrin 50%) control methods [9].

CONCLUSIONS

The domestic dog is the most important natural reservoir of Leishmania infantum and, therefore, it is crucial in the transmission of both canine leishmaniosis and zoonotic visceral leishmaniosis. A number of control methods of the L. infantum canine reservoir have been experimented, but at present the use of preventive tools directly applied on dogs seems to be the most successful one. Culling of infectious animals is now widely considered unacceptable from an ethical point of view: more and more countries are producing new "no-kill" laws with which control programs must necessarily deal. Moreover, it has been reported that this kind of approach often fails in achieving good results concerning its effects on reducing both the number of human and canine cases, particularly if applied without the contemporary use of repellent tools [86]. Treatment of symptomatic dogs could seem too costly to afford for many countries but, according to animal welfare laws and the new "humane" sensitivity of a large part of the population, the absence of therapies could be intended as maltreatment and therefore unacceptable [141]. The absence of treatments can also be a risk for public health, considering the correlation between infectiousness of dogs and parasite burden [89, 90]. The contemporary use of more than one control method has been repeatedly suggested in the past in order to enforce their efficacy [19, 25] and, in particular, the use of repellent tools can integrate the use of therapeutic treatments improving their effects and, therefore, their usefulness and affordability. Moreover, the community-wide use of repellent tools (spot-on or impregnated collars) could be a valid alternative or support to control programs based on dog euthanasia, both considered for their proven efficacy and limited costs. The anti-Leishmania vaccination has been successfully used [12] and it could be a valuable tool in order to implement efficient surveillance programs to control the L. infantum canine reservoir [3]. However, until a certain and commonly recognized diagnostic method will not be available to distinguish vaccinated from seropositive individuals, the use of this tool on large-scale-control programs should not be suggested yet. At present, repellent tools associated with the treatment of infectious dogs seems to be the most desirable and widely accepted approach in order to control the L. infantum canine reservoir.

REFERENCES

1. G. P. Borja-Cabrera, F. N. Santos, F. B. Santos et al., "Immunotherapy with the saponin enriched-Leishmune® vaccine versus immunochemotherapy in dogs with natural canine visceral leishmaniasis,"Vaccine, vol. 28, no. 3, pp. 597–603, 2010.
2. V. F. Manzillo, R. Paparcone, S. Cappiello, R. De Santo, P. Bianciardi, and G. Oliva, "Resolution of tongue lesions caused by Leishmania infantum in a dog treated with the association miltefosine-allopurinol,"Parasites and Vectors, vol. 2, supplement 1, article S6, 2009.
3. L. Gradoni, "An update on antileishmanial vaccine candidates and prospects for a canine Leishmaniavaccine," Veterinary Parasitology, vol. 100, no. 1-2, pp. 87–103, 2001.
4. I. L. Mauricio, J. R. Stothard, and M. A. Miles, "The strange case of Leishmania chagasi," Parasitology Today, vol. 16, no. 5, pp. 188–189, 2000.
5. R. J. Quinnell and O. Courtenay, "Transmission, reservoir hosts and control of zoonotic visceral leishmaniasis," Parasitology, vol. 136, no. 14, pp. 1915–1934, 2009.
6. V. Foglia Manzillo, G. Oliva, A. Pagano, L. Manna, M. Maroli, and L. Gradoni, "Deltamethrin-impregnated collars for the control of canine leishmaniasis: evaluation of the protective effect and influence on the clinical outcome of Leishmania infection in kennelled stray dogs," Veterinary Parasitology, vol. 142, no. 1-2, pp. 142–145, 2006.
7. D. Otranto, P. Paradies, R. P. Lia et al., "Efficacy of a combination of 10% imidacloprid/50% permethrin for the prevention of leishmaniasis in kennelled dogs in an endemic area," Veterinary Parasitology, vol. 144, no. 3-4, pp. 270–278, 2007.
8. D. Otranto, G. Testini, F. Dantas-Torres et al., "Diagnosis of canine vector-borne diseases in young dogs: a longitudinal study," Journal of Clinical Microbiology, vol. 48, no. 9, pp. 3316–3324, 2010.
9. M. Podaliri Vulpiani, L. Iannetti, T. Di Mattia, and P. Dalla Villa, "Leishmania infantum in a Central Italy dog shelter: retrospective study of serologic reactivity during a 4-year period in a confined dog population subjected to preventive and therapeutic treatment," Veterinary

Parasitology, vol. 160, no. 3-4, pp. 190–197, 2009.

10. D. A. Ashford, J. R. David, M. Freire et al., "Studies on control of visceral leishmaniasis: impact of dog control on canine and human visceral leishmaniasis in Jacobina, bahia, Brazil," The American Journal of Tropical Medicine and Hygiene, vol. 59, no. 1, pp. 53–57, 1998.
11. O. Courtenay, R. J. Quinnell, L. M. Garcez, J. J. Shaw, and C. Dye, "Infectiousness in a cohort of Brazilian dogs: why culling fails to control visceral leishmaniasis in areas of high transmission," Journal of Infectious Diseases, vol. 186, no. 9, pp. 1314–1320, 2002. ·
12. C. B. Palatnik-de-Sousa, I. Silva-Antunes, A. D. A. Morgado, I. Menz, M. Palatnik, and C. Lavor, "Decrease of the incidence of human and canine visceral leishmaniasis after dog vaccination with Leishmune® in Brazilian endemic areas," Vaccine, vol. 27, no. 27, pp. 3505–3512, 2009.·
13. G. Baneth and S. E. Shaw, "Chemotherapy of canine leishmaniosis," Veterinary Parasitology, vol. 106, no. 4, pp. 315–324, 2002.
14. A. B. Reis, R. C. Giunchetti, E. Carrillo, O. A. Martins-Filho, and J. Moreno, "Immunity to Leishmaniaand the rational search for vaccines against canine leishmaniasis," Trends in Parasitology, vol. 26, no. 7, pp. 341–349, 2010.
15. G. P. Borja-Cabrera, F. N. Santos, F. S. Bauer et al., "Immunogenicity assay of the Leishmune® vaccine against canine visceral leishmaniasis in Brazil," Vaccine, vol. 26, no. 39, pp. 4991–4997, 2008.
16. C. de Oliveira Mendes, E. Paraguai De Souza, G. P. Borja-Cabrera et al., "IgG1/IgG2 antibody dichotomy in sera of vaccinated or naturally infected dogs with visceral leishmaniosis," Vaccine, vol. 21, no. 19-20, pp. 2589–2597, 2003.
17. M. Gramiccia and L. Gradoni, "The current status of zoonotic leishmaniases and approaches to disease control," International Journal for Parasitology, vol. 35, no. 11-12, pp. 1169–1180, 2005. ·
18. F. F. Tuon, V. Amato Neto, and V. Sabbaga Amato, "Leishmania: origin, evolution and future since the Precambrian," FEMS Immunology and Medical Microbiology, vol. 54, no. 2, pp. 158–166, 2008.
19. L. Gradoni, M. Gramiccia, C. Khoury, and M. Maroli, "Linee guida per il controllo del serbatoio canino della leishmaniosi viscerale zoonotica in Italia," Rapporti ISTISAN 04/12, Istituto Superiore di Sanità, Dipartimento di Malattie Infettive, Parassitarie ed Immunomediate, Rome, Italy, 2004.
20. E. Mondino, G. Bottari, P. L. Caponcelli, C. Manfrinato, and A. Poggio, "Un caso autoctono di leishmaniosi viscerale in una regione alpina italiana," Giornale Italiano di Malattie Infettive, vol. 7, no. 1, supplement 1, article S125, 2001.
21. P. Desjeux, "Leishmaniasis: public health aspects and control," Clinics in Dermatology, vol. 14, no. 5, pp. 417–423, 1996.
22. R. B. Tesh, "Control of zoonotic visceral leishmaniasis: is it time to change strategies?" The American Journal of Tropical Medicine and Hygiene, vol. 52, no. 3, pp. 287–292, 1995. ·
23. H. Neuber, "Leishmaniasis," Journal der Deutschen Dermatologischen Gesellschaft, vol. 6, pp. 4754–765, 2008.
24. E. Bottero, M. Poggi, and M. Viglione, "Lesioni papulari indotte da Leishmania spp in 8 cani giovani,"Veterinaria, vol. 1, pp. 33–36, 2006.
25. L. Solano-Gallego, A. Koutinas, G. Miró et al., "Directions for the diagnosis, clinical staging, treatment and prevention of canine leishmaniosis," Veterinary Parasitology, vol. 165, no. 1-2, pp. 1–18, 2009.
26. S. Adler and O. Theodor, "Investigation on mediterranean kala-azar. VI—canine visceral Leishmaniasis,"Proceedings of the Royal Society of London, vol. 110, pp. 402–412, 1932.
27. L. Parrot, A. Donatien, and F. Lestoquard, "Sur le développement de la leishmaniose canine visceral chezPhlebotomus major var. perniciosus Newstead," Bulletin de la Societe de Pathologie Exotique, vol. 23, pp. 724–726, 1930.
28. M. Maroli, L. Rossi, R. Baldelli et al., "The northward spread of leishmaniasis in Italy: evidence from retrospective and ongoing studies on the canine reservoir and phlebotomine vectors," Tropical Medicine and International Health, vol. 13, no. 2, pp. 256–264, 2008. ·
29. R. De la Rosa, J. A. Pineda, J. Delgado et al., "Incidence of and risk factors for symptomatic visceral leishmaniasis among human immunodeficiency virus type 1-infected patients from Spain in the era of highly active antiretroviral therapy," Journal of Clinical Microbiology, vol. 40, no. 3, pp. 762–767, 2002. ·
30. L. Gradoni, A. Scalone, M. Gramiccia, and M. Troiani, "Epidemiological surveillance of leishmaniasis in HIV-1-infected individuals in Italy," AIDS, vol. 10, no. 7, pp. 785–791, 1996. ·
31. P. Paradies, G. Capelli, C. Cafarchia, D. De Caprariis, M. Sasanelli, and D. Otranto, "Incidences of canine leishmaniasis in an endemic area of southern Italy," Journal of Veterinary Medicine Series B: Infectious Diseases and Veterinary Public Health, vol. 53, no. 6, pp. 295–298, 2006.
32. R. Paredes, J. Muñoz, P. Domingo, M. Gurgui, and B. Clotet, "Leishmaniasis in HIV infection," Journal of Postgraduate Medicine, vol. 49, no. 1, pp. 39–49, 2003.
33. A. S. Mazloumi Gavgani, M. H. Hodjati, H. Mohite, and C. R. Davies, "Effect of insecticide-impregnated dog collars on incidence of zoonotic visceral leishmaniasis in Iranian children: a matched-cluster randomised trial," The Lancet, vol. 360, no. 9330, pp. 374–379, 2002.
34. U. Sharma and S. Singh, "Insect vectors of Leishmania: distribution, physiology and their control,"Journal of Vector Borne Diseases, vol. 45, no. 4, pp. 255–272, 2008.
35. R. Killick-Kendrick, "The biology and control of Phlebotomine sand flies," Clinics in Dermatology, vol. 17, no. 3, pp. 279–289, 1999.
36. J. Alvar, C. Cañavate, R. Molina, J. Moreno, and J. Nieto, "Canine leishmaniasis," Advances in Parasitology, vol. 57, pp. 1–88, 2004.

37. R. Molina, J. M. Lohse, F. Pulido, F. Laguna, R. López-Vélez, and J. Alvar, "Infection of sand flies by humans coinfected with Leishmania infantum and human immunodeficiency virus," The American Journal of Tropical Medicine and Hygiene, vol. 60, no. 1, pp. 51–53, 1999.
38. A. B. Reis, A. Teixeira-Carvalho, R. C. Giunchetti et al., "Phenotypic features of circulating leucocytes as immunological markers for clinical status and bone marrow parasite density in dogs naturally infected byLeishmania chagasi," Clinical and Experimental Immunology, vol. 146, no. 2, pp. 303–311, 2006.
39. A. B. Reis, O. A. Martins-Filho, A. Teixeira-Carvalho et al., "Systemic and compartmentalized immune response in canine visceral leishmaniasis," Veterinary Immunology and Immunopathology, vol. 128, no. 1–3, pp. 87–95, 2009.
40. A. P. da Costa-Val, R. R. Cavalcanti, N. de Figueiredo Gontijo et al., "Canine visceral leishmaniasis: relationships between clinical status, humoral immune response, haematology and Lutzomyia(Lutzomyia) longipalpis infectivity," Veterinary Journal, vol. 174, no. 3, pp. 636–643, 2007.
41. J. L. Guarga, J. Moreno, J. Lucientes et al., "Canine leishmaniasis transmission: higher infectivity amongst naturally infected dogs to sand flies is associated with lower proportions of T helper cells," Research in Veterinary Science, vol. 69, no. 3, pp. 249–253, 2000.
42. G. Baneth, A. F. Koutinas, L. Solano-Gallego, P. Bourdeau, and L. Ferrer, "Canine leishmaniosis—new concepts and insights on an expanding zoonosis: part one," Trends in Parasitology, vol. 24, no. 7, pp. 324–330, 2008.
43. F. A. L. Costa, H. Goto, L. C. B. Saldanha et al., "Histopathologic patterns of nephropathy in naturally acquired canine visceral leishmaniasis," Veterinary Pathology, vol. 40, no. 6, pp. 677–684, 2003.
44. L. Ordeix, L. Solano-Gallego, D. Fondevila, L. Ferrer, and A. Fondati, "Papular dermatitis due toLeishmania spp. infection in dogs with parasite-specific cellular immune responses," Veterinary Dermatology, vol. 16, no. 3, pp. 187–191, 2005.
45. G. B. Gaeta, L. Gradoni, M. Gramiccia, et al., "Leishmaniosi viscerale in Italia. Epidemiologia, clinica, terapia," Recenti Progressi di Medicina, vol. 85, pp. 340–347, 1994.
46. J. .A. Rioux, R. Killick-Kendrick, A. J. Leaney, D. P. Turner, M. Bailly, and C. J. Young, "Ecologie des leishmanioses dans le sud de la France. 11. La leishmaniose viscerale canine: succes de la transmission experimentale chien–phlebotome–chien par la piqure de Phlebotomus ariasi Tonnoir 1921," Annales de Parasitologie Humaine et Comparee, vol. 54, pp. 401–407, 1979.
47. R. J. Slappendel, "Canine leishmaniasis. A review based on 95 cases in The Netherlands," Veterinary Quarterly, vol. 10, no. 1, pp. 1–16, 1988.
48. P. Ciaramella, G. Oliva, R. De Luna et al., "A retrospective clinical study of canine leishmaniasis in 150 dogs naturally infected by Leishmania infantum," The Veterinary Record, vol. 141, no. 21, pp. 539–543, 1997.
49. A. Blavier, S. Keroack, P. Denerolle et al., "Atypical forms of canine Leishmaniosis," Veterinary Journal, vol. 162, no. 2, pp. 108–120, 2001.
50. S. J. Semiao-Santos, A. El Harith, E. Ferreira, C. A. Pires, C. Sousa, and R. Gusmao, "Evora district as a new focus for canine leishmaniasis in Portugal," Parasitology Research, vol. 81, no. 3, pp. 235–239, 1995. ·
51. A. F. Koutinas, Z. S. Polizopoulou, M. N. Saridomichelakis, D. Argyriadis, A. Fytianou, and K. G. Plevraki, "Clinical considerations on canine visceral leishmaniasis in Greece: a retrospective study of 158 cases (1989–1996)," Journal of the American Animal Hospital Association, vol. 35, no. 5, pp. 376–383, 1999.
52. C. L. Swenson, J. Silverman, P. C. Stromberg et al., "Visceral leishmaniasis in an English Foxhound from an Ohio research colony," Journal of the American Veterinary Medical Association, vol. 193, no. 9, pp. 1089–1092, 1988.
53. O. Cortadellas, M. J. F. del Palacio, A. Bayón, A. Albert, and J. Talavera, "Systemic hypertension in dogs with leishmaniasis: prevalence and clinical consequences," Journal of Veterinary Internal Medicine, vol. 20, no. 4, pp. 941–947, 2006.
54. K. Plevraki, A. F. Koutinas, H. Kaldrymidou et al., "Effects of allopurinol treatment on the progression of chronic nephritis in canine leishmaniosis (Leishmania infantum)," Journal of Veterinary Internal Medicine, vol. 20, no. 2, pp. 228–233, 2006.
55. T. Rallis, M. J. Day, M. N. Saridomichelakis et al., "Chronic hepatitis associated with canine leishmaniosis (Leishmania infantum): a clinicopathological study of 26 cases," Journal of Comparative Pathology, vol. 132, no. 2-3, pp. 145–152, 2005.
56. C. D. Vamvakidis, A. F. Koutinas, G. Kanakoudis, G. Georgiadis, and M. Saridomichelakis, "Masticatory and skeletal muscle myositis in canine leishmaniasis (Leishmania infantum)," The Veterinary Record, vol. 146, no. 24, pp. 698–703, 2000.
57. A. Passantino, "Medico-legal considerations of canine leishmaniosis in Italy: an overview of an emerging disease with reference to the buying and selling of dogs," OIE Revue Scientifique et Technique, vol. 25, no. 3, pp. 1111–1123, 2006.
58. OIE (World Organization for Animal Health), "Leishmaniosis. Diagnostic techniques," in Manual of Diagnostic Tests and Vaccines for Terrestrial Animals, pp. 240–250, 2008.
59. E. D. C. Ferreira, M. de Lana, M. Carneiro et al., "Comparison of serological assays for the diagnosis of canine visceral leishmaniasis in animals presenting different clinical manifestations," Veterinary Parasitology, vol. 146, no. 3-4, pp. 235–241, 2007.
60. M. Mettler, F. Grimm, G. Capelli, H. Camp, and P. Deplazes, "Evaluation of enzyme-linked immunosorbent assays, an immunofluorescent- antibody test, and two rapid tests (immunochromatographic-dipstick and gel tests) for serological diagnosis of symptomatic and

asymptomatic Leishmania infections in dogs," Journal of Clinical Microbiology, vol. 43, no. 11, pp. 5515–5519, 2005.

61. E. Ferroglio and F. Vitale, "Diagnosis of leishmaniosis: between old doubts and new uncertainties,"Veterinary Research Communications, vol. 30, no. 1, pp. 35–38, 2006.

62. P. Volf, J. Hostomska, and I. Rohousova, "Molecular crosstalks in Leishmania-sandfly-host relationships,"Parasite, vol. 15, no. 3, pp. 237–243, 2008.

63. S. Bettini and L. Gradoni, "Canine leishmaniasis in the Mediterranean area and its implication for human leishmaniasis," Insect Science and Its Application, vol. 7, pp. 241–245, 1986.

64. M. Maroli, M. Gramiccia, L. Gradoni, P. D. Ready, D. F. Smith, and C. Aquino, "Natural infections of phlebotomine sandflies with Trypanosomatidae in central and south Italy," Transactions of the Royal Society of Tropical Medicine and Hygiene, vol. 82, no. 2, pp. 227–228, 1988.

65. M. Maroli, M. Gramiccia, L. Gradoni, M. Troiani, and R. Ascione, "Natural infection of Phlebotomus perniciosus with MON 72 zymodeme of Leishmania infantum in the Campania region of Italy," Acta Tropica, vol. 57, no. 4, pp. 333–335, 1994.

66. E. Ferroglio, M. Maroli, S. Castaldo, et al., "Survey of phlebotomine sandflies in North-West Italy,"Parassitologia, vol. 44, supplement 1, p. 68, 2002.

67. M. Maroli, C. Khoury, R. Bianchi, E. Ferroglio, and A. Natale, "Recent findings of Phlebotomus neglectus Tonnoir, 1921 in Italy and its western limit of distribution," Parassitologia, vol. 44, no. 1-2, pp. 103–109, 2002.

68. G. Poglayen, S. Marangon, M. G. Manca, et al., "A new outbreak of canine leishmaniosis in the North-East of Italy," Acta Parasitologica Turcica, vol. 21, p. 143, 1997.

69. European Union, "The cCASHh Project: climate change and adaptation strategies for human health in Europe," 2011, http://ec.europa.eu/research/environment/pdf/env_health_projects/climate_change/cl-ccashh.pdf.

70. Ready PD. Leishmaniasis emergence in Europe. Euro Surveillance, 2010http://www.eurosurveillance.org/ViewArticle.aspx?ArticleId=19505.

71. European Union. The EDEN project, "Emerging diseases in a changing European environment," inAnnual Meeting 2008, Brno, Czech Republic, January 2008.

72. J. Martín-Sánchez, S. D. Barón, M. Morales-Yuste, V. Díaz, and F. Morillas-Márquez, "Leishmaniasis in southern Spain: changes over the past two decades and risk factors," in EDEN International Conference, Montpellier, France, May 2010.

73. H. Ertabaklar, C. Balcioglu, N. Sakru, S. Ozensoy Toz, and Y. Ozbel, "First epidemiological and entomological studies of canine leishmaniasis in Kırklareli province, northwestern part of Turkey," inEDEN International Conference, Montpellier, France, May 2010.

74. R. P. Brazil, U. Brazil-Rocha, and B. G. Brazil, "mpact of climatic changes and habitat degradation on Phlebotominae (Diptera: Psychodidae) distribution and leishmaniasis dispersion in Brazil," 2011, http://international-conference2010.eden-fp6project.net/var/eden_colloque/storage/fckeditor/file/Poster%20session_web.pdf.

75. S. D. Owens, D. A. Oakley, K. Marryott et al., "Transmission of visceral leishmaniasis through blood transfusions from infected English Foxhounds to anemic dogs," Journal of the American Veterinary Medical Association, vol. 219, no. 8, pp. 1076–1083, 2001.

76. J. Alvar, P. Aparicio, A. Aseffa et al., "The relationship between leishmaniasis and AIDS: the second 10 years," Clinical Microbiology Reviews, vol. 21, no. 2, pp. 334–359, 2008.

77. I. Cruz, M. A. Morales, I. Noguer, A. Rodríguez, and J. Alvar, "Leishmania in discarded syringes from intravenous drug users," The Lancet, vol. 359, no. 9312, pp. 1124–1125, 2002.

78. F. L. Silva, R. G. Oliveira, T. M. A. Silva, M. N. Xavier, E. F. Nascimento, and R. L. Santos, "Venereal transmission of canine visceral leishmaniasis," Veterinary Parasitology, vol. 160, no. 1-2, pp. 55–59, 2009. ·

79. M. Masucci, M. De Majo, R. B. Contarino, G. Borruto, F. Vitale, and M. G. Pennisi, "Canine leishmaniasis in the newborn puppy," Veterinary Research Communications, vol. 27, no. 1, pp. 771–774, 2003.

80. A. C. Rosypal, G. C. Troy, A. M. Zajac, G. Frank, and D. S. Lindsay, "Transplacental transmission of a North American isolate of Leishmania infantum in an experimentally infected beagle," The Journal of Parasitology, vol. 91, no. 4, pp. 970–972, 2005.

81. M. T. Zanatta Coutinho, L. L. Bueno, A. Sterzik et al., "Participation of Rhipicephalus sanguineus (Acari: Ixodidae) in the epidemiology of canine visceral leishmaniasis," Veterinary Parasitology, vol. 128, no. 1-2, pp. 149–155, 2005.

82. B. L. Travi, C. J. Tabares, H. Cadena, C. Ferro, and Y. Osorio, "Canine visceral leishmaniasis in colombia: relationship between clinical and parasitologic status and infectivity for sand flies," The American Journal of Tropical Medicine and Hygiene, vol. 64, no. 3-4, pp. 119–124, 2001.

83. L. Gradoni, M. Gramiccia, F. Mancianti, and S. Pieri, "Studies on canine leishmaniasis control. 2. Effectiveness of control measures against canine leishmaniasis in the Isle of Elba, Italy," Transactions of the Royal Society of Tropical Medicine and Hygiene, vol. 82, no. 4, pp. 568–571, 1988.

84. Q. F. Shao, "Surveillance of kala-azar following preliminary eradication," Chinese Journal of Entomology, vol. 3, no. 1, pp. 35–37, 1982.

85. J. Moreno and J. Alvar, "Canine leishmaniasis: epidemiological risk and the experimental model," Trends in Parasitology, vol. 18, no. 9, pp. 399–405, 2002.

86. C. B. Palatnik-de-Sousa, W. R. dos Santos, J. C. França-Silva et al., "Impact of canine control on the epidemiology of canine and human visceral leishmaniasis in Brazil," The American Journal of Tropical Medicine and Hygiene, vol. 65, no. 5, pp. 510–517, 2001.

87. C. Dye, "The logic of visceral leishmaniasis control," The American Journal of Tropical Medicine and Hygiene, vol. 55, no. 2, pp. 125–130, 1996.

88. M. D. M. Braga, I. C. B. Coelho, M. M. L. Pompeu, et al., "Canine kala-azar control: aftermath comparison of a fast deletion program of serum-reactive dogs by immuno-enzimatic essay with another of late deletion program of serum-reactive dogs by indirect immunofluorescence of filter paper eluate,"Revista da Sociedade Brasileira de Medicina Tropical, vol. 31, pp. 419–424, 1998.

89. L. Gradoni, M. Maroli, M. Gramiccia, and F. Mancianti, "Leishmania infantum infection rates in Phlebotomus perniciosus fed on naturally infected dogs under antimonial treatment," Medical and Veterinary Entomology, vol. 1, no. 4, pp. 339–342, 1987.

90. R. R. Ribeiro, E. P. Moura, V. M. Pimentel et al., "Reduced tissue parasitic load and infectivity to sand flies in dogs naturally infected by Leishmania (Leishmania) chagasi following treatment with a liposome formulation of meglumine antimoniate," Antimicrobial Agents and Chemotherapy, vol. 52, no. 7, pp. 2564–2572, 2008.

91. D. L. Looker, J. J. Marr, and R. L. Berens, "Mechanisms of action of pyrazolopyrimidines in Leishmania donovani," The Journal of Biological Chemistry, vol. 261, no. 20, pp. 9412–9415, 1986.

92. T. Cavaliero, P. Arnold, A. Mathis, T. Glaus, R. Hofmann-Lehmann, and P. Deplazes, "Clinical, serologic, and parasitologic follow-up after long-term allopurinol therapy of dogs naturally infected withLeishmania infantum," Journal of Veterinary Internal Medicine, vol. 13, no. 4, pp. 330–334, 1999.

93. M. G. Pennisi, S. Reale, S. Lo Giudice et al., "Real-time PCR in dogs treated for leishmaniasis with allopurinol," Veterinary Research Communications, vol. 29, supplement 2, pp. 301–303, 2005.

94. G. Oliva, X. Roura, A. Crotti et al., "Guidelines for treatment of leishmaniasis in dogs," Journal of the American Veterinary Medical Association, vol. 236, no. 11, pp. 1192–1198, 2010.

95. P. Denerolle and G. Bourdoiseau, "Combination allopurinol and antimony treatment versus antimony alone and allopurinol alone in the treatment of canine leishmaniasis (96 cases)," Journal of Veterinary Internal Medicine, vol. 13, no. 5, pp. 413–415, 1999.

96. F. A. Ikeda-Garcia, R. S. Lopes, F. J. Marques et al., "Clinical and parasitological evaluation of dogs naturally infected by Leishmania (Leishmania) chagasi submitted to treatment with meglumine antimoniate," Veterinary Parasitology, vol. 143, no. 3-4, pp. 254–259, 2007.

97. L. Manna, S. Reale, F. Vitale, E. Picillo, L. M. Pavone, and A. E. Gravino, "Real-time PCR assay inLeishmania-infected dogs treated with meglumine antimoniate and allopurinol," Veterinary Journal, vol. 177, no. 2, pp. 279–282, 2008.

98. G. Oliva, L. Gradoni, L. Cortese et al., "Comparative efficacy of meglumine antimoniate and aminosidine sulphate, alone or in combination, in canine leishmaniasis," Annals of Tropical Medicine and Parasitology, vol. 92, no. 2, pp. 165–171, 1998.

99. R. J. Slappendel and E. Teske, "The effect of intravenous or subcutaneous administration of meglumine antimonate (glucantime) in dogs with leishmaniasis. A randomized clinical trial," Veterinary Quarterly, vol. 19, no. 1, pp. 10–13, 1997.

100. J. D. Berman, "Human leishmaniasis: clinical, diagnostic, and chemotherapeutic developments in the last 10 years," Clinical Infectious Diseases, vol. 24, no. 4, pp. 684–703, 1997.

101. J. Lamothe, "Activity of amphotericin B in lipid emulsion in the initial treatment of canine leishmaniasis,"The Journal of Small Animal Practice, vol. 42, no. 4, pp. 170–175, 2001.

102. R. Malik, A. J. Craig, I. Wigney, P. Martin, and D. N. Love, "Combination chemotherapy of canine and feline cryptococcosis using subcutaneously administered amphotericin," Australian Veterinary Journal, vol. 73, no. 4, pp. 124–128, 1996.

103. S. I. Rubin, D. R. Krawiec, H. Gelberg, and R. D. Shanks, "Nephrotoxicity of Amphotericin B in dogs: a comparison of two methods of administration," Canadian Journal of Veterinary Research, vol. 53, no. 1, pp. 23–28, 1989.

104. J. .W. Hiemenz and T. J. Walsh, "Lipid formulations of amphptericin B: recent progress and future directions," Clinical Infectious Diseases, vol. 22, supplement 2, pp. 133–144, 1996.

105. G. Oliva, L. Gradoni, P. Ciaramella et al., "Activity of liposomal amphotericin B (AmBisome) in dogs naturally infected with Leishmania infantum," Journal of Antimicrobial Chemotherapy, vol. 36, no. 6, pp. 1013–1019, 1995.

106. C. Vischer, D. Grousson, and C. Medaille, "Preliminary safety study of the combination therapy of Mitelfosina and allopurinol in dogs," in Proceedings of the 32nd World Small Animal Veterinary Conference, Sydney, Australia, August 2007.

107. A. Kuhlencord, T. Maniera, H. Eibl, and C. Unger, "Hexadecylphosphocholine: oral treatment of visceral leishmaniasis in mice," Antimicrobial Agents and Chemotherapy, vol. 36, no. 8, pp. 1630–1634, 1992.

108. L. Manna, F. Vitale, S. Reale et al., "Study of efficacy of miltefosine and allopurinol in dogs with leishmaniosis," Veterinary Journal, vol. 182, no. 3, pp. 441–445, 2009.

109. S. Sundar, A. Makharia, D. K. More, et al., "Short-course of oral miltefosine treatment of visceral leishmaniasis," Clinical Infectious Diseases, vol. 31, pp. 1110–1113, 2000.

110. F. Janvier, M. Morillon, and P. Olliaro, "Clinical sensitivity and resistance to various therapeutic agents,"Médecine Tropicale, vol. 68, no. 1, pp. 89–101, 2008.

111. G. P. Borja-Cabrera, N. N. Correia Pontes, V. O. da Silva et al., "Long lasting protection against canine kala-azar using the FML-QuilA saponin vaccine in an endemic area of Brazil (São Gonçalo do Amarante)," Vaccine,

vol. 20, no. 27-28, pp. 3277–3284, 2002.

112. C. Carson, M. Antoniou, M. B. Ruiz-Argüello et al., "A prime/boost DNA/Modified vaccinia virus Ankara vaccine expressing recombinant Leishmania DNA encoding TRYP is safe and immunogenic in outbred dogs, the reservoir of zoonotic visceral leishmaniasis," Vaccine, vol. 27, no. 7, pp. 1080–1086, 2009.

113. V. O. da Silva, G. P. Borja-Cabrera, N. N. Correia Pontes et al., "A phase III trial of efficacy of the FML-vaccine against canine kala-azar in an endemic area of Brazil (São Gonçalo do Amaranto, RN)," Vaccine, vol. 19, no. 9-10, pp. 1082–1092, 2000.

114. R. T. Fujiwara, A. M. Vale, J. C. França da Silva et al., "Immunogenicity in dogs of three recombinant antigens (TSA, LeIF and LmSTI1) potential vaccine candidates for canine visceral leishmaniasis,"Veterinary Research, vol. 36, no. 5-6, pp. 827–838, 2005. ·

115. J.-L. Lemesre, P. Holzmuller, R. B. Gonçalves et al., "Long-lasting protection against canine visceral leishmaniasis using the LiESAp-MDP vaccine in endemic areas of France: double-blind randomised efficacy field trial," Vaccine, vol. 25, no. 21, pp. 4223–4234, 2007.

116. M. Mohebali, A. Khamesipour, I. Mobedi, Z. Zarei, and R. Hashemi-Fesharki, "Double-blind randomized efficacy field trial of alum precipitated autoclaved Leishmania major vaccine mixed with BCG against canine visceral leishmaniasis in Meshkin-Shahr district, I.R. Iran," Vaccine, vol. 22, no. 29-30, pp. 4097–4100, 2004.

117. A. Rodríguez-Cortés, A. Ojeda, L. López-Fuertes et al., "Vaccination with plasmid DNA encoding KMPII, TRYP, LACK and GP63 does not protect dogs against Leishmania infantum experimental challenge," Vaccine, vol. 25, no. 46, pp. 7962–7971, 2007. ·

118. A. P. Fernandes, M. M. S. Costa, E. A. F. Coelho et al., "Protective immunity against challenge withLeishmania (Leishmania) chagasi in beagle dogs vaccinated with recombinant A2 protein," Vaccine, vol. 26, no. 46, pp. 5888–5895, 2008.

119. F. Dantas-Torres, "Canine leishmaniosis in South America," Parasites and Vectors, vol. 2, supplement 1, article S1, 2009.

120. F. S. Nogueira, M. A. B. Moreira, G. P. Borja-Cabrera et al., "Leishmune® vaccine blocks the transmission of canine visceral leishmaniasis: absence of Leishmania parasites in blood, skin and lymph nodes of vaccinated exposed dogs," Vaccine, vol. 23, no. 40, pp. 4805–4810, 2005.

121. E. M. Saraiva, A. D. F. Barbosa, F. N. Santos et al., "The FML-vaccine (Leishmune®) against canine visceral leishmaniasis: a transmission blocking vaccine," Vaccine, vol. 24, no. 13, pp. 2423–2431, 2006. ·

122. E. Ferroglio, M. Poggi, and A. Trisciuoglio, "Evaluation of 65% permethrin spot-on and deltamethrin-impregnated collars for canine Leishmania infantum infection prevention," Zoonoses and Public Health, vol. 55, no. 3, pp. 145–148, 2008.

123. M. Maroli, L. Gradoni, G. Oliva et al., "Guidelines for prevention of leishmaniasis in dogs," Journal of the American Veterinary Medical Association, vol. 236, no. 11, pp. 1200–1206, 2010.

124. N. Mencke, P. Volf, V. Volfova, and D. Stanneck, "Repellent efficacy of a combination containing imidacloprid and permethrin against sand flies (Phlebotomus papatasi) in dogs," Parasitology Research, vol. 90, no. 3, pp. S108–S111, 2003.

125. G. Miró, R. Gálvez, M. Mateo, A. Montoya, M. A. Descalzo, and R. Molina, "Evaluation of the efficacy of a topically administered combination of imidacloprid and permethrin against Phlebotomus perniciosus in dog," Veterinary Parasitology, vol. 143, no. 3-4, pp. 375–379, 2007.

126. P. Mercier, P. Jasmin, and A. Sanquer, "Prevention of sand fly attack by topical application of a permethrin/pyriproxyfen combination on dogs," Veterinary Therapeutics: Research in Applied Veterinary Medicine, vol. 4, no. 3, pp. 309–316, 2003.

127. R. Molina, G. Miró, R. Gálvez, J. Nieto, and M. A. Descalzo, "Evaluation of a spray of permethrin and pyriproxyfen for the protection of dogs against Phlebotomus perniciosus," The Veterinary Record, vol. 159, no. 7, pp. 206–209, 2006.

128. A. S. Mazloumi Gavgani, H. Mohite, G. H. Edrissian, M. Mohebali, and C. R. Davies, "Domestic dog ownership in Iran is a risk factor for human infection with Leishmania infantum," The American Journal of Tropical Medicine and Hygiene, vol. 67, no. 5, pp. 511–515, 2002.

129. J. H. Giffoni, C. E. de Almeida, S. O. dos Santos, V. S. Ortega, and A. T. de Barros, "Evaluation of 65% permethrin spot-on for prevention of canine visceral leishmaniasis: effect on disease prevalence and the vectors (Diptera: Psychodidae) in a hyperendemic area," Veterinary Therapeutics: Research in Applied Veterinary Medicine, vol. 3, no. 4, pp. 485–492, 2002.

130. M. Maroli, V. Mizzoni, C. Siragusa, A. D›Orazi, and L. Gradoni, "Evidence for an impact on the incidence of canine leishmaniasis by the mass use of deltamethrin-impregnated dog collars in southern Italy,"Medical and Veterinary Entomology, vol. 15, no. 4, pp. 358–363, 2001.

131. D. D. Amalraj, N. Sivagnaname, and R. Srinivasan, "Susceptibility of Phlebotomus argentipes and P. papatasi (Diptera : Psychodidae) to insecticides," Journal of Communicable Diseases, vol. 31, no. 3, pp. 177–180, 1999.

132. A. M. Oliveira Filho and M. T. Melo, "Vectors control importance on leishmaniasis transmission,"Memorias do Instituto Oswaldo Cruz, vol. 89, no. 3, pp. 451–456, 1994.

133. B. Alexander and M. Maroli, "Control of phlebotomine sandflies," Medical and Veterinary Entomology, vol. 17, no. 1, pp. 1–18, 2003.

134. B. N. Chaniotis, R. E. Parsons, H. J. Harlan, and M. A. Correa, "A pilot study to control phlebotomine sand flies (Diptera: Psychodidae) in a neotropical rain

forest," Journal of Medical Entomology, vol. 19, no. 1, pp. 1–5, 1982.

135. B. Ostyn, V. Vanlerberghe, A. Picado et al., "Vector control by insecticide-treated nets in the fight against visceral leishmaniasis in the Indian subcontinent, what is the evidence?" Tropical Medicine and International Health, vol. 13, no. 8, pp. 1073–1085, 2008. ·

136. K. Ritmeijer, C. Davies, R. Van Zorge et al., "Evaluation of a mass distribution programme for fine-mesh impregnated bednets against visceral leishmaniasis in eastern Sudan," Tropical Medicine and International Health, vol. 12, no. 3, pp. 404–414, 2007.

137. S. Miranda, S. Martorell, M. Costa, L. Ferrer, and A. Ramis, "Characterization of circulating lymphocyte subpopulations in canine leishmaniasis throughout treatment with antimonials and allopurinol,"Veterinary Parasitology, vol. 144, no. 3-4, pp. 251–260, 2007. ·

138. P. Denerolle, "Leishmaniose canine : difficultés du diagnostic et du traitement (125 cas)," Pratique Médicale et Chirurgicale de l›Animal de Compagnie, vol. 31, no. 2, pp. 137–145, 1996.

139. I. Amusategui, Tratamiento de la leishmaniosis canina: valoracion, caracterizacion y comparacion de la respuesta a distintos protocolos a base de antimoniato de meglumina (asociado o no a alopurinol), Doctoral thesis, Departamento de Patologıa Animal II, Facultad de Veterinaria, Universidad Complutense de Madrid, Madrid, Spain, 1998.

140. P. J. Ginel, R. Lucena, R. López, and J. M. Molleda, "Use of allopurinol for maintenance of remission in dogs with leishmaniasis," The Journal of Small Animal Practice, vol. 39, no. 6, pp. 271–274, 1998.

141. F. Pezza, "La protezione ed il benessere animale," in Guida All'esercizio Professionale del Medico Veterinario Dipendente e Libero Professionista, Aggiornamento 2005, F. Pezza, Ed., pp. 519–612, C.G. Edizioni Medico Scientifiche, Torino, Italy, 2005.

CHAPTER 27

CANINE AND FELINE VECTOR-BORNE DISEASES IN ITALY: CURRENT SITUATION AND PERSPECTIVES

Domenico Otranto and Filipe Dantas-Torres

BACKGROUND

Canine and feline vector-borne diseases (VBDs) are caused by a wide range of pathogens, including viruses, bacteria, protozoa, and helminths, which are transmitted by a variety of vectors, such as ticks, fleas, mosquitoes, and phlebotomine sand flies. Some VBDs might be life-threatening in cats and dogs, they might develop after long incubation period making their diagnosis challenging, particularly because their clinical signs are not pathognomonic [1,2]. In addition, cats and dogs may eventually act as reservoirs of pathogens of zoonotic concern. A wide range of factors (e.g., climatic changes, human and animal population dynamics) may affect the occurrence and spread of VBDs [1]. However, the renewed interest on canine and feline VBDs of zoonotic concern is often not paralleled by publication of updated information on their distribution and ecology (e.g., seasonality and risk of exposure for susceptible hosts) in different geographical areas. This lack of knowledge, especially in cats, greatly impairs the development and implementation of effective preventive and control measures at national and regional levels.

In Italy, as well as in many other European countries, the aforementioned key information on parasitic arthropods and the pathogens they transmit is scant, anecdotic, and often outdated [3]. This is mainly due to the fact that most of the regional surveys or case reports on VBDs have been published in Italian journals or in proceedings of national scientific meetings, thus being in most of the cases not available to the international scientific community.

The present article reviews the current situation and perspectives of canine and feline VBDs in Italy. Additionally, the risk of transmission of vector-borne pathogens through different seasons is discussed in order to afford the implementation of effective control programs.

ITALY: GEOGRAPHY AND CLIMATE

Italy is located in southern Europe and comprises the long, boot-shaped Italian Peninsula, the land between the peninsula and the Alps, and two main islands (Sicily and Sardinia). The country has a territory of 301,230 sq km, of which 294,020 sq km is land. It is geographically differentiated into three main areas which include administrative regions, namely northern (Liguria, Piedmont, Aosta Valley, Lombardy, Emilia-Romagna, Veneto, Trentino-Alto Adige, and Friuli-Venezia Giulia), central (Tuscany, Abruzzo, Umbria, Marche, and Lazio), and southern Italy (Campania, Apulia, Basilicata, Molise, and Calabria) including Sicily and Sardinia islands (Figure1).

Citation: Domenico Otranto and Filipe Dantas-Torres, Canine and feline vector-borne diseases in Italy: current situation and perspectives, DOI: 10.1186/1756-3305-3-2.

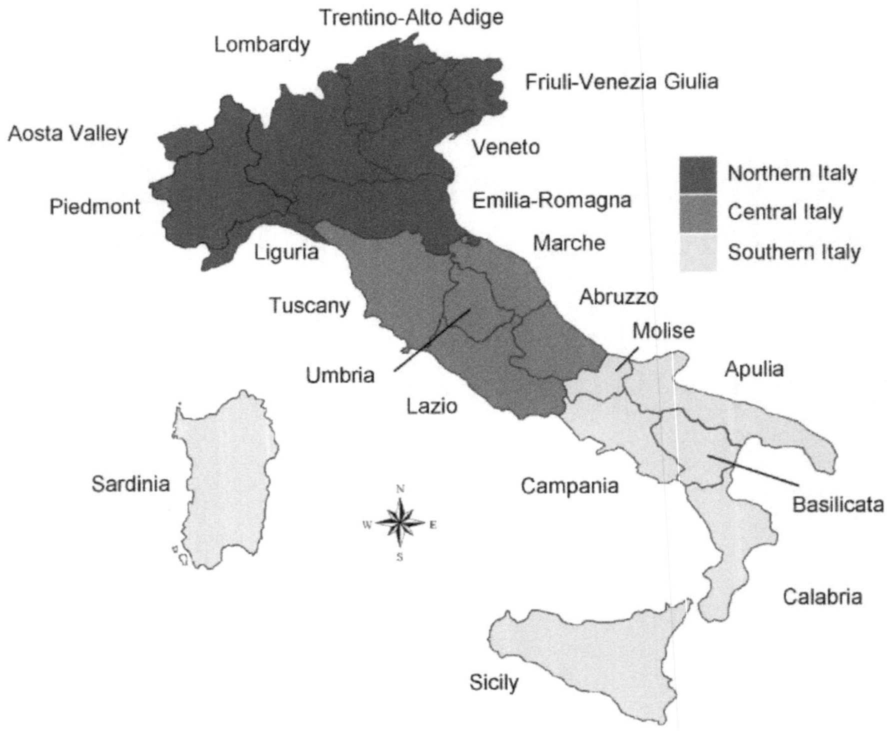

Figure 1: Italy. Three main areas with their respective administrative regions.

The climate of Italy is highly variable. Most of the inland northern areas have a continental humid climate whereas the coastal areas of the Liguria region and most of the peninsula have a typical Mediterranean temperate climate. The Italian peninsula has a large variety of habitats and environments, from the northern Alps through the Apennine Mountains to southern Italian and island regions. The geographical and climatic features, among other factors, contribute to the development of arthropod vectors, which may be present during most of the year, as is the case of ticks [4], fleas [5], and the Asian tiger mosquito*Aedes albopictus*[6].

Free-roaming Dogs and Cats and Risk of VBDs

Free-roaming (i.e., stray) dogs and cats are often present in urban and rural areas representing a public health concern in Italy [7]. Stray dogs have unrestricted movements and have been classified as neighbourhood (or community) and feral dogs on the basis of the level of dependence on human care [8]. It has been estimated that about one million stray cats and dogs live in Italy [7]. The high number of stray cats and dogs is probably due to the fact that their euthanasia is prohibited in Italy and animal abandoning is still a common practice. In fact, the current Italian legislation obligates public health authorities to maintain municipal shelters [7], where dogs are housed through their entire life, providing government protection and assistance for them.

Cats and dogs living in public shelters in Italy may be at high risk of acquiring vector-borne pathogens, mainly because they are often untreated against ectoparasites, thus, representing an easy feeding source for them. In addition, the general conditions of these animals (e.g., poor nutrition) may contribute to susceptibility to some VBDs. Likewise, when infected, free-roaming cats and dogs are often neither monitored nor treated against vector-borne pathogens.

Travelling of dogs and cats (e.g., for holidays) from VBD-endemic areas into Italy and*vice versa*poses a risk for the introduction and dissemination of exotic pathogens if competent vectors are present. In a recent study, it was found that 62% of dogs infected by*Babesia canis*had a history of travel to East European countries [9]. The above phenomenon highlights the importance of establishing effective surveillance systems to avoid the importation of infected cats and dogs into and from Italy.

Arthropod Vectors and Related Pathogens Affecting Dogs and Cats in Italy

Dogs and cats living in Italy are at risk of becoming infected by different vector-borne pathogens, including protozoa, bacteria, and nematodes (Tables1and2). Some vector-borne pathogens are widespread throughout the country and their occurrence in a given geographical area is affected by the presence of their competent arthropod vectors (i.e., ticks, fleas, lice, phlebotomine sand flies, mosquitoes, and secretophagous non-biting flies). Indeed, the likelihood of a dog or a cat becoming infected by a vector-borne pathogen in a given area is greatly influenced by vector population density as well as by the prevalence of the infection within the vector population. The closer is the contact between vectors and hosts, the higher will be the risk of infection. However, cases of VBDs have been diagnosed in cats and dogs in some areas where the presence of the proven vectors is unknown. This apparent absence of vectors in certain areas is likely to be the result of the limited number of studies conducted in these areas rather than the lack of the vectors themselves.

Table 1: Vector-borne pathogens affecting dogs in Italy.

Pathogen	Vector(s)[a]	Geographical distribution[b]
Anaplasma phagocytophilum	*Ixodes ricinus,Rhipicephalus sanguineus*(?)	C, Sardinia [16,82,83,84]
Anaplasma platys	*R.sanguineus*(?)	C, S [15,48,85,86]
Babesia canis	*Dermacentor reticulatus*(?),*R.sanguineus*(?)	C, N [14,54]
Babesia vogeli	*R.sanguineus,I.ricinus*(?)	C, S, N [54]
Babesia gibsoni	*R.sanguineus*(?)	S [52,87]
Bartonella henselae	*R.sanguineus*(?)	Sardinia [88]
Bartonella vinsonii berkhoffii	*R.sanguineus*(?)	S [17]
Borrelia burgdorferi	*I.ricinus*	C, N, S [20,21,22,24]
Dirofilaria immitis	*Anopheles maculipennis,Aedes albopictus,A. cinereus,A.geniculatus,A.detritus,A. punctor,Coquillettidia richiardii,Culex modestus,C.pipiens,C.torrentium*	C, N, S [33]
Dirofilaria repens	*A.albopictus,A.maculipennis,C.pipiens*	C, N, S [33]
Acanthocheilonema grassii	*R.sanguineus*	S [89]
Acanthocheilonema dracunculoides	*R.sanguineus*	S [90]
Acanthocheilonema reconditum	*R.sanguineus*	S [59]
Dipylidium caninum	*Ctenocephalides canis,C.felis*	C, N, S [91]
Ehrlichia canis	*R.sanguineus*	C, N, S, Sardinia [48,49,50]
Hepatozoon canis	*R.sanguineus*	C, N, S [14,92]
Leishmania infantum	*Phlebotomus ariasi,P.neglectus,P.perniciosus,P. perfiliewi,P.tobbi*(?)	C, N, S [33]
Rickettsia conorii	*R.sanguineus*	S [51,93]
Thelazia callipaeda	*Phortica variegata*	S, N [38,61]

Abbreviations: C, central Italy; N, northern Italy; S, southern Italy.

[a]Question mark (?) indicates "suspected vector" to dogs.

[b]Geographical distribution refers to the detection of pathogens either in dogs or in the vectors.

Table 2: Vector-borne pathogens affecting cats in Italy.

Pathogen	Vector(s)[a]	Geographical distribution
Anaplasma phagocytophilum	*Ixodes ricinus*(?),*Rhipicephalus sanguineus*(?)	S [86]
Bartonella henselae	*Ctenocephalides felis*(?)	N [94,95]
Bartonella clarridgeiae	*C.felis*(?)	N [72]
Dirofilaria immitis	*Culex*spp. (?)	N [34,96]
Dipylidium caninum	*C.felis*	C, S [97]
Acanthocheilonema grassii	*R.sanguineus*(?)	C [98]
Leishmania infantum	*Phlebotomus perniciosus*(?),*Phlebotomus*spp. (?)	C [31,32]
Rickettsia felis[b]	*C.felis*(?)	N [26]
Thelazia callipaeda	*Phortica variegata*(?)	N, S [61]

Abbreviations: C, central Italy; N, northern Italy; S, southern Italy.

[a]Question mark (?) indicates "suspected vector" to cats.

[b]*Rickettsia felis*DNA has been detected in*C.felis*fleas, but no evidence of infection in cats has been shown [26]. The pathogenic role of*R.felis*in cats is yet to be demonstrated [99].

The geographical distribution of the main vector-borne pathogens affecting cats and dogs in Italy is reported in Figures2and3. The maps have been elaborated based on data available in the literature, information provided by the Istituto Zooprofilattico della Sicilia (the reference centre for VBDs in Italy), and authors' unpublished data. Once again, the absence of certain pathogens in some regions (e.g.,*Babesia vogeli*in Basilicata and Calabria regions) might be due the lack of studies carried out in these regions.

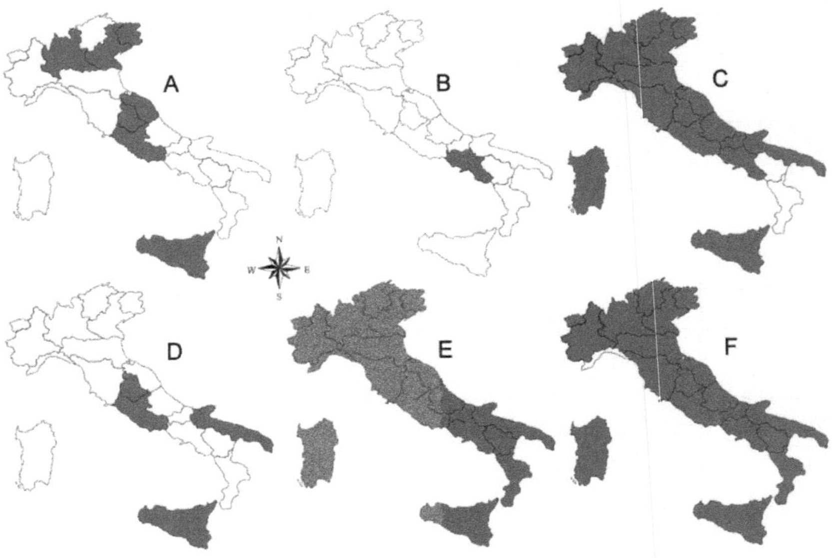

Figure 2: Distribution of major vector-borne protozoa and of*Dirofilaria immitis*infecting dogs in Italy. A,*Babesia canis*. B,*Babesia gibsoni*. C,*Babesia vogeli*. D,*Hepatoozon canis*. E,*Leishmania infantum*. F,*Dirofilaria immitis*.

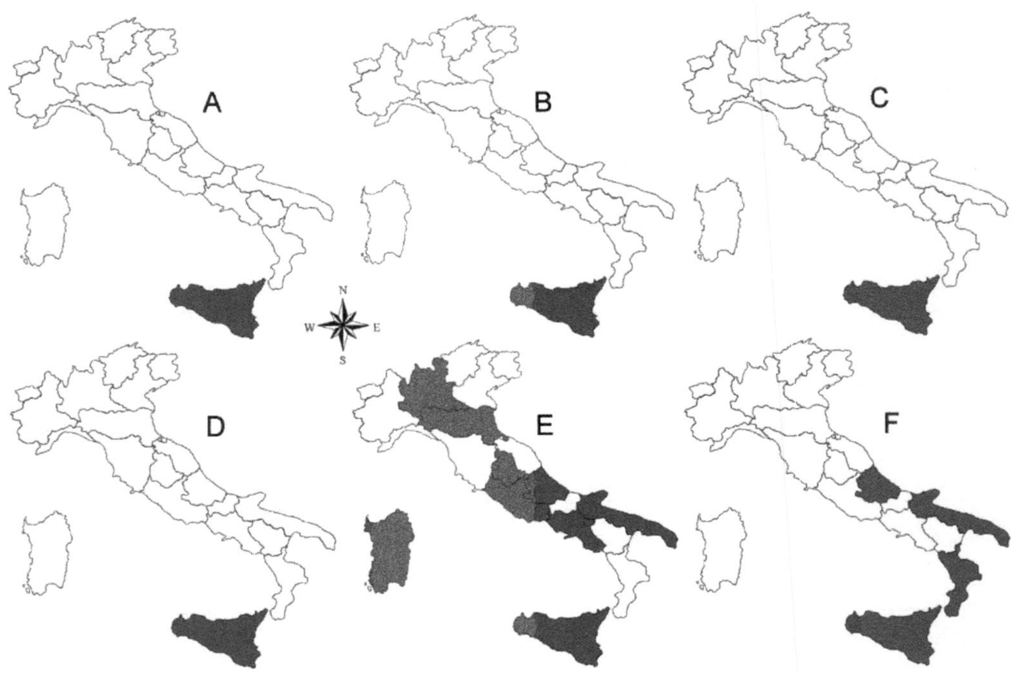

Figure 3: Distribution of major vector-borne bacteria infecting dogs in Italy. A,*Anaplasma phagocytophilum*. B,*Anaplasma platys*. C,*Borrelia burgdorferi*. D,*Coxiella burnetii*. E,*Ehrlichia canis*. F,*Rickettsia conorii*.

Rhipicephalus sanguineus(the brown dog tick) is among the most important arthropod vectors involved in the transmission of pathogens affecting dogs worldwide [10]. In Italy,*R.sanguineus*(Figure4) is the most common tick species infesting dogs [11,12,13,14]. It is the major vector of*B.vogeli*,*Ehrlichia canis*,*Hepatozoon canis*, and*Rickettsia conorii*and it is a putative vector of many other pathogens including*B.canis*,*Babesia microti*-like piroplasm (Spanish isolate),*Anaplasma platys*[14,15], and*Anaplasma phagocytophilum*[16]. Following the recent retrieval of*Bartonella vinsonii berkhoffii*genotypes II and III in dogs from southern Italy, a potentially new strain or species of*Bartonella*was detected in salivary glands of*R. sanguineus*ticks and in a dog [17]. Some of these pathogens (e.g.,*E.canis*) are passed to the subsequent tick developmental stage (i.e., from larvae to nymphs and from nymphs to adults) transstadially [18]. Additionally, certain pathogens, such as*R. conorii*, might be maintained over several tick generations by transovarial transmission [19]. In this case, not only nymphs and adults but also larvae might play a role in transmitting the infection.

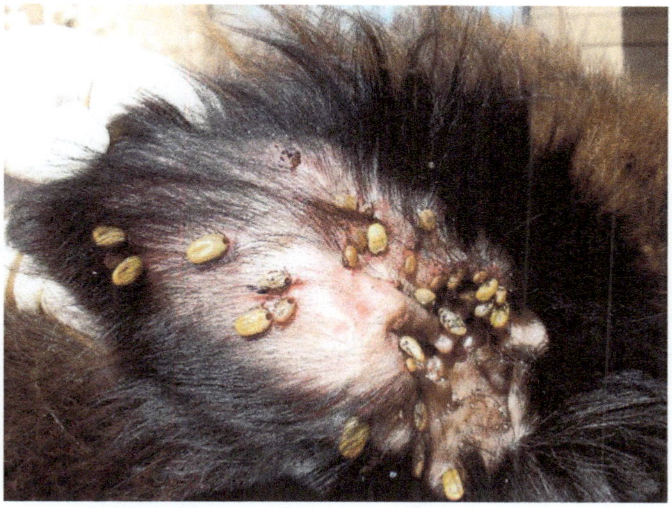

Figure 4: Rhipicephalus sanguineus. Several females attached to the ear of a dog from southern Italy.

Other tick species (e.g.,*Ixodes ricinus*, *Rhipicephalus turanicus*, *Hyalomma marginatum*, *Ixodes hexagonus*, *Rhipicephalus bursa*, *Dermacentor marginatus*, and *Dermacentor reticulatus*) have also been found on dogs in different Italian regions [4,14] and the potential role as vectors of some of them has been speculated upon. For instance, it has recently been suggested that*I.ricinus*could act as a vector of*B.vogeli*in central and northern Italy [14].*Ixodes ricinus*is the major vector of*Borrelia burgdorferi*sensu lato and different "genospecies" have been detected in ticks collected in northern and central Italy [20,21,22]. Although an early experimental study failed to demonstrate the pathogenicity of*B.burgdorferi*(BITs1 Italian strain) in four beagles [23], anti-*B.burgdorferi*antibodies have been detected by indirect immunofluorescence antibody assay in a dog from Sicily presenting with fever, gait abnormalities, and diffuse pain [24]. Cats have also been found infested by ticks (e.g.,*R.sanguineus*) in Italy [25] but the veterinary significance of this parasitism is largely unknown.

Fleas and lice are vectors of pathogens affecting dogs and cats worldwide [1], but little is known about their ecology and vectorial role in Italy.*Ctenocephalides felis*is the most common flea species infesting dogs and cats in Italy followed by*Ctenocephalides canis*[5,26]. Recent investigations have revealed the occurrence of*Rickettsia felis*DNA in*C. felis*collected from dogs and cats in different regions of Italy [26,27], pointing out the public health relevance of fleas infesting dogs and cats in this country. The prevalence of*R. felis*DNA in fleas was significantly higher in north-eastern (23.2% of 112 fleas) than in south-western (7.1% of 169) Italy [26]. Moreover, the positivity was higher among fleas collected from cats (17.6% of 74) than from dogs (10.2% of 246), although the number of fleas from cats tested was much lower when compared to those from dogs [26].

Lice (e.g.,*Trichodectes canis*) are intermediate hosts of*Dipylidium caninum*, but there is no information about their role as vectors of pathogens infecting dogs or cats in Italy.

Phlebotomine sand flies (e.g.,*Phlebotomus ariasi*,*Phlebotomus neglectus*,*Phlebotomus perniciosus*, and*Phlebotomus perfiliewi*) are vectors of*Leishmania infantum*[28], which is a pathogen of great zoonotic relevance affecting dogs [29] and occasionally cats [30,31,32] in Italy. By comparing recent entomological surveys with the historical data available, it has been recorded that there is an increase in terms of population density and geographical range of*P. perniciosus*and*P.neglectus*from southern and central to northern Italian areas [29]. The above phenomena might have ultimately contributed to the establishment of phlebotomine sand fly vectors of*L.infantum*into previously free areas in northern Italy and might represent an important issue to be considered while predicting the spread of phlebotomine sand flies northward through central European countries [33].

In Italy, about 16 species of mosquitoes (e.g.,*A. albopictus*and*Culex pipiens*) have been regarded as proven or suspected vectors of the filarid nematodes*Dirofilaria immitis*and*Dirofilaria repens*, the causative agents of cardiopulmonary and subcutaneous dirofilariosis, respectively, in cats and dogs [33,34,35]. The most common filarial species parasitizing dogs in Italy are*D.immitis*and*D.repens*whereas*Acanthocheilonema reconditum*,*Acanthocheilonema grassii*and*Acanthocheilonema dracunculoides*, which infest subcutaneous tissue and/or muscular fasciae, are less diffused and of minor zoonotic concern [33].

*Phortica variegata*flies feed on lachrymal secretions around the eyes of a wide range of hosts, including humans and wild and domestic carnivores [36]. Males of this drosophilid fly have been shown to act as vectors of*Thelazia callipaeda*eyeworms under both experimental and field conditions [37,38].

From the information above, it becomes clear that dogs and cats living in Italy are exposed to the risk of infection by different vector-borne pathogens, some of which are of public health concern. The occurrence of some arthropod vectors throughout the year (e.g., ticks) and of others during summer months indicates that the risk of infection by vector-borne pathogens can vary in different areas of Italy according to the seasonal activity of their respective vectors.

SEASONALITY OF VECTORS IN DIFFERENT ITALIAN REGIONS

The geographical distribution of VBDs is greatly influenced by the distribution and density of the different arthropod vectors which, in turn, is highly dependent on temperature and relative humidity of the different areas of Italy. For long time VBDs have been believed to be strictly linked to the seasonality in temperate areas and the role of climate and environmental factors on arthropod infection rate has been documented [39]. However, in the past decades, the 'seasonality paradigm' has been extensively debated and nowadays it cannot be considered more valid for many VBDs in the Mediterranean area [33]. In fact, there is evidence that microenvironment and climate changes have a significant impact on the distribution, transmission rates and prevalence of many VBDs. In the Mediterranean area, specifically in Italy, while some vectors (e.g., ticks, fleas, and some mosquito species) have been shown to be active throughout all the year [4,5,6], others (e.g., phlebotomine sand flies and*P.variegata*) display a typical seasonal activity [29,36]. This implies that dogs are at permanent risk of infection by certain tick-borne pathogens, such as*E.canis*. In the first case, a typical example is represented by*R.sanguineus*, the most widespread tick species in the world and probably the tick species transmitting the highest number of pathogens [10]. Due to its adaptability to human-modified ecosystems, this tick species is present through all the year in Italy [4]. Again, the presence of multiple tick species with overlapping seasonal patterns of activity in Italy (e.g.,*I.ricinus*in northern regions,*D.marginatus*and*R. sanguineus*throughout the country) represents a further risk for tick-borne infections through the whole year [4].

As far as fleas are concerned, the occurrence of*C.felis*has been investigated in southern Italy. Although the prevalence of flea infestation was higher during the period between June and October, dogs were infested throughout the year [5] indicating a constant risk for flea-borne pathogen transmission. The results of this study are likely to be representative of other Mediterranean countries being also confirmed by surveys carried out in central Europe [e.g., [40]].

For a long time, mosquito vectors of*D.immitis*were thought to be more active during the summer months, mainly in humid climate areas of northern Italy and, at a lesser extent, in the remaining part of the Peninsula [41]. However, the introduction of*A.albopictus*, a known vector of*D.immitis*and*D. repens*[41,42], during the 1990s has been implicated in the appearance of new autochthonous foci of heartworm disease that have recently been reported in previously non-endemic areas of southern Italy (i.e., Apulia and Calabria regions) [33]. In addition,*A.albopictus*has adapted to the relatively low winter temperatures of Italy, rapidly increasing its populations through the country, developing many generations over the year in central and southern regions and overwintering as eggs in colder northern regions [6]. In contrast to other vectors of filarid nematodes,*A.albopictus*has a diurnal activity pattern [6]. This poses an additional threat to animals and humans, making them proportionally more exposed to*Dirofilaria*spp. in areas where both*A.albopictus*and other nocturnal mosquitoes (e.g.,*C.pipiens*) occur in sympatry [41].

The occurrence and spread of canine leishmaniosis in a given area depends on several factors, including vector abundance and biting rates. In Italy, the activity of phlebotomine sand flies is seasonal and restricted to the summer months [43,44,45,46,47]. Indeed, recent entomological surveys carried out in northern [43], central [44] and southern regions [45] indicated that the activity of*P.perniciosus*(the most important vector of*L.infantum*in the Mediterranean area) is restricted to June and early October [29]. The activity of phlebotomine sand flies is predominantly nocturnal, but their biting activity pattern can vary according to species and foci [46,47].

The ecology and distribution of*P.variegata*has been studied in an area in southern Italy where*T.callipaeda*is highly endemic [36]. It has been shown that*P.variegata*has a seasonal pattern from May to October, being more active during July and August, at 20-25°C and 50-75% of relative humidity [36].

PREVALENCE OF INFECTION BY VECTOR-BORNE PATHOGENS IN CATS AND DOGS IN ITALY

It is difficult to assess the actual prevalence of infection by different vector-borne pathogens in cats and dogs in Italy due to the limited amount of data as well as to the difficulties in comparing information from studies using different diagnostic tools. Indeed, the prevalence of infection by vector-borne pathogens can also vary according to geographical region. For instance, the prevalence of*E.canis*infection in dogs estimated by serological surveys varied from 14.9% in southern Italy [48] to 46.7% in Sardinia [49]. Conversely, the overall prevalence of*E.canis*infection among 601 Italian dogs estimated by real-time PCR was lower than that recorded by serology, indicating that the infection is most prevalent in southern (9.7%) than in central (8%) and northern (2.9%) Italy [50]. Indeed, these discrepancies are due to the different methods used in each study, but also to the fact that the risk of*E.canis*infection varies among foci according to local factors (e.g., vector population density and activity patterns).*Anaplasma platys*infection has been molecularly detected in kennelled dogs in central (23%) [48] and southern Italy (11.3%) [15] as well as in dogs showing clinical signs of VDBs in southern Italy (4.3%) [51]. In addition, co-infection by*E.canis*and*A.platys*may also occur as recorded in a dog population from southern Italy where 44.4% of individuals infected by*A.platys*were co-infected with *E.canis*[48].*Rhipicephalus sanguineus*, a proven vector of*E.canis*, has been suspected to act a vector of*A.platys*in Italy [14,15] and the high frequency of co-infection by*E. canis*and*A.platys*adds weight to this hypothesis. Similarly, high prevalence rates of anti-*R.conorii*antibodies (up to 74%) have been detected in dogs [51]. A study carried out in different Italian areas reported the occurrence of antibodies to*R.conorii*(56%) and*A.phagocytophilum*(3.7%) in dogs [51]. In a recent investigation carried out in southern Italy, 11.6% of 60 healthy dogs were positive for*Bartonella*spp. DNA [17]. Moreover, an uncultured*Bartonella*sp. (strain HMD) has been detected in five dogs, one of which was co-infected with*B. vinsonii berkhoffii*(genotypes II and III) [17]. These data indicate that dogs are exposed to multiple*Bartonella*species, some of which being of human health concern (i.e.,*B.vinsonii berkhoffii*).

There are limited data on*Babesia*protozoa infecting dogs in Italy [51,52,53,54]. In a serological survey carried out in central and northern Italy it was recorded a mean prevalence of 34% of anti-*Babesia* antibodies in dogs with a decreasing trend from central to northern areas [14]. In the same survey, it has been recorded that 'kennel life style' and the age class 25-48 months represent risk factors for *Babesia* spp. infection [14]. The occurrence of *Babesia gibsoni* in Italy has recently been supported by molecular data [52]. Again, molecular investigations on *Babesia* spp. in blood samples from dogs with clinical signs compatible with VBDs have shown that *B. canis* is mainly detected in northern Italy (29.1%) whereas *B. vogeli* was detected mainly in central and southern Italy (16.3%) [54].

While canine dirofilariosis by *D. repens* has been considered for a long time to be mainly diffused in southern regions, *D. immitis* is endemic in northern regions with prevalence rates ranging from 22 to 80% [55,56] in dogs untreated with prophylactic drugs. In the past 20 years, *D. immitis* showed a relevant prevalence increase in endemic areas [56] and it was also recorded outside the main endemic area of the Po Valley, in provinces of north-eastern Italy previously regarded as non-endemic [57]. Furthermore, *D. immitis* has also become endemic in central regions such as Tuscany and Umbria [56,58]. A recent study carried out on dogs from southern Italy reported the occurrence of *A. reconditum* (16.5%) followed by *D. repens* (1.4%) and *D. immitis* (0.5%) in Campania [59]. The occurrence of *D. immitis* and *D. repens* has been also recorded in Apulia and Calabria with prevalence rates up to 1.6% [33]. The spread of *D. repens* in northern Italy [55] and the new foci of *D. immitis* recently detected in southern regions [33] indicate that dogs are at risk of both *Dirofilaria* spp. throughout the whole country. Until now, *D. immitis* infection in cats has been diagnosed mostly in northern Italy where the prevalence is about 18% in pet cats [60].

The highest prevalence of canine thelaziosis has been reported in some areas of southern Italy (Basilicata region), reaching up to 60% in certain municipalities [61]. In this area, *T. callipaeda* has also been found among different wildlife species, which have been implicated as its reservoirs [62].

For long time, stable endemic foci of canine leishmaniosis have been reported in southern and central Italy, with seroprevalence rates reaching up to 53.1% in some foci [63]. In a study conducted in the Apulia region (southern Italy), the yearly incidence rate of canine leishmaniosis among 168 dogs (92 farm and 76 kennel dogs) was calculated to be 9.5%, being higher (13.1%) among kennel dogs [64]. On the basis of recent data on phlebotomine sand fly collections and on human and canine leishmaniosis, new foci of canine leishmaniosis have been detected in northern regions where the disease was previously regarded as non-endemic [29]. As in the case of canine leishmaniosis, many other vector-borne pathogens infecting dogs and cats in Italy are not only important from a veterinary standpoint but might also represent a public health concern.

VECTOR-BORNE PATHOGENS OF ZOONOTIC CONCERN AFFECTING CATS AND DOGS IN ITALY

Many vector-borne pathogens infecting cats and dogs in Italy may also be a threat to human health. These include many bacteria (e.g., *A. phagocytophilum*, *Bartonella henselae*, *B. vinsonii berkhoffii*, *B. burgdorferi*, *Coxiella burnetii*, *R. conorii*, and *R. felis*), nematodes (e.g., *D. immitis*, *D. repens*, and *T. callipaeda*), tapeworms (*D. caninum*), and *L. infantum*. In most of the cases, cats and dogs are unlikely to represent important reservoir hosts and their role in the transmission of these pathogens to humans is probably minor. On the other hand, cats and dogs may play a key role in the zoonotic cycle of transmission of some pathogens, such as *B. henselae* and *L. infantum*, respectively.

Dogs are primary hosts of vector-borne pathogens that may occasionally affect humans in Italy, including *D. immitis*, *D. repens* [65,66], and *T. callipaeda* [67]. Most importantly, dogs have been regarded as the main domestic reservoirs of *L. infantum* [29,68,69], which affects about 200 people annually in Italy [70]. Although *D. immitis* and *D. repens* have long been regarded as pathogens of veterinary concern, only recently these nematodes have been recognized as emerging zoonotic agents in Italy [65,66]. In particular, Italy is the first country in the world in the number of case reports (246 cases, from 1885 to 1999) of human dirofilariosis by *D. repens* [65] and dogs have been regarded as natural reservoirs of this filarid [71]. Similarly, the first cases of human thelaziosis in Europe have been diagnosed in the Piedmont region (northern Italy) in patients coming from north-western Italy and south-eastern France and now *T. callipaeda* has been recognized as an emerging parasite of humans in Italy as well as in other European countries [67]. Although dogs have also been found naturally infected by other pathogens (e.g., *A. phagocytophilum*, *C. burnetii*, and *R. conorii*) of public health concern in Italy [51], their role in the zoonotic transmission of these pathogens in this country is yet to be determined.

Cats have been found infected by emerging human pathogens, such as *B. henselae* and *Bartonella clarridgeiae* in Italy [72], and might be involved in the zoonotic transmission of these pathogens to man. The role of cats as additional domestic reservoirs of *L. infantum* has long been discussed [73] and a recent study has demonstrated that they can act as a source of *L. infantum* infection to *P. perniciosus* under laboratory conditions [32]. Recent studies have revealed high infection rates by *R. felis* (the causative agent of flea-borne spotted fever in humans) in fleas (*C. felis* and *C. canis*) collected from cats [26,27]. However, the role of cats in the epidemiology of flea-borne spotted fever is still to be determined [27].

Considering the zoonotic relevance of many vector-borne pathogens infecting cats and dogs in Italy, the control of VBDs they cause should not be only of veterinary concern but also a public health priority.

CONTROL AND PREVENTION OF VBDS AFFECTING CATS AND DOGS IN ITALY

The control of VBDs requires a holistic approach, considering the distribution, and the ecology of the vectors and of pathogens they may transmit and the infection progression in infected animals. The current strategies for the control of arthropod vectors in dogs and cats have recently been reviewed elsewhere [2,74]. The control of ectoparasites on dogs and cats is largely based on the use of acaricides and/or insecticides (e.g., amitraz, fipronil, and permethrins) that are available in a number of formulations (e.g., pour-on, spot-on, baths, and insecticide-impregnated collars). Most of the commercially available ectoparasiticides for use in dogs and cats have a long-lasting effect, being safe for pets, their owners, and the environment. Moreover, they can present killing and/or anti-feeding effects, which may prevent pets from being bitten by arthropods for long periods, and thus from becoming infected by vector-borne pathogens [74]. The use of insecticides in combination with insect growth regulators (e.g., chitin synthesis inhibitors and juvenile hormone analogues) increases their ovicidal and/or larvicidal activity. When applied on dogs and cats, insect growth regulators also act in their sleeping areas which may be highly infested by fleas [74]. Indeed, the control of arthropod vectors such as fleas and ticks should be performed by using an integrated approach focusing on animals, but also on the environment.

The prevention of VBDs can be achieved by means of systematic application of acaricides and/or insecticides, prophylactic administration of drugs, and vaccination. However, as discussed previously in this review, the occurrence and the risk of acquiring VBDs in Italy can vary according to the geographical and seasonal distribution of their respective vectors. Thus, the success of any prevention strategy depends on the appropriate use of commercially available tools, which should not only consider the manufacturer's instructions but also the available information on the vector ecology in a given area or region.

In Italy, the chemoprophylatic use of ivermectin against third- and fourth-stage larvae of*D.immitis*and*D.repens*has long been recommended for dogs in highly endemic areas of northern regions [75]. In southern Italy, the same approach should be recommended only for dogs travelling to highly endemic areas. Ectoparasiticides with different modes of action and targeting different vector developmental stages have the potential to protect dogs and cats against infection by different vector-borne pathogens. For instance, field studies have shown the efficacy of different commercially available products in reducing the infection rate by*E.canis*[48] and*L.infantum*in dogs [45,76]. In Italy, vaccines against canine babesiosis are commercially available and should be recommended for dogs living in or travelling to endemic areas. Vaccines are also available against Lyme disease caused by*B.burgdorferi*sensu stricto, but not against the other species. The decision to vaccinate against Lyme borreliosis should be made based on a risk assessment of the individual dog that includes information about where the dog lives and how often it frequents a tick-infested area. As far as cats, no studies are available in the literature about the prevention of VBDs.

FINAL CONSIDERATIONS AND PERSPECTIVES

Undoubtedly, the general picture of the VBDs affecting dogs and cats in Italy is complex mainly due to the limited amount of published data on ecology and distribution of arthropod vectors and the pathogens they transmit in northern, central and southern areas of the country. Gaps in our knowledge are even worse for vector-borne pathogens infecting cats; for some of which (e.g.,*R.felis*) almost no information is available.

Among arthropods parasitizing dogs and cats in Italy, ticks are the most important vectors of pathogens. Indeed, ticks are proven vectors of a large number of pathogens, present in a wide geographical distribution and, most importantly, they are active during the whole year. In particular, due to its high degree of adaptability to different microenvironments and its capability to occasionally feed on hosts other than dogs,*R. sanguineus*represents one of the major threats not only to dogs, but also to cats and humans [4,11]. Furthermore, the role of this tick as a putative vector of many species of other pathogens is a currently debated issue. For instance, the transmission of*Leishmania*parasites by*R.sanguineus*or by*C.felis*has received a renewed attention from the scientific community in recent years [10,77]. For instance, there is experimental evidence indicating that ticks could act as mechanical vectors of*L. infantum*via their ingestion [78] and a recent study has reported the detection of*L.infantum*kinetoplast DNA in salivary glands of*R.sanguineus*ticks collected from a dog living in a rural area in southern Italy [79]. Further studies are needed to assess the competence of ticks as vectors of*Leishmania*parasites from dog to dog which ultimately could open new perspectives for the control of this infection in areas where canine leishmaniosis is endemic but the primary vectors have not been found. Again, the retrieval of new strains or species of pathogens (e.g.,*Bartonella*sp. strain HMD) [17] in salivary glands of*R. sanguineus*in southern Italysuggests that unrecognized vector-borne pathogens may exist, which could complicate the diagnosis and management of other endemic VBDs in dogs and cats. Furthermore, considering the importance of*R. sanguineus*as vectors of*R.conorii*and the medical relevance of*R.conorii*infection in Italy [80,81], further research on the role of dogs in the epidemiology of Mediterranean spotted fever should be carried out.

As a priority, it is necessary to establish effective national surveillance systems based on a regional level that, using standardized diagnostic procedures and protocols, could provide a clear picture on vector-borne pathogens circulating among dogs and cats (both pet and free-roaming ones) in different Italian regions. Data on the distribution of arthropod vectors (e.g., regional maps) and the pathogens they transmit would not only allow the assessment of the risk of the introduction of exotic pathogens into non-endemic areas but, more practically, could provide information to veterinarians and pet owners on timing and protocols that should be chosen for preventing VBDs in different Italian regions. In this regard, it is crucial to translate that data from research into changed practices by veterinarians and to ensure owners' compliance.

An affordable and reliable control of canine and feline VBDs should also be part of a strategy for the management of zoonotic infections in order to reduce the risk of pathogen circulation between pet animals and humans. However, these actions cannot be disconnected from political initiatives to reduce the number of free-roaming dogs and cats in Italy and to improve vector control programs in public kennels. Finally, it is crucial to implement a permanent surveillance system to prevent the entry and exit of exotic vector-borne pathogens through dogs and cats travelling with their owners to and from Italy.

DECLARATIONS

Acknowledgements

The authors are grateful to Alessandra Torina (Istituto Zooprofilattico della Sicilia, Italy), Laia Solano-Gallego (The Royal Veterinary College, London, UK) and Rudi

Cassini (Università degli Studi di Padova, Italy), for sharing information on the distribution of vector-borne pathogens in Italy and to Riccardo Lia (Università degli Studi di Bari, Italy) for his assistance in figure preparation.

Competing interests

The authors declare that they have no competing interests.

Authors' contributions

DO and FD-T contributed equally to conceiving and writing this article.

REFERENCES

1. Otranto D, Dantas-Torres F, Breitschwerdt EB: Managing canine vector-borne diseases of zoonotic concern: part one. Trends Parasitol. 2009, 25: 157-163. 10.1016/j.pt.2009.01.003.
2. Otranto D, Dantas-Torres F, Breitschwerdt EB: Managing canine vector-borne diseases of zoonotic concern: part two. Trends Parasitol. 2009, 25: 228-235. 10.1016/j.pt.2009.02.005.
3. Trotz-Williams LA, Trees AJ: Systematic review of the distribution of the major vector-borne parasitic infections in dogs and cats in Europe. Vet Rec. 2003, 152: 97-105.
4. Manilla G: Fauna d'Italia Vol. XXXVI Acari-Ixodida. Edizioni Calderini, Bologna. 1998
5. Rinaldi L, Spera G, Musella V, Carbone S, Veneziano V, Iori A, Cringoli G: A survey of fleas on dogs in southern Italy. Vet Parasitol. 2007, 148: 375-378. 10.1016/j.vetpar.2007.06.036.
6. Romi R, Majori G: An overview of the lesson learned in almost 20 years of fight against the "tiger mosquito". Parassitologia. 2008, 50: 117-119.
7. Slater MR, Di Nardo A, Pediconi O, Dalla Villa P, Candeloro L, Alessandrini B, Del Papa S: Free-roaming dogs and cats in central Italy: Public perceptions of the problem. Prev Vet Med. 2008, 84: 27-47. 10.1016/j.prevetmed.2007.10.002.
8. WHO and WSPA: Guidelines for dog population management. Technical Report WHO/ZOO/90.166. 1990, World Health Organization and The World Society for the Protection of Animals
9. Solano-Gallego L, Trotta M, Caldin M, Furlanello T: Molecular survey of*Rickettsia*spp. in sick dogs in Italy. Zoonoses Public Health. 2008, 55: 521-525.
10. Dantas-Torres F: The brown dog tick,*Rhipicephalus sanguineus*(Latreille, 1806) (Acari: Ixodidae): from taxonomy to control. Vet Parasitol. 2008, 152: 173-185. 10.1016/j.vetpar.2007.12.030.
11. Maroli M, Khoury C, Frusteri L, Manilla G: Distribution of dog ticks (*Rhipicephalus sanguineus*Latreille, 1806) in Italy: a public health problem. Ann Ist Super Sanita. 1996, 32: 387-397.
12. Iori A, Di Paolo M: Acarological studies in two protected areas of Central Italy. Parassitologia. 1999, 41 (Suppl 1): 53-55.
13. Otranto D, Lia RP, Cantacessi C, Galli G, Paradies P, Mallia E, Capelli G: Efficacy of a combination of imidacloprid 10%/permethrin 50% versus fipronil 10%/(S)-methoprene 12%, against ticks in naturally infected dogs. Vet Parasitol. 2005, 130: 293-304. 10.1016/j.vetpar.2005.04.014.
14. Cassini R, Zanutto S, di Regalbono AF, Gabrielli S, Calderini P, Moretti A, Tampieri MP, Pietrobelli M: Canine piroplasmosis in Italy: epidemiological aspects in vertebrate and invertebrate hosts. Vet Parasitol. 2009, 165: 30-35. 10.1016/j.vetpar.2009.06.044.
15. Sparagano OA, de Vos AP, Paoletti B, Cammà C, de Santis P, Otranto D, Giangaspero A: Molecular detection of*Anaplasma platys*in dogs using polymerase chain reaction and reverse line blot hybridization. J Vet Diagn Invest. 2003, 15: 527-534.
16. Alberti A, Addis MF, Sparagano O, Zobba R, Chessa B, Cubeddu T, Parpaglia ML, Ardu M, Pittau M:*Anaplasma phagocytophilum*, Sardinia, Italy. Emerg Infect Dis. 2005, 11: 1322-1324.
17. Diniz PP, Billeter SA, Otranto D, De Caprariis D, Petanides T, Mylonakis ME, Koutinas AF, Breitschwerdt EB: Molecular documentation of*Bartonella*infection in dogs in Greece and Italy. J Clin Microbiol. 2009, 47: 1565-1567. 10.1128/JCM.00082-09.
18. Bremer WG, Schaefer JJ, Wagner ER, Ewing SA, Rikihisa Y, Needham GR, Jittapalapong S, Moore DL, Stich RW: Transstadial and intrastadial experimental transmission of*Ehrlichia canis*by male*Rhipicephalus sanguineus*. Vet Parasitol. 2005, 131: 95-105. 10.1016/j.vetpar.2005.04.030.
19. Socolovschi C, Bitam I, Raoult D, Parola P: Transmission of*Rickettsia conorii conorii*in naturally infected*Rhipicephalus sanguineus*. Clin Microbiol Infect. 15 (Suppl 2): 319-321. 10.1111/j.1469-0691.2008.02257.x.
20. Cinco M, Padovan D, Murgia R, Poldini L, Frusteri L, Pol van de I, Verbeek-De Kruif N, Rijpkema S, Maroli M: Rate of infection of*Ixodes ricinus*ticks with*Borrelia burgdorferi*sensu stricto,*Borrelia garinii*,*Borrelia afzelii*and group VS116 in an endemic focus of Lyme disease in Italy. Eur J Clin Microbiol Infect Dis. 1998, 17: 90-94.
21. Bertolotti L, Tomassone L, Tramuta C, Grego E, Amore G, Ambrogi C, Nebbia P, Mannelli A:*Borrelia lusitaniae*and spotted fever group rickettsiae in*Ixodes ricinus*(Acari: Ixodidae) in Tuscany, central Italy. J Med Entomol. 2006, 43: 159-165. 10.1603/0022-2585(2006)043[0159:BLASFG]2.0.CO;2.
22. Pecchioli E, Hauffe HC, Tagliapietra V, Bandi C, Genchi C, Rizzoli A: Genospecies of*Borrelia burgdorferi*sensu lato in*Ixodes ricinus*ticks from the Autonomous Province of Trento, Italy. Int J Med Microbiol. 2007, 297: 53-59. 10.1016/j.ijmm.2006.07.003.
23. Cerri D, Farina R, Andreani E, Nuvoloni R, Pedrini A, Cardini G: Experimental infection of dogs with*Borrelia burgdorferi*. Res Vet Sci. 1994, 57: 256-258.
24. Giudice E, Domina F, Britti D, Di Pietro S, Pugliese A: Clinical findings associated with*Borrelia*

*burgdorferi*infection in the dog. Vet Res Commun. 2003, 27 (Suppl 1): 767-770. 10.1023/B:VERC.0000014267.25428.32.

25. Manfredi MT, Dini V, Piacenza S, Genchi C: Tick species parasitizing people in an area endemic for tick-borne diseases in north-western Italy. Parassitologia. 1999, 41: 555-560.

26. Capelli G, Montarsi F, Porcellato E, Maioli G, Furnari C, Rinaldi L, Oliva G, Otranto D: Occurrence of*Rickettsia felis*in dog and cat fleas (*Ctenocephalides felis*) from Italy. Parasit Vectors. 2009, 2 (Suppl 1): S8-10.1186/1756-3305-2-S1-S8.

27. Maioli G, Horta MC, Ogrzewalska M, Capelli G, Souza SO, Richtzenhain LJ, Labruna MB: First detection of*Rickettsia felis*in*Ctenocephalides felis*fleas in Italy. Clin Microbiol Infect. 15 (Suppl 2): 222-223.

28. Maroli M, Bigliocchi F, Khoury C: Sandflies in Italy: observations on their distribution and methods for control. Parassitologia. 1994, 36: 251-264.

29. Maroli M, Rossi L, Baldelli R, Capelli G, Ferroglio E, Genchi C, Gramiccia M, Mortarino M, Pietrobelli M, Gradoni L: The northward spread of leishmaniasis in Italy: evidence from retrospective and ongoing studies on the canine reservoir and phlebotomine vectors. Trop Med Int Health. 2008, 13: 256-264.

30. Poli A, Abramo F, Barsotti P, Leva S, Gramiccia M, Ludovisi A, Mancianti F: Feline leishmaniosis due to*Leishmania infantum*in Italy. Vet Parasitol. 2002, 106: 181-191. 10.1016/S0304-4017(02)00081-X.

31. Vita S, Santori D, Aguzzi I, Petrotta E, Luciani A: Feline leishmaniasis and ehrlichiosis: serological investigation in Abruzzo region. Vet Res Commun. 2005, 29 (Suppl 2): 319-321. 10.1007/s11259-005-0071-8.

32. Maroli M, Pennisi MG, Di Muccio T, Khoury C, Gradoni L, Gramiccia M: Infection of sandflies by a cat naturally infected with*Leishmania infantum*. Vet Parasitol. 2007, 145: 357-360. 10.1016/j.vetpar.2006.11.009.

33. Otranto D, Capelli G, Genchi C: Changing distribution patterns of canine vector borne diseases in Italy: leishmaniosis vs. dirofilariosis. Parasit Vectors. 2009, 2 (Suppl 1): S2-10.1186/1756-3305-2-S1-S2.

34. Kramer L, Genchi C: Feline heartworm infection: serological survey of asymptomatic cats living in northern Italy. Vet Parasitol. 2002, 104: 43-50. 10.1016/S0304-4017(01)00602-1.

35. Dantas-Torres F, Lia RP, Barbuto M, Casiraghi M, Crovace A, Caligiani L, Genchi C, Otranto D: Ocular dirofilariosis by*Dirofilaria immitis*in a dog: first case report from Europe. J Small Anim Pract. 2009, 50: 667-669. 10.1111/j.1748-5827.2009.00846.x.

36. Otranto D, Brianti E, Cantacessi C, Lia RP, Máca J: Morphology, ecology and biological niches of the zoophilic fruitfly,*Phortica variegata*. Med Vet Entomol. 2006, 20: 358-364. 10.1111/j.1365-2915.2006.00643.x.

37. Otranto D, Lia RP, Cantacessi C, Testini G, Troccoli A, Shen JL, Wang ZX: Nematode biology and larval development of*Thelazia callipaeda*(Spirurida, Thelaziidae) in the drosophilid intermediate host in Europe and China. Parasitology. 2005, 131: 847-855. 10.1017/S0031182005008395.

38. Otranto D, Cantacessi C, Testini G, Lia RP:*Phortica variegata*is an intermediate host of*Thelazia callipaeda*under natural conditions: evidence for pathogen transmission by a male arthropod vector. Int J Parasitol. 2006, 36: 1167-1173. 10.1016/j.ijpara.2006.06.006.

39. Rogers DJ, Randolph SE: Climate change and vector-borne diseases. Adv Parasitol. 2006, 62: 345-381. 10.1016/S0065-308X(05)62010-6.

40. Beck W, Boch K, Mackensen H, Wiegand B, Pfister K: Qualitative and quantitative observations on the flea population dynamics of dogs and cats in several areas of Germany. Vet Parasitol. 2006, 137: 130-136. 10.1016/j.vetpar.2005.12.021.

41. Cancrini G, Scaramozzino P, Gabrielli S, Di Paolo M, Toma L, Romi R:*Aedes albopictus*and*Culex pipiens*implicated as natural vectors of*Dirofilaria repens*in central Italy. J Med Entomol. 2007, 44: 1064-1066. 10.1603/0022-2585(2007)44[1064:AAACPI]2.0.CO;2.

42. Cancrini G, Frangipane di Regalbono A, Ricci I, Tessarin C, Gabrielli S, Pietrobelli M:*Aedes albopictus*is a natural vector of*Dirofilaria immitis*in Italy. Vet Parasitol. 2003, 118: 195-202. 10.1016/j.vetpar.2003.10.011.

43. Ferroglio E, Maroli M, Gastaldo S, Mignone W, Rossi L: Canine leishmaniasis, Italy. Emerg Infect Dis. 2005, 11: 1618-1620.

44. Rossi E, Bongiorno G, Ciolli E, Di Muccio T, Scalone A, Gramiccia M, Gradoni L, Maroli M: Seasonal phenology, host-blood feeding preferences and natural*Leishmania*infection of*Phlebotomus perniciosus*(Diptera, Psychodidae) in a high-endemic focus of canine leishmaniasis in Rome province, Italy. Acta Trop. 2008, 105: 158-165. 10.1016/j.actatropica.2007.10.005.

45. Otranto D, Paradies P, Lia RP, Latrofa MS, Testini G, Cantacessi C, Mencke N, Galli G, Capelli G, Stanneck D: Efficacy of a combination of 10% imidacloprid/50% permethrin for the prevention of leishmaniasis in kennelled dogs in an endemic area. Vet Parasitol. 2007, 144: 270-278. 10.1016/j.vetpar.2006.09.012.

46. Killick-Kendrick R, Ready PD, Pampiglione S: Notes on the prevalence and host preferences of*Phlebotomus perfiliewi*in Emilia-Romagna, Italy. Ecologie des Leishmanioses. Colloques Internationaux du C.N.R.S. 239: 169-175.

47. Maroli M, Gradoni L, Gramiccia M, Pozio E: Man-bait catch of*Phlebotomus perniciosus*(Diptera, Psycodidae) [sic] in a human and canine leishmaniasis focus in central Italy. Parassitologia. 1984, 26: 269-272.

48. Otranto D, Paradies P, Testini G, Latrofa MS, Weigl S, Cantacessi C, Mencke N, de Caprariis D, Parisi A, Capelli G, Stanneck D: Application of 10% imidacloprid/50% permethrin to prevent*Ehrlichia canis*exposure in dogs under natural conditions. Vet Parasitol. 2008, 153: 320-328. 10.1016/j.vetpar.2008.02.008.

49. Cocco R, Sanna G, Cillara MG, Tola S, Ximenes L, Pinnaparpaglia ML, Masala G: Ehrlichiosis and rickettsiosis in a canine population of Northern Sardinia. Ann N Y Acad Sci. 2003, 990: 126-130. 10.1111/j.1749-6632.2003.tb07350.x.

50. Solano-Gallego L, Trotta M, Razia L, Furlanello T, Caldin M: Molecular survey of*Ehrlichia canis*and*Anaplasma phagocytophilum*from blood of dogs in Italy. Ann N Y Acad Sci. 2006, 1078: 515-518. 10.1196/annals.1374.101.

51. Torina A, Caracappa S: Dog tick-borne disease in Sicily. Parassitologia. 2006, 48: 145-147.

52. Trotta M, Carli E, Novari G, Furlanello T, Solano-Gallego L: Clinicopathological findings, molecular detection and characterization of*Babesia gibsoni*infection in a sick dog from Italy. Vet Parasitol. 2009, 165: 318-322. 10.1016/j.vetpar.2009.07.022.

53. Puccini A, Fasanella A, Lia RP: La babesiosi nel cane in Puglia e Basilicata. Ob & Doc Vet. 1998, 9: 480-484.

54. Solano-Gallego L, Trotta M, Carli E, Carcy B, Caldin M, Furlanello T:*Babesia canis canis*and*Babesia canis vogeli*clinicopathological findings and DNA detection by means of PCR-RFLP in blood from Italian dogs suspected of tick-borne disease. Vet Parasitol. 2008, 157: 211-221. 10.1016/j.vetpar.2008.07.024.

55. Rossi L, Pollono F, Meneguz PG, Gribaudo L, Balbo T: An epidemiological study of canine filarioses in north-west Italy: what has changed in 25 years?. Vet Res Commun. 1996, 20: 308-315. 10.1007/BF00366536.

56. Genchi C, Kramer LH, Prieto G: Epidemiology of canine and feline Dirofilariosis: a global view. Heartworm infection in humans and animals. Edited by: Simon F, Genchi C Salamanca. 2001, 121-133.

57. Poglayen G, Martini M, Bomben L, Roda R: An updating of the occurrence of canine heartworm disease in northern Italy. Vet Res Commun. 1996, 20: 303-307. 10.1007/BF00366535.

58. Piergili Fioretti D, Diaferia M, Grelloni V, Maresca C: Canine filariosis in Umbria: an update of the occurrence one year after the first observation of autochthonous foci. Parassitologia. 2003, 45: 79-83.

59. Cringoli G, Rinaldi L, Veneziano V, Capelli G: A prevalence survey and risk analysis of filariosis in dogs from the Mt. Vesuvius area of southern Italy. Vet Parasitol. 2001, 102: 243-252. 10.1016/S0304-4017(01)00529-5.

60. Genchi C, Venco L, Ferrari N, Mortarino M, Genchi M: Feline heartworm (*Dirofilaria immitis*) infection: a statistical elaboration of the duration of the infection and life expectancy in asymptomatic cats. Vet Parasitol. 2008, 158: 177-182. 10.1016/j.vetpar.2008.09.005.

61. Otranto D, Ferroglio E, Lia RP, Traversa D, Rossi L: Current status and epidemiological observation of*Thelazia callipaeda*(Spirurida, Thelaziidae) in dogs, cats and foxes in Italy: a "coincidence" or a parasitic disease of the Old Continent?. Vet Parasitol. 2003, 116: 315-325. 10.1016/j.vetpar.2003.07.022.

62. Otranto D, Dantas-Torres F, Mallia E, Digeronimo PM, Brianti E, Testini G, Traversa D, Lia RP:*Thelazia callipaeda*(Spirurida, Thelaziidae) in wild animals: Report of new host species and ecological implications. Vet Parasitol. 2009, 166: 262-267. 10.1016/j.vetpar.2009.08.027.

63. Brandonisio O, Carelli G, Ceci L, Consenti B, Fasanella A, Puccini V: Canine leishmaniasis in the Gargano Promontory (Apulia, South Italy). Eur J Epidemiol. 1992, 8: 273-276. 10.1007/BF00144813.

64. Paradies P, Capelli G, Cafarchia C, de Caprariis D, Sasanelli MT, Otranto D: Incidence of canine leishmaniasis in an endemic area of Southern Italy. J Vet Med B Infect Dis Vet Public Health. 2006, 53: 295-298.

65. Pampiglione S, Rivasi F, Angeli G, Boldorini R, Incensati R, Pastormerlo M, Pavesi M, Ramponi A: Dirofilariasis due to*Dirofilaria repens*in Italy, an emergent zoonosis: report of 60 new cases. Histopathology. 2001, 38: 344-354. 10.1046/j.1365-2559.2001.01099.x.

66. Pampiglione S, Rivasi F, Gustinelli A: Dirofilarial human cases in the Old World, attributed to*Dirofilaria immitis*: a critical analysis. Histopathology. 2009, 54: 192-204. 10.1111/j.1365-2559.2008.03197_a.x.

67. Otranto D, Dutto M: Human thelaziasis, Europe. Emerg Infect. 2008, 14: 647-649. 10.3201/eid1404.071205.

68. Ferroglio E, Romano A, Passera S, D'Angelo A, Guiso P, Ghiggi E, Bolla C, Trisciuoglio A, Biglino A: Dogs' parasite and zoonotic risk: from old to new "emergencies" in the North-West of Italy. Parassitologia. 2006, 48: 115-116.

69. Maresca C, Scoccia E, Barizzone F, Catalano A, Mancini S, Pagliacci T, Porrini M, Principato M, Venditti G, Grelloni V: A survey on canine leishmaniasis and phlebotomine sand flies in central Italy. Res Vet Sci. 2009, 87: 36-38. 10.1016/j.rvsc.2008.11.009.

70. Gradoni L, Gramiccia M, Scalone A: Visceral leishmaniasis treatment, Italy. Emerg Infect Dis. 2003, 9: 1617-20.

71. Pampiglione S, Villani M, Fioravanti ML, Rivasi F: La dirofilariasi umana nel sud Italia. III regione Molise. Pathologica. 1995, 87: 139-141.

72. Fabbi M, Vicari N, Tranquillo M, Pozzi C, Prati P, De Meneghi D, Bertoletti I, Lauzi S, Guiso P, Genchi C: Prevalence of*Bartonella henselae*in stray and domestic cats in different Italian areas: evaluation of the potential risk of transmission of*Bartonella*to humans. Parassitologia. 2004, 46: 127-129.

73. Mancianti F: Feline leishmaniasis: what's the epidemiological role of the cat?. Parassitologia. 2004, 46: 203-206.

74. Otranto D, Wall R: New strategies for the control of arthropod vectors of disease in dogs and cats. Med Vet Entomol. 2008, 22: 291-302. 10.1111/j.1365-2915.2008.00741.x.

75. Venco L, McCall JW, Guerrero J, Genchi C: Efficacy of long-term monthly administration of ivermectin on the progress of naturally acquired heartworm infections in dogs. Vet Parasitol. 2004, 124: 259-268. 10.1016/j.vetpar.2004.06.024.

76. Maroli M, Mizzoni V, Siragusa C, D'Orazi A, Gradoni L: Evidence for an impact on the incidence of canine leishmaniasis by the mass use of deltamethrin-impregnated dog collars in Southern Italy. Med Vet Entomol. 2001, 15: 358-363. 10.1046/j.0269-283x.2001.00321.x.

77. Ferreira MG, Fattori KR, Souza F, Lima VM: Potential role for dog fleas in the cycle of*Leishmania*spp. Vet Parasitol. 2009, 165: 150-154. 10.1016/j.vetpar.2009.06.026.

78. Coutinho MT, Bueno LL, Sterzik A, Fujiwara RT, Botelho JR, De Maria M, Genaro O, Linardi PM: Participation of*Rhipicephalus sanguineus*(Acari: Ixodidae) in the epidemiology of canine visceral leishmaniasis. Vet Parasitol. 2005, 128: 149-155. 10.1016/j.vetpar.2004.11.011.

79. Dantas-Torres F, Lorusso V, Testini G, Paiva-Cavalcanti M, Figueredo L, Stanneck D, Mencke N, Brandão-Filho S, Alves L, Otranto D: Detection of*Leishmania infantum*in*Rhipicephalus sanguineus*ticks from Brazil and Italy. Parasitol Res. 10.1007/s00436-010-1722-4.

80. Tringali G, Intonazzo V, Perna AM, Mansueto S, Vitale G, Walker DH: Epidemiology of boutonneuse fever in western Sicily. Distribution and prevalence of spotted fever group rickettsial infection in dog ticks (*Rhipicephalus sanguineus*). Am J Epidemiol. 1986, 123: 721-727.

81. Cascio A, Iaria C: Epidemiology and clinical features of Mediterranean spotted fever in Italy. Parassitologia. 2006, 48: 131-133.

82. Alberti A, Sparagano OA: Molecular diagnosis of granulocytic anaplasmosis and infectious cyclic thrombocytopenia by PCR-RFLP. Ann N Y Acad Sci. 2006, 1081: 371-378. 10.1196/annals.1373.055.

83. Lillini E, Macrì G, Proietti G, Scarpulla M: New findings on anaplasmosis caused by infection with*Anaplasma phagocytophilum*. Ann N Y Acad Sci. 2006, 1081: 360-370. 10.1196/annals.1373.053.

84. Ebani V, Cerri D, Fratini F, Ampola M, Andreani E: Seroprevalence of*Anaplasma phagocytophilum*in domestic and wild animals from central Italy. New Microbiol. 2008, 31: 371-375.

85. de la Fuente J, Torina A, Naranjo V, Nicosia S, Alongi A, La Mantia F, Kocan KM: Molecular characterization of*Anaplasma platys*strains from dogs in Sicily, Italy. BMC Vet Res. 2006, 2: 24-10.1186/1746-6148-2-24.

86. Torina A, Alongi A, Naranjo V, Scimeca S, Nicosia S, Di Marco V, Caracappa S, Kocan K, de la Fuente J: Characterization of*Anaplasma*infections in Sicily, Italy. Ann NY Acad Sci. 2008, 1149: 90-93. 10.1196/annals.1428.065.

87. Casapulla R, Baldi L, Avallone V, Sannino R, Pazzanese L, Mizzoni V: Canine piroplasmosis due to*Babesia gibsoni*: clinical and morphological aspects. Vet Rec. 1998, 142: 168-169.

88. Pinna Parpaglia ML, Masu G, Masala G, Porcu R, Zobba R, Pintori G, Cocco R: Seroprevalence of*Bartonella henselae*in dogs and cats in Sassari. Vet Res. 2007, 31 (Suppl 1): 317-320.

89. Bain O, Aeschlimann A, Chatelanat P: Presence, in ticks from the Geneva region, of infective larvae which may be related to the dog filaria*Dipetalonema grassii*. Ann Parasitol Hum Comp. 1982, 57: 643-646.

90. Giannetto S, Poglayen G, Gaglio G, Brianti E, Ferlazzo M, Giudice E:*Dipetalonema dracunculoides*(Nematoda: Onchocercidae): first report in dog in Italy. Parasite. 2003, 10: 188-

91. Tassi P, Widenhorn O: Research on intestinal parasitic diseases in dogs of the city of Rome. Parassitologia. 1977, 19: 43-57.

92. Sasanelli M, Paradies P, Lubas G, Otranto D, de Caprariis D: Atypical clinical presentation of coinfection with*Ehr lichia*,*Babesia*and*Hepatozoon*species in a dog. Vet Rec. 2009, 164: 22-23.

93. Solano-Gallego L, Kidd L, Trotta M, Di Marco M, Caldin M, Furlanello T, Breitschwerdt E: Febrile illness associated with*Rickettsia conorii*infection in dogs from Sicily. Emerg Infect Dis. 2006, 12: 1985-1988.

94. Cabassi CS, Farnetti E, Casali B, Taddei S, Donofrio G, Galvani G, Cavirani S: Isolation of*Bartonella henselae*from domestic cats in an Italian urban area. New Microbiol. 2002, 25: 253-257.

95. Ciceroni L, Fabbi M, Ciarrocchi S, Pinto A, Ciervo A, Kasten RW, Chomel BB: Characterization of the first*Bartonella henselae*strain isolated from a cat in Italy. Comp Immunol Microbiol Infect Dis. 2002, 25: 217-228. 10.1016/S0147-9571(02)00013-9.

96. Cornegliani L, Vercelli A, Bo S, Colombo S: Two cases of cutaneous nodular dirofilariasis in the cat. J Small Anim Pract. 2003, 44: 316-318. 10.1111/j.1748-5827.2003.tb00161.x.

97. Poglayen G, Traldi G, Capelli G, Genchi C: Gastrointestinal parasitic fauna of cats in the cities of Bologna, Florence and Milan. Parassitologia. 1985, 27: 297-302.

98. Tarello W: Identification and treatment of*Dipetalonema grassii*microfilariae in a cat from central Italy. Vet Rec. 2004, 155: 565-566.

99. Bayliss DB, Morris AK, Horta MC, Labruna MB, Radecki SV, Hawley JR, Brewer MM, Lappin MR: Prevalence of*Rickettsia*species antibodies and*Rickettsia*species DNA in the blood of cats with and without fever. J Feline Med Surg. 2009, 11: 266-270. 10.1016/j.jfms.2008.06.007.

CHAPTER 28

CANINE BABESIOSIS: FROM MOLECULAR TAXONOMY TO CONTROL

Peter J Irwin

INTRODUCTION

Canine babesiosis is a common and clinically significant tick-borne haemoprotozoan disease with a worldwide distribution. *Babesia* species are often referred to as piroplasms, a collective term for phenotypically similar protozoan parasites that utilise mammalian erythrocytes in their life cycle. Piroplasms of domestic animals encompass two main genera, *Babesia* and *Theileria*, and have been subject of intense research interest and molecular-based re-classification during the last 10 years. In dogs, infection by these haemoparasites results in a wide range of clinical presentations; from subclinical disease to serious illness characterised by fever, pallor, jaundice, splenomegaly, weakness and collapse associated with intra- and extravascular haemolysis, hypoxic injury, systemic inflammation, thrombocytopenia and pigmenturia [1, 2, 3]. Although canine babesiosis is recognised as a tick-borne disease, transmitted by a variety of well-described Ixodid vectors around the world, *Babesia gibsoni* is an emerging disease with molecular evidence of clonal expansion due to non-vectored transmission by blood exchange during fighting and biting [4, 5, 6]. Recent research into canine babesiosis has focussed on determining the taxonomic status of well recognised and newly discovered canine piroplasms, developing improved diagnostic methods, investigating aspects of pathophysiology and searching for improved chemotherapeutic and immunoprophylactic protocols.

TAXONOMY AND MOLECULAR PHYLOGENY

The classification of *Babesia* spp. places them in order Piroplasmida within the phylum Apicomplexa. Two morphologically distinct forms of the erythrocytic stage in the canine host were recognised in early studies that led to the naming of the larger form, measuring approximately 3–5 μm as *B. canis*, and the smaller (1–3 μm) as *B. gibsoni*. Despite painstaking observation of the parasites in blood films by many early researchers, further understanding of the taxonomic classification of these parasites was hampered for the best part of one hundred years by the fact that within these general size ranges, their morphological features did not permit further differentiation. The first suggestion that all *B. canis* isolates were not identical species came from the German protozoologist Eduard Reichenow who recognised differences in pathogenicity of "*B. canis*" isolates from France and North Africa (these were most likely parasites that are currently known as *B. (canis) canis* and *B. (canis) vogeli*, respectively) [7, 8]. Further clarification did not come until the late 1980s with the advent of molecular tools for phylogenetic studies; molecular genotyping of canine piroplasms has resulted currently in the identification of four large and at least four

Citation: Peter J Irwin, Canine babesiosis: from molecular taxonomy to control, DOI: 10.1186/1756-3305-2-S1-S4.

small parasites, but it is likely that new species will be added as further isolates are characterised.

"*Babesia canis*" was reclassified into three sub-species (*B. canis canis*, *B. canis rossi* and *B. canis vogeli*) on the basis of cross-immunity, serological testing, vector specificity and molecular phylogeny; these parasites are now considered to be separate species in their own right [9, 10] (Table 1). A fourth 'large' (as yet unnamed)*Babesia* sp. has been described recently in a number of dogs with clinical signs and haematological parameters consistent with babesiosis in North Carolina [11, 12]. With regard to small piroplasms, three genetically and clinically distinct species are currently recognised to cause disease in dogs; *Babesia gibsoni*,*Babesia conradae* (reported in dogs in the western United States and described in original reports as "*B. gibsoni*") [13, 14], and a *Babesia microti*-like piroplasm (named *Theileria annae*) [15, 16].

Table 1: Piroplasm species of domestic dogs.

Size	Species	Synonyms	Vector in dog	Geographic Distribution	Comments
Large	*Babesia vogeli*	*Babesia canis vogeli*	*Rhipicephalus sanguineus*	Wide range:Tropical, subtropical and Mediterranean regions	
	Babesia canis	*Babesia canis canis*	*Dermacentor*spp.	Europe	
	Babesia rossi	*Babesia canis rossi*	*Haemaphysalis elliptica*(formerly *H. leachi*)	Sub-Saharan Africa, South Africa	
	*Babesia*sp.	Un-named large*Babesia* sp., North Carolina isolate	Unknown	North Carolina, USA	
Small	*Babesia gibsoni*	*Babesia gibsoni* Asia strain	*Haemaphysalis longicornis*	Asia including Japan, sporadic occurrence worldwide	Outside Asia this infection is often associated with Pit Bull Terriers and other fighting dogs
	Theileria annae	*Babesia microti*-like Spanish isolate/piroplasm/agent	*Ixodes hexagonus*(putative)	Spain, Portugal	
	*Theileria*sp.	Un-named *Theileria* sp., South African *Theileria*sp.	Unknown	South Africa	Molecular detection only
	Theileria annulata		Unknown	Africa, Europe, Asia	Molecular detection only
	Theileria equi	*Babesia equi*	Unknown	Africa, Europe, Asia	Molecular detection only

In addition, three *Theileria* species have been isolated in a small number of dogs' blood in Europe (*Theileria (Babesia) equi* and *Theileria annulata*) [17, 18] and from 82 dogs in South Africa (unnamed *Theileria* sp. related to an isolate obtained from antelope) [19] (Table 1). Until more information is available the competence of the dog as a host for these piroplasms is uncertain; the clinical correlation for these organisms is unknown, and neither intraerythrocytic nor extraerythrocytic stages have yet been visualised.

As with many taxonomic debates, the classification of canine piroplasms has not been without disagreement among parasitologists, especially concerning nomenclature of the smaller parasites. Furthermore, data from molecular analysis of the mammalian host stages have far outstripped our understanding of the life-cycle features of these organisms, notably identification of their vectors and other important biological data. Under light microscopy the intraerythrocytic stage of *Babesia* spp. is indistinguishable from *Theileria* spp. (In cats*Cytauxzoon* is also similar in appearance, but to date there has been no report of this genus affecting canines.) Historically these two genera, *Babesia* and *Theileria*, are separated on the basis of certain life-cycle stages and transovarial passage within the tick vector [20], yet to date the only piroplasm of companion animals known to have an extra-erythrocytic (schizogony) stage to its life cycle is *Cytauxzoon felis* in the cat.

The controversy focuses on whether all small canine piroplasm species should be classified as *Babesia* spp. or whether *Theileria* spp. infect dogs as part of their natural life cycle. To inform the debate, molecular studies of canine piroplasms have predominantly utilised the small subunit ribosomal 18S gene locus to infer phylogenetic relationships, favoured for its conserved nature and predictable rate of mutation, but other rRNA loci, *cytochrome b*, and genes encoding the heat-shock proteins have been also utilised for this purpose [6, 18,21].

As noted above, pre-erythrocytic parasite (schizont) stages in lymphocytes or macrophages, a defining feature of *Theileria*, have not been observed in dogs. However, the formation of distinct tetrad forms (the "Maltese cross"), considered as a feature of both *Theileria* spp. and *Babesia microti*, has been described in *Babesia conradae* [14, 22]. *Babesia conradae* appears to be most closely related to a group of piroplasms found in free-ranging ruminants (deer and sheep) and isolated from humans in the western United States – the 'western clade' [22]. This group is phylogenetically distinct from *Babesia microti*, a rodent piroplasm with a wide distribution throughout the Holarctic ecozone (see review [23]) in which schizogony in lymphocytes has been reported [24]. The piroplasm species reported in dogs from northern Spain forms into a clade with*Babesia microti* and was given the name *Theileria annae* [15], but is often referred to as the "*Babesia microti*-like" piroplasm or agent, or "Spanish isolate". Indisputably *Theileria* species (*Theileria annulata* and *Theileria equi*) have been detected in canine blood [17, 18] and the most recently reported canine piroplasm, in South Africa [19], is also phylogenetically aligned with recognised *Theileria* spp., yet as stated previously their significance is unclear at the present time.

GEOGRAPHICAL DISTRIBUTION

The distribution maps for canine vector-borne diseases are continually changing as new information about parasite infections and ranges comes to light. In general it may be useful to consider two levels of regional prevalence and incidence for specific diseases; those regions where the specific parasite is well established (i.e., endemic) and clinically recognised; and those regions where sporadic autochthonous infections or cases associated with travelling dogs have been reported.

Established Endemic Ranges

The established ranges for canine piroplasms are listed in Table 1; comprehensive and up-to-date canine vector-borne disease maps of Europe, and East and Southeast Asia are available [25]. As would be expected, the geographical distribution of these organisms is delineated largely by the ecological ranges of their vector ticks. Interestingly this generalisation seems not to apply to *Babesia gibsoni*, whose rapid recent global dispersion is now proposed to have been achieved predominantly by direct dog-to-dog transmission under unique ownership and management practices, without involvement of a vector (see later discussion) [4, 5].

Babesia vogeli is the most widespread canine piroplasm due to the cosmopolitan nature of its host, the brown dog tick *Rhipicephalus sanguineus* (Table 1). *Babesia vogeli* has a truly worldwide distribution throughout tropical and subtropical regions and extending into cooler latitudes where it potentially occurs alongside (and may be confused with) the other large *Babesia* spp. *Babesia canis* (*sensu strictu*) is transmitted by*Dermacentor* spp. and has been increasingly recognised throughout central Europe when it was once thought to be confined to France. *Babesia rossi* is the other African *Babesia* (with *B. vogeli* and *B. gibsoni*); originally recognised only in South Africa but has been reported recently in other regions of the African continent including Nigeria [26] and Sudan [27] where its vector ticks (*Haemaphysalis* spp.) are enzootic (Table 1).

The small canine piroplasm with the greatest geographical distribution is undoubtedly *B. gibsoni*. The type-species is referred to as the "Asia strain", reflecting its original molecular identification from a number of different southern, eastern and southeastern Asian countries. However, in the last 10 years *B. gibsoni*infections have been reported in many countries outside Asia, in American Pit Bull Terrier-type dogs predominantly, and there is now convincing evidence that these cases have arisen due to biting and fighting between infected and non-infected dogs [4, 28]. Gene sequence conservation has been noted in the ITS and 18S gene of *B. gibsoni* isolates originating in many disparate regions of the world [6, 22, 29]. This observation has led to the intriguing hypothesis that the lack of genetic diversity in *B. gibsoni* is a result of the absence of sexual reproduction (sporogony) in the tick; in other words a clonal expansion of a single strain is occurring within a susceptible host population. Therefore the dogs themselves are the reservoir for *B. gibsoni*, specific fighting dogs in particular, and not an endemic species of tick. Due to the worldwide popularity of this and similar breeds, it is speculated that *Babesia gibsoni* will be reported eventually from all countries where (usually illegal) dog fighting is practiced.

The three most recently characterised small piroplasm species of dogs occur, as previously mentioned, in the western United States, specifically California (*Babesia conradae*), southern Africa (*Theileria* sp.) and the Iberian peninsular (*Theileria annae*), where the latter is thought to be transmitted by *Ixodes hexagonus*. The vectors for *Babesia conradae* and the South African *Theileria* sp. are currently unknown and apart from a single case report of *Theileria annae* in the USA [28], these piroplasms have not been reported outside these fairly localised geographical boundaries.

Autochthonous Infections and other Single Infection Reports

Autochthonous infection refers to discovery of an infection that has originated in the place where it is found, usually in the context of a new, or unexpected finding in a location where the infection is generally not considered to occur. In the case of babesiosis, autochthonous cases are most likely to arise when dogs have come into contact with infected vectors which may themselves have been introduced by hosts returning from vector-endemic areas, or by extension of the vector range due to ecological changes. There have been a number of reports of autochthonous babesiosis and piroplasmosis in northern Europe (where vector-borne diseases have been considered unusual or exotic) and such cases have raised concern among the local veterinary and pet-owning fraternities. The importance of collecting travel history as an integral step during a veterinary consultation has been emphasised, together with concern about the risks of disease spread associated with deregulated pet travel, particularly in mainland Europe and the UK. The history of being a hunting dog or extensive rural exposure is a risk factor for canine babesiosis in Europe [30].

DIAGNOSIS OF BABESIOSIS

Microscopy remains the simplest and most accessible diagnostic test for most veterinarians and during acute infections microscopy is reasonably sensitive for detecting intraerythrocytic parasites in Giemsa or Wright's stained blood smears. Differentiation between large and small piroplasms is also relatively simple. Moreover, microscopy is still the only viable option available to veterinarians in many parts of the developing world where babesiosis is endemic. With large *Babesia* species at least, sampling from capillary beds (ear tip, toe nail) or examination of cells from beneath the buffy coat of a haematocrit tube may improve the probability of finding parasites [31, 32].

The diagnosis of piroplasmosis in chronically infected and carrier dogs however remains a significant challenge due to very low, often intermittent parasitaemias. Failure to detect *Babesia/Theileria* parasites in animals with hemolytic anaemia or thrombocytopenia has led to an incorrect diagnosis in documented cases, often when the clinical suspicion of babesiosis was also low. Given the possibility of direct horizontal transmission of *Babesia gibsoni*, veterinary clinicians should always ascertain whether the patient has been bitten by any other dog in the preceding 4–8 weeks, irrespective of its breed [4, 28].

Molecular diagnosis – conventional PCR and other Methods

Although PCR has greatly increased the sensitivity and specificity of parasite detection and is well suited to epidemiological and phylogenetic studies, access to molecular techniques for routine clinical diagnosis of babesiosis is still restricted to relatively few laboratories worldwide. Ribosomal RNA genes 18S, 5.8S, 28S and the internal transcribed spacer (ITS) sequences have been used for conventional PCR, but some researchers have chosen other loci such as the p18/BgTRAP [33]. Since parasite morphology is a poor guide to speciation, modifications of the PCR have been utilised to rapidly differentiate between piroplasm species; PCR-RFLP and nested PCR have been reported to differentiate *B. vogeli* and *B. gibsoni* in Australia [34], and between the large babesial species [9] and *B. gibsoni* in endemic regions [35]. In a clinicopathological study of large *Babesia*spp. infections in dogs in Italy using PCR-RFLP, *Babesia canis* was detected in 34/164 and *Babesia vogeli* in 11/164 dogs. Although a distinct geographical difference in the incidence of these infections is noted [30], many of the dogs with *B. canis* infection had recently returned from hunting trips in Eastern Europe. Further refinement in primer design was reported recently to clearly separate amplicons of 342 bp, 546 bp, and 746 bp target fragments of *B. canis rossi, B. canis vogeli, B. canis canis*, respectively [36]. Loop-mediated isothermal amplification (LAMP) was found to have advantages of speed and specificity for detecting *B. gibsoni*infections in Japan [37] and reverse-line blot (RLB) hybridisation was applied in epidemiological studies of arthropod-borne haemopathogens of dogs and cats in Trinidad [38] and dogs in Africa [19]. Real-time PCR enables quantification of pathogen levels within blood and tissue samples; the amount of final PCR product can be used to deduce the starting number of target molecules and infer parasite levels within a host. Quantitative PCR (qPCR) was used in an experimental infection of 3 dogs with *B. gibsoni* that concluded that the methodology might be adapted to the determination of vaccine or chemotherapeutic efficacy, or the elucidation of immunological responses [39]. Furthermore, a number of these PCR methods have been applied to filter-paper technologies such as FTA cards (Whatman Bioscience) and IsoCode Stix (Schleicher and Scheull) for ease of transport of samples to distant laboratories and for epidemiological and other diagnostic studies [34, 40]. Long-term storage and archival qualities of this methodology have not been investigated [40].

Whereas the detection limit of light microscopy is approximately 0.001% parasitaemia, PCR is capable of detecting parasite loads in the region of 50 organisms/ml [35] and 9 parasites/μl [39]. Yet despite its extraordinary sensitivity, PCR will clearly not detect target DNA when there are no organisms within the sample. “False negative” results may occur in chronic babesiosis and it is very important to recognise this limitation when screening potential carriers and other asymptomatic dogs such as blood donors. The ability of PCR to detect infected dogs in such situations, with and without treatment, has been investigated [41, 42]. In one study [42] clinical parameters, haematology, serologic titer (by IFAT) and the presence of *Babesia* DNA was monitored on a daily basis after experimental infection. All dogs (n = 3) made a full clinical recovery, as judged by normal clinical signs, absence of splenic enlargement, a normal haemogram and absence of piroplasms on microscopic examination by 30–50 days after peak parasitaemia. During this period of clinical normality, babesial DNA was inconsistently detected. This suggests a very low, fluctuating parasitaemia in these dogs, possibly analogous to chronic, asymptomatic natural infection.

The ability of PCR to detect parasite DNA in chronically infected animals can be improved by testing on more than one occasion, but the use of serology as an alternative, complementary diagnostic test is advisable in these situations [42, 43].

Serological testing – the IFAT and ELISA

Immunofluorescent antibody testing (IFAT) has been the most widely supported serological diagnostic test for canine babesiosis for the last 30 years [44, 45]. However, poor specificity due to cross-reactions between*Babesia* spp. and with other apicomplexan parasites, operator subjectivity and its inadequacy for large-scale screening have all been limiting factors [46]. Recent research by several groups in Japan directed towards finding specific immunodominant *Babesia gibsoni* antigens for use in recombinant protein enzyme-linked immunosorbent assays (ELISA) – and potential vaccine candidates in the future – has identified numerous promising compounds [46, 47, 48, 49, 50, 51, 52]. Thrombospondin-related adhesive proteins (TRAPs) comprise a group of highly conserved functional proteins identified in apicomplexan parasites, mooted to be associated with merozoite motility and invasion, and capable of inducing a host antibody response [49]. An ELISA using recombinant BgTRAP was reported to be more sensitive than other ELISAs using recombinant antigens rBgP50, rBgSA1, and rBgP32 [43], and Konishi et al. (2008) utilised a BgTRAP ELISA to test 1,206 randomly selected non-fighting breed dogs in Japan to test for exposure to *B. gibsoni* [53]. These authors reported higher infection rates in western Japan and concluded that having excluded fighting dogs, a history of tick (*Haemaphysalis longicornis*) exposure was a significant risk factor for anti-babesial antibody detection, thus demonstrating two distinct epidemiological patterns of *B. gibsoni* infection in that country.

A second major limitation of serological tests is their inability to differentiate acute from chronic infections, and interpretation of a positive titre is somewhat problematic for clinicians working in regions that are endemic for babesiosis. Nevertheless, for *B. gibsoni* in the USA and Australia, where cases are sporadic, the IFAT is a useful tool for detection of infected dogs, especially if combined with PCR [31, 38].

PATHOPHYSIOLOGY

The severity of babesiosis in dogs and cats ranges from subclinical infection, the development of mild anaemia to widespread organ failure and death. The critical determinant of this variable pathogenesis is the piroplasm species, yet other factors such as the age and immune status of the host and concurrent infections or illness also play a role. All species (Table 1) may cause pyrexia, anorexia, splenomegaly, anaemia and thrombocytopenia. Direct parasite-induced red-cell damage, increased osmotic fragility of infected cells, oxidative and secondary immune-mediated injury of the erythrocyte membrane result in a combination of intravascular and extravascular haemolysis.

The clinical features of babesiosis have been reviewed elsewhere [1, 2, 3]. In broad terms it is generally agreed that the least pathogenic of the well-recognised canine piroplasm species is *Babesia vogeli*, at least in adult dogs, and the most virulent is *Babesia rossi* in Africa [1, 30, 31]. With *Babesia rossi* infections a large proportion of dogs develop complications, some of which (hepatopathy, immune-mediated haemolysis) typically extend hospital stay but do not affect mortality if treated appropriately, while others (haemoconcentration, neurological signs, acute renal failure and pulmonary oedema) require early, aggressive and intensive therapy and carry a poor prognosis [32]. In contrast, *Babesia vogeli* is often subclinical (except in puppies less than 3–4 months old, in which infection may be fatal); it is occasionally observed in blood films of dogs with other primary disease or receiving medical treatment (e.g., immunosuppression or chemotherapy) or surgery (notably splenectomy), and in these potentially immunocompromised individuals the appearance of the parasite may be inconsequential to the outcome (and may not even warrant treatment).

The pathogenicity of *Babesia canis, Babesia gibsoni, Theileria annae* and *Babesia conradae* is moderate to severe in dogs, but it should be stressed again that a wide range of clinical signs of varying severity can be observed in individuals. *Babesia conradae* is considered to be more pathogenic than *B. gibsoni*, resulting in higher parasitaemias and more severe anaemia [14]. In Spain, *Theileria annae* infection is associated with severe haemolysis and azotaemia [16]. The unnamed *Babesia* sp. from North Carolina has been associated with non-specific illness (lethargy and anorexia), pigmenturia and mild fever, predominantly in splenectomised dogs [54]. Laboratory findings have included mild anaemia and severe thrombocytopenia, similar to *Babesia vogeli* infections [54].

The potential for renal involvement in dogs with babesiosis has received attention in recent years, with hypoxaemia, haemoglobinuric nephropathy and glomerulonephritis all considered possible mechanisms and supported by histological studies [55]. A clinicopathological study of *Theileria annae* infection in Northwest Spain reported 36% dogs (n = 58) were azotaemic at the time of diagnosis and that these dogs had a 10-fold higher risk of death from piroplasmosis than those that were not azotaemic [56]. Unfortunately neither urine-specific gravity nor urine osmolality was reported in these dogs, but elevated urine protein: creatinine ratios, hypoalbuminaemia and hypercholesterolaemia in affected dogs led the authors to suggest that glomerular injury was occurring and that renal failure was most likely a feature of *Theileria annae* infection [56]. In contrast, study of azotaemia associated with *B. rossi* infection concluded that urea and creatinine were unreliable indicators of renal damage or acute renal failure in acute babesiosis [57, 58]. Mortality of *B. rossi* was significantly associated with high cortisol and high ACTH concentrations and with low T4 and fT4 concentrations in a recent study investigating endocrine markers of disease [59].

The clinical consequences of chronic babesial infection are unclear and while most dogs appear to tolerate this state of premunity with few ill effects, theoretically they remain at risk of developing immune-mediated complications and recrudescence of clinical disease (and parasitaemia) if immunocompromised at a later time. Chronic infection may be inconsequential in some dogs and may be even beneficial for hosts living in endemic regions by protecting them from further disease [60].

RECENT ADVANCES IN THE TREATMENT AND PREVENTION OF BABESIOSIS

Despite a plethora of anecdotal reports and uncontrolled experimental data, there is a paucity of scientifically robust evidence regarding the efficacy of drugs that have been used to treat canine babesiosis over the last 100 years. Early treatment studies were hampered by the need to rely on clinical signs and blood films to determine parasite clearance. More recently the limitations have been the cost of establishing controlled infections and the relatively small numbers of experimental dogs permitted by animal ethics committees. In order to determinate the efficacy of an anti-piroplasm drug with reasonable confidence, necropsy-obtained tissues from all organs need to be tested by validated PCR at the end of the experiment; clearance of the parasite DNA from peripheral blood alone is insufficient evidence of cure.

Imidocarb dipropionate and diminazine aceturate are widely used anti-piroplasm drugs, but other compounds that have been used for many years and have enjoyed varying degrees of success in managing the clinical signs of piroplasmosis include quinuronium sulphate, trypan blue, pentamidine, phenamidine and parvaquone. National registration authorities have restricted access to some of these drugs in certain countries, and some, notably the diamidine derivative diminazine, are associated with a high rate of toxic side effects. At best these drugs result in amelioration of clinical signs; rarely do they achieve true sterilisation of the infection.

The successful treatment of the small piroplasm infections, notably *B. gibsoni*, has been especially challenging. Clindamycin at 25 mg/kg q12 h PO induced morphological changes and reduced the parasitaemia in an experimental infection compared with untreated controls, but did not eliminate the parasite, and piroplasms were still observed in low numbers 108 days after infection [61]. Recently, the apparent cure of *B. gibsoni* was reported in 3 out of 4 experimental dogs that had not responded to repeated diminazine treatment, with a combination of clindamycin, metronidazole (15 mg/kg q12 h PO) and doxycycline (5 mg/kg q12 h PO) [62]. Successful treatment in these dogs was determined by a combination of normal clinical signs and the absence of *B. gibsoni* DNA in peripheral blood. More recently, a combination of azithromycin (10 mg/kg q24 h PO) and atovaquone (13.3 mg/kg q8 h PO) for 10 days has been used for treating *B. gibsoni* and appears to combine reasonable clinical efficacy with great safety [41]; the expense of atovaquone limits widespread acceptance of this therapy where it is most needed, in Asia. Cheaper formulations of atovaquone with proguanil cause an unacceptably high incidence of gastrointestinal side effects in dogs. Unfortunately this drug combination also does not result in a cure in some dogs, and rapid development of resistance to atovaquone caused by mutation of the *cytochrome b* gene has been reported [42, 63].

In vitro studies of numerous rainforest plant extracts for their antibabesial properties have been published recently [64, 65, 66], but to date no clinical trials have been reported with these compounds. A *Haemaphysalis longicornis* tick-derived peptide reduced parasitaemias of *B. microti* in BALB/c mice and directly kills *B. gibsoni*parasites in ticks [67].

Prevention of babesiosis, as with any tick-transmitted disease, is best achieved by removing the possibility of exposure to the vector. This is rarely achievable in endemic areas despite attentive ectoparasite control.

Several drugs have been investigated for their prophylactic potential against babesiosis, yet none has been consistently reliable in this regard. Experimental studies suggested that a single dose of imidocarb dipropionate (6 mg/kg) protects dogs from *B. canis* challenge for up to 8 weeks [68] and that doxycycline at 5 mg/kg/day ameliorates the severity of disease when challenged with virulent *B. canis* [69].

In vitro culture-derived soluble parasite antigens (SPA) have been used to protect dogs in European against *B. canis* (*sensu strictu*) challenge in a commercially available vaccine since the 1980s, and it was reported in one study that the incidence of babesiosis decreased from 16% to near zero in populations of vaccinated dogs living in endemic regions over the three-year period of study (reviewed in [70]). However, variable efficacy of the SPA vaccine during homologous challenge has been attributed to strain variation [71] and it was clear from early studies that *B. canis*-derived SPA did not protect dogs from heterologous challenge with *B. rossi* [72], which led to the development of a vaccine containing a mixture of SPA from both European *B. canis* and South African *B. rossi* that offered greater protection against heterologous challenge [73]. Current research is also conducted in Japan in search of suitable immunodominant and protective antigens for use in vaccines against*Babesia gibsoni* [74].

CONCLUSION

Canine babesiosis/piroplasmosis remains as a significant disease that despite considerable advances during the last decade in our knowledge and understanding of the pathogens themselves, the intricacies of transmission, and their pathophysiological mechanisms, still poses significant diagnostic and therapeutics challenges for veterinary practitioners around the world. New species of piroplasm will almost certainly be described, and the geographical range of established piroplasms will expand due to international movements of dogs and expansion of vector tick habitats. The challenges for the researchers are to provide practitioners with readily accessible and accurate diagnostic tools, safer and more efficacious anti-babesial drugs, and the "Holy Grail" of this applied research – effective immunologicals for the prevention or, at least, amelioration of the clinical signs of canine babesiosis.

DECLARATIONS

Acknowledgements

This article is published as part of *Parasites & Vectors* Volume 2 Supplement 1, 2009: Proceedings of the 4th International Canine Vector-Borne Disease Symposium. The full contents of the supplement are available online at http://www.parasitesandvectors.com/supplements/2/S1.

Publication of the supplement has been sponsored by Bayer Animal Health GmbH.

Competing Interests

The author declares that they have no competing interests.

REFERENCES

1. Lobetti RG: Canine babesiosis. Comp Cont Ed Pract Vet. 1998, 20: 418-431.
2. Irwin PJ: Babesiosis and Cytauxzoonosis. Arthropod-borne infectious diseases of the dog and cat. Edited by: Shaw SE, Day MJ. 2005, London: Manson Publishing/ The Veterinary Press, 63-77.
3. Jacobsen LS: The South African form of severe and complicated canine babesiosis: clinical advances 1994–2004. Vet Parasitol. 2006, 138: 126-139. 10.1016/j.vetpar.2006.01.047.
4. Birkenheuer AJ, Correa MT, Levy MG, Breitschwerdt EB: Geographic distribution of babesiosis among dogs in the United States and association with dog bites: 150 cases (2000–2003). J Am Vet Med Assoc. 2005, 227: 942-947. 10.2460/javma.2005.227.942.
5. Jefferies R, Ryan UM, Jardine J, Broughton DK, Robertson ID, Irwin PJ: Blood, bull terriers and babesiosis: further evidence for direct transmission of *Babesia gibsoni* in dogs. Aust Vet J. 2007, 85: 459-463. 10.1111/j.1751-0813.2007.00220.x.
6. Bostrom B, Wolf C, Greene C, Peterson DS: Sequence conservation in the rRNA first internal transcribed spacer region of*Babesia gibsoni* genotype Asia isolates. Vet Parasitol. 2008, 152: 152-157. 10.1016/j.vetpar.2007.11.024.
7. Reichenow E: Übertagungsweise und Entwicklung der Piroplasmen. Zbl Bakt I Orig. 1935, 135: 108-199.
8. Reichenow E: Über die Entwicklung von *Theileria parva*, dem Erreger des Küstenfiebers der Rinder, in *Rhipicephalus appendiculatus*. Zbl Bakt I Orig. 1937, 140: 223-226.

9. Zahler M, Schein E, Rinder H, Gothe R: Characteristic genotypes discriminate between *Babesia canis* isolates of differing vector specificity and pathogenicity in dogs. Parasitol Res. 1998, 84: 544-548. 10.1007/s004360050445.

10. Carret C, Walas F, Carcy B, Grande N, Précigout É, Moubri K, Schetters T, Gorenflot A: *Babesia canis canis*, *Babesia canis vogeli*, *Babesia canis rossi*: Differentiation of three subspecies by restriction fragment length polymorphism analysis on amplified small subunit ribosomal RNA genes. J Eukaryot Microbiol. 1999, 46: 298-303. 10.1111/j.1550-7408.1999.tb05128.x.

11. Birkenheuer AJ, Neel J, Ruslander D, Levy MG, Breitschwerdt EB: Detection and molecular characterization of a novel large *Babesia* species in a dog. Vet Parasitol. 2004, 124: 151-160. 10.1016/j.vetpar.2004.07.008.

12. Lehtinen LE, Birkenheuer AJ, Drolesky RE, Holman PJ: In vitro cultivation of a newly recognised *Babesia* sp. in dogs in North Carolina. Vet Parasitol. 2008, 151: 150-157. 10.1016/j.vetpar.2007.10.022.

13. Conrad P, Thomford J, Yamane I, Whiting J, Bosma L, Uno T, Holshuh HJ, Shelley S: Hemolytic anemia caused by *Babesia gibsoni* infections in dogs. J Am Vet Med Assoc. 1991, 199: 601-605.

14. Kjemtrup AM, Wainwright K, Miller M, Penzhorn BL, Carreno RA: *Babesia conradae*, sp. nov., a small canine *Babesia*identified in California. Vet Parasitol. 2006, 138: 103-111. 10.1016/j.vetpar.2006.01.044.

15. Zahler M, Rinder H, Schein E, Gothe R: Detection of a new pathogenic *Babesia microti*-like species in dogs. Vet Parasitol. 2000, 89: 241-248. 10.1016/S0304-4017(00)00202-8.

16. Camacho AT, Pallas E, Gestal JJ, Guitiàn FJ, Olmeda AS, Goethert HK, Telford SR: Infection of dogs in north-west Spain with a *Babesia microti*-like agent. Vet Rec. 2001, 149: 552-555.

17. Criado-Fornelio A, Martinez-Marcos A, Buling-Saraña A, Barba-Carretero JC: Molecular studies on *Babesia, Theileria* and*Hepatozoon* in southern Europe Part I: Epizootiological aspects. Vet Parasitol. 2003, 113: 189-201. 10.1016/S0304-4017(03)00078-5.

18. Criado A, Martinez J, Buling A, Barba JC, Merino S, Jefferies R, Irwin PJ: New data on epizootiology and genetics of piroplasms based on sequences of small ribosomal subunit and cytochrome b genes. Vet Parasitol. 2006, 142: 238-247. 10.1016/j.vetpar.2006.07.004.

19. Matjila PT, Leisewitz AL, Ooshuizen MC, Jongejan F, Penzhorn B: Detection of a *Theileria* species in dogs in South Africa. Vet Parasitol. 2008, 157: 34-40. 10.1016/j.vetpar.2008.06.025.

20. Uilenberg G: *Babesia* – a historical overview. Vet Parasitol. 2006, 138: 3-10. 10.1016/j.vetpar.2006.01.035.

21. Yamasaki M, Inokuma H, Sugimoto C, Shaw S, Aktas M, Yabsley MJ, Yamato O, Maede Y: Comparison and phylogenetic analysis of the heat shock protein 70 gene of *Babesia* parasites from dogs. Vet Parasitol. 2007, 145: 217-227. 10.1016/j.vetpar.2007.01.003.

22. Kjemtrup AM, Kocan AA, Whitworth L, Meinkoth J, Birkenheuer AJ, Cummings J, Boudreaux MK, Stockham SL, Irizarry-Rovira A, Conrad P: There are at least three genetically distinct small piroplasms from dogs. Int J Parasitol. 2000, 30: 1501-1505. 10.1016/S0020-7519(00)00120-X.

23. Goethert HK, Telford SR: What is *Babesia microti*?. Parasitology. 2003, 127: 301-309. 10.1017/S0031182003003822.

24. Mehlhorn H, Raether W, Schein E, Weber M, Uphoff M: Licht-und elektronenmikroskopische Untersuchungen zum Entwick-lungszyklus und Einfluss von Pentamidin auf die Morphologie der intraerythrocytären Stadien von *Babesia microti*. Dtsch Tierärztl Wochenschr. 1986, 93: 400-405.

25. [http://www.cvbd.org/4627.0.html]

26. Sasaki M, Omobowale O, Tozuka M, Ohta K, Matsuu A, Nottidge HO, Hirata H, Ikadai H, Oyamada T: Molecular survey of*Babesia canis* in dogs in Nigeria. J Vet Med Sci. 2007, 69: 1191-1193. 10.1292/jvms.69.1191.

27. Oyamada M, Davoust B, Boni M, Dereure J, Bucheton B, Hammad A, Itamoto K, Okuda M, Inokuma H: Detection of*Babesia canis rossi*, *B. canis vogeli*, and *Hepatozoon canis* in dogs in a village of Eastern Sudan by using a screening PCR and sequencing methodologies. Clin Diagn Lab Immunol. 2005, 12: 1343-1346. 10.1128/CDLI.12.11.1343-1346.2005.

28. Yeagley TJ, Reichard MV, Hempstead JE, Allen KE, Parsons LM, White MA, Little SE, Meinkoth JH: Detection of *Babesia gibsoni* and the small *Babesia* sp. 'Spanish isolate' in confiscated pit bull terriers. J Am Vet Med Assoc.

29. Trapp SM, Messick JB, Vidotto O, Jojima FS, Autran de Morais HS: *Babesia gibsoni* genotype Asia in dogs from Brazil. Vet Parasitol. 2006, 141: 177-180. 10.1016/j.vetpar.2006.04.036.

30. Solano-Gallego L, Trotta M, Carli E, Carcy B, Caldin M, Furlanello T: *Babesia canis canis* and *Babesia canis vogeli*clinicopathological findings and DNA detection by means of PCR-RFLP in blood from Italian dogs suspected of tick-borne disease. Vet Parasitol. 2008, 157: 211-221. 10.1016/j.vetpar.2008.07.024.

31. Irwin PJ, Hutchinson GW: Clinical and pathological findings of *Babesia* infection in dogs. Aust Vet J. 1991, 68: 204-209. 10.1111/j.1751-0813.1991.tb03194.x.

32. Böhm M, Leisewitz AL, Thompson PN, Schoeman JP: Capillary and venous *Babesia canis rossi* parasitaemias and their association with outcome of infection and circulatory compromise. Vet Parasitol. 2006, 141: 18-29. 10.1016/j.vetpar.2006.05.002.

33. Fukumoto S, Xuan X, Shigeno S, Kimbita E, Igarashi I, Nagasawa H, Fujisaki K, Mikami T: Development of a polymerase chain reaction methods for diagnosing *Babesia gibsoni* infection in dogs. J Vet Med Sci. 2001, 63: 977-981. 10.1292/jvms.63.977.

34. Jefferies R, Ryan U, Irwin P: PCR-RFLP for the detection and differentiation of the canine piroplasm species and its use with filter paper-based technologies. Vet Parasitol. 2007, 144: 20-27. 10.1016/j.vetpar.2006.09.022.

35. Birkenheuer AJ, Levy MG, Breitschwerdt EB: Development and evaluation of a seminested PCR for detection and differentiation of *Babesia gibsoni* (Asian genotype) and *B. canis* DNA in canine blood samples. J Clin Microbiol. 2003, 41: 4172-4177. 10.1128/JCM.41.9.4172-4177.2003.

36. Duarte SC, Linhares GFC, Romanowsky TN, Neto O, Borges LMF: Assessment of primers designed for the subspecies-specific discrimination among *Babesia canis canis, Babesia canis vogeli* and *Babesia canis rossi* by PCR assay. Vet Parasitol. 2008, 152: 16-20. 10.1016/j.vetpar.2007.12.013.

37. Ikadai H, Tanaka H, Shibahara N, Matsuu A, Uechi M, Itoh N, Oshiro S, Kudo N, Igarashi I, Oyamada T: Molecular evidence of infections with *Babesia gibsoni* parasites in Japan and evaluation of the diagnostic potential of a loop-mediated isothermal amplification method. J Clin Microbiol. 2004, 42: 2465-2469. 10.1128/JCM.42.6.2465-2469.2004.

38. Georges K, Ezeokoli CD, Newaj-Fyzul A, Campbell M, Mootoo N, Mutani A, Sparagano OAE: The application of PCR and reverse line blot hybridization to detect arthropod-borne haemopathogens of dogs and cats in Trinidad. Ann N Y Acad Sci. 2008, 1149: 196-199.

39. Matsuu A, Ono S, Ikadai H, Uchide T, Imamura S, Onuma M, Okanao S, Higuchi S: Development of a SYBR green real-time polymerase chain reaction assay for quantitative detection of *Babesia gibsoni* (Asian genotype) DNA. J Vet Diagn Invest. 2005, 17: 569-573.

40. Tani H, Tada Y, Sasai K, Baba E: Improvement of DNA extraction method for dried blood spots and comparison of four methods for detection of *Babesia gibsoni* (Asian genotype) infection in canine blood samples. J Vet Med Sci. 2008, 70: 461-467. 10.1292/jvms.70.461.

41. Birkenheuer AJ, Levy MG, Breitschwerdt EB: Efficacy of combined atovaquone and azithromycin for therapy of chronic*Babesia gibsoni* (Asian genotype) infections in dogs. J Vet Intern Med. 2004, 18: 494-498. 10.1892/0891-6640(2004)18<494:EOCAAA>2.0.CO;2.

42. Jefferies R, Ryan UM, Jardine J, Robertson ID, Irwin PJ: *Babesia gibsoni*: Detection during experimental infections and after combined atovaquone and azithromycin therapy. Exp Parasitol. 2007, 117: 115-123. 10.1016/j.exppara.2007.03.016.

43. Goo Y, Jia H, Aboge GO, Terkawi MA, Kuriki K, Nakamura C, Kumagai A, Zhou J, Lee EG, Nishikawa Y: *Babesia gibsoni*: Serodiagnosis of infection in dogs by an enzyme-linked immunosorbent assay with recombinant BgTRAP. Exp Parasitol. 2008, 118: 555-560. 10.1016/j.exppara.2007.11.010.

44. Anderson JF, Magnarelli LA, Sulzer AJ: Canine babesiosis: Indirect fluorescent antibody test for a North American isolate of *Babesia gibsoni*. Am J Vet Res. 1980, 41: 2102-2105.

45. Levy MG, Breitschwerdt EB, Moncol DJ: Antibody activity to *Babesia canis* in dogs in North Carolina. Am J Vet Res. 1987, 48: 339-341.

46. Aboge GO, Jia H, Terkawi MA, Goo Y, Kuriki K, Nishikawa Y, Igarashi I, Suzuki H, Xuan X: A novel 57-kDa merozoite protein of *Babesia gibsoni* is a prospective antigen for diagnosis and serosurvey of canine babesiosis by enzyme-linked immunosorbent assay. Vet Parasitol. 2007, 149: 85-94. 10.1016/j.vetpar.2007.06.025.

47. Fukumoto S, Xuan X, Nishikawa Y, Inoue N, Igarashi I, Nagasawa H, Fujisaki K, Mikami T: Identification and expression of a 50-kilodalton surface antigen of *Babesia gibsoni* and evaluation of its diagnostic potential in an enzyme-linked immunosorbent assay. J Clin Microbiol. 2001, 39: 2603-2609. 10.1128/JCM.39.7.2603-2609.2001.

48. Fukumoto S, Xuan X, Inoue N, Igarashi I, Sugimoto C, Fujisaki K, Nagasawa H, Mikami T, Suzuki H: Molecular characterization of a gene encoding a 29-kDa cytoplasmic protein of *Babesia gibsoni* and evalution of its diagnostic potentiality. Mol Biochem Parasitol. 2003, 131: 129-136. 10.1016/S0166-6851(03)00199-3.

49. Zhou J, Fukumoto S, Jia H, Yokoyama N, Zhang G, Fujisaki K, Lin J, Xuan X: Characterization of the *Babesia gibsoni* P18 as a homologue of thrombospondin related adhesive protein. Mol Biochem Parasitol. 2006, 148: 190-198. 10.1016/j.molbiopara.2006.03.015.

50. Jia H, Zhou J, Ikadai H, Matsuu A, Suzuki H, Igarashi I, Fujisaki K, Xuan X: Identification of a novel gene encoding a secreted antigen 1 of *Babesia gibsoni* and evaluation of its use in Serodiagnosis. Am J Trop Med Hyg. 2006, 75: 843-850.

51. Aboge GO, Jia H, Kuriki K, Zhou J, Nishikawa Y, Igarashi I, Fujisaki K, Suzuki H, Xuan X: Molecular characterization of a novel 32-kDa merozoite antigen of *Babesia gibsoni* with a better diagnostic performance by enzyme-linked immunosorbent assay. Parasitology. 2007, 134: 1185-1194. 10.1017/S0031182007002594.

52. Zhou J, Jia H, Nishikawa Y, Fujisaki K, Xuan X: *Babesia gibsoni* rhoptry-associated protein 1 and its potential use as a diagnostic antigen. Vet Parasitol. 2007, 145: 16-20. 10.1016/j.vetpar.2006.10.022.

53. Konishi K, Sakata Y, Miyazaki N, Jia H, Goo YK, Xuan X, Inokuma H: Epidemiological survey of *Babesia gibsoni* infection in dogs in Japan by enzyme-linked immunosorbent assay using *B. gibsoni* thrombospondin-related adhesive protein antigen. Vet Parasitol. 2008, 155: 204-208. 10.1016/j.vetpar.2008.04.025.

54. Birkenheuer AJ: Personal communication. 2009

55. Máthé A, Dobos-Kovacs M, Voros K: Histological and ultra-structural studies of renal lesions in *Babesia canis* infected dogs treated with imidocarb. Acta Vet Hung. 2007, 55: 511-523. 10.1556/AVet.55.2007.4.10.

56. Camacho AT, Guitian FJ, Pallas E, Gestal JJ, Olmeda AS, Goethert HK, Telford SR, Spielman A: Azotaemia and mortality among *Babesia-microti*-like infected dogs. J Vet Int Med. 2004, 18: 141-146. 10.1892/0891-6640(2004)18<141:AAMABM>2.0.CO;2.

57. Lobetti RG, Jacobsen LS: Renal involvement in dogs with babesiosis. J Sth Afr Vet Assoc. 2001, 72: 23-28.

58. de Scally MP, Lobetti RG, Reyers F, Humphris D: Are urea and creatinine values reliable indicators of azotaemia in canine babesiosis?. J Sth Afr Vet Assoc.

2004, 75: 121-124.

59. Schoeman JP, Rees P, Herrtage ME: Endocrine predictors of mortality in canine babesiosis caused by *Babesia canis rossi*. Vet Parasitol. 2007, 148: 75-82. 10.1016/j.vetpar.2007.06.010.

60. Brandao LP, Hagiwara MK, Myiashiro SI: Humoral immunity and reinfection resistance in dogs experimentally inoculated with *Babesia canis* and either treated or untreated with imidocarb dipropionate. Vet Parasitol. 2003, 114: 253-265. 10.1016/S0304-4017(03)00130-4.

61. Wulansari R, Wijaya A, Ano H, Horii Y, Nasu T, Yamane S, Makimura S: Clindamycin in the treatment of *Babesia gibsoni*infections in dogs. J Am Anim Hosp Assoc. 2003, 39: 558-562.

62. Suzuki K, Wakabyashi H, Takahashi M, Fukushima K, Yabuki A, Endo Y: A possible treatment strategy and clinical factors to estimate the treatment response in *Babesia gibsoni* infection. J Vet Med Sci. 2007, 69: 563-568. 10.1292/jvms.69.563.

63. Matsuu A, Miyamato K, Ikada H, Okano S, Higuchi S: Short Report: Cloning of the *Babesia gibsoni cytochrome B* gene and isolation of three single nucleotide polymorphisms from parasites present after atovaquone treatment. Am J Trop Med. 2006, 74: 593-597.

64. Subeki , Matsuura H, Yamasaki M, Yamato O, Maede Y, Katakura K, Suzuki M, Trimurningsih , Chairul , Yoshihara T: Effects of central Kalimantan plant extracts on intraerythrocytic *Babesia gibsoni* in culture. J Vet Med Sci. 2004, 66: 871-874. 10.1292/jvms.66.871.

65. Subeki , Matsuura H, Takahashi K, Yamasaki M, Yamato O, Maede Y, Katakura K, Suzuki M, Trimurningsih , Chairul , Yoshihara T: Antibabesial activity of protoberberine alkaloids and 20-hydroxyecdysone from *Arcangelisia flava* against*Babesia gibsoni* in culture. J Vet Med Sci. 2005, 67: 223-227. 10.1292/jvms.67.223.

66. Subeki , Matsuura H, Takahashi K, Yamasaki M, Yamato O, Maede Y, Katakura K, Kobayashi S, Trimurningsih , Chairul , Yoshihara T: Anti-babesial and anti-plasmodial compounds from *Phyllanthus niruri*. J Nat Prod. 2005, 68: 537-539. 10.1021/np0497245.

67. Tsuji N, Battsetseg B, Boldbaatar D, Miyoshi T, Xuan X, Oliver J, Fujisaki K: Babesial vector tick defensin against *Babesia*sp. parasites. Infect Immun. 2007, 75: 3633-3640. 10.1128/IAI.00256-07.

68. Uilenberg G, Verdiesen AHM, Zwart D: Imidocarb: A chemoprophylactic experiment with *Babesia canis*. The Vet Quarterly. 1981, 3: 118-123.

69. Vercammen F, de Deken R, Maes L: Prophylactic treatment of experimental canine babesiosis (*Babesia canis*) with doxy-cycline. Vet Parasitol. 1996, 66: 251-255. 10.1016/S0304-4017(96)01016-3.

70. Schetters T: Vaccination against canine babesiosis. Trends in Parasitol. 2005, 21: 179-184. 10.1016/j.pt.2005.02.006.

71. Carcy B, Precigout E, Schetters T, Gorenflot A: Genetic basis for GPI-anchor merozoite surface antigen polymorphism of*Babesia* and resulting antigenic diversity. Vet Parasitol. 2006, 138: 33-49. 10.1016/j.vetpar.2006.01.038.

72. Schetters T, Kleuskens J, Scholtes N, Bos HJ: Strain variation limits protective activity of vaccines based on soluble*Babesia canis* antigens. Parasite Immunol. 1995, 17: 215-218. 10.1111/j.1365-3024.1995.tb00891.x.

73. Schetters TPM, Kleuskens JAGM, Scholtes NC, Gorefnflot A, Moubri K, Vermeulen AN: Vaccination of dogs against heterologous *Babesia canis* infection using antigens from culture supernatants. Vet Parasitol. 2001, 100: 75-86. 10.1016/S0304-4017(01)00485-X.

74. Fukumoto S, Tamaki Y, Shirafuji H, Harakawa S, Suzuki H, Xuan X: Immunization with recombinant surface antigen P50 of *Babesia gibsoni* expressed in insect cells induced parasite growth inhibition in dogs. Clin Diagn Lab Immunol. 2005, 12: 557-559. 10.1128/CDLI.12.4.557-559.2005.

SECTION VII: PARASITES OF UNGULATES

CHAPTER 29

SOME PROTOZOAN PARASITES INFECTING BLOOD OF CAMELS (CAMELUS DROMEDARIUS) AT ASSIUT LOCALITY, UPPER EGYPT

Barakat Shehata Abd-Elmaleck, Gamal Hassan Abed and Ahmed Mohammad Mandour

Keywords: Camelus dormaderius, Surra, Babesia, Piroplasms, Theileria

INTRODUCTION

Camel (Camelus dromedarius) is an important multipurpose animal in arid and semi-arid areas of the world [1]. Protozoal diseases particularly trypanosomosis, cause remarkable losses on animal production in all the tropical and subtropical area. Trypanosomosis in camels is caused by Trypanosoma evansi and is transmitted from camel to camel by a number of species of haematophagous biting flies including Tabanus, Stomoxys, Lyperosiaand Haematobia [2]. Animal African trypanosomosis is a serious constraint to livestock sector development in sub-Saharan Africa. The disease, mainly caused by T. congolense, has a limitation in its diagnosis and treatment [3]. Trypanosomosis caused by T. evansi is the most recognized protozoan disease of camels and causes a disease known as Surra [4]. Surra has been reported in Pakistan [5], Jordan [6], Kenya [7], and many African countries. An outbreak of abortion and neonatal mortality associated with T. evansi infection in dromedary camels has been reported in Canary Islands [8].

Equine babesiosis is an infectious disease of horses and other equips caused by the protozoan hemoparasites B. equi and B. caballi [9]. B. equi infects 90% of the world equine populations [10], and transmitted naturally by the ticks of the Genera Hyalomma, Dermacentor and Rhipicephalus [11], and experimentally by Boophilus microplus [12]. B. equi was first isolated in Brazil by Ribeiro, et al. [13] from naturally infected horses to produce an antigen for serologicaly purposes. Babesiosis is vectored to humans by ticks that are ectoparasites of rodents [14]. Human babesiosis caused by B. microti was first described from sites along the North Eastern United States terminal moraine [15] and later from Minnesota and Wisconsin [16]. B. bovis and B. bigemina, exhibit a typical apicomplexan life cycle characterized by merogony, gametogony and sporogony [17].

The disease caused by the apicomplexan protozoan parasite Theileriaparva, known as East Coast fever or Corridor disease, is one of the most serious cattle diseases in Eastern, Central, and Southern Africa [18]. Hemoparasites known to infect bovine erythrocytes and cause anemia include organisms from the genera Anaplasma, Eperythrozoon, B., and Th. [19].

Accordingly the aim of the present work is to differentiate between different forms of T. evansi, to describe Th. and B. sp. as new species Infecting Camelus dromedaries using light and electron microscopy and to examine the zoonotic importance for these parasites on the experimental animals (White rates and mices).

Citation: Abd-Elmaleck BS, Abed GH, Mandourt AM (2014) Some Protozoan Parasites Infecting Blood of Camels (Camelus dromedarius) at Assiut Locality, Upper Egypt. J Bacteriol Parasitol 5: 184. doi: 10.4172/2155-9597.1000184.

MATERIALS AND METHODS

Out of 98 blood samples of camels (Camelus dromedarius) examined for blood protozoan parasites collected from different localities of Sloughter houses at Assiut city, Egypt (Dairout, Beni Ady, El ethamna). These freshly collected blood samples were divided in two groups one in a tube coated with EDTA, and the other in a test tube for centrifugation to obtain sera. Thick and thin blood smears were made for morphological examination of some protozoan blood parasites.

Electron microscopic Studies

TEM: Few drops from blood which is highly infected with Trypanosoma, Babesia and Theileria immediately fixed in 3 ml. of 3% glutaraldehyde solution in phosphate buffer (PH 7.2), for 24 hours and kept at 4°C in refrigerator. The samples were post fixed in 1% Osmium tetroxide in phosphate buffer (PH 7.2, 300 mom), for 30 minutes. They were washed several times with phosphate buffer solution. The samples were then embedded in Epon which can preserve fine structure from distortion during processing then ultra-thin sections were cut by an Ultra microtome and examined by JEOL, 100 CXII operating at 80 KV(TEM).

SEM: For scanning electron microscope of blood; few dropswere fixed in 3 % Glutaraldehyde in buffer for 24 hours. Specimens were washed three times in Phosphate buffer and post fixed in 1% Osmium tetroxide for 2 hours and then washed in the same buffer. They were dehydrated in different grades of ethyl alcohol and then mounted on special holders and coated with gold. Then they were examined in a JSM-T 200 L.V. 5400 Scanning Electron Microscopy (SEM). Experimental infection: Two groups of laboratory animals representing in five white from both rates and mices were dispensed with freshly infected blood camels by Babesia and Theileria in three doses each dose 3 ml blood to examine the zoonotic importance for these parasites. Blood examination was performed daily for determine the infection of these laboratory animals.

RESULTS

Out of ninety eight camels, (Camelus dromedaries) collected from different parts of Assiut (Benny Adie, El-atamna and Dairout). They revealed three genera of parasites including Trypanosoma, Theileria and Babesia.

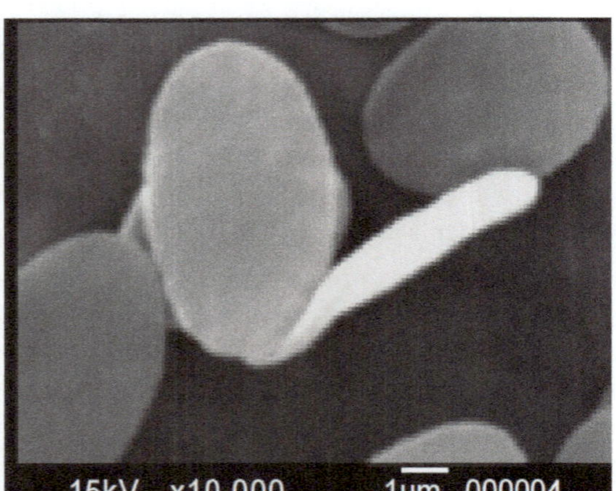

Figure 1: Presence of developmental stages Stumpy forms, Trypomastigote stage with free flagellum, undulating membrane and longitudinal binary fission.

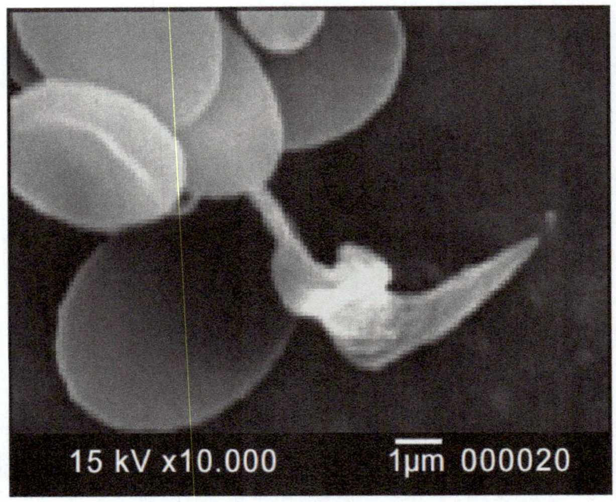

Figure 2: Presence of developmental stages Stumpy forms, Trypomastigote stage with free flagellum, undulating membrane and longitudinal binary fission.

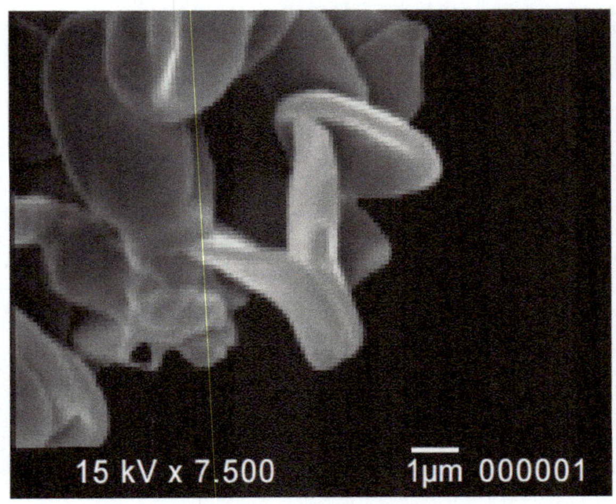

Figure 3: Presence of developmental stages Stumpy forms, Trypomastigote stage with free flagellum, undulating membrane and longitudinal binary fission.

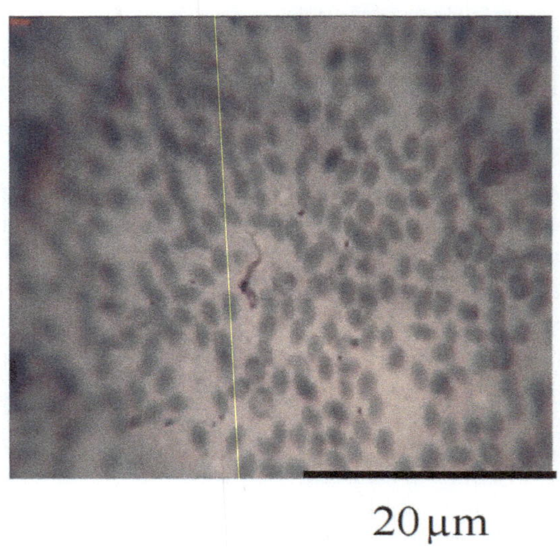

Figure 4: Free flagellum length 7 μm with two small folds of undulating membrane.

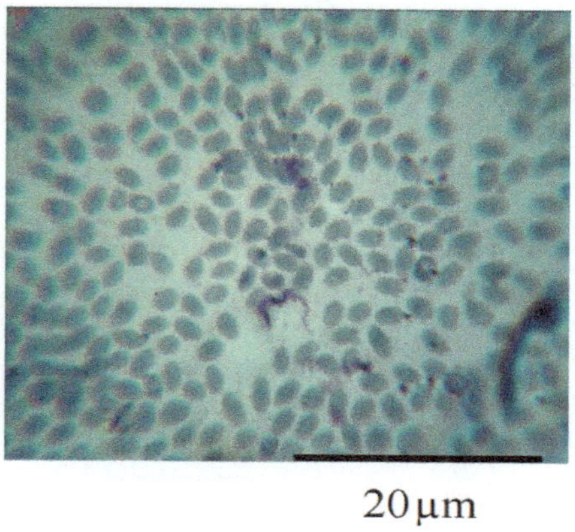

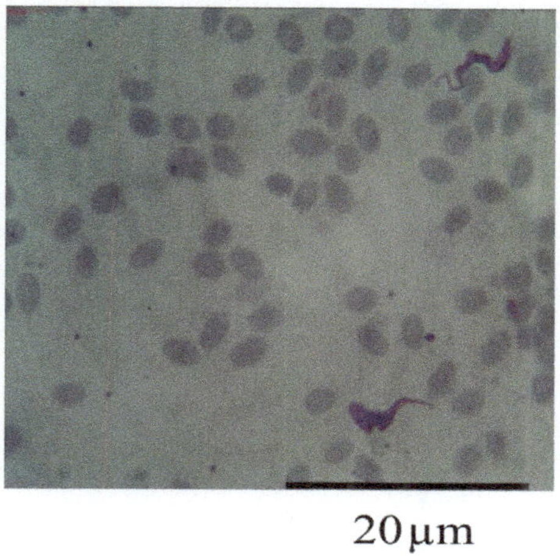

Figure 6: Eight with no folds.

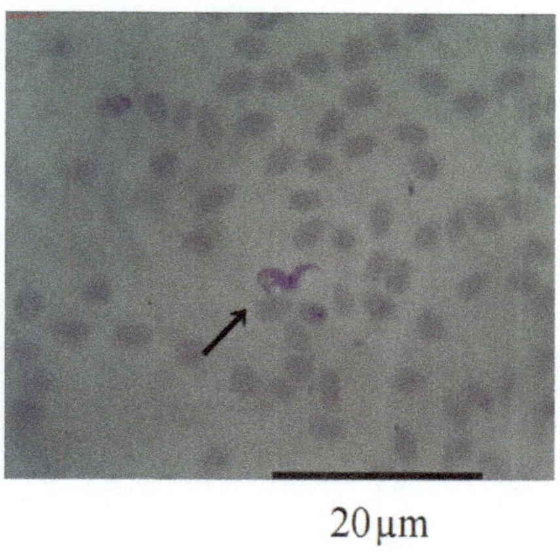

Figure 7: 17-20 with pulp body shape.

Trypanosoma sp.

Trypanosoma evansi is similar in shape with T. evansi in all mammals although it is different in size. Three camels from 98 (3.06 %) were infected. SEM revealed that presence of developmental stages Stumpy forms, Trypomastigote stage with free flagellum, undulating membrane and longitudinal binary fission as in Figures 1-3 respectively. They are five different forms according to the different morphological features (Total length, Total width, Nucleus index, the distance between (Kinetoplast to the posterior end, Nucleus to the anterior end, Nucleus to the posterior end),Presence of free flagellum, Presence of undulating membrane and the shape of posterior end) Figures 4-8 as in Table 1.

Babesia sp.

Forty six from ninety eight examined of Camellus dromedaries (46.9 %) were found infected with Babesia sp. It infects the camels by ticks with heavy infections as Figure 9 in the intra and extra of the red blood corpuscles (Figures 10 and 11) respectively and showing that different stages as ray body (Figures 12). The infection by the parasite sometimes accompanied by the infection with Theileria sp. SEM and TEM, reveal the sporokinetes of B. have elongate shape, 3.12 µm long and 1.56 µm wide, being wider at the anterior end and containing a single nucleus, large endoplasmic reticulum and abundant micronemes which was concentrated at the anterior end as in Figures 13 and 14. The Encephalitozoon – like microsporidia are present within the same specimen in which sporokinetes of B. caballiare found. They presented different morphological stages, suggesting a sequential phases of development. All stages contained a single nucleus. Sporonts have thicker and more electron-dense walls due to deposition of granules on the surface of the parasite. They have oval or elongate shapes (Figure 15). The sporonts multiplied producing the sporoblasts with polar filament. In the transverse sections, four coils of the polar tube and two food vacuoles were observed (Figure 16). Also, the scanning electron microscope show the trophozoites located very close to the erythrocyte membrane presented a tubular feeding structure, which emerged from the interior of the parasite and extended to the blood plasma, the tubular feeding structure was formed by the concomitant invaginations of the plasma membranes of the erythrocyte and the parasite Figure 17.

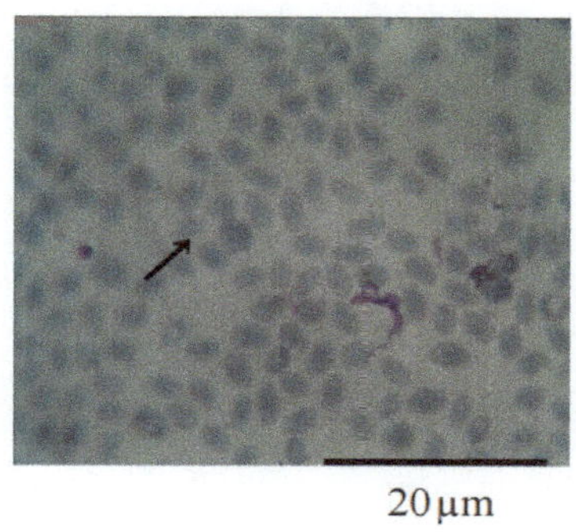

Figure 8: 10-12 with well-developed undulating membrane with two to four folds.

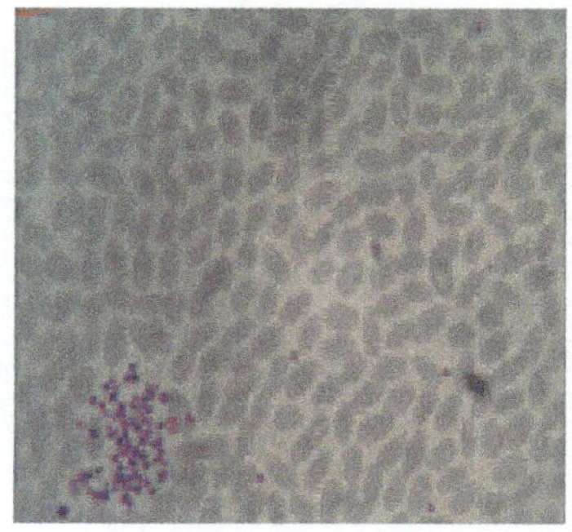

Figure 9: Babesia sp infects the camels by ticks with heavy infections in the intra and extra of the red blood corpuscles.

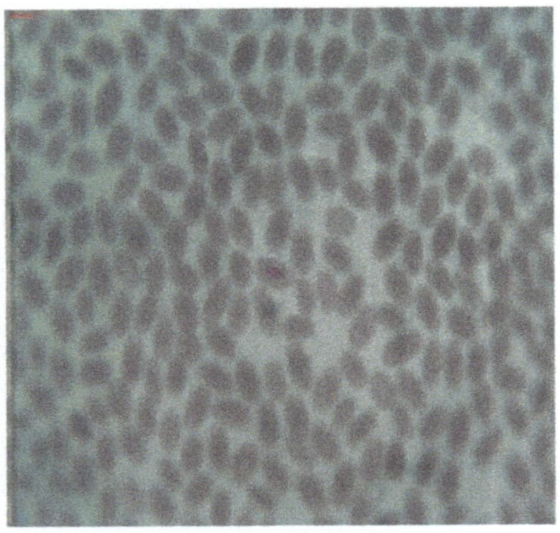

Figure 10: Babesia sp infects the camels by ticks with heavy infections in the intra and extra of the red blood corpuscles.

Figure 11: Babesia sp infects the camels by ticks with heavy infections in the intra and extra of the red blood corpuscles.

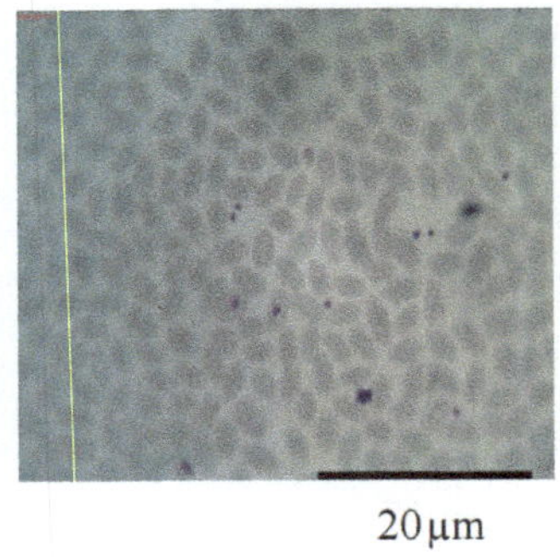

Figure 12: Different stages as ray body.

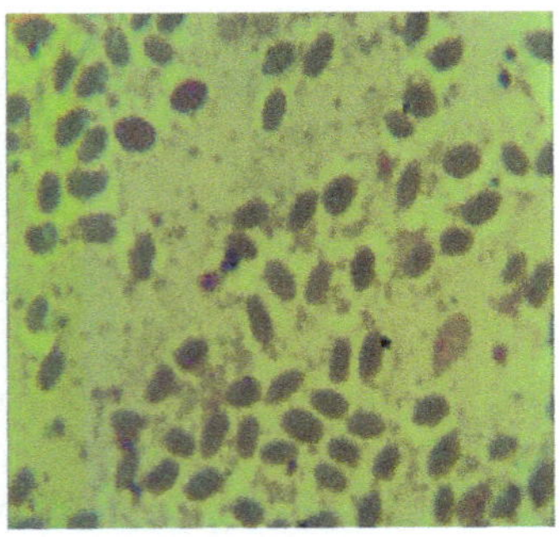

Table 1: Showing differences between different forms of T. evansi (measurements with µm).

Type or form No	1	2	3	4	5
Total length	23-30	20-27	28-30	20-30	36-44
Total width	2.5-5	4-Mar	6-Apr	13.5-20	7-May
Nucleus index	6 x 2.5	2 x 5	2.5 x 4	4 x 4	3 x 6
Kinetoplast to the posterior end	2	4	Contact with it	13-Oct	5-Mar
Free flagellum and undulating membrane	Free flagellum length 7 µm with two small folds of undulating membrane	Free flagellum 8 µm with one to two small folds	8 with no folds	17-20 with pulp body shape	10-12 with well-developed undulating membrane with two to four folds
Shape of the posterior end	Pointed posterior end	Sharp posterior end	Truncated posterior end	Vacoulated like structure with granules	Normal posterior end
Nucleus to posterior end	15	15	8	3	15
Nucleus to anterior end	7	13	8	12	10
Figs. no.	Figure (4)	Figure (5)	Figure (6)	Figure (7)	Figure (8)

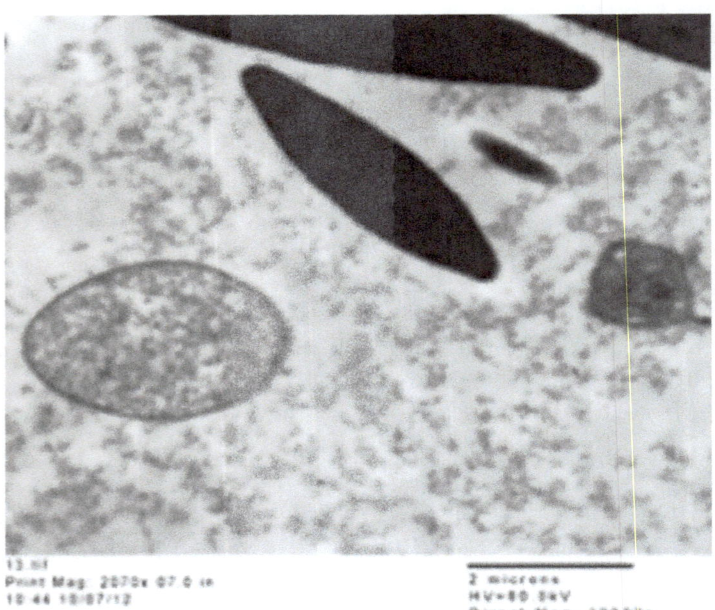

Figure 13: SEM and TEM, reveal the sporokinetes.

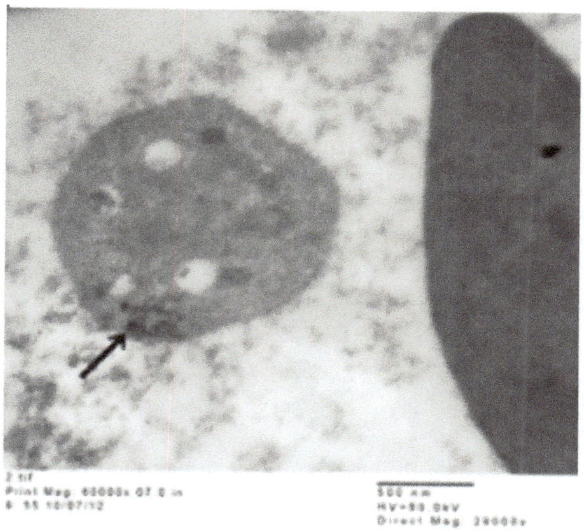

Figure 14: SEM and TEM, reveal the sporokinetes.

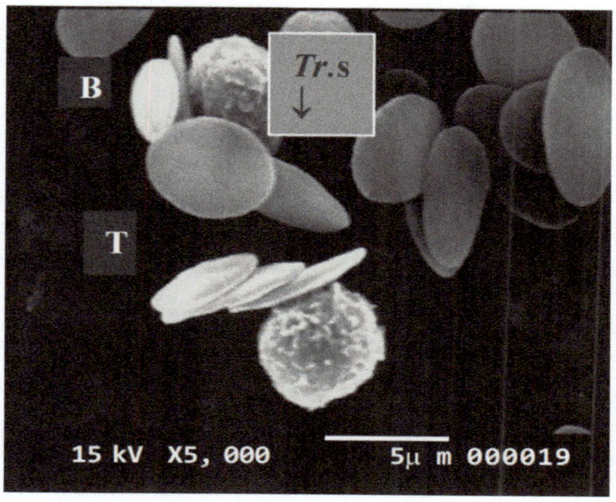

Figure 15: Sporokinetes having oval or elongate shapes.

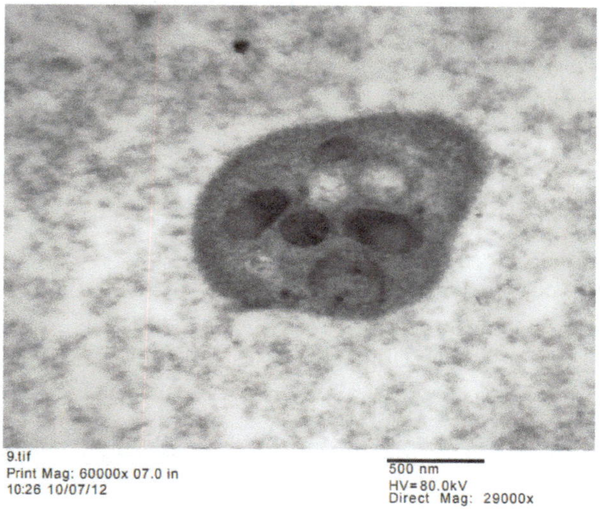

Figure 16: Transverse sections of sporokinetes.

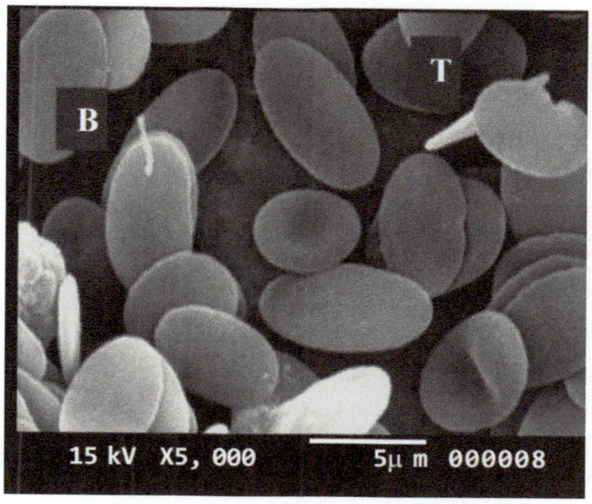

Figure 17: Concomitant invaginations of the plasma membranes of the erythrocyte and the parasite.

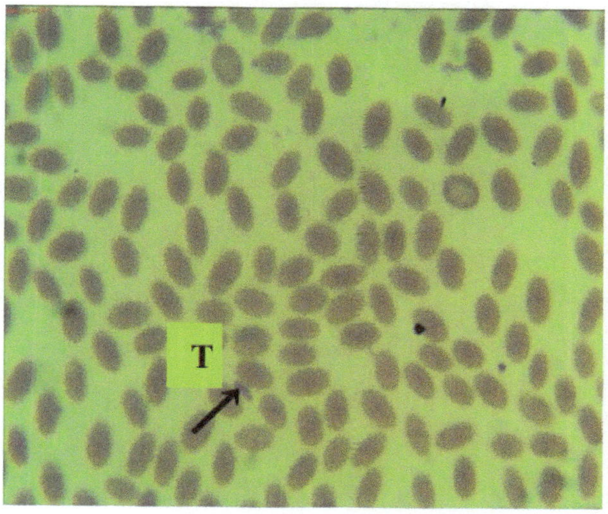

20 µm

Figure 18: Trophozoite stages intra and extra of the red blood corpuscles.

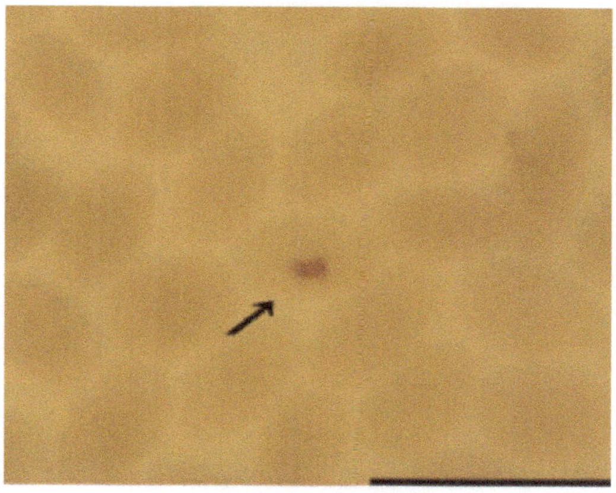

20 µm

Figure 19: Blood films which stained with Giemsa contained Th. piroplasms including, cocci and comma shaped.

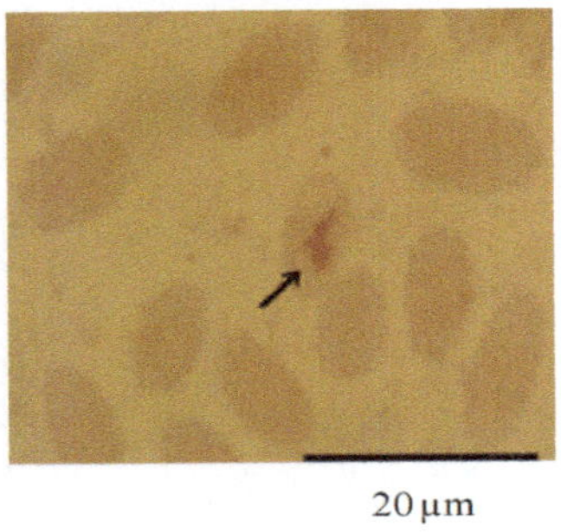

Figure 20: Blood films which stained with Giemsa contained Th. piroplasms including, cocci and comma shaped.

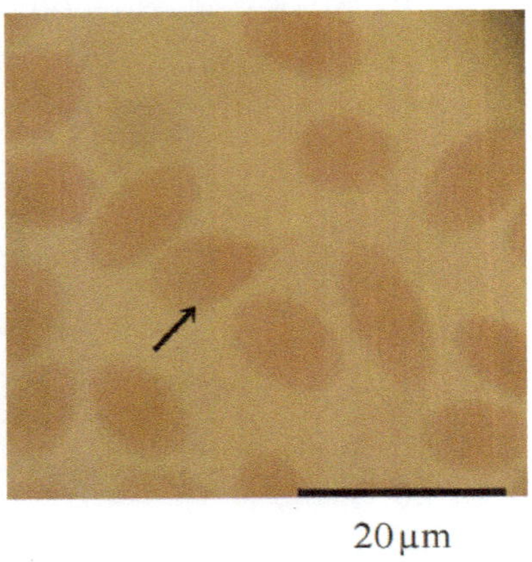

Figure 21: Abnormalities in erythrocyte structure included acanthocytosis.

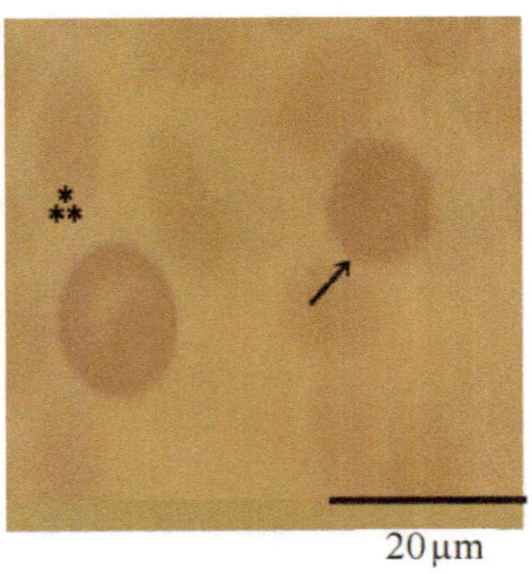

Figure 22: Spherocytosis and basophilic stippling.

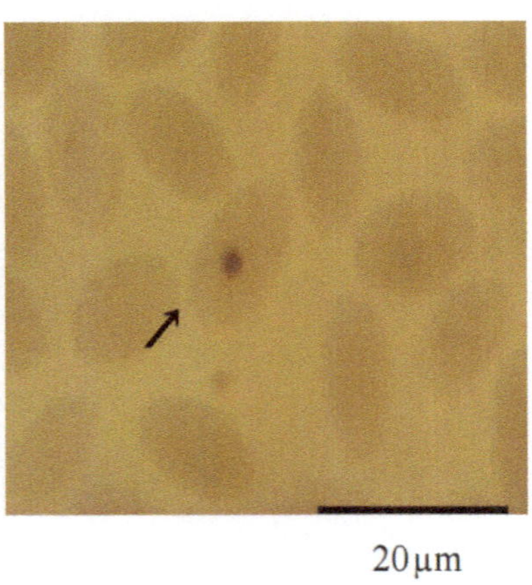

Figure 23: Howell-jolly body.

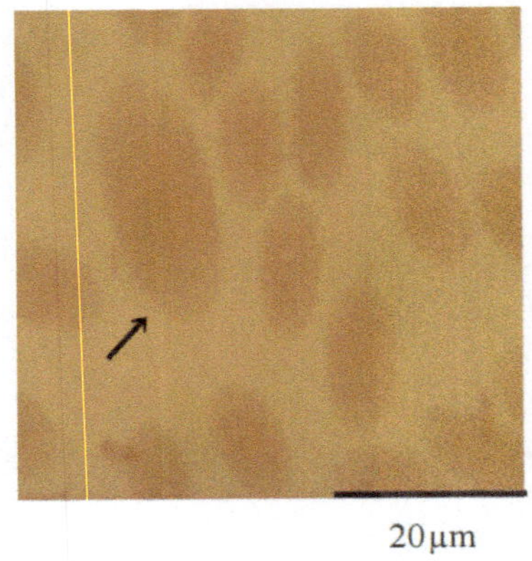

Figure 24: Macrocyte.

Theileria sp.

Only nine from ninety eight Camelus dromedarius (9.18%) are infected with the parasite. Trophozoite is a cigarette shaped and the light microscope shows some stages intra and extra of the red blood corpuscles as in Figure 18. Initial blood films examination revealed anemia, thrombocytosis and leukocytosis. Also, blood films which stained with Giemsa contained Th. piroplasms including, cocci Figure 19 and comma shaped Figure 20. Other abnormalities in erythrocyte structure included acanthocytosis Figure 21, spherocytosis and basophilic stippling, Figure 22, Howell-jolly body's Figure 23 and macrocyteas in Figure 24. Scanning electron microscopy also shows many different developmental stages.

Experimental Infection

Theileria and Babesia were appeared in both of the white rates and mice after 24 days of infection but 3 mice died after 80 days of infection. Rates could tolerate the infection with appearing of some symptoms such as diarrhea and a very reddish color for rates eyes. Some different stages of both parasites at different times appeared after 44, 59 and 74 days of infection as in Figures 25 A-D. This experimental infection had been proved that both of Theileria and Babesia have zoonotic importance whatever for that, of a very economic importance in the life experimental field.

DISCUSSION

Trypanosomaevansi

Trypanosomes of the section salivaria might or might not possess a free flagellum, their kinetoplast is terminal or subterminal in position and the posterior end of the parasite is usually rounded [20]. Several studies have observed a significant morphological difference in some T. evansi isolates [21,22]. The presence of vacuoles in T. evansi has been reported (ID and International Medicine Parasitology Volume 1 for web, 2008). In the present work T. evansi measured 20-44 µm in length, agreement with some species described by Hoare CA [23]. Although the main morphological parameters (total length with flagellum, total width, nuclear index, posterior end to the kinetoplast, free flagellum, shape of the posterior end, posterior end to the nucleus, and the nucleus to the anterior end) show some few differences with other data reported by authors Silva RAS, et al. and Sarataphan N, et al. [10,24]. The subgenus Duttonella trypanosomes have feebly developed undulating membranes and a large kinetoplast. The latter feature could resemble those of form 5 in the present study, but the undulating membrane contains two or three big fold sand its pointed posterior end is different from T. vivax [8,23,25]. By contrast, forms 3 and 4 showed rounded posterior extremity but the most important feature the Duttonella trypanosomes, the large kinetoplast, was absent [23]. The results obtained in the present study would indicate that biometrically distinct T. evansi could also be found in the same area and even in the same animal species.

Babesia sp.

Ticks are widespread in camel habitats. They cause serious adverse effects such as anemia, dermatitis, mastitis reduced meat and milk production and low quality hides [26]. Camels were infected with Babesia caballi for the first record in Sudan [26]. So, that the infection of Camelus dromedaries by Babesia sp. is the first record in Egypt. Babesia caballi is a hemoparasitic protozoan of the Phylum Apicomplexa that is transmitted naturally in New World by Anocentor nitens ticks [2]. Few papers have reported the multiplication of B. caballi in ticks and most of them were based on optic microscopy [27]. Only one paper on ultrastructure has used transmission electron microscopy to describe the development of B. caballi in salivary glands of Hyalomma truncayum [28]. The forms of B. sp. which are found in Camelus dromedarius in the present study are in agreement with those describe by Ribeiro, et al. [13] within the same cells infected with B. caballi sporokinetes or in other neighbor cells, it was observed that microsporidia organisms were undergoing different stages of development. Ultra-structural analysis showed that all stages of development of microsporidia with a single nucleus, while the stages of the sporoblast and spore had four coils of the polar tubes. Based on these findings, the microsporidia could be classified as Encephalitozoon cuniculi [29]. Encephalitozoon cuniculi infections were described in mammals, including horses, causing asymptomatic infections in immunocompetent hosts [4]. So that, according to the present work there are two species of B. one is B. caballi and the other B. equi. Which have two vacuoles.

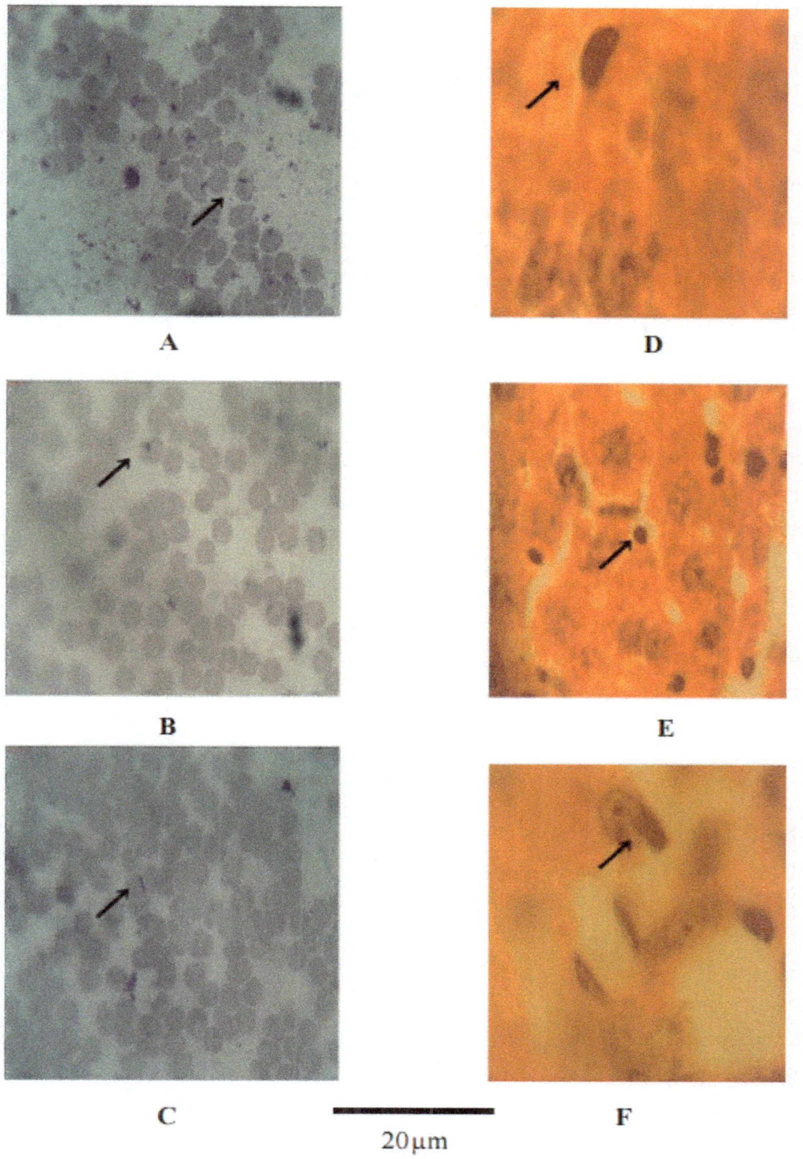

Figure 25: Different stages of both parasites at different times appeared after 44, 59 and 74 days of infection.

Theileria sp.

Taxonomic classification of Theileria sp. was based on microscopic appearance of intraerythrocytic piroplasms, geographical location of the infected animal apparent pathogenicity of the organism and serologic testing [30,31] Most theilerial organisms of cattle that had low pathogenicity were called Th. Mutans [14]. As more Th. sp. were isolated and studied, some organisms were reclassified. For example, the US theilerial organism reported to be T. mutans was renamed T. orientalis in 1985 [31].These authors also considered some isolates of Th. orientalis to be the same stocks of T. sergenti, the name given to a more pathogenic species found in Southeastern Asia. So that, the presence of basophilic stippling indicateda regenerative response consistent with a hemolyticanemia. A combination of spherocytosis and acanthocytosis indicated intravascular erythrocyte fragmentation. Spherocytes can also be formed by immune-mediated processes. There is no evidence of blood loss, but there was a hypoprotienemia. For the first time theilerial infection in camels occurs in Egypt but intraerythrocytic piroplasms were highly pleomorphic, and rod forms were most common. Piroplasms shape may vary with stage of an infection and thus is not a reliable criterion of species differentiation [31]. Thus, the present study suggests that this Species is Theileria camelli.

CONCLUSIONS

The higher incidence of the infected camels with protozoan parasites in Egypt is (48.9%) due to some environmental conditions. It is the first time in Egypt to record infections of camels with both B. sp and Th. sp. with higher incidence (46.9% and 9.18%) respectively resulting from their habitat with other animals (cattle's and sheep's).

REFERENCES

1. Roby TO, Anthony DW (1963) Transmission of equine piroplasmosis by Dermacentornitens Neumann. J Am Vet Med Assoc 142: 768-769.
2. Stewart NP, Uilenberg G, de Vos AJ (1996) Review of Australian species of Theileria, with special reference to Theileriabuffeli of cattle. Trop Anim Health Prod 28: 81-90.
3. Levkutová M, Hípiková V, Faitelzon S, Benath G, Paulík S, et al. (2004) Prevalence of antibodies to Encephalitozooncuniculi in horses in the Israel. Ann Agric Environ Med 11: 265-267.
4. Gutierrez C, Corbera JA, Juste MC, Doreste F, Morales I (2005) An outbreak of abortions and high neonatal mortality associated with Trypanosomaevansi infection in dromedary camels in the Canary Islands. Vet Parasitol 130: 163-168.
5. Abo-Shehada MN, Anshassi H, Mustafa G, Amr Z (1999) Prevalence of Surra among camels and horses in Jordan. Prev Vet Med 38: 289-293.
6. Luckins AG (1992) Protozoan diseases of Camels. In. Proc 6: 23-27.
7. Guerra NC, Junior AB, Santos HP, Abreu-Silva AL, Santos AC (2008) Biometry of Trypanosomavivax found in a calf in the State of Maranhao, Brazil. Ciencia Rural 38: 833-835.
8. de Waal DT (1992) Equine piroplasmosis: a review. Br Vet J 148: 6-14.
9. Sarataphan N, Vongpakorn M, Nuansrichay B, Autarkool N, Keowkarnkah T, et al. (2007) Diagnosis of a Trypanosomalewisi-like (Herpetosoma) infection in a sick infant from Thailand. J Med Microbiol 56: 1118-1121.
10. FriedhoffKT (1988) Transmission of Babesia, babesiosis of domestic animals and man. CRC Press, Flor 23-52
11. Hooshmand-Rad JA, Roux JP, Toccalino PA, Navias JC, Cayo DO (1976) The pathogenesis of anaemia in Theileriaannulata infection. Res Vet Sci 20: 324-329.
12. Ribeiro MF, Passos LM (2006) Natural co-infection of Babesiacaballi and Encephalitozoon-like microsporidia in the tick Anocentornitens (Acari: Ixodidae). J InvertebrPathol 93: 183-185.
13. Steketee RW, Eckman MR, Burgess EC, Kuritsky JN, Dickerson J, et al. (1985) Babesiosis in Wisconsin. A new focus of disease transmission. JAMA 253: 2675-2678.
14. Schein E (1988) Equine babesiosis, In: Ristic M. (ed.) Babesiosis of Domestic Animals and Man. CRC Press, Florida 198-208.
15. Spielman A, Wilson ML, Levine JF, Piesman J (1985) Ecology of Ixodesdammini-borne human babesiosis and Lyme disease. Annu Rev Entomol 30: 439-460.
16. Chauvin A, Moreau E, Bonnet S, Plantard O, Malandrin L (2009) Babesia and its hosts: adaptation to long-lasting interactions as a way to achieve efficient transmission. Vet Res 40: 37.
17. Hayashida K, Abe T, Weir W, Nakao R, Ito K, et al. (2013) Whole-genome sequencing of Theileriaparva strains provides insight into parasite migration and diversification in the African continent. DNA Res 20: 209-220.
18. Conrad PA, Waldrup KA (1993) Babesiosis and theileriosis in free-ranging and captive artiodactylids. Zoo Wild Anim Med 3: 506-511.
19. Hoare CA (1964) Morphological and Taxonomic Studies on Mammalian Trypanosomes. X. Revision of the Systematics. J Protozool 11: 200-207.
20. Dávila AM, Ramirez L, Silva RA (1998) Biometrical alterations of Trypanosomaevansi isolate in laboratory rodents. Vet Parasitol 76: 149-152.
21. Gonzalez JA, Gonzalez AO, Santa Cruz AC, Ortiz JC, Comolli JA, et al. (2003) (Hydrochaerishydrochaeris) en cautiverlo, de la Provin de comunicationesCientificas y TechnologicasPNUnisersiteded Nacional del Nordest.
22. Hoare CA (1972) The Trypanosomes of Mammals. J small AnimPract 1: 749.
23. Shiota T, Kurimoto H, Haguma N, Yoshida Y (1984) Studies on babesia first found in murine in Japan: epidemiology, morphology and experimental infection. ZentralblBakteriolMikrobiolHyg A 256: 347-355.
24. Dávila A, Ramirez L, Silva R (1997) Morphological and biometrical differences among Trypanosomavivax isolates from Brazil and Bolivia. MemInst Oswaldo Cruz 92: 357-358.

25. Abdelrahim IA, Ismail AA, Majiid AM, Mohammed AS, Ibrahim AM, et al. (2009) Detection of Babesiacaballi in the one- humped Camel (Camelus dromedaries) using the Reverse Line Block (RLB) in Sudan. Sudan J Vet Res 24: 69-72.

26. Holbrook AA, Anthony DW, Johnson AJ (1968) Observations on the development of Babesiacaballi (Nuttall) in the tropical horse tick Dermacentornitens Neumann. J Protozool 15: 391-396.

27. Blouin EF, De Waal DT (1989) The fine structure of developmental stages of Babesiacaballi in the salivary glands of Hyalommatruncatum. Onderstepoort J Vet Res 56: 189-193.

28. SPLITTER EJ (1950) Theileriamutans associated with bovine anaplasmosis in the United States. J Am Vet Med Assoc 117: 134-135.

29. Irvin AD (1987) Characterization of species and strains of Theileria. AdvParasitol 26: 145-197.

30. Telford SR 3rd, Korenberg EI, Goethert HK, KovalevskiÄIuV, Gorelova NB, et al. (2002) [Detection of natural foci of babesiosis and granulocytic ehrlichiosis in Russia]. ZhMikrobiolEpidemiolImmunobiol : 21-25.

31. Kuttler KL, Craig TM (1975) Isolation of a bovine Theileria. Am J Vet Res 36: 323-325.

SECTION VIII: VETERINARY ENTOMOLOGY

CHAPTER 30

SURVEILLANCE OF ARTHROPOD VECTOR-BORNE INFECTIOUS DISEASES USING REMOTE SENSING TECHNIQUES: A REVIEW

Satya Kalluri, Peter Gilruth, David Rogers, Martha Szczur

INTRODUCTION

Hematophagous arthropod vectors such as mosquitoes, ticks, and flies are responsible for transmitting bacteria, viruses, and protozoa between vertebrate hosts, causing such deadly diseases as malaria, dengue fever, and trypanosomiasis. Until the early 20th century, vector-borne diseases were responsible for more deaths in humans than all other causes combined. These diseases prevented the development of large areas of the tropics, especially in Africa [1]. Table 1 provides a list of common arthropod vectors, the diseases they carry, and the type of pathogen responsible for the disease. Floods and other natural disasters create environments conducive to the spread of communicable diseases such as malaria, diarrhea, and cholera. Some studies suggest that climate change and increased climate variability are fostering the spread of infectious diseases beyond their traditional geographic domains [2]. For example, West Nile virus, which was previously confined to Africa, Asia, and Europe (i.e., the Old World), has recently spread to North America. The mosquito Aedes albopictus, a vector of both dengue fever and West Nile virus and a native to Asia, has recently established in North America [3]. The "burden" of prominent infectious diseases worldwide transmitted by arthropod vectors is given in Table 2 [4]. Disease burden is expressed in Disability Adjusted Life Years (DALYs), which is the sum of years lost prematurely due to mortality and disability for incidence cases of the disease [5]. One DALY represents the loss of a year of healthy life.

Table 1. Common Arthropod Vectors, Diseases, and the Type of Pathogen Responsible for the Disease

Vector	Disease	Pathogen Type
Mosquitoes	Filariasis	Helminth
	Malaria	Protozoa
	Dengue fever	Virus
	Yellow fever	Virus
	St. Louis encephalitis	Virus
	Eastern equine encephalitis	Virus
	Western equine encephalitis	Virus
	West Nile	Virus
	Rift Valley fever	Virus
Ticks	Lyme disease	Bacteria
	Rocky Mountain spotted fever	Bacteria
	Q fever	Bacteria
	Tularemia	Bacteria
	Relapsing fever	Bacteria
	Ehrlichiosis	Bacteria
	Colorado tick fever	Virus
	Crimean hemorrhagic fever	Virus
	Babesiosis	Protozoa
Mites	Q fever	Bacteria
	Rickettsioses/rickettsialpox	Bacteria
Deerflies	Tularemia	Bacteria
Tsetse flies	Sleeping sickness (African trypanosomiasis)	Protozoa
Blackflies	Onchocerciasis	Helminth
Muscoid flies	Yaws	Bacteria
Sandflies	Leishmaniasis	Protozoa
	Sandfly fever	Virus
	Vesicular stomatitis	Virus
Lice	Epidemic typhus	Bacteria
	Trench fever	Bacteria
Fleas	Endemic typhus	Bacteria
	Bubonic plague	Bacteria
Reduviids (also known as bed bugs, kissing bugs, cone-nose bugs)	Chagas disease (American trypanosomiasis)	Protozoa

doi:10.1371/journal.ppat.0030116.t001

Citation: Kalluri S, Gilruth P, Rogers D, Szczur M (2007) Surveillance of Arthropod Vector-Borne Infectious Diseases Using Remote Sensing Techniques: A Review. PLoS Pathog 3(10): e116. doi:10.1371/journal.ppat.0030116.

Table 2. Global Burden of Infectious Diseases Caused Due to Arthropod Vectors [4]

Disease	Disease Burden (DALYs[a]) in Thousands	Mortality in Thousands
Malaria	42,280	1,124
African trypanosomiasis	1,598	50
Lymphatic filariasis	5,644	0
Dengue fever	653	21
Leishmaniasis	2,357	59
Chagas disease	649	13
Onchocerciasis	987	0

[a]DALYs – Disability Adjusted Life Years (the number of healthy years of life lost due to premature death and disability).

doi:10.1371/journal.ppat.0030116.t002

Passive disease surveillance involves voluntary reporting by people who are ill enough to go to a treatment center; such centers are therefore only effective for detection and mitigation after a person has been infected. On the other hand, active disease surveillance, which involves "searching" for evidence of disease proactively through routine and continuous monitoring in endemic areas, could help prevent an outbreak, or slow transmission at an earlier stage of an epidemic. Improved methods are required for forecasting, early detection, and prevention of vector-borne diseases due to the increasing trend of large-scale epidemics such as malaria [6]. Of late, satellite remote sensing technology has shown promising results in assessing the risk of various vector-borne diseases at different spatial scales. Satellite measurements and other remote sensing techniques cannot identify the vectors themselves, but may be used to characterize the environment in which the vectors thrive. Environmental variables such as land and sea surface temperature and amount, type, and health of vegetation can be identified and measured from space. A list of environmental factors that can be mapped through remote sensing and their potential linkages with various diseases has been previously described [7]. Satellites have the ability to detect anomalies and deviations from the normal climate patterns that are conducive to the breeding of disease-carrying vectors such as mosquitoes. Techniques to map disease occurrence and risk from satellite data therefore require at least some understanding of the relationships between a vector-borne disease and the air, land, and water environment in which it occurs. The objectives of this review are to summarize developments in the application of remote sensing techniques for studying infectious diseases in humans due to arthropod vectors and to identify future opportunities for further research.

Remote Sensing of the Vector Environment

Remote sensing satellites provide continuous measurements of the earth and its environment, and offer a synoptic monitoring capability. Satellite measurements have distinct advantages over ground measurements since they can be collected repeatedly and automatically. In the United States, the National Aeronautics and Space Administration (NASA) is the prime agency responsible for developing new remote sensing technologies and remote sensing satellites, collecting earth system science data to study global change, and developing applications to use remotely sensed data. The National Oceanic and Atmospheric Administration (NOAA) operates a series of weather satellites that collect operational data for weather forecasting and climate prediction. Besides NASA and NOAA, several European Union countries, Japan, Canada, and India have remote sensing satellites that provide global observations. A list of different Earth-observing satellite sensors that are discussed in this paper and their spectral, spatial, and temporal characteristics are given in Table 3.

The use of remote sensing techniques to map vector species distribution and disease risk has evolved considerably during the past two decades. The complexity of techniques range from using simple correlations between spectral signatures from different land use–land cover types and species abundance (e.g., [8,9]) to complex techniques that link satellite-derived seasonal environmental variables to vector biology [10]. While a variety of numerical techniques to create maps of vector distribution in time and space from satellite data are available, only those techniques that aid our understanding of biological processes provide meaningful information in epidemiology and vector control. A review of different modeling approaches for mapping vector and vector-borne diseases is discussed by Rogers [11]. The typical modeling approach is to use either logistic regression or discriminant analysis techniques that investigate associations between multivariate environmental data and patterns of vector presence or absence for mapping vectors and vector-borne diseases. Both of these methods are capable of predicting the a posteriori probability of the presence of the dependent variable (e.g., either the vector or the disease) from a set of independent variables (e.g., climate and land cover data) and can be used to make risk maps from sample data sets (i.e., training datasets) based on the observed similarity of environmental conditions to sites. The choice of techniques should be able to accommodate both categorical (e.g., disease presence or absence) as well as continuous data (e.g., surface temperature data) spatial data.

Table 3. Characteristics of Different Earth-Observing Satellite Instruments Discussed in This Paper That Have Potential Applications in Epidemiology

Satellite	Instrument	Spectral Bands (μm)	Spatial Resolution	Temporal Resolution
Landsat-5 (USGS)	**MSS**	2 visible	57 m × 79 m	16 days
		2 NIR	57 m × 79 m	
	TM	3 visible	30 m	
		1 NIR	30 m	
		2 SWIR	30 m	
		1 LWIR	120 m	
Landsat-7 (USGS)	**ETM+**	3 visible	30 m	16 days
		1 NIR	30 m	
		2 SWIR	30 m	
		1 LWIR	60 m	
		1 panchromatic (B&W)	15 m	
NOAA-K, L, M, N (NOAA)	**AVHRR**	1 visible	All at 1.1 km	Daily
		1 NIR		
		1 SWIR		
		1 MIR		
		2 LWIR		
Terra, Aqua (NASA)	**MODIS**	1 visible and 1 NIR	250 m	1–2 days
		5 visible, NIR, SWIR	500 m	
		29 visible, NIR, SWIR, MIR, TIR	1 km	
Terra (NASA)	**ASTER**	2 visible	15 m	16 days
		1 NIR	15 m	
		6 SWIR	30 m	
		5 TIR	90 m	
IKONOS (GeoEye)	**IKONOS**	1 panchromatic (B&W)	1 m	3 days
		3 visible	4 m	
		1 NIR	4 m	
SPOT 1, 2, 3 (Spot Image)	**HRV**	1 panchromatic (B&W)	10 m	26 days
		2 visible	20 m	
		1 NIR	20 m	
SPOT 4 (Spot Image)	**HRVIR**	1 panchromatic (B&W)	10 m	26 days
		2 visible	20 m	
		1 NIR	20 m	
		1 SWIR	20 m	
	VEGETATION	2 visible	1 km	Daily
		1 NIR	1 km	
		1 SWIR	1 km	
SPOT 5 (Spot Image)	**HRG**	1 panchromatic (B&W)	5 m	26 days
		2 visible	10 m	
		1 NIR	10 m	
		1 SWIR	20 m	
	VEGETATION	Same as the one on SPOT4		
GOES (NOAA)	**GOES Imager**	1 visible	1 km	30 min
		1 MIR	4 km	
		1 LWIR	8 km	
		2 LWIR	4 km	
IRS 1C, IRS 1D, IRS P6 (ISRO)	**PAN**	1 panchromatic (B&W)	5.8 m	25 days
	LISS-III	2 visible	23.5 m	
		1 NIR	23.5 m	
		1 SWIR	70 m	
Meteosat Second Generation (MSG) (ESA)	**SEVIRI**	1 panchromatic (B&W)	1 km	15 min
		1 visible	3 km	
		2 NIR	3 km	
		1 MIR	3 km	
		7 LWIR	3 km	

Visible = 0.4–0.7 μm; NIR = 0.7–1.3 μm; SWIR = 1.3–3 μm; MIR = 3–5 μm; LWIR (thermal) = 5–14 μm.
ASTER = Advanced Spaceborne Thermal Emission and Reflection Radiometer; ETM+ = Enhanced Thematic Mapper+; IRS = Indian Remote Sensing Satellite; GOES = Geostationary Operational Environmental Satellite; HRG = High Resolution Geometric; HRV = High Resolution Visible; HRVIR = High Resolution Visible Infrared; LISS = Linear Imaging Self-Scanning System; MODIS = Moderate Resolution Imaging Spectroradiometer; MSS, Multispectral Scanner; SEVIRI = Spinning Enhanced Visible and InfraRed Imager; SPOT = Satellite Probatoire d'Observation de la Terre.
European Organisation for the Exploitation of Meteorological Satellites (EUMETSAT) (Europe): http://www.eumetsat.int/Home/index.htm.
European Space Agency: http://www.esa.int/esaEO/GGGH88WTGEC_index_0.html.
GeoEye: http://www.geoeye.com/.
Japan Aerospace Exploration Agency (JAXA): http://www.jaxa.jp/index_e.html.
Indian Space Research Organization (ISRO): http://www.isro.org/.
National Aeronautics and Space Administration (NASA) (USA): http://www.earth.nasa.gov/.
National Oceanic and Atmospheric Administration (NOAA) (USA): http://www.noaa.gov/.
National Remote Sensing Agency (NRSA) (India): http://www.nrsa.gov.in/satellites/satellites.html.
Spot Image: http://www.spotimage.fr/web/en/.
US Geological Survey (USGS): http://www.usgs.gov/.
doi:10.1371/journal.ppat.0030116.t003

The approach in developing remote sensing applications in epidemiology depends on the spectral, spatial, and temporal characteristics of remote sensing measurements. Environmental satellites that collect earth observations daily or several times a day of the same geographic region (e.g., NOAA's Polar Operational Environmental Satellites and Geostationary Operational Environmental Satellites) are ideally suited for collecting rapidly changing meteorological variables such as atmospheric moisture and surface temperature. Data from these satellites are valuable in modeling the climate-dependent vector life cycles and sustainability. In general, operational environmental satellites collect more frequent observations at a coarser spatial resolution (~1 km), over large geographic regions, and are cheaper to acquire compared to images from other land imaging satellites such as Landsat or IKONOS that have less frequent revisit capability but have a higher spatial resolution (30 m or higher). A summary of the availability of environmental satellite data for mapping infectious diseases can be found in [12]. A combination of high spatial resolution data for land use and land cover classification and frequent coarse resolution environmental satellite data for monitoring environmental variability would be ideal for studying surface climate conditions for modeling vector populations.

Application of remote sensing data in epidemiology involves retrieving environmental variables that characterize the vector ecosystem such as land cover, temperature, humidity or vapor pressure, and precipitation. Measurements of Earth's surface reflectances and temperature can be made directly from satellites. However, measuring meteorological and climate variables near the surface is more difficult, and frequently, empirical methods are used. Because of complexities and limitations in estimating meteorological variables through remote sensing, proxy variables such as vegetation indices that measure the abundance, spatial extent, and dynamics of vegetation are used as a surrogate indicator of climate variability in epidemiological studies (e.g., [13]). The Normalized Difference Vegetation Index (NDVI), which exploits the strong contrast in the reflectance of vegetation in the red and near infrared wavelengths, is a commonly used index to study vegetation dynamics (e.g., [14]). Since vegetation dynamics are influenced by variations in climate, strong correlations between vegetation indices and climate variables can be found. A combination of vegetation indices, surface reflectance, and temperature measurements have been used by epidemiologists to model vector ecosystems (e.g., [10]). An earlier discussion of remote sensing techniques used in the study and control of invertebrate hosts and vectors for diseases can be found in [15].

REMOTE SENSING STUDIES IN ARTHROPOD VECTOR-BORNE DISEASES

Mosquitoes

Diseases and vector habitats. Mosquitoes (Figure 1) are found throughout the world, and mosquito-borne diseases are among the world's leading causes of illness and death. Despite great strides over the last 50 years, the World Health Organization estimates that more than 300 million clinical cases of mosquito-borne illnesses occur each year. There is a long history of developing disease transmission models by mosquitoes (e.g., [16,17]) and a good summary is provided by Anderson and May [18]. Several factors, such as seasonality, proximity to breeding grounds, vector density, biting rates, and proportion of infectious mosquitoes, contribute to the spread of mosquito-borne diseases.

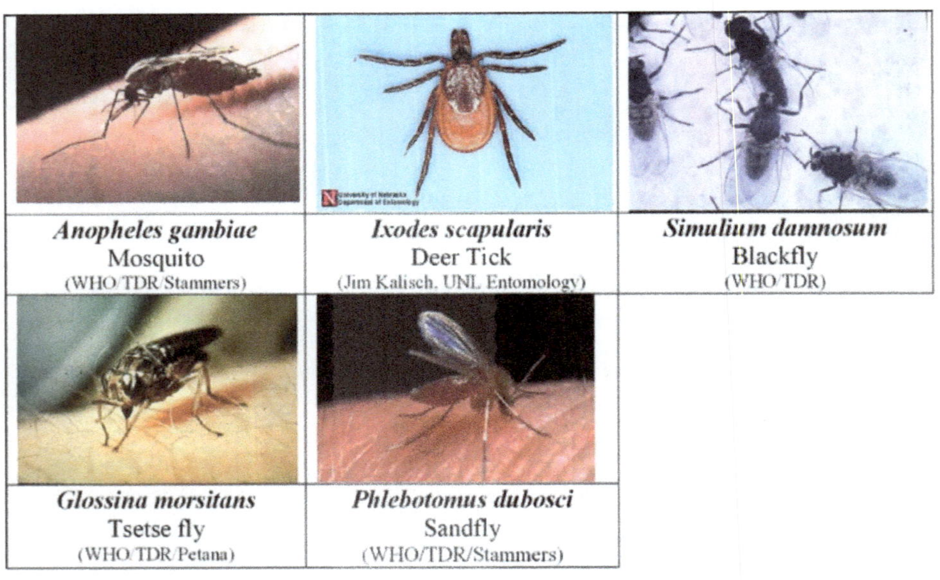

doi:10.1371/journal.ppat.0030116.g001

Figure 1. Arthropod Vectors That Are Discussed in This Paper.

Mosquitoes require still or slow moving water for completing the larval and pupal stages of their life cycle. Both natural as well as man-made environments of stagnant water are conducive to their breeding. For example, in Asia and America, Aedes aegypti breeds primarily in man-made water containers such as automobile tyres, metal drums, recycling containers, and domestic water storage containers, whereas in Africa, they breed in tree holes and leaf axils [19,20]. Temperature, precipitation, and relative humidity are the three main factors that determine the abundance of mosquitoes and the prevalence of mosquito-borne diseases such as malaria [21]. The optimum temperature for mosquito development of tropical species is 25–27 °C [22], and there is a strong temperature dependence of the development of the parasites within the mosquito vectors. For example, the time needed for the sporozoites of Plasmodium falciparum to reach the salivary glands of mosquitoes is inversely proportional to the air temperature with a difference of 14 days between 30 °C and 10 °C [23]. Mosquito-borne diseases such as malaria are seasonal and case numbers correlate well with rainfall patterns [23]. However, too little rainfall creates fewer breeding habitats, and too much rainfall tends to wash away the mosquito eggs [24]. Irrigated agricultural areas such as paddy fields in Asia and inland tidal waters are also very favorable for the breeding of some mosquito species.

Remote sensing studies of mosquito-borne diseases. Mosquito-borne diseases are prevalent throughout the world, and remote sensing applications in epidemiology have been most widely used to study mosquito-borne diseases. A good summary of mosquito biology and methods to map their habitats from satellites can be found in [25].

Initial studies largely focused on identifying mosquito breeding habitats such as marshes and wetlands through land-use and land-cover mapping using remote sensing data (e.g., [26–31]). For example, Landsat data was used to determine green leaf area index (LAI) over 104 rice fields, and these measurements were compared to larval counts of Aedes freeborni at the edge of the fields and the minimum distance from the center of each field to the nearest livestock pastures that provide the blood-meal source [8,32]. This analysis showed that fields that are near pastures that have high LAI and tiller density produce large numbers of mosquitoes, and fields with low LAI that are further from the pastures have lower numbers of mosquitoes. A combination of spectral measurements from the satellite data and distance measurements to pastures were used in discriminant analysis to identify high mosquito producing areas with 90% accuracy.

Multispectral data from the SPOT (Satellite Probatoire d'Observation de la Terre) satellite was used to map the probability of mosquito presence in Belize by Roberts et al. [33]. This study measured the distance of houses from waterways, altitude above specified waterways, and amount of forest between houses and waterways. Each site was then ranked as high, medium, or low for probability of mosquito infestation based on thresholds of distance, elevation, and forest cover. Areas that were closest to the water in both distance and altitude with no intervening forests were assigned the highest probability of mosquito presence around humans. Their results showed that Anopheles pseudopunctipennis was present in 50% of all the high probability locations and absent in all the low probability locations.

Anopheles darlingi larval habitats were surveyed in Belize by sampling along the Sibun River in Belize and compared with land cover classification from SPOT and IKONOS data [34]. Ground survey showed a strong correlation between positive larval habitats and debris from trees such as fallen trunks, branches, and root systems compared to other landscape features. However, no such correlations could be made between positive larval habitats and different land cover types such as forests and orchards or landscape features such as river bends where one would expect to find fallen tree detritus. Overhanging spiny bamboo trees were one of the major sources of floating detritus mats for larval breeding, but the satellite imagery did poorly in discriminating bamboos from other vegetation during classification in this study. The only association between positive and negative A. darlingi sampling sites was their distance to the nearest houses, where the negative sites were 162 m further away from homes compared to the positive sites. The authors conclude that the high cost of high spatial resolution imagery to identify houses along a river would make this technique unsuitable for developing countries. Nevertheless, the use of high spatial resolution data for mapping land use, land cover, and hydrological features to identify suitable vector habitats continues to be a popular approach (e.g., [35]).

Advances in understanding of correlations between multispectral satellite measurements and meteorological variables such as rainfall and temperature have led to the development of statistical models of mapping vector habitats using relationships between satellite-derived climatology and vector ecology. Rift Valley fever (RVF) is a mosquito-borne disease that affects humans and animals in various parts of Africa. Mosquito breeding habitats in East Africa, known locally as "dambos", are frequently flooded during periods of heavy rainfall, which leads to a build-up of mosquito populations and subsequent RVF outbreaks. Since NDVI is known to be correlated with variations in rainfall, variability of NDVI has been shown to be associated with RVF incidence [36]. A discussion on the use of temporal profiles of NDVI and cold cloud duration (CCD) measurements from satellites in models of mosquito distribution and malaria in Africa is found in [37]. Sea surface temperature (SST) variations indicate that El Niño Southern Oscillation and concurrent SST elevations in the Pacific and Indian oceans are correlated with increased rainfall in Eastern Africa. When SST data and NDVI were used together as the predictor variables, the incidence of RVF could be forecast up to 5 months in advance [38,39].

Temporal Fourier processed measurements of NDVI, land surface temperature, and CCD were used by Rogers et al. [10] to capture the seasonal climatology of the African landscape. Fourier processing of these variables reduces the dimensionality of the data set while retaining crucial information about habitat seasonality (information that is lost by other methods of data reduction, such as Principal Components Analysis). The Fourier processed images were used in discriminant analytical models to describe both the distribution of five important species in the Anopheles gambiae complex of species in Africa and the risk of malaria as captured by the entomological inoculation rate (EIR, the number of infectious bites per person per year). Relationships observed between EIR and satellite data were used to make a predictive map of EIR across the continent. Similar techniques were used to create risk maps of West Nile virus in the United States [40] and maps of global distributions of yellow fever and dengue [41]. The predicted risk maps showing the maximum likelihood, posterior probability of disease presence or absence had an average kappa index between model predictions and observations of 0.742 for yellow fever and 0.700 for dengue.

Figure 2 shows the potential distribution of four species of West Nile virus–carrying mosquitoes in the United States derived using the techniques described by Rogers et al. [40]. Note the close agreement between the geographic extent of distribution derived from satellite data and the recorded distribution on the ground.

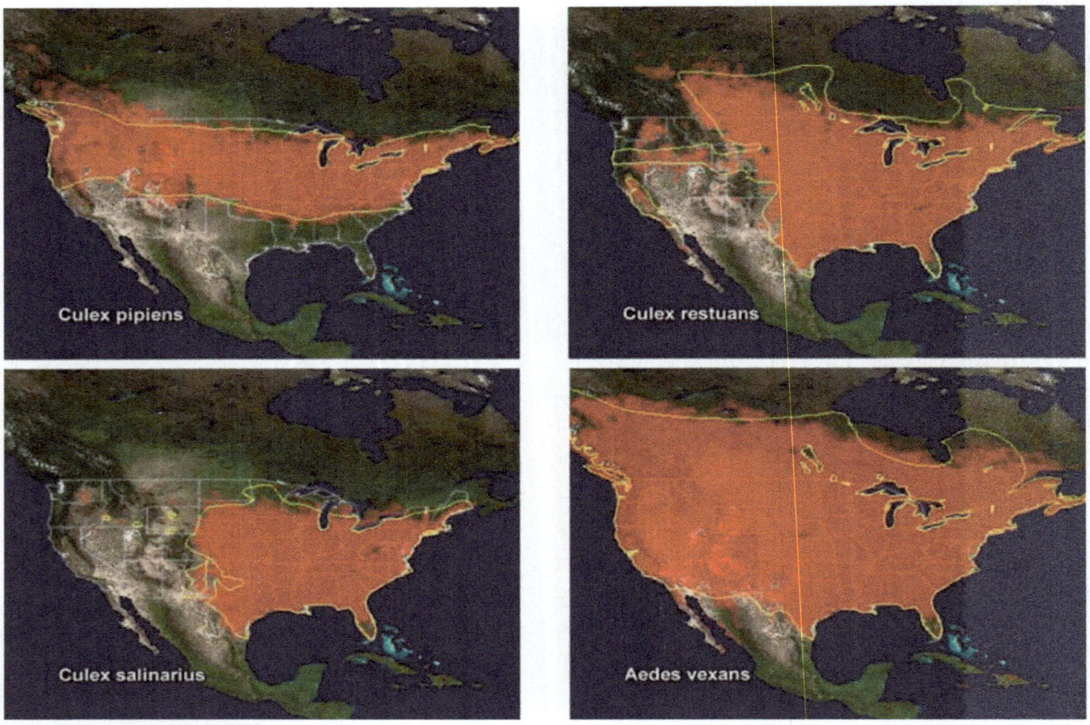

doi:10.1371/journal.ppat.0030116.g002

Figure 2. Maps Showing the Potential Distribution of Four Species of Mosquitoes in the United States Distribution predicted using satellite derived environmental data is in red, and recorded distribution is outlined in yellow. Image courtesy: TALA Research Group–University of Oxford.

Ticks

Diseases and vector habitats. Ticks are responsible for transmitting a variety of pathogens, including protozoa, rickettsia, bacteria, and viruses, to both humans and livestock [42], which causes substantial economic damage worldwide [43,44]. Lyme disease, Rocky Mountain spotted fever, ehrlichiosis, and babesiosis are some of the more common diseases in humans that are transmitted by ticks. Lyme disease is the most common vector-borne disease of humans in the United States and Europe [45,46].

Unlike other arthropod vectors such as mosquitoes, ticks are hematophagous only once per life cycle stage, taking large blood meals equivalent to 10–100 times their body weight [47]. The primary hosts of Ixodes scapularis (Figure 1), the black-legged tick that carries the bacteria Borrelia burgdorferi, which causes Lyme disease in humans, are the white-footed mice (Peromyscus leucopus) and white-tailed deer (Odocoileus virginianus) [45]. During their life cycle, different Ixodid tick species may use one, two, or three different host species [48]. In their free-living stages, most tick species have specific requirements in terms of microclimate and tend therefore to be picked up only by those hosts that frequent the habitats providing such conditions [48–51]. Tick populations are abundant in deciduous forests with leaf litter and ecosystems with shrubs and tall grasses in temperate climates with high relative humidity. Lyme disease shows strong seasonality, with peaks occurring during the summer and fall months when the nymphs are most active [52]. However, changes in the incidence of tick-borne diseases cannot always be related to climate change; changes in other elements of complex epidemiological cycles may also play a part. For example, Lyme disease within the United States is concentrated mostly in the northeastern Atlantic states [53], and the spread of this disease seems to be closely related to an increase in the population of the white-tailed deer [54], an increase due to a diminution of hunting pressure and an increase in woodland in close proximity to human habitation.

Remote sensing studies of tick-borne diseases. A land cover map derived from a Landsat Thematic Mapper (TM) image of Guadeloupe, French Windward Islands, was used by Hugh-Jones [55,56] to discriminate four grazing regions with different levels of cattle tickAmblyomma variegatum infestation in 103 cattle herds. The four classes were lightly infested dry meadows, moderately infested foothills, heavily infested dry scrub, and rocky grasslands. The spatial variability of pixel values within individual grazing fields also correlated well with tick density; areas where the landscape was variable had more ticks compared to homogenous areas.

Ticks exhibit strong seasonal dependence of mortality and disease transmission, which can be related to temperature and vegetation conditions [47]. A critical factor for egg laying and larval development is temperature and humidity. Since these factors can be related to NDVI, multitemporal NDVI measurements from the Advanced Very High Resolution Radiometer (AVHRR) have been correlated with mean mortality during the life cycle between the adult female and subsequent larval stages in Burundi, Uganda, and Tanzania [57].

Using environmental variables obtained at the residences of Lyme disease patients in Baltimore County, Maryland, from 1989 through 1990 within a geographic information system (GIS), Glass et al. [58] showed that many suitable tick habitats in the northeastern United States coincide with residential properties close to wooded areas. Brightness, greenness, and wetness determined from Landsat data [59] were used along with elevation and land cover classes to determine risk for Lyme disease on 337 residential properties in two communities of suburban Westchester County, New York [60]. Spatial analysis of Lyme disease risk indicated that high-risk properties had a greater abundance of green vegetation and/or a higher proportion of woods than lower and no-risk properties, which is consistent with field-based studies of the landscape ecology of Lyme disease.

Ticks are not highly mobile in nature, and they depend on their hosts (e.g., the white-footed mouse) for movement over large distances. However, not all environments that a host might inhabit are suitable for ticks to survive and reproduce. Therefore, the presence of an adequate host population by itself is not a risk factor for the transmission of Lyme disease. To determine what specific environments are conducive for the survival of I. scapularis in the upper Midwest, a survey was conducted of tick populations by collecting samples from vertebrate hosts on the ground, and environmental data from each collection site was compared with tick abundance [61]. Land cover data derived from Landsat TM data was used with maps of soils, geology, elevation, and climate to determine significant associations between tick presence and environmental variables. Discriminant analysis was used to determine the significant environmental factors that differentiate positive and negative tick sites. Logistic regression analysis was used to create maps of habitat suitability for I. scapularis. Areas that had high suitability coincided with the incidence of Lyme disease in Wisconsin. The results of the logistic regression (83.9% classification accuracy) were in agreement with the discriminant analysis (85.7% classification accuracy) and both techniques showed that soil order and land cover were the dominant factors for tick presence.

Using NDVI and surface temperature measurement from AVHRR between 1982 and 2000, Estrada-Pena [62] showed that favorable tick habitats within the United States are increasing. A reduction in biodiversity due to deforestation and forest fragmentation could lead to an increase in the density of the white-footed mouse, and ticks feeding on the white-footed mouse have a higher probability of being infected with B. burgdorferi than any other host [63].

Environmental data derived from satellites was used by Randolph and Rogers [64] to differentiate the eco-climatic zones of six tick-borne flaviviruses. Since only certain environments that can sustain the appropriate natural life cycles of the vector can support the virus transmission cycles, this study suggests that climate may have played a role in directing the evolution of the flaviviruses. By understanding the biotic and abiotic constraints imposed on the evolution and mutation of vector-borne microbes, it may be possible to predict the non-evolutionary emergence of vector-borne diseases under dynamic eco-climatic conditions with a detailed knowledge of vector biology and transmission conditions.

Black Flies

Diseases and vector habitats. Blackflies are about 1–6 mm in length and are amongst the smallest blood-sucking Dipterans. They usually breed in well-aerated water bodies such as swiftly moving shallow mountain torrents [48], or sunlit, fast flowing rivers in the tropics [65]. Onchocerciasis or river blindness is caused by the helminth Onchocerca volvulus of the family Filariidae, whose larvae are transmitted between humans by blackflies of the family Simuliidae (Figure 1). Onchocerciasis is the second leading cause of blindness in the world with 96% of the affected people living in 30 countries in sub-Saharan Africa (and Yemen), with the remainder in six countries in Latin America [66]. Several programs such as the Onchocerciasis Control Programme in West Africa [67], the Onchocerciasis Elimination Program for the Americas [68], and the African Programme for Onchocerciasis Control [69] target this dreadful disease which, because its impact is greatest in mature individuals (i.e., the agriculturally productive sector of societies), has a disproportionate effect on human communities.

Remote sensing studies of diseases due to black flies. The African Programme for Onchocerciasis Control developed a program called Rapid Epidemiological Mapping of Onchocerciasis (REMO) to enable communities at high risk to be quickly and cheaply identified and mapped for priority treatment. However, when ivermectin, the drug used to treat onchocerciasis is administered to patients who are also infected with Loa loa, fatal complications have been reported [70]. Therefore, before Ivermectin could be distributed, WHO wanted to map areas with L. loa infection so that drug administration protocols could be modified to avoid complications. Flies of the genus *Chrysops* (family Tabanidae) that carry the cutaneous filarial parasite L. loa, causing Calabar swellings in humans, are associated with forest and forest fringe habitats with larval stages restricted to wet, organically rich and muddy low-lying areas within the forests [71]. Using forest cover and landcover classes derived from AVHRR along with soil and topography data, the prevalence of L. loa in six African countries was predicted, and the results were compared with priority areas defined by the REMO project [71]. About 50% of the variation in prevalence rates of the infection could be explained by the satellite-derived environmental factors. There were extensive areas of agreement between the satellite derived maps and areas that were identified by REMO as high priority treatment areas in Cameroon and the Democratic Republic of Congo.

Tsetse Flies

Diseases and vector habitats. Tsetse flies (genus *Glossina*), which are found only in Africa, transmit various protozoan parasites of the genus *Trypanosoma*, which cause sleeping sickness in humans and "nagana" in domestic animals. There are 30 species or subspecies of tsetse, classified into three groups: the *fusca* group, found mostly in forests, the *palpalis*group, found in forests and riverine vegetation, and the *morsitans* group, found in woodland areas of savannah regions. Human sleeping sickness is caused by *Trypanosoma brucei gambiense* and *Trypanosoma brucei rhodesiense*, which threaten up to 60 million people in 36 countries of sub-Saharan Africa [72]. *T. b. gambiense* is usually transmitted by tsetse of the *palpalis* group and occurs mostly in cultivated lands within proximity of pools of water in western and central Africa; it is a disease adapted to humans, although other animals—especially domestic ones—may be important reservoir hosts. *T. b. rhodesiense*, which is the more virulent of the two, is usually transmitted by tsetse of the *morsitans* group and occurs primarily in the savannah woodlands of eastern and central/southern Africa [13,73]; it is a disease that occurs naturally in a large number of domestic and wildlife hosts [74]. In humans, as the disease progresses, the parasite crosses the blood–brain barrier and invades the central nervous system, causing neurological problems [75]. Compared to other arthropod vectors such as mosquitoes, tsetse flies have a very low reproductive rate and a longer life expectancy. The mortality and reproductive rates of tsetse flies are highly dependent upon microclimatic conditions, with high survival rates in cool, moist areas [76]. Animal trypanosomiasis occurs more or less throughout the area of Africa inhabited by one or more species of tsetse (an area of approximately 10 million km^2), while human sleeping sickness, which has a much higher threshold for transmission [77], occurs only in a relatively few, but very persistent, disease foci.

Remote sensing studies of diseases due to tsetse flies. Predictive, process-based models of disease transmission based on the biology of the insect vectors are in general more robust than statistical models, which do not necessarily describe causal relationships between the predictor variables and the predicted phenomena. Air temperature and vapor pressure deficit from climatology records have been successfully used to model the birth and death rates, and density, of tsetse flies over Africa [76]. Since these environmental variables can be related to NDVI, land surface temperature, and cold cloud top temperature duration (CCD) observed from meteorological satellites, techniques have been developed for modeling tsetse distribution in Africa using multi-temporal satellite data [78–80]. The techniques used in these analyses include Fourier analysis of the time series data to reduce the dimensionality while capturing the seasonality of variables, and classifying the images using linear and non-linear discriminant analysis to predict species distribution. These methods were able to predict the distribution of tsetse with accuracies of greater than 80%. Among the different variables used in modeling tsetse distribution, NDVI was considered to be the most important variable, followed by CCD, surface temperature, and elevation. Analysis of habitats and species' distributions from these studies indicated that different species of tsetse flies are differently but closely adapted to local climate conditions. In some cases, the presence or absence of flies was shown to be dependent upon temperature differences of 1 °C or less, and the importance and number of environmental variables in determining tsetse distribution differed from region to region. A review of different methods used in tsetse modeling from satellite data is provided by Rogers [80], and this review contains the first ever satellite-driven, process-based model of disease transmission (trypanosomiasis) based upon a satellite-driven, processed-based model for its insect vector (tsetse flies).

Sandflies

Diseases and vector habitats. Visceral leishmaniasis (kala-azar), mucocutaneous leishmaniasis, and cutaneous leishmaniasis are three diseases caused by *Leishmania*protozoa (close relatives of trypanosomes) that are spread through the bite of about 30 different species of sandflies of the subfamily Phlebotominae (super-family Psychodoidea) [81]. Sandflies feed mostly at night, when they are most active, and breed in dark, humid environments with organic matter that serves as food for the larvae [48]. Studying their life cycle is difficult because the larvae, which are tiny, are very hard to find, even in areas of high disease prevalence [82]. Sandflies are restricted to tropical and temperate climates (hot and humid), and therefore leishmaniasis is endemic to these areas, which include northern Africa, the Middle East, parts of Europe, and central South America [73]. Leishmaniasis is primarily a zoonotic disease, affecting mostly rodents and dogs, and humans are incidental hosts. Factors such as deforestation, population migration from endemic rural areas, and increased population in areas with low sanitation have caused a resurgence of leishmaniasis by increasing the contact between the vectors and the hosts [83].

Remote sensing studies of diseases due to sandflies. Leishmaniasis transmitted by sandflies was reported as a health hazard for troops deployed in the Middle East both during World War II and in the 1991 Persian Gulf War. The spatial distribution of sandflies is, however, not well understood, mainly because the larvae are so difficult to find. The distribution of Phlebotomus papatasi using NDVI and meteorological data in the Middle East has been modeled [84]. In this study [84], published reports of leishmaniasis and sandfly fever in the Middle East were used to determine the presence of sandflies and their location. Meteorological data were collected on the ground from 114 weather stations in nine countries, including Saudi Arabia, Kuwait, Iran, and Iraq. Meteorological data were not available for all of the locations that had leishmaniasis and sandfly fever. The objective, therefore, was to develop a technique that would determine the probability of disease for those areas where there were no weather data. Using discriminant analysis, the probability of vector occurrence was determined for all 114 locations that had weather data. For those areas that were determined to be positive for sandfly presence, NDVI measurements from AVHRR were analyzed for a 12-year period from 1982. Analysis indicated that the range of NDVI that was associated with vector presence was 0.0–0.06, and this information was used to create a map showing the areas where sandflies could be present. This map was able to identify accurately all the areas where sandflies were present, including those areas that had no meteorological data.

Comparison of sandfly (P. argentipes) densities with different land use land cover types derived from IRS LISS3 (Indian Remote Sensing Satellite Linear Imaging Self-Scanning System 3) data over two are areas that were endemic and non-endemic to visceral leishmaniasis (kala-azar) in Northern India showed that the endemic areas had a higher percentage of water bodies [85]. The endemic areas also had a higher proportion of marshes compared to the non-endemic areas, and there were also significant differences in vegetation and soil types among the two areas. Succulent vegetation was more prominent in endemic areas, whereas non-endemic areas had predominantly thorny and hard-stemmed plants. In endemic areas, the vector density (as described by the man hour density) was higher during the summer (March–June) and rainy seasons (July–October) compared to non-endemic areas. This study was useful for the health authorities in prioritizing their visits to specific sites.

FUTURE PROSPECTS

Improvements in both sensor capabilities and data processing algorithms are enabling estimates of parameters such as precipitation from space directly rather than using surrogate variables. The availability of moderate resolution imagery from new NASA satellites such as Terra and Aqua at up to 250-m spatial resolution offers improved capabilities in modeling epidemiology from space at a finer spatial resolution than AVHRR. Technologies such as global positioning systems and GIS provide geolocation and mapping capabilities on the ground at unprecedented accuracies, making it possible to merge more accurately ground observations of vector demographics and disease incidence with satellite data. A wide choice of powerful image processing, GIS and statistical software packages are available within an affordable desktop computing environment, making it feasible for epidemiologists and biologists to experiment with new spatial analysis techniques. Anthropogenic factors such as land cover conversion and increase in greenhouse gases are resulting in global climate change, which could expand the ecosystem boundaries of disease-carrying vectors, resulting in an increase in infectious diseases [86]. Maps showing seasonal risks of vector-borne diseases will be necessary to monitor the impacts of global change on vector ecologies. Our ability to forecast climate trends and events such as El Niño and La Niña and their impact on rainfall patterns in regional environments, combined with an understanding of vector-environmental relationships, will help us to improve forecasts of epidemics. Automation of satellite data processing could lead to the generation of risk maps in near real-time to warn local health care professionals.

A complex set of biotic and abiotic factors influence the emergence and spread of vector-borne diseases. While it is not possible to predict the evolution of new vector-borne pathogens, remote sensing techniques can aid in determining the influence of abiotic environmental factors on their spread. Although multitemporal satellite data are available for an extended time period, the availability of georeferenced and spatially explicit disease data for the same temporal record is still less common, especially in developing countries that have a high burden of vector-borne diseases. Other issues that are impacting the routine use of remote sensing in epidemiology include accessibility to high resolution and low-cost imagery [87,88], as well as issues with data continuity in terms of consistencies in spatial, spectral, and temporal resolutions among satellite sensors during different years. Unforeseen problems, such as the failure of Landsat 7 satellite and delays in the launch of new earth observing satellites such as the National Polar-orbiting Operational Environmental Satellite System, as well as shifting priorities of space agencies, could impact our ability to routinely use satellite data in epidemiology and other applications [89]. However, these issues with remote sensing data are not unique to epidemiological applications alone. It should be noted that the use of remote sensing techniques for modeling and forecasting vector-borne diseases is an emerging field, and a sustained use of these applications could be ensured by collaboration between remote sensing scientists and epidemiologists from the onset of research projects [87].

Remotely sensed environmental variables such as air temperature, humidity, and rainfall should be processed and made available to epidemiologists in real-time and in a format that they can readily use as inputs to their modeling by agencies and organizations that collect and archive satellite data. Within the United States, remote sensing data have potential applications in modeling risk from West Nile fever, dengue fever, and Lyme disease. The potential for epidemic dengue transmission within the United States still exists because of the presence of A. albopictus and *A. aegypti* mosquitoes that transmit the disease [1]. Application of remote sensing techniques to map areas at risk for dengue fever within the United States is yet to be done. The predictive maps of diseases need to be verified on the ground for accuracy. While several studies have shown correlations between global climate change and variations in the number of people infected with a particular vector-borne disease, it not yet clear how much change in disease would have occurred without environmental change. Efforts therefore should also focus on the development of stochastic, process-based models that rely on vector biology as predictors of diseases and their risk, instead of statistical models that do not clearly explain causal relationships between satellite data and disease. Nevertheless, simple statistical models could be a good starting point for linking the limited number of environmental variables that can be derived from satellite data with spatial and temporal patterns of diseases and vectors. Simple statistical models could help deduce the epidemiological processes from an analysis of the observed spatial patterns of the disease and the environment.

Remote sensing of vector ecosystems and interpretation of these patterns is likely to provide both challenges and opportunities in epidemiology. In addition to vector biology, social and behavioral patterns such as the time spent outside, which increases risk of exposure to anthropophilic vectors, types of house constructions, the use of nets and other repellents, as well as the availability of basic sanitation and primary healthcare facilities, which are related to socioeconomic conditions, are important in disease prevention and control. Disease patterns have been shown to be closely linked to poverty and social inequalities [90]. These factors cannot be inferred from remote sensing techniques alone.

While the studies reviewed in this paper demonstrate the efficacy of remote sensing and other geospatial technologies in disease surveillance, there are however, several factors that need to be considered for these technologies to be routinely adopted for public health management. These include the availability of resources for gathering, processing, and modeling geospatial data, training of personnel on the proper interpretation of results, cost effectiveness of these surveillance techniques, and the continuous availability of remote sensing data in a timely manner. It should also be emphasized that the allocation of resources for these novel monitoring techniques should not come at the cost of basic disease prevention and management activities at the community level.

ACKNOWLEDGMENTS

We thank the three anonymous reviewers for their valuable comments on the manuscript. Mehmet Dondurur and Steve Marley contributed to this work through literature search and database development.

AUTHOR CONTRIBUTIONS

SK and DR designed the study. DR performed the experiments. SK, PG, and DR analyzed the data. SK, DR, and MS contributed reagents/tools to this study. SK and PG contributed to writing the paper.

REFERENCES

1. Gubler DJ (1998) Resurgent vector-borne diseases as a global health problemEmerg Infect Dis 4: 442–450.
2. Davis JR, Lederberg J, editors(2001) Emerging infectious diseases from the global to the local perspectiveWashington (D. C.): National Academy Press134 p.
3. Madon MB, Mulla MS, Shaw MW, Kluh S, Hazelrigg JE (2002) Introduction of Aedes albopictus (Skuse) in Southern California and potential for its establishmentJ Vect Ecol 27: 149–154.
4. World Health Organization (2002) The world health reportGeneva: World Health Organization.
5. World Health Organization (2007) Disability adjusted life yearsAvailable:http://www. who. int/healthinfo/boddaly/en/Accessed 13 September 2007.
6. Teklehaimanot A, Singer B, Spielman A, Tozan Y, Schapira A (2005) Coming to grips with malaria in the new millenniumUN Millennium ProjectLondon: Earthscan.
7. Beck LR, Lobitz BM, Wood BL (2000) Remote sensing and human health: New sensors and new opportunitiesEmerg Infect Dis 6: 217–226.
8. Wood BL, Beck LR, Washino RK, Palchick SM, Sebesta D (1991) Spectral and spatial characterization of rice field mosquito habitatInt J Remote Sens 12: 621–626.
9. Sithiprasasna R, Lee WJ, Ugsang DM, Linthicum KJ (2005) Identification and characterization of larval and adult anopheline mosquito habitats in the Republic of Korea: potential use of remotely sensed data to estimate mosquito distributionsInt J of Health Geogr 4: 17Available: http://www. ij-healthgeographics. com/content/4/1/17Accessed 13 September 2007.
10. Rogers DL, Randolph SE, Snow RW, Hay SI, (2002) Satellite imagery in the study and forecast of malariaNature 415: 710–715.
11. Rogers DJ (2006) Models for vectors and vector-borne diseasesAdv Parasitol 62: 1–35.
12. Hay SI, Tatem AJ, Graham AJ, Goetz SJ, Rogers DJ (2006) Global environmental data for mapping infectious disease distributionAdv Parasitol 62: 37–77.
13. Rogers DJ (1991) Satellite imagery tsetse and trypanosomiasis in AfricaPrev Vet Med 11: 201–220.
14. Townshend JRG, Justice CO (1986) Analysis of the dynamics of African vegetation using the normalized difference vegetation indexInt J Remote Sens 7: 1435–1445.
15. Hay SI, Packer MJ, Rogers DJ (1997) The impact of remote sensing on the study and control of invertebrate intermediate hosts and vectors for diseaseInt J Remote Sens 18: 2899–2930.
16. Ross R (1916) An application of the theory of probabilities to the study of a priori pathometry-IProc R Soc Lond A92: 204–230.
17. Macdonald G (1957) The epidemiology and control of malariaLondon: Oxford University Press.
18. Anderson RM, May RM (1991) Infectious diseases of humansNew York: Oxford University Press757 p.
19. World Health Organization (1997) Dengue haemorrhagic fever: diagnosis treatment prevention and control2nd editionGeneva: World Health Organization.
20. World Health Organization (2002) Dengue and dengue haemorrhagic fever fact sheet number 117Geneva: World Health Organization.
21. Pampana E (1969) A textbook of malaria eradicationLondon: Oxford University Press.
22. McMichael AJ, Haines A, Sloof R, Kovats S, editors(1996) Climate change and human health technical report WHO/EHG/967Geneva: World Health Organization305 p.
23. Oaks SC Jr, Mitchell VS, Pearson GW, Carpenter CCJ, editors(1991) Malaria: obstacles and opportunities: A report of the Committee for the Study on Malaria Prevention and Control: Status review and alternative strategiesDivision of International Health, Institute of MedicineWashington (D. C.): National Academy Press328 p.
24. Srivatsava A, Nagpal BN, Saxena R, Subbarao SK (2001) Predictive habitat modeling for forest malaria vector species *An Dirus* in India–a GIS based approachCurr Sci 80: 1129–1134.
25. Hay SI, Omumbo JA, Kraig MH, Snow RW (2000) Earth observation geographic information systems and Plasmodium falciparum malaria in Sub-Saharan AfricaAdv Parasitol 47: 174–206.
26. Barnes CM, Cibula CG (1979) Some implications of remote sensing technology in insect control programs including mosquitoesMosquito News 39: 271–282.
27. Wagner VE, Hill-Rowley R, Newson H D (1979) Remote sensing: A rapid and accurate method of data acquisition for a newly formed mosquito control districtMosquito News 39: 271–282.
28. Pope KO, Sheffner EJ, Linthicum KJ, Bailey CL, Logan

TM, et al(1992) Identification of central Kenyan Rift Valley Fever virus vector habitats with Landsat TM and evaluation of their flooding status with airborne imaging radarRemote Sens Environ 40: 185–196.

29. Beck LR, Rodríguez MH, Dister SW, Rodríguez AD, Rejmánková E, et al(1994) Remote sensing as a landscape epidemiologic tool to identify villages at high risk for malaria transmissionAm J Trop Med Hyg 51: 271–280.

30. Rejmankova E, Savage HM, Rodriguez MH, Roberts DR, Rejmanek M (1992) Aquatic vegetation as a basis for classification of Anopheles albimanus Wiedemann (Diptera: Culcidae) larval habitatsEnviron Entomol 21: 598–603.

31. Rejmankova E, Roberts DR, Pawley A, Manguin S, Polanco J (1995) Predictions of adult Anopheles albimanus densities in villages based on distances to remotely-sensed larval habitatsAm J Trop Med Hyg 53: 482–488.

32. Wood B, Washino R, Beck L, Hibbard K, Pitcairn M, et al(1991) Distinguishing high and low Anopheline-producing rice fields using remote sensing and GIS technologiesPrev Vet Med 11: 277–288.

33. Roberts DR, Paris JF, Manguin S, Harbach RE, Woodruff R, et al(1996) Predictions of malaria vector distribution in Belize based on multispectral satellite dataAm J Trop Med Hyg 57: 304–308.

34. Achee NL, Grieco JP, Masuoka P, Andre RG, Roberts DR, et al(2006) Use of remote sensing and geographic information systems to predict locations of Anopheles darlingi-positive breeding sites within the Sibun River in Belize Central AmericaJ Med Entomol 43: 382–392.

35. Mushinzimana E, Munga S, Minakawa N, Li L, Feng CC, et al(2006) Landscape determinants and remote sensing of anopheline mosquito larval habitats in the western Kenya highlandsMalaria J 16: 5–13.

36. Linthicum KJ, Bailey CL, Tucker CJ, Angleberger DR, Cannon T, et al(1991) Towards real-time prediction of Rift-Valley fever epidemics in AfricaPrev Vet Med 11: 325–334.

37. Thomson MC, Connor SJ, Milligan PJM, Flasse SP (1996) The ecology of malaria seen by earth-observation satellitesAnn Trop Med Parasitol 90: 243–264.

38. Linthicum KJ, Anyamba A, Tucker CJ, Kelley PW, Myers MF, et al(1999) Climate and satellite indicators to forecast Rift Valley fever epidemics in KenyaScience 285: 397–4000.

39. Anyamba A, Linthicum KJ, Tucker CJ (2001) Climate-disease connections: Rift Valley Fever in KenyaCad Saude Publica 17: 133–140.

40. Rogers DJ, Myers MF, Tucker CJ, Smith PF, White DJ, et al(2002) Predicting the distribution of West Nile fever in North America using satellite sensor dataPhotogramm Eng Rem S 68: 112–114.

41. Rogers DJ, Wilson AJ, Hay SI, Graham AJ (2006) The global distribution of yellow fever and dengueAdv Parasitol 62: 181–220.

42. Sonenshine DE, Mather TN, editors(1994) Ecological dynamics of tick-borne zoonosesNew York: Oxford University Press464 p.

43. Bram RA (1983) Tick-borne live stock diseases and their vectorsFAO Animal Production and Health Paper 36Rome: Food and Agricultural Organization.

44. Bram RA, Gray JH (1983) Eradication–an alternative to tick and tick-borne disease controlFAO Animal Production and Health Paper 36Rome: Food and Agricultural Organization.

45. Barbour AG, Fish D (1993) The biological and social phenomenon of Lyme diseaseScience 260: 1610–1616.

46. Nocton JJ, Steere AC (1995) Lyme diseaseAdv Intern Med 40: 69–117.

47. Randolph SE (2000) Ticks and tick-borne disease systems in space and from spaceAdv Parasitol 47: 217–240.

48. Aiello SE, editor(2002) The Merck veterinary manual8th editionWhitehouse Station (New Jersey): Merck & Co.

49. Sonenshine DE (1991) Tick life cyclesBiology of ticksVolume 1 New York: Oxford University Press51–66.

50. Sonenshine DE (1993) Ecology of non-nidocolous ticksBiology of ticksVolume 2New York: Oxford University Presspp3–65.

51. Jones CG, Ostfeld RS, Richard MP, Schauber EM, Wolff JO (1998) Chain reactions linking acrons to gypsy moth outbreaks and lyme disease riskScience 279: 1023–1026.

52. Falco RC, McKenna DF, Daniels TJ, Nadelman RB, Nowakowski J, et al(1999) Temporal relation between Ixodes scapularis abundance and risk for Lyme disease associated with erythema migransAm J Epidemiol 149: 771–776.

53. Centers For Disease Control and Prevention (1999) Notice to readers availability of Lyme disease vaccineMMWR Morb Mortal Wkly Rep 48(2): 35–36Available:http:// www. cdc. gov/mmwr/preview/mmwrhtml/00056299. htmAccessed 28 September 2007.

54. Wilson MI, Adler GH, Spielman A (1985) Correlation between abundance of deer and that of the deer tick Ixodes dammini (Acari: Ixodidae)Ann Entomol Soc Am 7: 172–176.

55. Hugh-Jones M (1991) Landsat-TM identification of the habitats of the cattle tick Amblyomma variegatum in Guadeloupe French Windward IslandsPrev Vet Med 11: 355–356.

56. Hugh-Jones M (1991) The remote sensing of tick habitatsJ Agr Entomol 8: 309–315.

57. Randolph SE (1994) Population dynamics and density-dependent seasonal mortality indices of the tick Rhipicephalus appendiculatus in eastern and southern AfricaMed Vet Entomol 8: 351–368.

58. Glass GE, Schwartz BS, Morgan JM III, Johnson DT, Noy PM, et al(1995) Environmental risk factors for Lyme disease identified with geographic information systemsAm J Public Health 85: 944–948.

59. Kauth RJ, Thomas GS (1976) The tasseled cap–a graphic description of spectral-temporal development of agricultural crops as seen by LandsatProceedings of

the International Symposium on Machine Processing of Remotely Sensed DataPurdue UniversityWest Lafayette, Indiana, United StatesJune 29–July 1 1976;.

60. Dister SW, Fish D, Bros SM, Frank DH, Wood BL (1997) Landscape characterization of peridomestic risk for lyme disease using satellite imageryAm J Trop Med Hyg 57: 687–692.

61. Guerra M, Walker E, Jones C, Paskewitz S, Cortinas MR, et al(2002) Predicting the risk of lyme disease: habitat suitability for Ixodes scapularis in the North United StatesEmerg Infect Dis 8: 289–297.

62. Estrada-Pena A (2002) Increasing habitat suitability in the United States for the tick that transmits Lyme disease: a remote sensing approachEnviron Health Perspect 110: 635–640.

63. Allan BF, Keesing F, Ostfeld RS (2003) Effect of forest fragmentation on Lyme disease riskConserv Biol 17: 267–272.

64. Randolph SE, Rogers DJ (2006) Tick-borne disease systems: mapping geographic and phylogenetic spaceAdv Parasitol 62: 263–291.

65. Shelly AJ (2002) Human onchocerciasis in Brazil: an overviewCad Saúde Pública 18: 1167–1177.

66. World Health Organization (2000) Onchocerciasis (river blindness)WHO fact sheet number 95Geneva: World Health Organization.

67. Molyneux DH (1995) Onchocerciasis control in West Africa: current status and future of the Onchocerciasis Control ProgrammeParasitol Today 11: 399–401.

68. Blanks J, Richards F, Beltran F, Collins R, Alvarez E, et al(1998) The Onchocerciasis Elimination Program for the Americas: a history of partnershipRev Panam Salud Publica (Panamerican Journal of Public Health) 36: 367–374.

69. Remme JHF (1995) The African Programme for Onchocerciasis Control: preparing to launchParasitol Today 11: 403–406.

70. Gardon J, Gardon-Wendel N, Demanga-Ngangue , Kamgno J, Chippaux JP, Boussinesq M (1997) Serious reactions after mass treatment of onchocerciasis with ivermectin in an area endemic for Loa loa infectionLancet 350: 18–22.

71. Thomson MC, Obsomer V, Dunne M, Connor SJ, Molyneux DH (2000) Satellite mapping of Loa loa prevalence in relation to ivermectin use in west and central AfricaLancet 356: 1077–1078.

72. World Health Organization (2001) African trypanosomiasis or sleeping sicknessWHO fact sheet number 259Geneva: World Health Organization.

73. World Health Organization (2000) WHO Report on global surveillance of epidemic-prone infectious diseasesWHO/CDS/CSR/ISR/20001Geneva: World Health Organization.

74. Hutchinson OC, Fevre EM, Carrington M, Welburn SC (2003) Lessons learned from the emergence of a new Trypanosoma brucei rhodesiense sleeping sickness focus in UgandaLancet Infect Dis 3: 42–45.

75. Enanga B, Burchmore RJ, Stewart ML, Barrett MP (2002) Sleeping sickness and the brainCell Mol Life Sci 59: 845–58.

76. Rogers D (1979) Tsetse population dynamics and distribution: a new analytical approachJ Anim Ecol 48: 825–849.

77. Rogers DJ (1988) The dynamics of vector-transmitted diseases in human communitiesPhilos Trans R Soc Lond B Biol Sci B321: 513–537.

78. Green RM, Hay SI (2002) The potential of Pathfinder AVHRR data for providing surrogate climatic variables across Africa and Europe for epidemiological applicationsRemote Sens Environ 79: 166–175.

79. Rogers DJ, Hay SI, Packer MJ (1996) Predicting the distribution of tsetse flies in West Africa using Fourier processed meteorological satellite dataAnn Trop Med Parasitol 90: 225–241.

80. Rogers DJ (2000) Satellites space time and the African trypanosomiasisAdv Parasitol 47: 129–171.

81. World Health Organization (2000) The leishmaniasis and Leishmania/HIV co-infections fact sheet number 116Geneva: World Health Organization.

82. Lane RP (1993) Sandflies (Phlebotominae)In: Lane R, Crosskey RW, editorsMedical insects and arachnidsLondon: Chapman and Hallpp78–119.

83. Machado-Coelho GLL, Assuncao R, Mayrink W, Caiaffa WT (1999) American cutaneous leishmaniasis in Southern-Brazil: space time clusteringInt J Epidemiol 28: 982–989.

84. Cross ER, Newcomb WW, Tucker CJ (1996) Use of weather data and remote sensing to predict the seasonal distribution of Phlebotomus papatasi in southwestern AsiaAm J Trop Med Hyg 54: 530–536.

85. Sudhakar S, Srinivas T, Palit A, Kar SK, Battacharya SK (2006) Mapping of risk prone areas of kala-azar (visceral leishmaniasis) in parts of Bihar State India: an RS and GIS approachJ Vector Borne Dis 43: 115–122.

86. Patz JA, Reisen WK (2001) Immunology, climate change and vector-borne diseasesTrends Immunol 22: 171–172.

87. Herbreteau V, Salem G, Souris M, Hugot JP, Gonzalez JP (2005) Sizing up human health through remote sensing: uses and misusesParassitologia 47: 63–79.

88. Herbreteau V, Salem G, Souris M, Hugot JP, Gonzalez JP (2007) Thirty years of use and improvement of remote sensing applied to epidemiology: from early promises to lasting frustrationHealth Place 13: 400–403.

89. Goetz S (2007) Crisis in earth observationScience 315: 1767.

90. Heggenhougen HK, Hackethal V, Vivek P (2003) The behavioural and social aspects of malaria and its control: An introduction and annotated bibliographyGeneva: UNDP/World Bank/WHO Special Programme for Research and Training in Tropical Diseases (TDR) Available:http://www. who. int/tdr/publications/ publications/seb-malaria. htmAccessed 13 September 2007.

SECTION IX: ANTIPARASITICS, ANTIPROTOZOALS AND ECTOPARASITICIDES

CHAPTER 31

BODY SURFACE CHANGES IN GASTROINTESTINAL HELMINTHES FOLLOWING IN VITRO TREATMENT WITH ALLIUM SATIVUM OIL

Hatem A Shalaby and Tarek K Farag

Keywords: Haemonchus contortus, Moniezia expansa, Allium sativum oil, In vitro

INTRODUCTION

Gastrointestinal helminthes are the highest disease cost to small ruminants industry. The costs associated with parasite infection are categorised as direct and in-direct. The direct cost is the cost of treatment such as the anthelmintic, labour and animal deaths. The in-direct cost of parasitism is the loss of productivity such as reduced growth and live weight of infected animals, reduced milk production and reductions in wool growth and quality [1]. Small ruminants have numerous internal parasites; two of the most economic significance are the nematode Haemonchus contortus [2] and the cestode Moniezia expansa [3]. These two parasites have more reported cases of anthelmintic resistance around the world than other gastrointestinal parasites as well their prevalence and effects on the host [4]. The development of parasite anthelmintic resistance has been influenced by producers' over-reliance on these chemicals to control parasites as well as poor management practices such as under-dosing [5]. With the increased occurrence of multiple drug resistant parasites, other more sustainable methods are being investigated, including the use of medicinal plant extracts with anthelmintic properties, such as garlic.

Garlic (Allium sativum) is one of the oldest, most common medicinal herbs still used today. It has been reported to be a parasiticide, amebicide, acarifuge, vermifuge, larvicide, fungicide, and immuno-stimulant besides other properties [6]. It has been used to treat animals that suffer from gastrointestinal parasitism [7]. Garlic oil has a broad-antimicrobial spectrum; as it has antibacterial, antifungal, antiviral, and antiparasitic effects. Further, it influences the growth of at least 12 different human and nonhuman parasites [8].

The external surfaces of helminths serve as a barrier that shields the organism from external conditions. These surfaces are also vital for nutrient uptake, osmoregulation, immunoprotection and structural support [9]. Since the integrity of the external surfaces of helminths is essential for the nutritive and protective functions, scanning electron microscopic study was undertaken to assess, for the first time, whether the garlic oil had any effect on the cuticle of H. contortus and the tegument of M. expansa following incubation in vitro.

MATERIALS AND METHODS

Preparation of A. Sativum Oil Extract

Bulbs of fully grown A. sativum cultivated locally were used in the study. The dried bulbs were pounded and then steam distilled. The essential oil was extracted using solvent ether.

Anthelmintic effects of A. sativum oil

Adult worms of H. contortus (nematode) and M. expansa (cestode) were collected from abomasum and intestine, respectively, of naturally infected sheep slaughtered in a local abattoir in Cairo province, Egypt. After recovery, the

Citation: Shalaby HA, Farag TK (2014) Body Surface Changes in Gastrointestinal Helminthes Following in vitro Treatment with Allium sativum Oil. J Veterinar Sci Technol 5: 153. doi:10.4172/2157-7579.1000153.

worms were washed and transferred to Ringer solution, as recommended by Hanser et al. [10] containing ASO at concentrations of 10, 50 and 100 μg/ml. The worms were incubated for 24 h at 37°C in an atmosphere of 5% CO2. The ASO was initially prepared as a stock solution in DMSO and added to the culture medium to give a final solvent concentration of 0.01% (v/v). Solvent control worms were incubated for 24 h in Ringer solution containing 0.01% (v/v) DMSO. Fresh control worms at 0 h were fixed immediately following the initial washing. Five worms were examined for each group.

Scanning Electron Microscopy (SEM)

Following incubation, the anterior end of adult worms was fixed intact for 12 h in a 3:1 mixture of 4% (w/v) glutaraldehyde in 0.12 M-Millonig's buffer, pH 7.4 and 1% aqueous osmium tetroxide. Then specimens were processed for SEM following a method previously reported [11].

RESULTS

Scanning electron microscopic observations of the anterior end of adult H. contortus

Normal freshl worms

The mouth of the normal fresh worm was hexagonal with six semicircular rudimentary lips, lateral amphids and papillae. A pair of cervical papillae was prominent and spine-like (Figure 1a). The cuticle was transversally striated and with lateral ridges (Figure 1b).

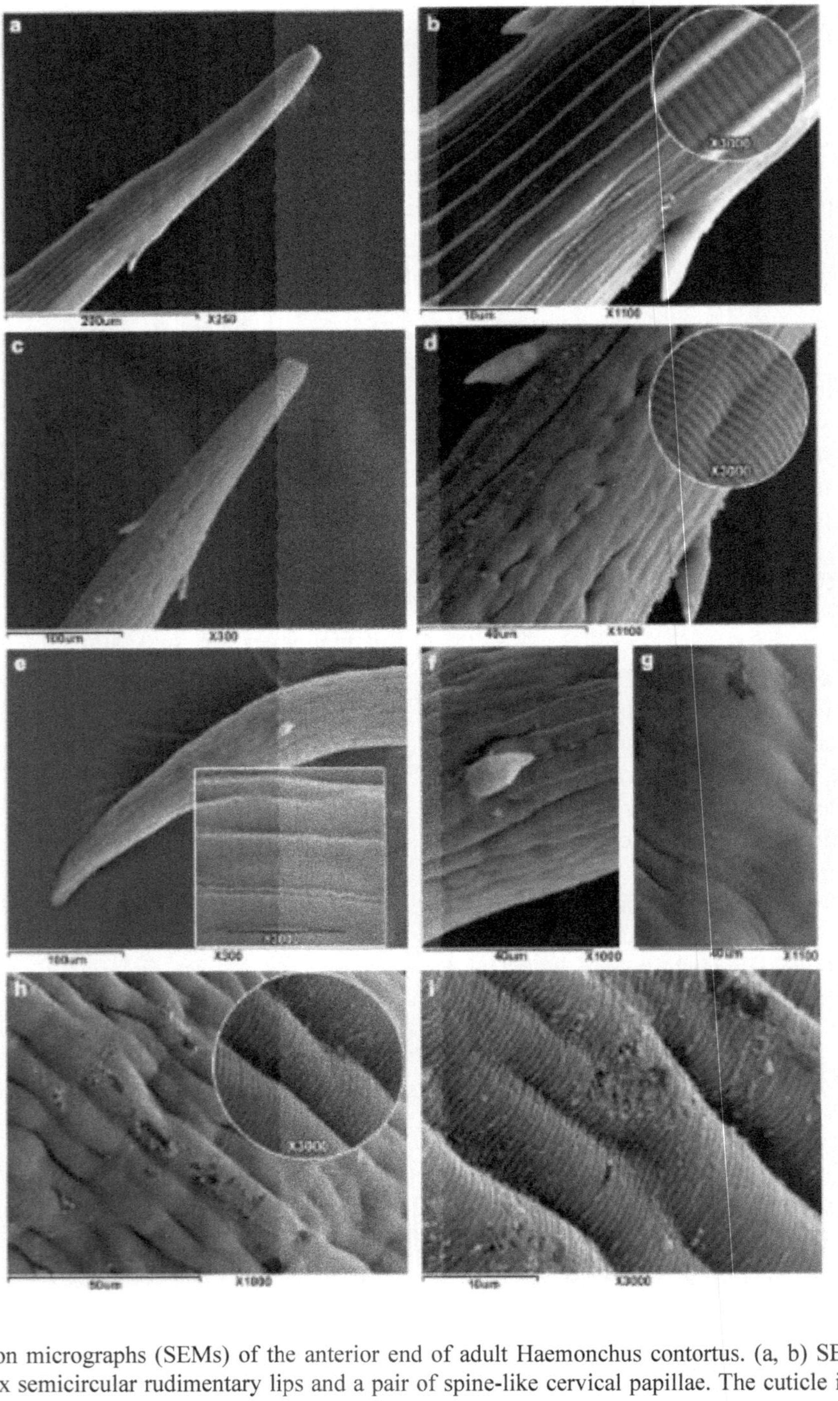

Figure 1: Scanning electron micrographs (SEMs) of the anterior end of adult Haemonchus contortus. (a, b) SEMs of normal fresh worm showing the mouth with six semicircular rudimentary lips and a pair of spine-like cervical papillae. The cuticle is transversally striated and

with lateral ridges (Inset). (c, d) Following 24 h of incubation with 10 μg/ml ASO, showing slightly more swollen cuticle than normal with less pronounced transverse striations (Inset). (e-g) Following 24 h of incubation with 50 μg/ml ASO, revealing wrinkled and corrugated cuticular surface with ill distinguished cuticular striations. (h, i) Following 24 h of incubation with 100 μg/ml ASO, showing severely folded and corrugated cuticle (Inset) and small areas of lesions scattered over its surface.

Treated Worms

After 24 h incubation with 10 μg/ml ASO, the cuticle appeared to be more swollen than normal so that the transverse striations became less pronounced and lost their normal aspect showing longitudinal wrinkles (Figure 1c and 1d). The cuticular swelling became pronounced with wrinkling of the cuticular ridges, on increasing the concentration to 50 μg/ml ASO (Figure 1e). Besides, the cuticular surface had a wrinkled, corrugated appearance (Figure 1f). In extreme cases, the cuticular swelling became so severe so that the cuticular striations were ill distinguished (Figure 1g). With higher concentration of 100 μg/ml ASO, the distortion of the cuticle was similar to that described for the previous concentration, except it was more extensive. But what was apparent in this region was the presence of small areas of lesions scattered over the cuticular surface (Figure 1h and 1i).

Scanning Electron Microscopic Observations of the Anterior end of Adult M. expansa

Normal Fresh Worms

The scolex appeared globular and was provided with four oval suckers radially located around the proximal end of the scolex (Figure 2a). The strobila was an elongated ribbon-like structure composed of series of segments (proglottids) which were broader than longer (Figure 2b).

Treated Worms

After 24 h incubation with 10 μg/ml ASO, the changes in adult cestodes concerned the proglottides other than the scolex which retained its normal morphology (Figure 2c). The proglottides lost their normal aspect showing wrinkled tegumental surface throughout the strobila (Figure 2d). On increasing the concentration to 50 μg/ml ASO, the changes concerned the whole-body surface.The scolex appeared to be more swollen than normal with contractions to the sucker's opening (Figure 2e). The proglottides appeared deformed with circular areas of pronounced swelling occurred along their margins (Figure 2f). With higher concentration of 100 μg/ml ASO, the adult cestodes showed shrunken scolex with severely distorted and folded tegument around the suckers so that a complete closure of their openings had occurred (Figure 2g). In the proglottides, the tegument was swollen and severely distorted (Figure 2h).

In all of the experiments, no significant differences were observed between fresh and control worms incubated for 24 h in solvent, 0.1% (v/v) DMSO.

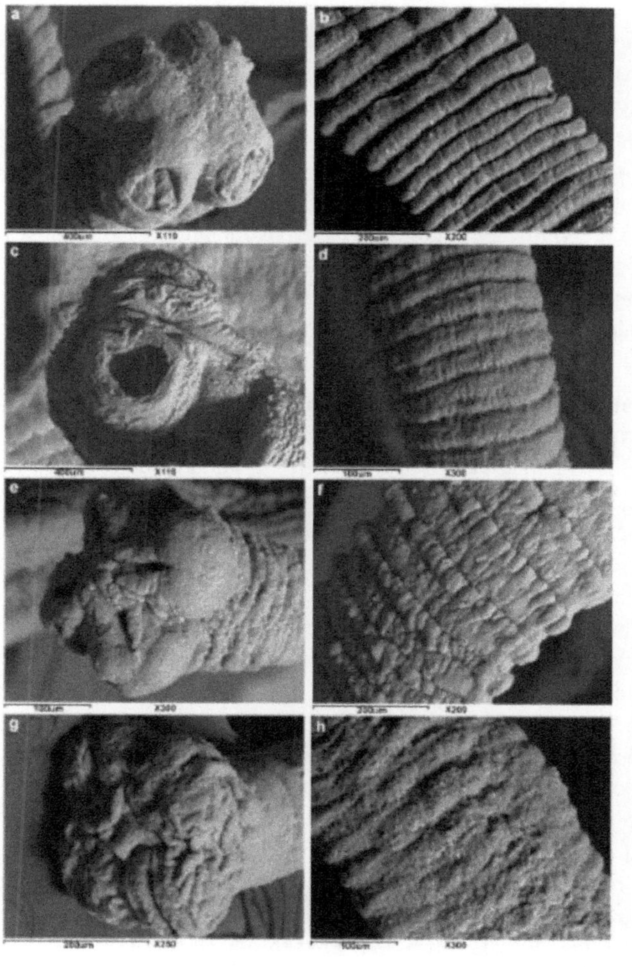

Figure 2: SEMs of the anterior end of adult Moniezia expansa. (a, b) SEMs of normal fresh worm showing a globular scolex with four oval suckers and an elongated ribbon-like structure called strobila. (c, d) Following 24 h of incubation with 10 μg/ml ASO, showing wrinkled tegumental surface throughout the strobila. (e, f) Following 24 h of incubation with 50 μg/ml ASO. The scolex becomes more swollen than normal with narrowing of sucker's opening. The proglottides appear deformed with circular areas of pronounced swelling occurred along their margins. (g, h) Following 24 h of incubation with 100 μg/ml ASO, showing shrunken scolex with severely distorted and folded tegument.

DISCUSSION

The present study demonstrated the effect of ASO on gastrointestinal helminthes. Scanning electron microscopic observations could be used to determine, for the first time, the target of ASO as morphological changes could be observed. These changes were concentration dependent, and consisted of destructive alterations and deformity in the cuticle of H. contortus and also in the tegumental architecture of M. expansa. The cuticle of nematodes is metabolically active and morphologically specialized for selective absorption of nutrients and osmoregulation. Thus, passive diffusion of anthelmintics through the cuticle [9] would probably be responsible for destructive changes and deformation of the nematode body surface [12]. In cestodes, the general body surface acts as an absorptive surface [3]. In the present investigation, the body surface of these helminthes was observed to be affected and altered by ASO. Similar to the present observations, the surface cuticle or tegument was found to be a principal target site for different synthetic drugs and natural anthelmintic products as proved by histomorphological and ultrastructural studies [4,11,13,14]. The swelling and distortion of the body surface of H. contortus and M. expansa induced by ASO had been described for these helminthes by Nigella sativa oil [4]. In Fasciola hepatica, a similar pattern of tegumental swelling had been described following incubation with a number of anthelmintics, as summarized by Hegazi et al. [15]. This was a common feature of drug treated parasites and considered to be an indicator of a stress reaction by the parasite, in an attempt to replace damaged surface membrane [16].

The literature survey of A. sativum suggested that it had anthelmintic action in vitro against H. contortus [17], Heterakis gallinae and Ascaridia galli [18], a free-living nematode of Rhabditis sp, larvae of Nippostrongylus brasiliensis, and eggs of Ascaris sum [19]. Besides, it had antiprotozoal [20] and acaricidal [21] effects. The bioactive property of garlic was formed by the interaction of the non-protein amino acid alliin and the enzyme alliinase [22]. Thiosulfinates were produced through interaction, most commonly induced by crushing the mature garlic clove, of which around 70% of the bioactive compounds produced was allicin (diallylthiosulphinate) [22,23]. Allicin was responsible for garlic's pungent odour and the many medicinal health benefits associated with the consumption of garlic [24]. Garlic essential oil was produced by grinding whole garlic cloves in water; the oil fraction was then obtained by either heat distilling or extraction with an organic solvent. Seventy to eighty percent of the thiosulphinates produced in this oil were made up of allicin (diallylthiosulfinate) [25,26]. Garlic oil was reported to inhibit the growth of more than 12 human and nonhuman parasites [8]. The mode of action of allicin varied depending on the species of parasite. Williams and Lamprecht [27] and Anthony et al. [8] stated that some of actions on parasites were inhabit/blocking of receptor sites of cysteine proteinases, phosphatidylcholine biosynthesis, and the synthesis of coenzyme Q and cell lysis. Other parasitic modes of action were the interactions with thiol-containing enzymes, alcohol dehydrogenases, thioredoxin reductases, as well as the alteration of intracellular membranous structures. When allicin broke down, one of the chemicals, ajoene, was reported to be antiparasitic, which interfered with lipid and protein absorption in the parasite and resulted in a broke down in the intracellular membrane system and cell lysis [8]. There were also reports of garlic being ineffective as an anthelmintic in experimental procedures both in vitro and in vivo which could be due to the preparation methods. The failure of garlic as an anthelmintic to donkeys in the trial by Sutton and Haik [28] was attributed to an inappropriate extraction method and/ or the dose rate, while in a trial by Pena et al. [29] where no extraction method was used and the garlic was fed intact there was a 100% reduction in worm burdens.

The current study and those cited above indicate that an alternative, effective and natural anthelmintic can be developed using garlic that could offer a suitable and cheaper alternative for the more expensive anthelmintics. Further studies with in vivo effect of ASO on gastrointestinal helminthes are clearly warranted.

REFERENCES

1. Ijaz M, Khan MS, Avais M, Ashraf K, Ali MM, et al. (2008) Infection rate and chemotherapy of various helminths in goats in and around Lahore. Pakistan Vet J 28: 167-170.
2. Dai YB, Liu XY, Liu M, Tao JP (2006) Pathogenic effects of the coccidium Eimeria ninakohlyakimovae in goats. Vet Res Commun 30: 149-160.
3. Bashtar AR, Hassanein M, Abdel-Ghaffar F, Al-Rasheid K, Hassan S, et al. (2011) Studies on monieziasis of sheep I. Prevalence and antihelminthic effects of some plant extracts, a light and electron microscopic study. Parasitol Res 108: 177-186.
4. Shalaby HA, Abu El Ezz NMT, Farag TK, Abou-Zeina HAA (2012) In vitro efficacy of a combination of ivermectin and Nigella sativa oil against helminth parasites. Global Veterinaria 9: 465-473
5. Shalaby HA (2013) Anthelmintics Resistance; How to Overcome it? Iran J Parasitol 8: 18-32.
6. Duke J A (2002) Handbook of Medicinal Herbs. CRC Press, Boca Raton, FL, USA.
7. Guarrera PM (1999) Traditional antihelmintic, antiparasitic and repellent uses of plants in Central Italy. J Ethnopharmacol 68: 183-192.
8. Anthony JP, Fyfe L, Smith H (2005) Plant active components - a resource for antiparasitic agents? Trends Parasitol 21: 462-468.
9. Alvarez LI, Mottier ML, Lanusse CE (2007) Drug transfer into target helminth parasites. Trends Parasitol 23: 97-104.
10. Hanser E, Mehlhorn H, Hoeben D, Vlaminck K (2003) In vitro studies on the effects of flubendazole against Toxocara canis and Ascaris suum. Parasitol Res 89: 63-74.
11. Shalaby HA, El Namaky AH, Kamel RO (2009) In vitro effect of artemether and triclabendazole on adult Fasciola gigantica. Vet Parasitol 160: 76-82.
12. Schmahl G, Mehlhorn H, Klimpel S, Krieger KJ (2007) Efficacy of a combination of imidacloprid plus moxidectin against larva and adult stages of nematodes (Trichuris muris, Angiostrongylus cantonensis) in rodents. Parasitol Res 101: 85-92
13. Martin RJ, Robertson AP, Bjorn H (1997) Target sites of anthelmintics. Parasitology 114 Suppl: S111-124.
14. Roy B, Lalchhandama K, Dutta BK (2008) Scanning electron microscopic observations on the in vitro anthelmintic effects of Millettia pachycarpa on Raillietina echinobothrida. Pharmacognosy Magazine 4: 20-26
15. Hegazi AG, Abd El Hady FK, Shalaby HA (2007) An in vitro effect of propolis on adult worms of Fasciola gigantica. Vet Parasitol 144: 279-286.
16. Stitt AW, Fairweather I (1993) Fasciola hepatica: tegumental surface changes in adult and juvenile flukes following treatment in vitro with the sulphoxide metabolite of triclabendazole (Fasinex). Parasitol Res 79: 529-536

17. Zafar-Iqbal, Nadeem QK, Khan MN, Akhtar MS, Waraich FN (2001) In vitro anthelmintic activity of Allium sativum, Zingiber officinale, Cucurbita Mexicana and Ficus religiosa. Int J Agric Biol 3: 454-457

18. Nagaich SS (2000) Studies on the anthelmintic activity of Allium sativum (Garlic) oil on common poultry worms Ascaridia galli and Heterakis gallinae. J Parasitol App Anim Biol 9: 47-52

19. Chybowski J (1997) Study of the anthelmintic activity of garlic extracts. Herba Polonica 43: 383-387

20. Yakoob J, Abbas Z, Beg MA, Naz S, Awan S, et al. (2011) In vitro sensitivity of Blastocystis hominis to garlic, ginger, white cumin, and black pepper used in diet. Parasitol Res 109: 379-385.

21. Aboelhadid SM, Kamel AA, Arafa WM, Shokier KA (2013) Effect of Allium sativum and Allium cepa oils on different stages of Boophilus annulatus. Parasitol Res 112: 1883-1890.

22. Miron T, Shin I, Feigenblat G, Weiner L, Mirelman D, et al. (2002) A spectrophotometric assay for allicin, alliin, and alliinase (alliin lyase) with a chromogenic thiol: reaction of 4-mercaptopyridine with thiosulfinates. Anal Biochem 307: 76-83.

23. Shadkchan Y, Shemesh E, Mirelman D, Miron T, Rabinkov A, et al. (2004) Efficacy of allicin, the reactive molecule of garlic, in inhibiting Aspergillus spp. in vitro, and in a murine model of disseminated aspergillosis. J Antimicrob Chemother 53: 832-836.

24. Amagase H, Petesch BL, Matsuura H, Kasuga S, Itakura Y (2001) Recent advances on the nutritional effects associated with the use of garlic as a supplement: Intake of garlic and its bioactive components. J Nutr 22: 995-962

25. Busquet M, Calsamiglia S, Ferret A, Carro MD, Kamel C (2005) Effect of garlic oil and four of its compounds on rumen microbial fermentation. J Dairy Sci 88: 4393-4404.

26. Kamel C, Greathead HMR, Tejido ML, Ranilla MJ, Carro MD (2008) Effects of allicin and diallyl disulfide on in vitro rumen fermentation of a mixed diet. Anim Feed Sci Technol 145: 351-363

27. Williams CA, Lamprecht ED (2008) Some commonly fed herbs and other functional foods in equine nutrition: a review. Vet J 178: 21-31.

28. Sutton GA, Haik R (1999) Efficacy of garlic as an anthelmintic in donkeys. Israel J Vet Med 54: 23-27

29. Peña N, Auró A, Sumano H (1988) A comparative trial of garlic, its extract and ammonium-potassium tartrate as anthelmintics in carp. J Ethnopharmacol 24: 199-203.

CHAPTER 32

ANTHELMINTIC TREATMENT ALTERS THE PARASITE COMMUNITY IN A WILD MOUSE HOST

Amy B. Pedersen and Janis Antonovics

Keywords: Helminths, community ecology, within-host interactions

INTRODUCTION

Infectious diseases play a key role in the dynamics and regulation of wild populations through negative effects on host survival and fecundity [**1**]. It is becoming clear that individuals are often simultaneously co-infected with multiple parasite species and that those parasites may interact within a host [**2–9**]. This dynamic and complex parasite community may be structured either via direct interactions or indirectly through shared resources or immune responses [**4**,**5**]. From an applied perspective, understanding the role of such parasite interactions in shaping disease dynamics is crucial for optimizing intervention strategies.

To date, most evidence of interspecific parasite interactions from wild populations has been observational and based on cross-sectional or longitudinal surveys which correlate parasite infections to infer interactions [**3**,**10**]. However, as is well known in community ecology, only a more direct, experimental approach can ascertain the consequences of these interactions for disease dynamics [**7**].

In this study, we investigate the effects of removing one taxonomic group of parasites on the prevalence and intensity of other non-target parasite species, as well as on host recapture rates under natural conditions. We experimentally reduced nematode infections in wild populations of *Peromyscus leucopus* (white-footed mouse) and *Peromyscus maniculatus* (deer mouse) and monitored the intestinal parasite and ectoparasite community. We show that nematodes may exert a strong, yet unexpected, antagonistic force on non-target parasites, with important potential consequences for parasite community composition, dynamics and host health.

MATERIAL AND METHODS

This study was conducted in an oak–maple forest at Mountain Lake Biological Station (MLBS) in Virginia, where populations of *Peromyscus* have been studied for more than 25 years [**11**,**12**]. In this locality, *Peromyscus* species share more than 10 species of intestinal parasites (including*Aspicularis americana*, *Capillaria americana*, *Syphacia peromysci*, *Eimeria* spp., *Hymenolepis dimunata* and *H. citelli*), several ectoparasites (including ticks, fleas and *Cutebra* sp.) and co-infection is common ([**13**] and electronic supplementary material, table S1).

Six 0.5 ha trapping grids (8 × 8 arrays with 10 m spacing) were established and mice were trapped for three consecutive nights every two weeks in June–August 2003. Sherman folding traps were set at dusk, baited with crimped oats and checked the following morning. Grids were separated by more than 70 m. In four randomly selected 'experimental' grids, individuals at first capture were randomly assigned to receive either a single oral dose of ivermectin (200 μg kg^{-1}) or an equal volume of water. Ivermectin removes nematode infections and some ectoparasites, yet has no known negative effects on host fitness [**9**,**12**]. In two 'control' grids, all individuals were given water.

At each capture, individuals were ear-tagged and their species, sex, age, weight, length and reproductive condition

Citation: Pedersen AB, Antonovics J. 2013 Anthelmintic treatment alters the parasite community in a wild mouse host. Biol Lett 9: 20130205. http://dx.doi.org/10.1098/rsbl.2013.0205.

were recorded. *Peromyscus maniculatus* was distinguished from *P. leucopus* based on tail length exceeding body length, sharply bicoloured tail and a hair tuft at the end of the tail. Developmental age (juvenile, subadult and adult) was determined by pelage colour. Males with testes greater than 6 × 4 mm, and females with a perforate vagina, lactating nipples or who were pregnant, were considered to be reproductive.

Peromyscus abundance was measured as the minimum number known alive by summing the individuals caught in the session with those trapped at prior and later sessions. Faecal samples were taken from every capture, and individuals were scanned for ectoparasites (presence/absence). All traps were then cleaned and sterilized with a hospital-grade detergent.

Faecal samples were weighed and stored in 10 per cent buffered formalin at 4°C. All samples were analysed within four months of capture. Salt flotations and microscopy were used to count eggs/oocysts [**14**]. Two measures were used to describe intestinal parasite infection: (i) prevalence and (ii) intensity of infection (eggs/oocysts per gram faeces), a common proxy for worm burden [**15**].

We analysed the effect of ivermectin on target and non-target parasites using generalized linear models (GLMs) and generalized linear mixed models (GLMMS) in R v. 2.13 [**16**]. We tested fixed effects: time, treatment, grid, date of first capture, age, sex, species, interactions and importantly treatment × time. Mouse ID was included as a random effect to control for multiple samples per mouse over time. GLMs and GLMMs gave very similar results, likely due to low captures/mouse (mean = 1.7). Conclusions were unaffected by model type. GLMs are usually more robust, especially for non-normal response variables and unbalanced data [**17**], thus the GLMMs are presented in the electronic supplementary material. For prevalence, we used a binomial error structure, and for parasite intensity (log-transformed as the data were eggs per gram of faeces), we used a Gaussian error structure. Full models were simplified by backward stepwise elimination of non-significant terms ($p > 0.1$) to obtain the minimum adequate model. To measure the effect of ivermectin treatment on survival (weeks recaptured post-treatment), we used a GLM, with Poisson error structure and the fixed effects listed above, and capture–mark–recapture methods to measure survival and recapture probabilities in the program Mark [**18**].

Data will be made available after a 1 year embargo. Until this time, data are available upon request from the authors.

RESULTS

During the experiment, 270 individuals were tagged and treated (90 with water on control grids; 88 were treated with ivermectin and 86 with water on experimental grids, totalling 453 captures (see the electronic supplementary material, figure S1 for demographic patterns). There were no significant differences in species composition, sex or parasite prevalence of untreated animals between control and experimental grids; these data were therefore combined for further analyses.

(a) Effects on target and non-target parasites

Ten intestinal parasite species were identified to taxonomic class: coccidia (three spp.), nematodes (five spp.) and cestodes (two spp.); as well as three ectoparasites (see the electronic supplementary material, table S1); because not all parasites could be identified to species, analyses were at the class level.

Ivermectin treatment reduced the prevalence of intestinal nematodes by more than 28 per cent; whereas in control mice prevalence decreased by only 8 per cent (treatment × time: $F_{1,390} = 6.42$, $p = 0.0112$; **table 1** and **figure 1***a*). Treated individuals tended to have lower ectoparasite prevalence than controls, although this was not significant (treatment × time: $F_{1,390} = 2.18$, $p = 0.13$; **table 1** and **figure 1***b*). Prevalence of ectoparasites (primarily driven by botfly infections) increased by more than 15 per cent in controls, but was unchanged in ivermectin-treated mice.

Table 1. Results from the minimum adequate binomial GLMs on the change in parasite prevalence post-ivermectin treatment. Statistics show the chi-squared value, d.f. and *p*-value, with $n = 397$. The treatment × time interaction is the test of the experimental effect of ivermectin (italicized). Models are plotted in **figure 1**.

	nematode prevalence	ectoparasite prevalence	coccidia prevalence	cestode prevalence
grid	—	9.86_5 (0.08)	—	—
first capture	—	*13.2_2 (0.001)*	—	—
age	*4.17_1 (0.041)*	—	—	2.0_1 (0.16)
sex	*4.189_1 (0.041)*	—	2.52_1 (0.11)	1.48_1 (0.22)
species	1.68_1 (0.195)	—	*6.8_1 (0.009)*	—
treatment × time	*6.42_1 (0.0112)*	2.18_1 (0.13)	*4.17_1 (0.04)*	*5.49_1 (0.02)*

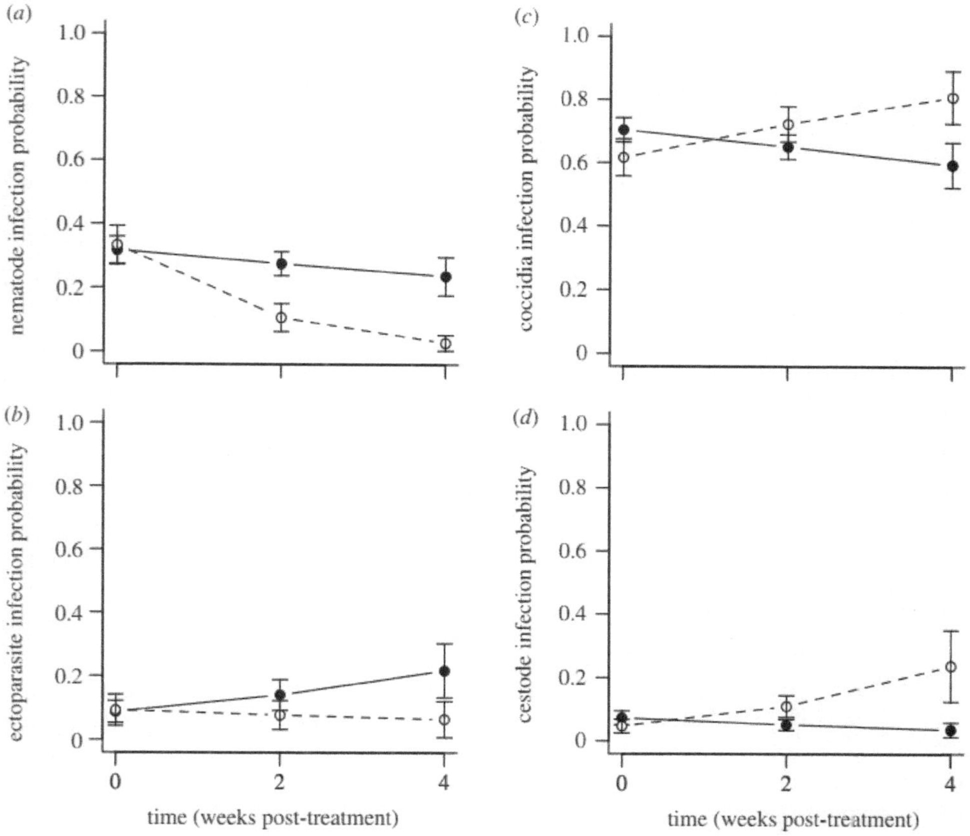

Figure 1. The effect of ivermectin on the probability of infection of drug-target parasites: (*a*) nematodes and (*b*) ectoparasites; and non-target parasites: (*c*) coccidial protozoans and (*d*) cestodes of ivermectin-treated (dashed line; open circles) and control (water; solid line; filled circles) mice from the GLM models (**table 1**). Week 0 represents pre-treatment infection probability, and week 2 and 4 represent recaptured individuals after treatment. Bars represent s.e.

Ivermectin-treated mice had a significantly higher prevalence of coccidia than control mice (treatment × time: $F_{1,390}$ = 4.17, p = 0.04; **table 1** and **figure 1***c*), increasing by more than 20 per cent four-weeks post-treatment, while decreasing in control individuals by 10 per cent over the same period. Cestode prevalence also significantly increased by approximately 20 per cent in ivermectin-treated mice, whereas prevalence remained relatively constant in controls (treatment × time: $F_{1,390}$ = 5.49, p = 0.02; **table 1** and **figure 1***d*).

Among untreated nematode-infected individuals, the average infection intensity was 226.6 eggs per gram (see the electronic supplementary material, table S1). Ivermectin treatment did not significantly reduce nematode intensity, however all treated-mice were uninfected by four-weeks. There was also no significant effect of ivermectin treatment on non-target parasite intensity.

(b) Effects on host fitness

The encounter rates for control and ivermectin-treated mice were more than 95 per cent. Ivermectin-treated mice were recaptured for, on average, 1.35 weeks after treatment, whereas control mice were recaptured for 1.57 weeks; this difference was not significant (p > 0.1; see the electronic supplementary material for more details). Ivermectin-treated or control groups did not differ significantly in the proportion of reproductive male or female mice post-treatment.

DISCUSSION

These results suggest the presence of antagonistic interspecific parasite interactions in a natural population of mice. Removing one group of intestinal parasites had significant, and unexpected, effects on the parasite community within an individual. Ivermectin treatment successfully decreased intestinal nematode infection, but this was accompanied by increases in non-target coccidia and cestodes. The mechanisms driving these interactions are currently unknown. They may be due to either a 'bottom-up' process (via competition for space/resources) because all parasite groups inhabit the gastrointestinal tract or a 'top-down' (via shared immune responses) interaction, owing to immune-mediated mechanisms such as enterocyte turnover, which is a host response elicited by helminth infection that can reduce resources available to coccidia [**18**]. Nematode and coccidia infection, but not intensity, were affected by ivermectin treatment, which may suggest that the interaction affects parasite establishment and not within-host replication. In addition, it is possible that ivermectin treatment increased exposure to non-target parasites via changes in behaviour or dietary habits; further experiments are needed to determine the specific mechanisms.

Quite unexpectedly, there was no evidence that reducing nematode infection increased the fitness of treated mice. In fact, ivermectin-treated mice had lower recapture rates than control mice. Although this effect was not significant, our results are counter to studies showing increased fitness following removal of a single dominant nematode parasite

[**12,19,20**]. In this study, ivermectin treatment increased the prevalence of non-target gastrointestinal parasites, especially coccidia, which have been associated with decreased mass and lower over-wintering survival in *P. maniculatus* [**21**] and with high juvenile mortality in other mammals [**22**]. We found no difference in reproductive condition between treated and control individuals. However, a larger-scale experiment that targets different parasite groups and tracks the longer-term host–parasite dynamics would provide a clearer picture of the network of interspecific interactions within the parasite community and their consequences for host health.

In conclusion, we find that interspecific parasite interactions can be assessed through a field-experimental approach, rather than through classical indirect observational studies using parasite infection data. It is clear that parasite–host dynamics cannot always be understood within a single-host–single-parasite framework. Like ecological communities of free-living species, parasite communities are dynamic and structured by interactions that determine species presence/absence and intensity. This is consistent with the increasingly accepted view that parasite control strategies need to take parasite community structure into account for effective disease management of human and animal diseases [**23**].

ACKNOWLEDGEMENTS

We thank A. Fenton, M. E. Hood, S. Knowles, G. Devevey, A. L. Graham, H. M. Wilbur, D. Taylor, M. Bowers, C. Lively and S. Altizer for feedback, and J. Abbate, D. Streicker, A. Jones and K. Dexter for field/laboratory assistance. MLBS provided land/facilities. A.B.P. was supported by grants from NSF-DIG, Sigma Xi, MLBS and the American Society of Mammalogy, and is currently supported by an Advanced Fellowship (Wellcome Trust Strategic grant to the CIIE, 095831) and a Chancellors Fellowship.

REFERENCES

1. Anderson RM, May RM. 1992 Infectious diseases of humans: dynamics and control. Oxford, UK: Oxford University Press.
2. Cox FEG. 2001 Concomitant infections, parasites and immune responses. Parasitology 122, S23– S38. (doi:10.1017/S003118200001698X)
3. Lello J, Boag B, Fenton A, Stevenson IR, Hudson PJ. 2004 Competition and mutualism among the gut helminthes of a mammalian host. Nature 428, 840–844.
4. Pedersen AB, Fenton A. 2007 Emphasizing the ecology in parasite community ecology. Trends Ecol. Evol. 22, 133 – 139. (doi:10.1016/j.tree.2006.11.005)
5. Graham AL. 2008 Ecological rules governing helminth–microparasite coinfection. Proc. Natl Acad. Sci. USA 105, 566– 570. (doi:10.1073/pnas. 0707221105)
6. Telfer S, Lambin X, Birtles R, Beldomenico P, Burthe S, Paterson S, Begon M. 2010 Species interactions in a parasite community drive infection risk in a wildlife population. Science 330, 243– 246. (doi:10. 1126/science.1190333)
7. Johnson PTJ, Buller ID. 2011 Parasite competition hidden by correlated coinfection: using surveys and experiments to understand parasite interactions. Ecology 92, 535– 541. (doi:10.1890/10-0570.1)
8. Griffiths EC, Pedersen AB, Fenton A, Petchey OL. 2011 The nature and consequences of coinfection in humans. J. Infect. 63, 200– 206. (doi:10.1016/j.jinf. 2011.06.005)
9. Ferrari N, Cattadori IM, Nespereira J, Rizzoli A, Hudson PJ. 2004 The role of host sex in parasite dynamics: field experiments on the yellow-necked mouse Apodemus flavicollis. Ecol. Lett. 7, 88 – 94. (doi:10.1046/j.1461-0248.2003.00552.x)
10. Behnke J, Gilbert FS, Abu-Madi MA, Lewis JW. 2005 Do the helminth parasites of wood mice interact? J. Anim. Ecol. 74, 982– 993. (doi:10.1111/j.1365-2656.2005.00995.x)
11. Wolff JO. 1996 Population fluctuations of masteating rodents are correlated with production of acorns. J. Mammal. 77, 850 – 856. (doi:10.2307/ 1382690)
12. Pedersen AB, Greives TJ. 2008 The interaction of parasites and resources cause crashes in a wild mouse population. J. Anim. Ecol. 77, 370– 377. (doi:10.1111/j.1365-2656.2007.01321.x)
13. Pedersen AB. 2005 Intestinal parasites, acorn masts and population dynamics of Peromyscus. PhD dissertation. Department of Biology, University of Virginia, Charlottesville, VA.
14. Pritchard MH, Kruse GOW. 1982 The collection and preservation of animal parasites. Lincoln, NE: University of Nebraska Press.
15. Scott ME, Dobson A. 1989 The role of parasites in regulating host abundance. Parasitol. Today 5, 176 – 183. (doi:10.1016/0169-4758(89)90140-3)
16. R Development Core Team. 2011 R: a language and environment for statistical computing. Vienna, Austria: R Foundation for Statistical Computing.
17. Bolker BM, Brooks ME, Clark CJ, Geange SW, Poulsen JR, Stevens HH, White J-SS. 2009 Generalized linear mixed models: a practical guide for ecology and evolution. Trends Ecol. Evol. 24, 127– 135. (doi:10.1016/j.tree. 2008.10.008)
18. White GC, Burnham KP. 1999 Program MARK: survival estimation from populations of marked animals. Bird Study 46S, 120– 138. (doi:10.1080/00063659909477239)
19. Artis D, Grencis RK. 2008 The intestinal epithelium: sensors to effectors in nematode infection. Mucosal Immunol. 1, 252. (doi:10.1038/mi.2008.21)
20. Hudson PJ, Dobson AP, Newborn D. 1998 Prevention of population cycles by parasite removal. Science 282, 2256– 2258. (doi:10.1126/science.282. 5397.2256)
21. Vandegrift KJ, Raffel TR, Hudson PJ. 2008 Parasites prevent summer breeding in white-footed mice, Peromyscus leucopus. Ecology 89, 2251 – 2258. (doi:10.1890/07-1935.1)
22. Fuller CA, Blaustein AR. 1996 Effects of the parasite Eimeria arizonensis on survival of deer mice (Peromyscus maniculatus). Ecology 77, 2196 – 2202. (doi:10.2307/2265712)

23. Catchpole J, Norton CC, Joyner LP. 1976 Experiments with defined multispecific coccidial infections in lambs. Parasitology 72, 137– 147. (doi:10.1017/S0031182000048447)

24. Jolles AE, Ezenwa VO, Etienne RS, Turner WC, Olff H. 2008 Interactions between macroparasites and microparasites drive infection patterns in freeranging African buffalo. Ecology 89, 2239 – 2250. (doi:10.1890/07-0995.1)

CHAPTER 33

MARKED ANTIGIARDIAL ACTIVITY OF YUCCA BACCATA EXTRACTS: A POTENTIAL NATURAL ALTERNATIVE FOR TREATING PROTOZOAN INFECTIONS

Luis Quihui-Cota, Rocio León-Trujillo, Humberto Astiazarán-García, Julián Esparza-Romero, María del Refugio Robles, Ramón E. Robles-Zepeda, Rafael Canett, and Jesús Sánchez-Escalante

INTRODUCTION

One of the most important intestinal protozoans responsible for human infections worldwide is Giardia duodenalis. In 2000, it was estimated that 200 million people in Asia, Africa, and Latin America showed symptomatic giardiosis and 500,000 new cases were diagnosed annually [1]. Later estimations showed that it could be responsible for one billion cases annually and is accompanied by an overall worldwide prevalence of 30% [2]. Acute symptoms include diarrhea, gas, abdominal cramps, nausea or vomiting, and dehydration [3, 4]. In some areas of Mexico, the prevalence of giardiosis can reach up to 68% [5] and now G. duodenalis is the most important protozoan parasite causing human intestinal infection in Northwestern Mexico [6]. Currently, this infection is treated with conventional and effective drugs (quinacrine, nitroimidazoles, and nitrofurans) [7]; however, people reject them because of their undesirable side effects [8]. Otherwise, a meta-analysis review [9] concluded that safety, effectiveness, and low cost make of albendazole an alternative and/or replacement for the metronidazole in the treatment of giardiosis in humans. However, the development of resistant strains due to overuse of any drug and the possibility of finding a drug to be used in shorter treatment times than those of the conventional drugs are some reasons for considering alternative therapies. One of them being investigated for the treatment of giardiosis consists of new antigiardialcompounds with different structures and mechanisms of action compared to conventional drugs. Since ancient times, people have used plants to treat common infectious diseases, and some of them have been integrated as a cure for diverse pathologies [10]. Yucca was one of the plants used as an important natural resource by Indians of the American Southwest, Mexico, and Latin America for thousands of years against arthritis, fever, headaches, ulcers, and appendicitis [11]. Extracts ofYucca contain a variety of compounds such as saponins, alkaloids, tannin, terpenoids, and reducing sugars [12]. Saponins of Yucca schidigera, a plant of the family Agavaceae and native to the southwestern United States and Baja California in Mexico [13], have been investigated as defaunation agents. In addition, extracts of Y. schidigera have been shown to reduce the rumen protozoal population in vitro [14] and in vivo [15]. Based on that information, the present study was conducted to investigate whether extracts of another species, Y. baccata,which is native to the desert on the Mexican side (Northwestern Mexico), possess antigiardial activity and to consider it as a potential agent for controlling giardiosis could be potential agents for controlling giardiosis.

Citation: Luis Quihui-Cota, Rocio León-Trujillo, Humberto Astiazarán-García, et al., "Marked Antigiardial Activity of Yucca baccata Extracts: A Potential Natural Alternative for Treating Protozoan Infections" BioMed Research International, vol. 2014, Article ID 823492, 6 pages, 2014. doi:10.1155/2014/823492.

MATERIALS AND METHODS

Plant Material

Samples of Yucca baccata were collected at the Rancho El Aribabi located in northeastern Sonora, Mexico. The samples were placed in bags and transported to the herbarium of the University of Sonora (Herbarium USON) for their taxonomic authentication. The material used in this study was backed up with a specimen of reference (USON 18607, J. Sánchez 2011-095) that is currently deposited in the USON collection.

Yucca baccata Extract Preparation

Once the Yucca stem was dried under sunny conditions (25°C–35°C), it was pulverized using a Wiley Mill (Thomas-Wiley Mill, Model 4, Laboratory Mill, USA) to obtain a coarse powder (2 mm particle size). The preparation of the extracts was performed based on the method described by Newbold et al. [16] for Sesbania sesban. An aqueous suspension of the pulverized material of the stem of Y. baccata (33 g/L) was left overnight at room temperature (25°C–30°C). The aqueous material was filtered and shaken in equal volumes of n-butanol for 30 minutes at room temperature. Extractions were repeated with n-butanol. The resulting organic layers from each extraction process were pooled and dried using a rotavapor (ROTAVAPOR BUCHI 461 Water Bath, Pace Analytical Services, Minneapolis, MN, USA) at 40°C, and the residue was weighed and resuspended in PBS at a 1 : 15 ratio. The solution was clarified by filtration through preweighed Whatman no. 1 filter paper. Solid residues were scraped from the filter paper and washed three times with n-butanol, and the liquid extractant was rotoevaporated. The residue was weighed and stored at 4°C in 15 mL centrifuge tubes prior to use in the preparation of extracts with 3 different concentrations before their administration to the treatment groups.

Animals

Forty-two female Mongolian gerbils of the strain Meriones unguiculatus, aged 6–12 weeks old and weighing 41 g–64 g, from the Animal Bioterium Center of the National Autonomous University of Mexico (acronym in Spanish UNAM), were used in this study. We decided to work with this number of gerbils on the basis of our previous findings with Y. schidigera [17]. The gerbil is susceptible to G. duodenalis infection [18].

Ethical Considerations

This study was approved by the ethical committee of the Centro de Investigación en Alimentación y Desarrollo A.C. (Centre of Research in Food and Development) to be carried out in strict accordance with the recommendations in the Guide for the Care and Use of Laboratory Animals of the Mexican Official Regulations [19] and the Committee on Care and Use of Laboratory Animals of the Institute of Laboratory Animals Resources [20]. All surgery was performed under chloroform anesthesia, and efforts to minimize animal suffering were made during the study course.

Bioterium Area Conditions

The bioterium was sanitized with sodium 10% hypochlorite. The temperature was maintained between 20°C and 26°C (mean 22°C ± 1°C) and humidity between 40% and 70%; there were 10 to 14 air-room changes per h and 12-12 h-light/dark cycles. The gerbils were housed in individual sanitized stainless-steel cages (60 × 40 × 30) and bedded on sterilized sawdust that was replaced daily. Cages were arranged on racks and their sanitation was continuously monitored. Biohazard bags [21] were used to autoclave infective biological materials at the end of the study (urine, feces, and carcass) [22].

Maintenance Diet and Supplied Water

Gerbils were given a commercial diet for a 20-day period based on their daily nutritional requirements. It was composed of casein, corn oil, fiber, mineral mixture, zinc gluconate, vitamins mixture, choline, corn starch, and sucrose [23]. Both diet and commercial pure water were supplied ad libitum to the gerbils throughout the entire study.

Culture, Preparation, and Administration of G. duodenalis Inoculum

The Giardia isolate used in this study was G. duodenalis strain GS/M83-H7. Giardia trophozoites culture (1×10^6 trophozoites/mL, 250 µL) was added in 15 mL glass screw-capped test tubes containing 7 mL of TYI-S-33 medium supplemented with 10% bovine serum. Subculturing was performed every 72–96 h by incubation in an anaerobic chamber (18% CO_2 atmosphere) at 37°C for 24 h [24]. After incubation, the plates were placed on ice and rocked gently (20 min) to suspend nonadherent trophozoites, and the liquid was quickly discharged to avoid contamination using a purifier [25]. Trophozoites were washed 3 times in PBS pH 7.2 (GIBCO PBS pH 7.2, Life Technologies, Thermo Fisher Scientific Inc., Waltham, MA, USA) by centrifuging at 800 g for 10 min at 4°C. The pellet was resuspended in 500 µL of PBS and further diluted 1 : 15 with PBS and 1 : 2 with 0.4% Trypan Blue (Solution Trypan Blue, SIGMA Aldrich Company, ST Louis MO, USA) for microscopic analysis and trophozoite counting in a Neubauer chamber at 40x magnification. Washed pellets were adjusted to a concentration of 5×10^6 trophozoites in 200 µL. Experimental infections with Giardia GS/M-83-H7 were established by orogastric inoculation with 5×10^6 trophozoites suspended in 500 µL of PBS [18].

Bioassay

Previous to the bioassay, the 42 female gerbils were weighed and gastric inoculation was performed with G. duodenalis trophozoites. A couple of inoculated gerbils were randomly selected, anaesthetized with chloroform, and euthanized for examination to confirm establishment of the infection via trophozoite detection in the duodenum and the proximal intestine at day 6 of postinfection [18]. Forty gerbils were randomly allocated into 5 treatment groups (8 per group). The treatments were randomly assigned to the 5 groups, and they comprised 0.5 mL oral doses of PBS (negative control), metronidazole (2 mg/mL in PBS or 1 mg per dose, positive control), or 1 of 3 different Y. baccata extracts with different concentrations (24.4 mg/mL, 12.2 mg/mL, and 6.1 mg/mL).

Treatments were administered once daily for 3 days from day 7 of postinfection to day 9 of postinfection, and the weight of each gerbil was recorded again before euthanasia. After asepsis, 5 cm each of the proximal (midsection) and duodenum segments were removed and cut from fixed locations along the intestine length. Each segment was slit longitudinally and washed with PBS (shaking at 130 rpm) and the washing solutions were transferred to 3 mL vials and kept at 4°C until we counted the trophozoites. After homogenization, the solutions were transferred to conical tubes and centrifuged at 800 g at 4°C for 10 min. The supernatant was discharged and sediment was homogenized. An aliquot of the sediment (0.5 μL) was diluted 1 : 20 with PBS, and 0.5 μL of the dilution was placed in a Neubauer chamber. Trophozoites on each 1 mm^2 square (4 in total) were microscopically counted at 40x magnification (Microscope Olympus, CKX41, Center Valley, PA, USA). The total number of trophozoites per mL was calculated as follows: (Number of trophozoites/4 squares) × (500/100) × 10000 [26].

Study Design

This was a ten-day bioassay with a completely randomized design, in which the treatments consisted of different concentrations of Yucca extract and the experimental units were the gerbil groups infected with 5×10^6 trophozoites of the G. intestinalis clone GS/M-83-H7. The assignment of gerbils to each experimental unit (groups) and the assignment of the treatments to each experimental unit (groups) were completely random (Figure 1).

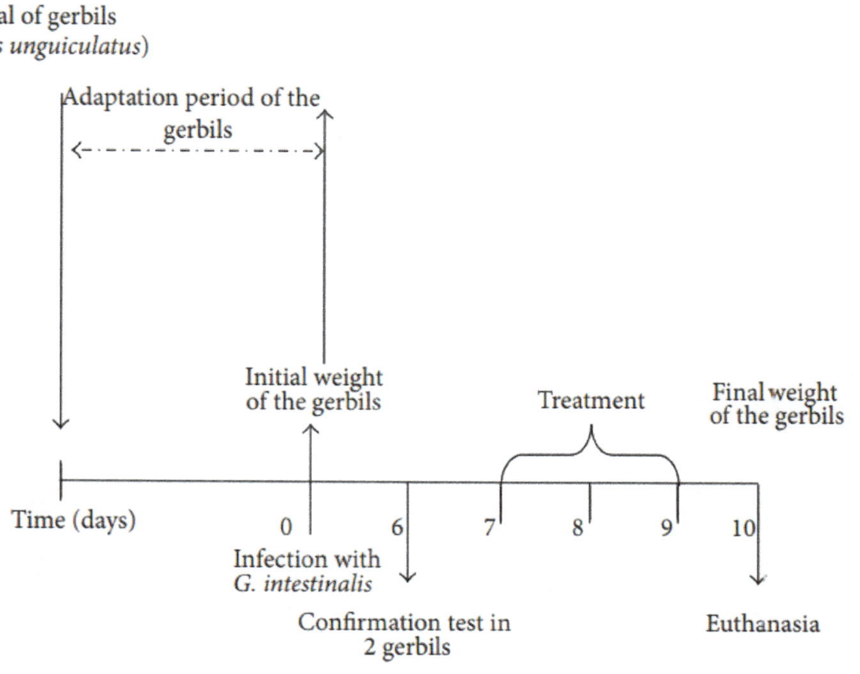

Figure 1: Design of the bioassay based on five treatments and 42 gerbils to test the antigiardial activity of the Y. baccata extracts.

Statistical Analysis

Descriptive statistics were generated for the weight and trophozoite count data from the study gerbils. The Wilcoxon matched-pairs signed rank test was used to compare the change of weight in the gerbil groups between the baseline and day 10 of postinfection. The effect of the 3 different concentrations of Yucca's extracts on G. intestinalis trophozoites were measured based on the geometric median of the active trophozoite counts observed in the intestinal tissue of the Giardia infected gerbils in each experimental unit after treatment, and the significance of the differences among log-transformed geometric medians was calculated with the nonparametric Kruskal-Wallis one-way and Tukey-Kramer (post hoc) tests. The Mann Whitney U test was used to test the difference in the geometric mean trophozoite counts between those from the duodenum and those from the proximal segments of the intestine of the infected gerbils. All analyses were performed using the STATA (Stata Corp LP, 4905 Lakeway Drive, College Station, TX 77845, USA), and statistical significance was established at $P \leq 0.05$.

RESULTS AND DISCUSSION

This study investigated the activity of extracts of Y. baccata from the desert area of Northwestern Mexico against G. duodenalis. Our study gerbils were 6–12 weeks of age and weighed 52 to 56 grams. This weight and age combination is proper for bioassays in gerbils to test their susceptibility to Giardia infection. McAllister et al. [17] successfully developed bioassays using gerbils that were 6–9 weeks of age and weighing 50 to 60 g. In this study, infection with G. duodenalis in Mongolian gerbils (Meriones unguiculatus) was established by orogastric inoculation with 5×10^6 trophozoites/500 μL of PBS, and the test confirming infection in 2 gerbils at day 6 of postinfection revealed median trophozoite counts of 120,000 trophozoites/mL PBS and 85,000 trophozoites/mL PBS in the duodenum and the proximal segments, respectively. McAllister et al. [17] used 2×10^5 Giardia trophozoites in 0.5 mL of PBS to infect, by orogastric inoculation, the same strain of gerbils as those used in this study. They found that, at day 6 after inoculation, the trophozoite counts tended to be higher in the duodenum than those in the jejunum or ileum. In this study, the trophozoite counts always tended to be higher in the duodenum than those in the proximal intestine of the infected gerbils (P≥0.05) (data not shown). Most likely, the different configuration of the intestinal membrane at the bottom of the villus and the villus: crypt ratios play an important role in trophozoite attachment in the different sections of the small intestine sections [27]. The median weights at preinfection (baseline) and at day 10 of postinfection for 31 gerbils randomly allocated to 5 experimental groups are shown in Table 1. Over the course of the study, each experimental group showed weight loss, but it was not significant (Table 1). Bénéré et al. [28] published that the overall weight gain in 24 gerbils was significantly lower for 16 Giardia infected gerbils (0.491±0.0167g) than 8 gerbils free ofGiardia intestinalis (0.769±0.059g) at day 18 of postinfection. It is well recognized that giardiosis may be asymptomatic or associated with acute and chronic diarrhea. Giardia trophozoites may cause intestinal lesions, leading to nutrient malabsorption that may explain the weight loss in infected humans [29] or animals [30]. Most likely, this 10-day bioassay was not sufficiently long to observe differences in the pre- and postinfection gerbil weights. In addition, the orogastric administration of the 24.4 mg/mL, 12.2 mg/mL, and 6.1 mg/mL butanol extracts did not significantly reduce the trophozoite counts in the duodenum segment of the infected gerbils compared to the untreated group at day 10 of postinfection. In addition, no difference was observed in the trophozoite count reductions among the 3 extract-treated groups (P≥0.05) (Figure 2).

Table 1: Median weight of 35 gerbils allocated in 5 treatment groups at preinfection and day 10 of postinfection during the bioassay.

Butanol extract	n	Weight at preinfection (g) Median (SE)	Weight at day 10 of postinfection (g) Median (SE)	n	ΔWeight (g)	P^*
24.4 mg/mL of extract[&]	5	52.7 (1.44)	50.3 (1.84)	5	−2.4	0.293
12.2 mg/mL of extract[&]	5	48.7 (3.1)	47.5 (3.87)	5	−1.2	0.403
6.1 mg/mL of extract[&]	5	56.6 (1.2)	55.6 (1.18)	5	−1.0	0.400
Metronidazole	8	56.0 (2.71)	55.3 (2.62)	8	−0.7	0.636
Untreated	8	52.6 (2.25)	49.9 (2.21)	8	−2.7	0.372

(SE): (Standard error); P: *Wilcoxon matched-paired-sum test; Significance at $P \le 0.05$.
[&]3 gerbils died per extract-treated group during the bioassay course.

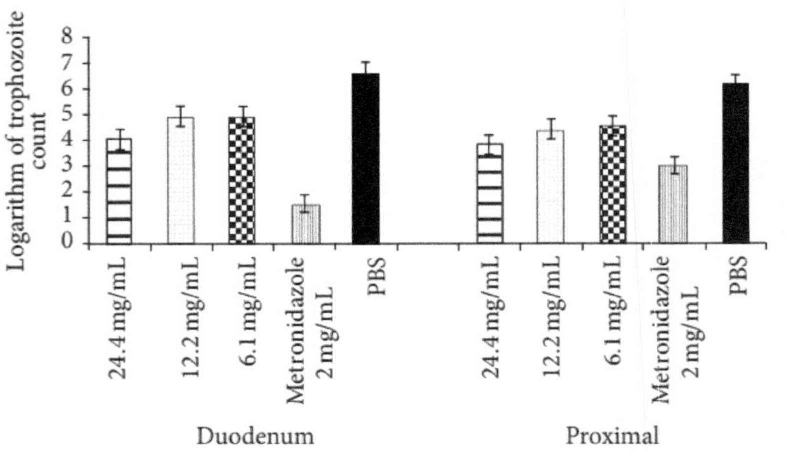

Figure 2: Effect of the extracts with 3 different concentrations of extracts per dose of Y. baccata, of metronidazole, and phosphate buffered saline (PBS) on the trophozoite counts in the duodenum and proximal of Giardia infected Mongolian gerbils.

In contrast, the high concentration extract (24.4 mg/mL) alone significantly reduced (P<0.05) the trophozoite counts in the proximal segment of the infected gerbils compared to the untreated infected gerbils (Figure 2). There was no difference in the trophozoite count reductions between the group treated with the high extract concentration and the group treated with metronidazole (P>0.05). The trophozoite count was significantly lower for the high concentration extract (P<0.05) than that for the medium and low extract concentrations (Figure 2). The geometric mean of the trophozoite counts remained unchanged in the untreated infected gerbils at day 10 of postinfection in both the duodenum and proximal segments (Figure 2). In contrast, metronidazole significantly reduced the trophozoite counts in both the upper and lower intestine of the infected gerbils (P=001) (Figure 1). McAllister et al. [17] found that the oral administration of 6.1 mg/mL of schidigeraextracts using the same treatment regime as that used in the present study significantly reduced the number of trophozoites in the lower region (jejunum and ileum) but not the number in the duodenum of the infected gerbils. Those authors explained that the extract's compounds may form complexes with bile salts released in the duodenum [17, 31, 32], reducing their antigiardial properties in the upper regions of the small intestine. However, only the higher extract concentration was capable of significantly reducing the trophozoite counts in the lower region. Gerbils exhibited toxic reactions to the different administered concentrations in this study. Three gerbils per group that received Yucca extracts died. McAllister et al. [17] found that a higher extract concentration than the concentrations in this study (50 mg of butanol extract in eight doses over the 3 day period) had a negative impact on the overall health of the gerbils. Although metronidazole failed to eradicate the trophozoite populations, it was more effective at eliminating trophozoites from the proximal segment than from the duodenum segment of the intestine.

CONCLUSION

The butanol extracts of Y. baccata exhibited antigiardial activity by reducing, although not significantly, the trophozoite counts in the duodenum, and the higher extract concentration showed a similar antigiardial activity to that of metronidazole in the proximal segment. The effective antigiardial activity in the proximal segment and the toxic effects observed in the gerbils in this study have encouraged us to study the chemical characterization, mechanism of action, and degree of toxicity of the components with antigiardial properties and to compare their antigiardial efficacy against Y. schidigera under similar laboratory conditions. Extracts ofY. baccata may represent an effective and economical alternative to treat intestinal parasitism in humans.

Conflict of Interests

The authors declare that there is no conflict of interests regarding the publication of this paper.

ACKNOWLEDGMENTS

The first and second authors in this paper developed work activities which make them deserve the same recognition level. The authors appreciate the support provided by the Q.B. Carmen María Lugo Flores and the M. in Sc. Gloria Guadalupe Morales Figueroa in preparing the paper. They also thank Carlos Robles Elias, owner of Rancho El Aribabi, for his permission to collect samples of Yucca from his property. The assistance of the professional technicians Berthita Pacheco, Bianca Vargas, and Orlando Tortoledo is also appreciatively acknowledged. The authors appreciate the support granted by the Consejo Nacional de Ciencia y Tecnología and the Centro de Investigación en Alimentación y Desarrollo A.C.

REFERENCES

1. R. C. A. Thompson, R. M. Hopkins, and W. L. Homan, "Nomenclature and genetic groupings of giardia infecting mammals," Parasitology Today, vol. 16, no. 5, pp. 210–213, 2000.
2. Ishatva, "Disease Symptoms & Treatment. Giardiasi," 2013, http://disease-symptoms-treatment.com/disclaimers.html.
3. T. B. Gardner and D. R. Hill, "Treatment of giardiasis," Clinical Microbiology Reviews, vol. 14, no. 1, pp. 114–128, 2001.
4. L. J. Robertson, K. Hanevik, A. A. Escobedo, K. Mørch, and N. Langeland, "Giardiasis—why do the symptoms sometimes never stop?" Trends in Parasitology, vol. 26, no. 2, pp. 75–82, 2010.
5. M. Ponce-Macotela, G. E. Peralta-Abarca, and M. N. Martínez-Gordillo, "Giardia intestinalis and other zoonotic parasites: prevalence in adult dogs from the southern part of Mexico City," Veterinary Parasitology, vol. 131, no. 1-2, pp. 1–4, 2005.
6. L. Quihui-Cota and G. G. Morales-Figueroa, "Intestinal parasitism in school children periodically treated with albendazole in 2 sampling periods," The International Journal of Mathematics and Mathematical Sciences, vol. 5, no. 2, pp. 43–47, 2013.
7. R. Romero-Cabello and I. F. Herrera-Benavente, Síndrome Diarreico Infeccioso, Yucatán, México, 2002.
8. Y. Chin, M. J. Balunas, H. B. Chai, and A. D. Kinghorn, "Drug discovery from natural sources," AAPS Journal, vol. 8, no. 2, article 28, pp. E239–E253, 2006.
9. S. Solaymani-Mohammadi, J. M. Genkinger, C. A. Loffredo, and S. M. Singer, "A meta-analysis of the effectiveness of albendazole compared with metronidazole as treatments for infections with Giardia duodenalis," PLoS Neglected Tropical Diseases, vol. 4, no. 5, article e682, 2010.
10. J. L. Rios and M. C. Recio, "Medicinal plants and antimicrobial activity," Journal of Ethnopharmacology, vol. 100, no. 1-2, pp. 80–84, 2005.
11. altMD, "Yucca," http://www.altmd.com/Articles/Yucca–Encyclopedia-of-Alternative-Medicine.
12. M. S. Ishaq, M. M. Hussain, M. S. Afridi, et al., "In vitro phytochemical, antibacterial, and antifungal activities of leaf, stem, and root extracts of Adiantum capillus veneris," The Scientific World Journal, vol. 2014, Article ID 269793, 7 pages, 2014.
13. Innes, Fire Effects Information System: Yucca Schidigera, U.S. Department of Agriculture, Forest Service, Rocky Mountain Research Station, Fire Sciences Laboratory, Missiola, Mont, USA, 2013.
14. Y. Wang, T. A. McAllister, L. J. Yanke, and P. R. Cheeke, "Effect of steroidal saponin from Yucca schidigeraextract on ruminal microbes," Journal of Applied Microbiology, vol. 88, no. 5, pp. 887–896, 2000.
15. A. N. Hristov, T. A. McAllister, F. H. van Herk, K. J. Cheng, C. J. Newbold, and P. R. Cheeke, "Effect of Yucca schidigera on ruminal fermentation and nutrient digestion in heifers," Journal of Animal Science, vol. 77, no. 9, pp. 2554–2563, 1999.
16. C. J. Newbold, S. M. El Hassan, J. Wang, M. E. Ortega, and R. J. Wallace, "Influence of foliage from African multipurpose trees on activity of rumen protozoa and bacteria," The British Journal of Nutrition, vol. 78, no. 2, pp. 237–249, 1997.
17. T. A. McAllister, C. B. Annett, C. L. Cockwill, M. E. Olson, Y. Wang, and P. R. Cheeke, "Studies on the use of Yucca schidigera to control giardiosis," Veterinary Parasitology, vol. 97, no. 2, pp. 85–99, 2001.
18. H. Astiazarán-García, M. Espinosa-Cantellano, G. Castaón, B. Chávez-Munguía, and A. Martínez-Palomo, "Giardia lamblia: effect of infection with symptomatic and asymptomatic isolates on the growth of gerbils (Meriones unguiculatus)," Experimental Parasitology, vol. 95, no. 2, pp. 128–135, 2000.
19. SENASICA, "NORMA Oficial Mexicana NOM-062-ZOO-1999, Especificaciones técnicas para la producción, cuidado y uso de los animales de laboratorio," Servicio Nacional de Sanidad, Inocuidad y Calidad Agroalimentaria, 1999.

20. NRC, National Research Council. Guide for the Care and Use of Laboratory Animals, The National Academies Press, 8th edition, 2011.

21. VWR, “VWR 1.5 mil Autoclavable Biohazard Bags,” 2004.

22. CDC, Biosafety in Microbiological and Biomedical Laboratories, Centers for Disease Control and Prevention, National Institutes of Health, Department of Health and Human Services, Public Health Service, Atlanta, Ga, USA, 2009.

23. Harlan, Harlan Laboratories. Teklad Rodent Diet, 2010.

24. C. A. Bell, C. C. Dykstra, N. A. Naiman, M. Cory, T. A. Fairley, and R. R. Tidwell, “Structure-activity studies of dicationically substituted bis-benzimidazoles against Giardia lamblia: correlation of antigiardial activity with DNA binding affinity and giardial topoisomerase II inhibition,” Antimicrobial Agents and Chemotherapy, vol. 37, no. 12, pp. 2668–2673, 1993.

25. LABCONCO, “Purifier Logic+ Class II, Type A2 Biosafety Cabinets,” 2013.

26. L. Quihui-Cota, R. O. Méndez Estrada, H. Astiazarán-García et al., “Changes in serum zinc levels associated with giardiasis and dietary zinc intake in mice,” Biological Trace Element Research, vol. 145, no. 3, pp. 396–402, 2012.

27. W. Jakunowski and J. C. Hoff, Waterborne Transmission of Giardiasis, 1978.

28. E. Bénéré, T. Van Assche, C. Van Ginneken, O. Peulen, P. Cos, and L. Maes, “Intestinal growth and pathology of Giardia duodenalis assemblage subtype A_I, A_{II}, B and e in the gerbil model,” Parasitology, vol. 139, no. 4, pp. 424–433, 2012.

29. A. Celiksoz, M. Acioz, S. Degerli, Z. Cinar, N. Elaldi, and M. Erandaç, “Effects of giardiasis on school success, weight and height indices of primary school children in Turkey,” Pediatrics International, vol. 47, no. 5, pp. 567–571, 2005.

30. F. Aloisio, G. Filippini, P. Antenucci et al., “Severe weight loss in lambs infected with Giardia duodenalis assemblage B,” Veterinary Parasitology, vol. 142, no. 1-2, pp. 154–158, 2006.

31. J. M. Gee and I. T. Johnston, “Interactions between hemolytic saponins, bile salts and small intestinal mucosa in the rat,” Journal of Nutrition, vol. 118, no. 11, pp. 1391–1397, 1988.

32. G. S. Sidhu and D. G. Oakenfull, “A mechanism for the hypocholesterolaemic activity of saponins,”British Journal of Nutrition, vol. 55, no. 3, pp. 643–649, 1986. ·

CHAPTER 34

DEVELOPMENTS IN DIAGNOSIS AND ANTILEISHMANIAL DRUGS

Prachi Bhargava and Rajni Singh

INTRODUCTION

Protozoan parasitic diseases remain a major concerned public health problem, especially in tropical regions. The major death toll is due to malaria, African and American trypanosomiasis, and leishmaniasis, whose high mortality rates in underdeveloped developing countries are associated to poor hygienic conditions and lack of efficient prophylactic measures [1].

For many years, the public health impacts of the parasitic diseases have been grossly underestimated, mainly due to lack of awareness of its serious impact on health. Protozoan parasites of the genus Leishmania cause severe diseases that threaten human beings, both for the high death rates involved and the economic loss resulting from morbidity, primarily in the tropical and subtropical areas [2]. It ranks the second only to malaria, and the control of leishmaniasis remains a serious problem with ever increasing cases worldwide. It has become a major focus of concern and a serious third world problem affecting the poorer sections of the society [3].

Leishmaniasis is included in the list of neglected tropical diseases (NTDs) [4] and has a strong link to poverty [5]. The disease has been reported in 88 countries in five continents—Africa, Asia, Europe, North America, and South America out of the seven continents (22 in the new world and 66 in the old world) [6], out of which 16 are developed countries, 72 are developing, and 13 of them are among the least developed [7]. Approximately, 350 million individuals are at risk of leishmaniasis and 20 million people are infected worldwide, and an estimated 2.0 million new cases occur each year [8] with an incidence of 1.5 million cases per annum of the disfiguring cutaneous leishmaniasis (CL) and 0.5 million cases per annum of the potentially fatal visceral leishmaniasis (VL) [9, 10]. However, with increasing travel to and from endemic regions, there is an increase in the number of patients suffering from leishmaniasis [10–12]. The importance of this parasitic disease is further stressed out by the rise of Leishmania/HIV coinfection in many parts of the world including European countries such as Spain, Italy, France, and Portugal where up to 9% of the AIDS patients suffer from fatal visceral leishmaniasis [13]. However, due to underreporting and misdiagnosis, the number of actual cases is expected to be higher.

No effective vaccines are available against Leishmania infections as yet and the treatment relies solely on chemotherapy, with pentavalent antimonials as first-line drugs and amphotericin B and pentamidine as second-line agents [10, 11]. Miltefosine is the first recognized oral treatment for leishmaniasis, but resistance to miltefosine may emerge easily during treatment due to single point mutation [14]. There is a pressing need for the identification of novel drug targets, virulence factors, and development of vaccines to expand our understanding of the prevention and treatment of leishmaniasis.

Epidemiology: Impact and Geographical Distribution

Leishmaniases cause considerable morbidity and mortality and are a typical example of an anthropozoonosis. The majority of infections are originally zoonotic, although some cases of transmission of L. donovani from human to human are also known. The different epidemiological cycles are (i) a primitive

Citation: Prachi Bhargava and Rajni Singh, "Developments in Diagnosis and Antileishmanial Drugs," Interdisciplinary Perspectives on Infectious Diseases, vol. 2012, Article ID 626838, 13 pages, 2012. doi:10.1155/2012/626838.

or sylvatic cycle (human infection is accidental, transmission occurring in wild foci), for example, L. braziliensis; (ii) a secondary or peridomestic cycle (the reservoir is a peridomestic or domestic animal, the parasite being transmitted to humans by anthropophilic sand flies), for example, L. infantum; (iii) a tertiary, strictly anthroponotic cycle (in which the animal reservoir has disappeared or has not yet been identified, and the sand fly vectors are totally anthroponotic), for example, L. donovani. Nevertheless, many unknown factors remain. For example, the main animal reservoir of L. braziliensis is still unknown [15]. L. tropica was considered to be a strict anthroponosis, but several cases of canine infection have been described [16–18].

Leishmaniasis is a complex disease caused by haemoflagellate obligate intracellular protozoa belonging to the genus Leishmania, family Trypanosomatidae of the order Kinetoplastida. Visceral leishmaniasis (VL), cutaneous leishmaniasis (CL), and rarer manifestations such as mucosal leishmaniasis and post-kala-azar dermal leishmaniasis (PKDL) are the major forms of this disease. Parasites are transmitted by female sandflies via anthroponotic or zoonotic cycles [19]. Theparasites have a dimorphic lifecycle; flagellated promastigotes develop in the gut of female Phlebotomine sandflies to infectious forms that are transmitted to mammalian hosts [20, 21]. Inside the host, the parasites survive and multiply as amastigotes within parasitophorous vacuoles (PVs) of macrophages [22, 23].

Depending on the transmission cycle, VL and CL are considered to be either anthroponotic (AVL/ACL) or zoonotic (ZVL/ZCL). Anthroponotic VL is caused by Leishmania donovani and is mainly distributed in the Indian subcontinent where it accounts for 70% of the burden of VL with estimated annual incidence of 500,000 and 50,000 deaths each year [24], a death toll that is surpassed among the parasitic diseases only by malaria.

Both figures are approximations as VL is frequently not recognized or not reported [25, 26]. The majority (>90%) of cases occur in just six countries—Bangladesh, India, Nepal, Sudan, Ethiopia, and Brazil (Figure 1). Severe VL epidemics have been reported in the past in southern Sudan; in context of civil war and famine, VL killed an estimated 100,000 people out of a population of 280,000 between 1984 and 1998 [27]. As India, Nepal, and Bangladesh harbor an estimated 67% of the global VL disease burden [28], the commitment of the government of these countries to launch regional VL elimination programme is welcome. The target of this programme is to eliminate VL as a public health problem by 2015, by using a local approach to reduce the annual incidence of VL to less than one case per ten thousand individuals. Visceral leishmaniasis (VL) results in death if not treated, the majority of leishmaniasis deaths go unrecognized, and even with treatment access, VL may result in case-fatality rates of 10–20% [29–31]. In East Africa, it causes around 50,000 annual cases, in the form of epidemic outbreaks distributed in scattered displaced populations with a high death rate. Post-kala-azar dermal leishmaniasis (PKDL), which is developed in 5–50% of AVL patients depending on geographical areas, requires lengthy and costly treatment with a low efficacy [32, 33]. The most relevant factors behind the spread of AVL are the increasing transmission in urban areas with large numbers of immigrants living in poor conditions, the breakdown of social and health structures, malnutrition inducing weakening of the immune system, and finally HIV-Leishmania coinfection. The HIV-VL coinfection is characterized by frequent relapses and a high fatality rate, and cases are considered to constitute an important infectious reservoir [34]. Zoonotic VL is caused by L. infantum and is widely distributed in Central Asia, Middle East, the Mediterranean, and Brazil. Up to 50,000 annual cases may be caused by this form worldwide, with a scattered distribution.

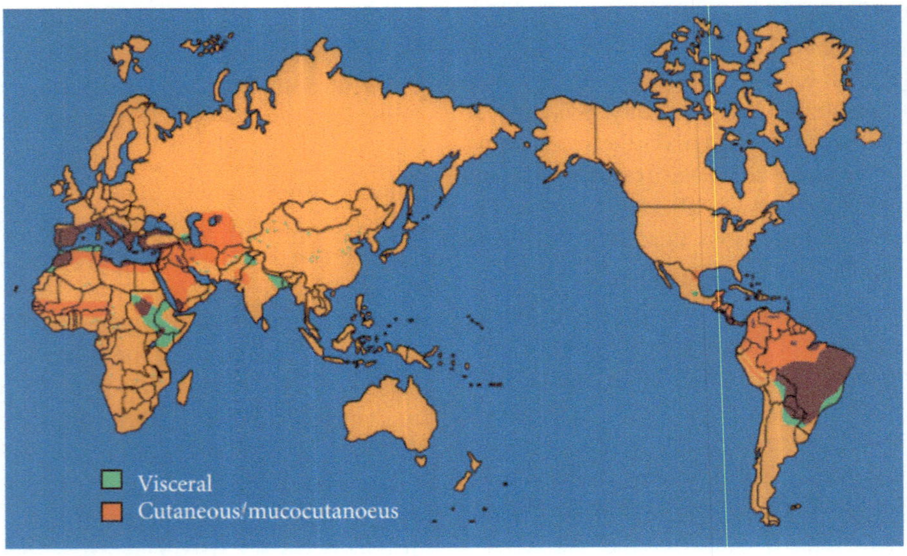

Figure 1: Geographical distribution of leishmaniasis worldwide [37].

CL is commonly known as oriental sore. Its causative agents are Leishmania major, L. tropica, L. aethiopica, andL infantum in old world and L. mexicana, L. venezuelensis, L. amazonensis, L. braziliensis, L. panamensis, L. guyanensis, L. peruviana, and L. chagasi in new world. It produces skin lesions mainly on the face, arms, and legs. It is frequently self-healing in the old world but when the lesions are multiple and disabling with disfiguring scars, it creates a lifelong aesthetic stigma. In Central Asia, the Middle East, North Africa, and some sub-Saharan countries, ZCL caused by L. major accounts for 500,000 cases every year. Outbreaks are typical in rural areas and depend on fluctuations in the rodent population. ACL caused by L. tropica is transmitted in urban zones and affects around 400,000 patients annually. Massive outbreaks have occurred in overcrowded suburbs with poor housing and deteriorated environmental conditions [35]. ZCL caused by L. aethiopica is present in Ethiopia and is the most neglected form of CL despite 50,000 annual cases and a potential serious clinical progression, including diffuse CL and to a lesser degree mucocutaneous leishmaniasis. In South America, around 300,000 new cases of ZCL occur annually. Leishmania braziliensis is responsible for nearly 90% of all CL cases. Species belonging to the subgenus Viannia (L. braziliensis, L. panamensis, L. peruviana, andL. guyanensis) are capable of causing mucocutaneous leishmaniasis. No or incomplete treatment of CL is associated with the subsequent development of mucocutaneous leishmaniasis. It is estimated that there are 4000 new mucocutaneous leishmaniasis cases every year [36]. The subgenus Leishmania groups comprise two main species, L. mexicana, causing a form of CL that heals spontaneously but can sometimes cause necrosis of the external ear (the "chiclero" ulcer), and L. amazonensis, which can in some cases manifest as diffuse CL in patients with weak immune systems.

Although leishmaniasis affect 98 countries in the world, it should be stressed that 90% of VL cases occur in India, Bangladesh, Sudan, Brazil, Nepal, and Ethiopia, and 90% of CL cases occur in Afghanistan, Algeria, Ethiopia, Sudan, Iran, Iraq, Saudi Arabia, Syria, Brazil, and Peru [6]. Apart from VL and CL, diffused cutaneous leishmaniasis is also a type which is difficult to treat due to disseminated lesions that resemble leprosy and do not heal spontaneously. This form is especially related to a defective immune system and it is often characterized by relapses after treatment.

Mucocutanoeus leishmaniasis is also called "espundia" in South America. Causative agents of MCL in old world are Leishmania aethiopica (rare) L. major and in new world are L. mexicana, L. amazonensis, L. braziliensis, L. guyanensis, and L. panamensis. The parasite invades the mucocutaneous region of the body and spreads to the oronasal/pharyngeal mucosa. The soft tissues and cartilage of the oronasal/pharyngeal cavity undergo progressive erosion. In contrast to cutaneous leishmaniasis, these lesions do not heal spontaneously. Suffering and mutilation are severe, and death occurs as a result of bronchopneumonia or malnutrition. There is always a large danger of bacteria infecting the already open sores. Reconstructive surgery of deformities is an important part of therapy [36].

The classification of Leishmania was initially based on ecobiological criteria such as vectors, geographical distribution, tropism, antigenic properties, and clinical manifestations [38–41]. However, biochemical and molecular analysis showed that pathological and geographical criteria were often inadequate and thus, other criteria such as the patterns of polymorphism exhibited by kinetoplastid DNA (k-DNA) markers, proteins, or antigens came to be used to classify Leishmania [42–49].

The genus Leishmania comes under subkingdom Protozoa, order Kinetoplastida, and family Trypanosomatidae. Initially, species classification was based on various extrinsic criteria such as clinical, geographical, and biological characteristics, for example, L. guyanensis (isolated in Guyana), L. peruviana(isolated in Peru), L. infantum (isolated from a child in Tunisia), and L. gerbilli (isolated from gerbils). Since the 1970s, intrinsic criteria such as immunological, biochemical, and genetic data have been used to define species of Leishmania. Use of these molecular techniques led to the publication of a taxonomic scheme by the World Health Organization [50]. New methods of detection, isolation, and genetic identification resulted in a massive increase in the number of species are described. Today, 30 species are known and approximately 20 are pathogenic for humans. These species generally present different epidemiological and clinical characteristics related to different genetic and phenotypic profiles. The validity of the classification scheme, considered by some workers as too arbitrary, has been questioned several times. Debate has centered on L. panamensis, L. peruviana, L. chagasi, L. infantum, L. archibaldi, L. garnhami, L. pifanoi, L. venezuelensis, and L. forattinii [15,51, 52]. Different studies have already clarified the status of some of these species; for example, L. chagasi is accepted as a synonym of L. infantum [51] and L. peruviana has been validated as an independent species [53].

Very recently, Fraga and his team [54] used sequences of the highly conserved 70-kDa heat shock protein (hsp70 gene) to analyze isolates and strains of different geographic origin, showing that only eight monophyletic groups were detectable against the 17 examined (Table 1).

Table 1: Nomenclature of Leishmania species based on heat shock protein 70 (hsp 70) gene sequences [54].

Name of the organism	Geographical distribution
L. donovani	China, Indian subcontinent, Ethiopia, Sudan, Kenya, Iran, Saudi Arabia, and Yemen
L. infantum/L. Chagasi As given [51]	Albania, Algeria, France, Greece, Italy, Morocco, Portugal, Spain, Syria, Tunisia, Turkey, Yemen, Argentina, Bolivia, Brazil, Colombia, Ecuador, El Salvador, Guadalupe, Guatemala, Honduras, Martinique, Mexico, Nicaragua, Paraguay, Suriname, and Venezuela
L. archibaldi	India, Sudan, Ethiopia, Lebanon, and Israel
L. tropica	Afghanistan, Algeria, Azerbaijan, Greece, Iran, Iraq, Israel, Morocco, Tunisia, Turkey, and Yemen
L. aethiopica	Ethiopia, Kenya
L. major	Afghanistan, Algeria, Chad, Iran, Iraq, Israel, Libya, Mauritania, Morocco, Syria, and Sudan
L. mexicana	Belize, Colombia, Costa Rica, Dominican Republic, Ecuador, Guatemala, Honduras, Mexico, Panama, and Venezuela
L. amazonensis	Bolivia, Brazil, Colombia, Costa Rica, Ecuador, French Guyana, Panama, Peru, and Venezuela
L. garnhami	Venezuela
L. guyanensis	Brazil, Colombia, Ecuador, French Guyana, Peru, Suriname, and Venezuela
L. panamensis	Belize, Colombia, Costa Rica, Ecuador, Honduras, Nicaragua, Panama, and Venezuela
L. naiffi	Brazil, French Guyana, Ecuador, and Peru
L. braziliansis	Argentina, Belize, Bolivia, Brazil, Colombia, Costa Rica, Ecuador, Guatemala, Honduras, and Nicaragua
L. peruviana	Peru

DIAGNOSIS

The reason behind the diagnostic challenges for leishmaniasis is the wide spectrum of clinical manifestations that they present: ulcerative skin lesions developing at the site of the sand fly bite (localized cutaneous leishmaniasis); multiple nonulcerative nodules (diffuse cutaneous leishmaniasis); destructive mucosal inflammation (mucosal leishmaniasis (ML)); disseminated, potentially fatal, and visceral infection (visceral leishmaniasis (VL)) [55]. However, differential diagnosis is important because diseases of other etiologies with a clinical spectrum similar to that of the leishmaniases (e.g., leprosy, skin cancers, and tuberculosis for CL and malaria and schistosomiasis for VL) are often present in areas of endemicity. These main manifestations may themselves deviate, complicating definitive clinical diagnosis even further. Cutaneous leishmaniasis (CL) lesions, for example, may vary in severity (e.g., in lesion size), clinical appearance (e.g., open ulcer versus flat plaques versus wart-like lesions), and duration (e.g., in time of evolution or in time to spontaneous cure). Patient management, screening of asymptomatic infections, surveillance including verification of elimination, and epidemiological studies are some of the areas where diagnostic tests play a major role.

In all cases, it is desirable to have the diagnosis of leishmaniasis confirmed by the finding of the etiological agent or its antigen or molecule in the sample obtained from the lesion. When these approaches fail, immunological tests are used to provide indirect parameters for the diagnosis.

Ideally, a test should make the distinction between acute disease and asymptomatic infection, as most of the antileishmanial drugs are toxic. Moreover, such tests should be highly sensitive and specific, simple and affordable, but unfortunately some commonly used serological tests like DAT carry some significant drawbacks: the inability to differentiate between clinically active and asymptomatic infections and showing positive long after cure. Molecular diagnostic tools like PCR and real-time PCR are quite sensitive and specific but are cumbersome to perform and have a high cost. DNA-based tests are available in strip formats but these cannot be used in the field [56]. Compared to other diagnostic techniques available, the molecular approaches remain expensive and require technological expertise, and efforts should be made to make PCR platforms more user-friendly and cost-effective, especially in remote areas where leishmaniasis is endemic.

Parasitological Methods

Demonstration of the amastigote form of the parasite by light microscopic examination of tissue aspirates from spleen, bone marrow, or lymph nodes is regarded as the most suitable diagnostic instrument. In preparations stained with Giemsa or Leishman stain, the cytoplasm appears to be pale blue, with a relatively large nucleus that stains with red. In the same plane as the nucleus, but at a right angle to it, is a deep red or violet rod-like body called a kinetoplast. The sensitivity of the direct examination is low, in case of cutaneous and mucocutaneous leishmaniasis, with a range of approximately 15–70% in the old and the new world [57, 58]. In case of visceral leishmaniasis, the specificity of this technique is high, although the sensitivity varies depending on the tissue used, being higher for spleen (93–99%) than for bone marrow (53–86%) or lymph node (53–65%) aspirates [59]. However, the procedure for splenic aspiration is risky for fatal internal bleeding, so the results are totally dependent on technical expertise and quality of prepared slides/reagents, both of which are often not available in field settings [60].

The microculture method (MCM) is a good method for the diagnosis of visceral leishmaniasis (VL) with samples from both the bone marrow (BM) and peripheral blood (PB). The MCM is superior to the traditional culture method (TCM) as determined by its higher sensitivity in the detection of promastigotes and the more rapid time for emergence of promastigotes. The sensitivity of MCM (100% in BMs and 77.8–100% in PB) is considerably higher than that of the TCM (37.5–100% in BMs and 0–100% in PB) according to decreasing parasite density ($P<0.05$) [61].

Serological Methods

The serological diagnosis is based on the presence of specific humoral response for which identification of antibodies in the sera of patients is done. Serum-based direct agglutination tests (DATs) using lyophilized promastigotes or urine-based latex agglutination tests (LATs) are used for determining antileishmanial antibodies or antigens in leishmaniasis patients. DAT has a high sensitivity (90–100%) and specificity (95–100%) [62, 63]. However, the major disadvantage of DAT is the need of multiple pipetting, relatively long incubation time, high cost of antigen, and limited production facility of quality controlled antigen. As with any antibody-based test, DAT remains positive for a long time after the disease is cured, thus cannot be used as a test of cure or for diagnosis of relapses [64].

Detecting antigen directly is an excellent method of diagnosing an infection and is more specific than antibody-based immunodiagnostic tests. Agglutination test to detect the antigen has been evaluated extensively in clinical trials, using urine collected from well-defined cases and controls from endemic and nonendemic regions. This test showed 79.1–94.1% specificity and sensitivity of 60.4–71.6% in India [65].

Several surface antigens, ribosomal proteins, nuclear proteins, histones, and kinesin-related proteins elicit specific humoral immune responses in VL patients. Recombinant antigens have considerably improved the sensitivity and specificity of immunological diagnosis over crude/total antigens. They are more preferred than other antigens both in immunoblotting as well as ELISA.

Immunochromatographic strips using K39 antigen have been a quite promising method that has been tested widely. K39 (recombinant) antigen contains 39 amino acids encoded in the highly conserved kinesin region ofL. chagasi. Using its recombinant product, an immunochromatographic-based strip test is used in which rK39 is fixed on a nitrocellulose paper, and colloidal gold-protein A is used for detection. In the initial clinical evaluation, 100% sensitivity and 98% specificity was observed. ICT suffers from the same disadvantage as DAT, being positive in a significant proportion of healthy individuals in endemic regions and for long periods after cure of VL.

ELISA has also been used in the serodiagnosis of all types of leishmaniasis but the sensitivity and specificity of ELISA depends upon the antigen used. Most promising results are shown by antigen RK39 with sensitivity and specificity of 100% and 96%, respectively. The antibody titres to this antigen directly correlate with active disease and have potential in monitoring the chemotherapy and in predicting the clinical relapse [66]. Due to the requirement of skilled personnel, sophisticated equipment, and electricity, ELISA is not used in the endemic regions for the diagnosis of VL [67].

Molecular Methods

PCR-based assays form the mainstay of molecular diagnosis of leishmanial infection as they enhance sensitivity, reliability, and rapidity for the benefit of researchers and health professionals. The primers target several multicopy sequences for the diagnosis of human and canine VL which include ribosomal RNA genes [68]; kinetoplast DNA (kDNA) [69]; miniexon-derived RNA (med RNA) genes and genomic repeats [70], the β-tubulin gene region [71], glycoprotein 63 (gp63) gene locus [72], and internal transcribed spacer (ITS) regions [73].

ThePCR-ELISAhas shown promising results for diagnosing visceral leishmaniasis (VL) in blood samples. However, the method has been validated mostly with HIV-positive patients who are known to have high levels of parasitaemia. As far as blood samples are concerned,PCR-ELISAis more sensitive (83.9%) than conventional PCR (73.2%) and demonstrated 100% and 87.2% specificity when healthy controls who had never travelled to a VL-endemic area and controls from a VL-endemic area as references, respectively, were used [74].

RT-PCR simply refers to amplification of DNA (by PCR) that is monitored while the amplification is occurring. The benefit of this RT-PCR is that it allows the researcher to better determine the amount of starting DNA in the sample before the amplification by PCR. Also real-time PCR can distinguish specific sequences from a complex mixture of DNA. However, its application requires the availability of primers and probes that must be selected according to very rigid conditions, which cannot always be easily applied [75]. Table 2 depicts the properties of few generally used diagnostic tools for leishmaniasis and PKDL.

Table 2: Diagnostic methods for leishmaniasis and PKDL.

Diagnostic methods	Test name	Clinical specimen	Sensitivity	References
Parasitic detection methods	LD bodies	Lymph node, bone marrow, splenic, and slit aspirates	spleen (93–99%) than for bone marrow (53–86%) or lymph node (53–65%) aspirates	[59, 76]
	Culture (MCM)	Blood, lymph node, bone marrow, splenic, and slit aspirates	100% in bone marrow and 77.8–100% in peripheral blood	[77]
	Culture (TCM)	Blood, lymph node, bone marrow, splenic, and slit aspirates	37.5–100% in bone marrow and 0–100% in peripheral blood	[77]
Serological methods	DAT	Serum, urine	94.8%	[78–81]
	ELISA/immunoblotting soluble antigens	Serum, urine	100%	[82–84]
	Recombinant antigens (rK39, rK26, rHSP70)	Blood, serum, and antigens	100%	[85–88]
Molecular methods	PCR	Blood, serum, urine, lymph node, bone marrow,splenic, and slit aspirates	73.2%	[89, 90]
	PCR-ELISA	Blood, serum	83.9%	[90]
	Real-time PCR	Lymph node, bone marrow, splenic, and slit aspirates	90–100%	[75]

Developments in Antileishmanial Drugs

Pentavalent antimonials were developed in 1945; the generic sodium stibogluconate (pentosan) and branded meglumine antimoniate, and so forth, are the first choice in the treatment of both visceral and cutaneous leishmaniases over more than five decades where resistance is not reported [91]. To overcome the challenge of clinical resistance to antimony, pentamidine has been tried for the treatment of visceral leishmaniasis and was the first drug to be used for patients refractory to pentavalent antimony (SbV) [92]. This drug is associated with serious adverse events like insulin-dependent diabetes mellitus, shock, and hypoglycaemia and death in significant proportion of patients. The declining efficacy, resistance, and serious toxicity associated with the drugs have made it unsuitable as a viable alternative to SbV for kala-azar patients [93, 94]. Amphotericin B is one of the most effective antileishmanial drug, which induces high cure rates. Use of formulation of amphotericin B, a polyene antifungal drug for treatment of leishmaniasis is biochemically rational because the target of the drug is ergosterol, which is the major membrane sterol of Leishmania species. Due to high affinity of amphotericin B for sterols, aqueous pores are formed in the membrane leading to increased membrane permeability and killing of Leishmania [95]. The need to develop less toxic, more effective formulation of amphotericin B has led to new clinical formulation of amphotericin B in which deoxycholate has been replaced by other lipids. Miltefosine, an alkyl phospholipids developed as an antitumor agent, has an excellent antileishmanial activity.Paromomycin is an aminoglycoside antibiotic with unique antileishmanials activity. Paromomycin is currently in phase IV clinical trials against leishmaniasis [96]. Sitamaquine, a primaquine analogue (8-aminoquinolene), is another orally administrable compound (Table 3). To date, little is known about its efficacy and toxicity. However, there is a need to go for combitorial chemotherapies which are under process and provide better outputs.

Table 3: Current scenario of available chemotherapy drugs.

Drug	Properties and administration	Comments	Reactions in patients with CL/VL
Pentavalent antimonials	Polymeric organometallic complexes, intravenous, or intramuscular	For VL and CL. Drug resistance in Bihar, India. Variable response in different forms of CL. Generic sodium stibogluconate (SSG) has made treatment cheaper	Pain, erythema, oedema, abdominal pain, nausea, and thrombocytopenia
Amphotericin B fungizone	Polyene antibiotic, Fermentation product of Streptomyces nodus, intravenous	For VL, CL, and complex forms of CL, for example, MCL. first-line drug for VL in India where there is antimonial resistance	Infusion related, azotemia, anemia, or hypokalemia
Amphotericin B ambisome	Unilamellar liposome, intravenous	Most effective lipid formulation for VL and available at $18/50 mg ampoule via WHO used for complex forms, such as PKDL and MCL	Hypotension, anorexia, nausea, vomiting, and headache generalized weakness.
Miltefosine	Hexadecylphosphocholine, oral	First oral drug for VL. Effective against some forms of CL contraindicated in pregnancy	Nausea, vomiting and/or diarrhea, raised creatinine, and raised LFT's
Amphotericin B formulations	Lipidic formulations, intravenous	Other lipid formulations, including Abelcet, Amphocil, Amphomul, and multilamellar liposomes have been in clinical studies, mainly for VL	Shaking chills, nausea, hypotension, anorexia, headache, and vomiting,
Paromomycin	Aminoglycoside (also known as aminosidine or monomycin), fermentation product of *Streptomyces rimosus*. Supplied as sulphate. Intramuscular for VL and topical for CL	Registered for VL in India, completed Phase III trials for VL in East Africa where less effective in Sudan. Topical formulation (12%) with methyl benzethonium chloride available for CL. Topical with gentamicin and surfactants in Phase III trial	Pain, erythema, oedema, blisters, and ototoxicity
Pentamidine	Diamidine, as isethionate salt, intramuscular	For specific forms of CL in South America only	Nausea, vomiting, diarrhea, hyperglycemia, and cardiotoxicity
Sitamaquine	8-aminoquinoline analog, orally active	Tested in VL patients in Kenya and Brazil with limited success	Abdominal pain, headache, vomiting, dyspepsia, and cyanosis

NEW POTENTIAL DRUG TARGETS

The irony of the disease leishmaniasis is that it is the only tropical disease, which is being treated by nonleishmanial drugs [97]. Much of the focus till recent times was being made only on drug trials/combination therapy of available nonleishmanial drugs, evaluation of diagnostic and prognostic capability of available tools, and very little emphasis was being paid on other aspects by leishmanial biologists and researchers. Recently much emphasis has been given on novel control strategies in terms of new drug targets and vaccine candidates.

The route to drug target identification has been through comparative biochemistry of host and parasite enzymes, metabolites or protein identified in parasite. Biochemical analysis, genome sequencing of threeLeishmania species (L. major, L. braziliensis, and L. infantum) has identified potentially useful target enzymes, transporters, metabolites, and hypothetical proteins that are distinct to parasite and their mammalian host. The genome mining will also aid in large scale proteomics studies generating expression profiles of Leishmaniaparasites and gene targets for treatment development. Search of new potential drug targets mainly focuses on biochemical and metabolic pathways essential for parasite survival. The target enzymes of these pathways should have significant structural and functional differences from their mammalian counterparts for selective inhibition of target sites. Further, strategies to target more than one enzyme of a metabolic pathway simultaneously may prove more usefulness and effectiveness. Biological studies for the function of 50% ofLeishmania genes are lacking. The comparative genome study would provide a route to find those that might be essential to each species [98].

THIOL METABOLISM

The enzymes of thiol metabolism/thiols, of parasitic protozoa, are different from those of mammals in many ways. Trypanosoma and Leishmania are most remarkable in that they have trypanothione reductase (TR) instead of glutathione reductase (GR). This enzyme is responsible for maintaining the parasites, reducing intracellular milieu by keeping trypanothione [N[1], N8-bis-(glutathionyl) spermidine] in the dithiol state. The crucial role of TR for thiol homeostasis and its absence from mammalian cells suggest that it might be well suited as a target molecule for rational drug development. The trypanothione system, which replaces the nearly ubiquitous glutathione/glutathione reductase (GR) system, protects the parasites from oxidative damage and toxic heavy metals and delivers the reducing equivalents for DNA synthesis. The parasite system is far less efficient than mammalian glutathione peroxidases in detoxifying hydroperoxide, but has the advantage of much broader substrate specificity, with lipid hydroperoxides also being reduced. The relatively low activity of the tryparedoxin peroxidase system is in accordance with the high sensitivity of the parasites to oxidative stress. Trypanosomes and Leishmania have superoxide dismutase (SOD), but lack catalase and glutathione peroxidase. Thus, the trypanothione system seems to be the only mechanism to detoxify hydrogen peroxides.

Trypanothione is kept reduced by the flavoenzyme TR. Several reverse genetic approaches have undoubtedly shown that TR is essential in different Leishmania species as well as in bloodstream of T. brucei [99] and is thus an attractive target molecule for structure-based drug design. Castro-Pinto et al. [100] have reported the cloning, sequencing, and expression of the TR encoding gene from L. (L.) amazonensis. A 3D homology model for L. amazonensis TR was constructed based on the previously reported Crithidia fasciculata structure. Within the past 15 years, numerous compounds have been elucidated that inhibit TR, but not human GR, which is the closest related host enzyme. Despite knowledge of the three-dimensional structure of the protein and of complexes with its substrates and an inhibitor, as well as several high-throughput and virtual screening approaches, inhibitors of TR that are suitable to enter the clinical phase are still elusive. This lack of success might be attributable to several factors. The extremely wide active site of the parasite enzyme represents an obstacle for a structure-based drug design. In addition, the pharmacokinetic properties of the potential inhibitors are crucial because insufficient uptake, rapid extrusion, or metabolism plays significant roles in determining the in vivo efficacy of a drug. Recently, the biological activities of a series of mesoionic 1,3,4-thiadiazolium-2-aminide derivatives were evaluated to determine their effect on trypanothione reductase (TryR) activity in Leishmania sp. and Trypanosoma cruzi. MI-4-NO(2) showed enzyme inhibition effect on extracts from different cultures of parasites, which was confirmed using the recombinant enzyme from T. cruzi(TcTryR) and Leishmania infantum (LiTryR) [101]

Thioredoxin reductase (TrxR) is a pyridine nucleotide-disulphide oxidoreductase as GR, TR, and lipoamide dehydrogenase. TrxR maintains the levels of reduced thioredoxin, a protein involved in the activity of ribonucleotide reductase, transcription factors, and cell signaling and the detoxification of reactive oxygen species. Most studies to date on TrxR of parasitic protozoa have concerned the enzyme of P. falciparum. Current evidence suggests that it is a promising drug target, although validation is awaited. The absence of this pathway in mammalian host and trypanosomatids sensitivity towards oxidative stress, trypanothione reductase, and enzymes of trypanothione metabolism is an attractive drug target for antileishmanial drug designing [102]. Homology modeling of Leishmania infantum, TR, and mammalian glutathione reductase shows a remarkable difference in their three-dimensional and catalytic active sites. Hence, specific inhibitors designed against TR may be an ideal drug that will stop parasite growth without altering host glutathione reductase (GR) activity.

Sterol Biosynthetic Pathway

The enzymes of this pathway are attractive targets for the specific treatment of leishmaniasis, because the etiological agents for the disease, that is, the leishmanial parasites have a strict requirement for specific endogenous sterols (ergosterol and analogs) for survival and growth and cannot use the abundant supply of cholesterol present in their mammalian host. There are differences in the enzymes in the biosynthetic pathways of ergosterol and cholesterol. A number of enzymes in the ergosterol biosynthetic pathway have been investigated as potential drug targets for these organisms and have shown great promise. Thus, C14-demethylase, sterol 24-methyltransferase, 3-hydroxy-3-methylglutaryl CoA reductase, squalene epoxide, squalene synthase, and farnesyl pyrophosphate synthase have been studied both individually and in combination, with varying degrees of success [103, 104]. Ergosterol biosynthesis inhibitors with potent in vitroactivity and special pharmacokinetic properties in mammals can induce radical parasitological cure in animal models of several forms of leishmaniasis [105].

Trypanosomatids contain predominantly ergostane-based sterols, which differ from cholesterol, the main sterol in mammalian cells, in the presence of a methyl group in the 24 position. The methylation is initiated by S-adenosyl-L-methionine: Delta (24 (25))-sterol methenyltransferase, an enzyme present in protozoa, but absent in mammals. The importance of this enzyme is underscored by its potential as a drug target in the treatment of the leishmaniasis [106]. The C-24 transmethylation reactions involving S-adenosyl-L-methionine as the methyl donor and a $\Delta^{24(25)}$-sterol or $\Delta^{24(24')}$-sterol substrate can be inhibited by various azasterols with a nitrogen substitution in the side chain and such compounds have been tested against trypanosomatids [107].

Polyamine Biosynthetic Pathway

The polyamine pathway of protozoan parasites has been successfully targeted in antiparasitic therapies. Polyamines are ubiquitous organic cations found in all eukaryotic cells and play critical role in key cellular processes such as growth, differentiation, and macromolecular biosynthesis. During the course of inhibition of any of the polyamine, the parasite cannot synthesize trypanothione, a conjugate of spermidine and glutathione that is unique to Trypanosoma and Leishmania. Trypanothione is a reducing agent with many protective and regulatory functions and consequently its depletion proves detrimental to the parasites. Recent studies on polyamine supplementation show that L. donovani lacks an intact back conversion pathway, thus the pathways operating in promastigote stage of parasite differ crucially from that in the host. Inhibitors of polyamine biosynthetic pathway have shown antileishmanial activity. Adomet DC inhibitor cures animal leishmanises but has not been tested on humans and seeks further experimental studies [108]. Arginase provides a building block for production of polyamines so it has been touted as a potential antileishmanial drug target, because N(omega)-hydroxyarginine, an inhibitor of arginase that is produced by the macrophages during the formation of nitric oxide, can reduce polyamine levels in Leishmania amastigotes and lowers parasitic loads [109, 110]. Other enzymes of this pathway which are under study as antileishmanial target are ornithine decarboxylases, S-adenosylmethionione, and Spermidine synthase.

Glycosomal Machinery

In all kinetoplastida studied so far the majority of the glycolytic enzymes are localized in organelles called glycosomes, whereas in other organisms these are cytosolic. As a result of this compartmentation, many regulatory mechanisms operating in other cell types cannot work in trypanosomes as reflected by the insensitivity of the glycosomal hexokinase (HK) and phosphofructokinase (PFK) to compounds that act as activity regulators in other cell types [111, 112]. Blocking of parasite enzyme without producing damage to glycolysis in host remains challenging. Several approaches have been considered—(1) exploitation of metabolic differences; (2) exploitation of differences in 3D structure; (3) exploitation of unique reactive residue in or near the active site of the parasite enzyme

Leishmania like other trypanosomatids depends solely on its host for carbon source to fulfill its energy requirements. The amastigotes uptake blood glucose from mammalian blood stream and receive other essential components like fatty acids, amino acids from phagolysosome of macrophages. Due to the result of the metabolic activities of glycosomes, superoxide radicals are generated as side products in large amount. To protect glycosomal enzymes from superoxide radical toxicity, Fe-superoxide dismutases (FeSods) are evolved inLeishmania species. More importantly, FeSod is absent in mammalian counterpart, so it could be used as effective drug target.

Cyclin-Dependent Kinases

Cyclin-dependent kinases (cdks) play crucial role in cell division cycle, transcription, apoptosis, and differentiation. In Leishmania mexicana, disruption of cdk-related kinase 3 (CRK3) leads to change ploidy level of the cell, though it was avoided when extra copy of CRK3 was expressed from episome, ensuring that CRK3 is essential [113]. The chemical inhibitors of class indirubin of CRK3 hampers the parasite viability within macrophage, proving the validity of CRK3 as potential drug target [114]. In Leishmania donovani, it was recently shown that glycogen synthase kinase (LdGSK3) is also involved in cell cycle control and apoptosis as validations based on indirubin test [115], exploiting the LdGSK3 as potential drug target in combination with CRK3. Likewise, other cdk may also be explored as possible targets.

Folate Metabolism

Dihydrofolate reductase (DHFR) is a key enzyme in folate metabolism, linked to the production of thymidine. DHFR reduces dihydrofolate to tetrahydrofolate using NADPH as cofactor. Therefore, inhibition of DHFR prevents biosynthesis of thymidine and as a consequence, DNA biosynthesis. Fortunately, this enzyme fromLeishmania major and Trypanosoma cruzi has been crystallized and the structural data can be used to exploit structural difference between parasite and human enzymes that may help to design selective DHFR inhibitors [116, 117]. An approach to discover novel parasite DHFR inhibitors using database mining has also been made to search the Cambridge structural database but DHFR as drug target requires more attention [118, 119]. In addition, it has been shown that the enzyme dihydrofolate reductase-thymidylate (DHFR-TS) that catalyzes conversion of dihydrofolate from methyhylene tetrahydrofolate (M-THF) and thymidine, which is related to parasite survival and the parasite lacking this enzyme is not able to survive in animals [120].

MITOCHONDRIA

The unique mitochondrial features of Leishmania make this organelle an ideal drug target while minimizing toxicity. Leishmania has a single large mitochondrion which is distributed in branches under the subpelicullar microtubes and a specialized region rich in DNA called the kinetoplast. Fonseca-Silva et al. demonstrated that the effect of the quercetin is associated with ROS production leading to mitochondrial dysfunction, ultimately causing parasite death [121]. The effects of several drugs that interfere directly with mitochondrial physiology in parasites such as Leishmania are under study. The unique mitochondrial features of Leishmania make this organelle an ideal drug target while minimizing toxicity.

CONCLUSIONS

All the neglected tropical diseases together take the toll of millions of lives every year. Leishmaniasis is a fatal disease which affects the people living below poverty line. The recent years have witnessed extraordinary progress in diagnosing and treating Leishmania infection. Lack of efficiency, high price, and growing resistance of the current antileishmanials imply the importance of search for new targets to be focused for making drugs against Leishmania. The challenge is to convert such studies in effective strategic programmes aimed to control and eradicate the disease.

REFERENCES

1. R. Pink, A. Hudson, M. A. Mouriès, and M. Bendig, “Opportunities and challenges in antiparasitic drug discovery,” Nature Reviews Drug Discovery, vol. 4, no. 9, pp. 727–740, 2005.
2. H. K. Majumder, B. B. Das, and A. Ganguly, “DNA topoisomerases of Leishmania: the Potential targets for anti-leishmanial therapy,” Advances in Experimental Medicine and Biology, vol. 625, pp. 103–115, 2008.
3. WHO, The world health report—reducing risks, promoting healthy life, World Health Organization, Geneva, Switzerland, 2002.

4. J. Alvar, S. Yactayo, and C. Bern, "Leishmaniasis and poverty," Trends in Parasitology, vol. 22, no. 12, pp. 552–557, 2006.

5. N. Feasey, M. Wansbrough-Jones, D. C. W. Mabey, and A. W. Solomon, "Neglected tropical diseases,"British Medical Bulletin, vol. 93, no. 1, pp. 179–200, 2010.

6. P. Desjeux, "Leishmaniasis: current situation and new perspectives," Comparative Immunology, Microbiology and Infectious Diseases, vol. 27, no. 5, pp. 305–318, 2004.

7. TDR/WHO, "Leishmaniasis," 2012, http://www.who.int/tdr/diseases/leish/info/en/index.html.

8. Leishmaniasis Control, 2007, http://www.who.int/topics/leishmaniasis/en/.

9. J. Alvar, I. D. Velez, C. Bern et al., "Leishmaniasis worldwide and global estimates of its incidence," PloS One, vol. 7, no. 5, pp. e35671–e356712.

10. B. L. Herwaldt, "Leishmaniasis," The Lancet, vol. 354, no. 9185, pp. 1191–1199, 1999.

11. H. W. Murray, J. Pépin, T. B. Nutman, S. L. Hoffman, and A. A. F. Mahmoud, "Recent advances: tropical medicine," British Medical Journal, vol. 320, no. 7233, pp. 490–494, 2000.

12. P. J. Guerin, P. Olliaro, S. Sundar et al., "Visceral leishmaniasis: current status of control, diagnosis, and treatment, and a proposed research and development agenda," Lancet Infectious Diseases, vol. 2, no. 8, pp. 494–501, 2002.

13. N. Berhe, D. Wolday, A. Hailu et al., "HIV viral load and response to antileishmanial chemotherapy in co-infected patients," AIDS, vol. 13, no. 14, pp. 1921–1925, 1999.

14. K. Seifert, F. J. Pérez-Victoria, M. Stettler et al., "Inactivation of the miltefosine transporter, LdMT, causes miltefosine resistance that is conferred to the amastigote stage of Leishmania donovani and persists in vivo," International Journal of Antimicrobial Agents, vol. 30, no. 3, pp. 229–235, 2007.

15. E. Cupolillo, L. R. Brahim, C. B. Toaldo et al., "Genetic polymorphism and molecular epidemiology ofLeishmania (Viannia) braziliensis from different hosts and geographic areas in Brazil," Journal of Clinical Microbiology, vol. 41, no. 7, pp. 3126–3132, 2003.

16. J. Dereure, J. A. Rioux, M. Gallego et al., "Leishmania tropica in Morocco: infection in dogs," Transactions of the Royal Society of Tropical Medicine and Hygiene, vol. 85, no. 5, p. 595, 1991.

17. J. Dereure, J. A. Rioux, A. Khiami, F. Pratlong, J. Périères, and A. Martini, "Ecoepidemiology of leishmaniases in Syria. 2—Presence, in dogs, of Leishmania infantum Nicolle and Leishmania tropica(Wright) (Kinetoplastida-Trypanonomatidae)," Annales de Parasitologie Humaine et Comparee, vol. 66, no. 6, pp. 252–255, 1991.

18. H. Yahia, P. D. Ready, A. Hamdani, J. M. Testa, and N. Guessous-Idrissi, "Regional genetic differentiation of Phlebotomus sergenti in three Moroccan foci of cutaneous leishmaniasis caused by Leishmania tropica," Parasite, vol. 11, no. 2, pp. 189–199, 2004.

19. R. Reithinger, J. C. Dujardin, H. Louzir, C. Pirmez, B. Alexander, and S. Brooker, "Cutaneous leishmaniasis," Lancet Infectious Diseases, vol. 7, no. 9, pp. 581–596, 2007.

20. P. A. Bates, "Transmission of Leishmania metacyclic promastigotes by phlebotomine sand flies,"International Journal for Parasitology, vol. 37, no. 10, pp. 1097–1106, 2007.

21. M. E. Rogers, T. Ilg, A. V. Nikolaev, M. A. J. Ferguson, and P. A. Bates, "Transmission of cutaneous leishmaniasis by sand flies is enhanced by regurgitation of fPPG," Nature, vol. 430, no. 6998, pp. 463–467, 2004.

22. E. Handman and D. V. R. Bullen, "Interaction of Leishmania with the host macrophage," Trends in Parasitology, vol. 18, no. 8, pp. 332–334, 2002.

23. R. J. S. Burchmore and M. P. Barrett, "Life in vacuoles—nutrient acquisition by Leishmania amastigotes,"International Journal for Parasitology, vol. 31, no. 12, pp. 1311–1320, 2001.

24. P. Desjeux, "Leishmaniasis: current situation and new perspectives," Comparative Immunology, Microbiology and Infectious Diseases, vol. 27, no. 5, pp. 305–318, 2004.

25. S. M. Collin, P. G. Coleman, K. Ritmeijer, and R. N. Davidson, "Unseen Kala-azar deaths in south Sudan (1999-2002)," Tropical Medicine and International Health, vol. 11, no. 4, pp. 509–512, 2006.

26. S. P. Singh, D. C. S. Reddy, M. Rai, and S. Sundar, "Serious underreporting of visceral leishmaniasis through passive case reporting in Bihar, India," Tropical Medicine and International Health, vol. 11, no. 6, pp. 899–905, 2006.

27. D. Jacquet, M. Boelaert, J. Seaman et al., "Comparative evaluation of freeze-dried and liquid antigens in the direct agglutination test for serodiagnosis of visceral leishmaniasis (ITMA-DAT/VL)," Tropical Medicine and International Health, vol. 11, no. 12, pp. 1777–1784, 2006.

28. P. J. Hotez, J. H. F. Remme, P. Buss, G. Alleyne, C. Morel, and J. G. Breman, "Combating tropical infectious diseases: report of the Disease Control Priorities in Developing Countries Project," Clinical Infectious Diseases, vol. 38, no. 6, pp. 871–878, 2004.

29. C. Bern, A. W. Hightower, R. Chowdhury et al., "Risk factors for kala-azar in Bangladesh," Emerging Infectious Diseases, vol. 11, no. 5, pp. 655–662, 2005.

30. S. Collin, R. Davidson, K. Ritmeijer et al., "Conflict and kala-azar: determinants of adverse outcomes of kala-azar among patients in southern Sudan," Clinical Infectious Diseases, vol. 38, no. 5, pp. 612–619, 2004.

31. L. C. Rey, C. V. Martins, H. B. Ribeiro, and A. A. M. Lima, "American visceral leishmaniasis (kala-azar) in hospitalized children from an endemic area," Jornal de Pediatria, vol. 81, no. 1, pp. 73–78, 2005.

32. E. E. Zijlstra, A. M. Musa, E. A. G. Khalil, I. M. El Hassan, and A. M. El-Hassan, "Post-kala-azar dermal leishmaniasis," Lancet Infectious Diseases, vol. 3, no. 2, pp. 87–98, 2003.

33. P. R. V. Desjeux, "Post-kala-azar dermal leishmaniasis: facing the challenge of eliminating kala-azar from South Asia," in Kala Azar in South Asia: Current Status and Challenges Ahead, pp. 111–124, Springer Science + Business Media B.V., 2011.
34. J. Alvar, P. Aparicio, A. Aseffa et al., "The relationship between leishmaniasis and AIDS: the second 10 years," Clinical Microbiology Reviews, vol. 21, no. 2, pp. 334–359, 2008.
35. H. Reyburn, M. Rowland, M. Mohsen, B. Khan, and C. Davies, "The prolonged epidemic of anthroponotic cutaneous leishmaniasis in Kabul, Afghanistan: "Bringing down the neighbourgood","Transactions of the Royal Society of Tropical Medicine and Hygiene, vol. 97, no. 2, pp. 170–176, 2003.
36. H. Goto and J. A. L. Lindosc, "Current diagnosis and treatment of cutaneous and mucocutaneous leishmaniasis," Expert Review of Anti-Infective Therapy, vol. 8, no. 4, pp. 419–433, 2010. ·
37. http://www.fp7-rapsodi.eu/150/.
38. P. D. Marsden and W. H. Lumsden, "Trypanosomiasis and leishmaniasis," Practitioner, vol. 207, no. 238, pp. 181–185, 1971.
39. R. S. Bray, "Leishmania," Annual Review of Microbiology, vol. 28, pp. 189–217, 1974.
40. D. M. Pratt and J. R. David, "Monoclonal antibodies that distinguish between New World species of Leishmania," Nature, vol. 291, no. 5816, pp. 581–583, 1981.
41. L. Ryan, A. Vexenat, P. D. Marsden, R. Lainson, and J. J. Shaw, "The importance of rapid diagnosis of new cases of cutaneous leishmaniasis in pin-pointing the sandfly vector," Transactions of the Royal Society of Tropical Medicine and Hygiene, vol. 84, no. 6, p. 786, 1990.
42. D. E. Arnot and D. C. Barker, "Biochemical identification of cutaneous leishmanias by analysis of kinetoplast DNA. II. Sequence homologies in Leishmania kDNA," Molecular and Biochemical Parasitology, vol. 3, no. 1, pp. 47–56, 1981.
43. M. A. Miles, R. Lainson, J. J. Shaw, M. Povoa, and A. A. de Souza, "Leishmaniasis in Brazil: XV. Biochemical distinction of Leishmania mexicana amazonensis, L. braziliensis braziliensis and L. braziliensis guyanensis—aetiological agents of cutaneous leishmaniasis in the Amazon Basin of Brazil,"Transactions of the Royal Society of Tropical Medicine and Hygiene, vol. 75, no. 4, pp. 524–529, 1981.
44. A. A. L. De Ibarra, J. G. Howard, and D. Snary, "Monoclonal antibodies to Leishmania tropica major: specificities and antigen location," Parasitology, vol. 85, no. 3, pp. 523–531, 1982.
45. E. Handman and J. M. Curtis, "Leishmania tropica: surface antigens of intracellular and flagellate forms,"Experimental Parasitology, vol. 54, no. 2, pp. 243–249, 1982.
46. D. F. Wirth and D. M. Pratt, "Rapid identification of Leishmania species by specific hybridization of kinetoplast DNA in cutaneous lesions," Proceedings of the National Academy of Sciences of the United States of America, vol. 79, no. 22, pp. 6999–7003, 1982.
47. G. C. Brainard and P. L. Podolin, "Near-ultraviolet radiation suppresses pineal melatonin content,"Endocrinology, vol. 119, no. 5, pp. 2201–2205, 1986.
48. S. M. Le Blancq and W. Peters, "Leishmania in the Old World: 2. Heterogeneity among L. tropica zymodemes," Transactions of the Royal Society of Tropical Medicine and Hygiene, vol. 80, no. 1, pp. 113–119, 1986.
49. B. L. Travi, Y. Osorio, P. C. Melby, B. Chandrasekar, L. Arteaga, and N. G. Saravia, "Gender is a major determinant of the clinical evolution and immune response in hamsters infected with Leishmania spp,"Infection and Immunity, vol. 70, no. 5, pp. 2288–2296, 2002.
50. WHO, "Control of the Leishmaniasis," Technical Report Series 793, 1990.
51. I. L. Mauricio, J. R. Stothard, and M. A. Miles, "The strange case of Leishmania chagasi," Parasitology Today, vol. 16, no. 5, pp. 188–189, 2000.
52. N. L. Sharma, V. K. Mahajan, A. Kanga et al., "Localized cutaneous leishmaniasis due to Leishmania donovani and Leishmania tropica: preliminary findings of the study of 161 new cases from a new endemic focus in Himachal Pradesh, India," American Journal of Tropical Medicine and Hygiene, vol. 72, no. 6, pp. 819–824, 2005.
53. A. L. Bañuls, J. C. Dujardin, F. Guerrini et al., "Is Leishmania (Viannia) peruviana a distinct species? A MLEE/RAPD evolutionary genetics answer," Journal of Eukaryotic Microbiology, vol. 47, no. 3, pp. 197–207, 2000.
54. J. Fraga, A. M. Montalvo, S. De Doncker, J. C. Dujardin, and G. Van der Auwera, "Phylogeny ofLeishmania species based on the heat-shock protein 70 gene," Infection, Genetics and Evolution, vol. 10, no. 2, pp. 238–245, 2010.
55. H. W. Murray, J. D. Berman, C. R. Davies, and N. G. Saravia, "Advances in leishmaniasis," The Lancet, vol. 366, no. 9496, pp. 1561–1577, 2005.
56. S. Deborggraeve, T. Laurent, D. Espinosa et al., "A simplified and standardized polymerase chain reaction format for the diagnosis of leishmaniasis," Journal of Infectious Diseases, vol. 198, no. 10, pp. 1565–1572, 2008.
57. F. Vega-Lopez, "Diagnosis of cutaneous leishmaniasis," Current Opinion in Infectious Diseases, vol. 16, pp. 97–101, 2003.
58. S. N. Al-Hucheimi, B. A. Sultan, and M. A. Al-Dhalimi, "A comparative study of the diagnosis of Old World cutaneous leishmaniasis in Iraq by polymerase chain reaction and microbiologic and histopathologic methods," International Journal of Dermatology, vol. 48, no. 4, pp. 404–408, 2009.
59. M. Siddig, H. Ghalib, D. C. Shillington, and E. A. Petersen, "Visceral leishmaniasis in the Sudan: comparative

parasitological methods of diagnosis," Transactions of the Royal Society of Tropical Medicine and Hygiene, vol. 82, no. 1, pp. 66–68, 1988.

60. G. Srividya, A. Kulshrestha, R. Singh, and P. Salotra, "Diagnosis of visceral leishmaniasis: developments over the last decade," Parasitology Research, vol. 110, pp. 1065–1078, 2012.

61. A. M. Allahverdiyev, M. Bagirova, S. Uzun et al., "The value of a new microculture method for diagnosis of visceral leishmaniasis by using bone marrow and peripheral blood," American Journal of Tropical Medicine and Hygiene, vol. 73, no. 2, pp. 276–280, 2005.

62. G. Sreenivas, N. A. Ansari, R. Singh et al., "Diagnosis of visceral leishmaniasis: comparative potential of amastigote antigen, recombinant antigen and PCR," British Journal of Biomedical Science, vol. 59, no. 4, pp. 218–222, 2002.

63. D. Jacquet, M. Boelaert, J. Seaman et al., "Comparative evaluation of freeze-dried and liquid antigens in the direct agglutination test for serodiagnosis of visceral leishmaniasis (ITMA-DAT/VL)," Tropical Medicine and International Health, vol. 11, no. 12, pp. 1777–1784, 2006.

64. S. Sundar, R. K. Singh, R. Maurya et al., "Serological diagnosis of Indian visceral leishmaniasis: direct agglutination test versus rK39 strip test," Transactions of the Royal Society of Tropical Medicine and Hygiene, vol. 100, no. 6, pp. 533–537, 2006.

65. M. Boelaert, S. El-Safi, A. Hailu et al., "Diagnostic tests for kala-azar: a multi-centre study of the freeze-dried DAT, rK39 strip test and KAtex in East Africa and the Indian subcontinent," Transactions of the Royal Society of Tropical Medicine and Hygiene, vol. 102, no. 1, pp. 32–40, 2008.

66. R. Kumar, K. Pai, K. Pathak, and S. Sundar, "Enzyme-linked immunosorbent assay for recombinant K39 antigen in diagnosis and prognosis of Indian visceral leishmaniasis," Clinical and Diagnostic Laboratory Immunology, vol. 8, no. 6, pp. 1220–1224, 2001.

67. P. Srivastava, A. Dayama, S. Mehrotra, and S. Sundar, "Diagnosis of visceral leishmaniasis," Transactions of the Royal Society of Tropical Medicine and Hygiene, vol. 105, no. 1, pp. 1–6, 2011.

68. P. Srivastava, S. Mehrotra, P. Tiwary, J. Chakravarty, and S. Sundar, "Diagnosis of indian visceral leishmaniasis by nucleic acid detection using PCR," PLoS ONE, vol. 6, no. 4, article e19304, 2011.

69. R. Maurya, R. K. Singh, B. Kumar, P. Salotra, M. Rai, and S. Sundar, "Evaluation of PCR for diagnosis of Indian kala-azar and assessment of cure," Journal of Clinical Microbiology, vol. 43, no. 7, pp. 3038–3041, 2005.

70. K. Kuhls, L. Keilonat, S. Ochsenreither et al., "Multilocus microsatellite typing (MLMT) reveals genetically isolated populations between and within the main endemic regions of visceral leishmaniasis,"Microbes and Infection, vol. 9, no. 3, pp. 334–343, 2007.

71. A. Dey and S. Singh, "Genetic heterogeneity among visceral and post-Kala-Azar dermal leishmaniasis strains from eastern India," Infection, Genetics and Evolution, vol. 7, no. 2, pp. 219–222, 2007.

72. K. W. Q. Tintaya, X. Ying, J. P. Dedet, S. Rijal, X. De Bolle, and J. C. Dujardin, "Antigen genes for molecular epidemiology of leishmaniasis: polymorphism of cysteine proteinase B and surface metalloprotease glycoprotein 63 in the Leishmania donovani complex," Journal of Infectious Diseases, vol. 189, no. 6, pp. 1035–1043, 2004.

73. I. L. Mauricio, J. R. Stothard, and M. A. Miles, "Leishmania donovani complex: genotyping with the ribosomal internal transcribed spacer and the mini-exon," Parasitology, vol. 128, no. 3, pp. 263–267, 2004.

74. S. De Doncker, V. Hutse, S. Abdellati et al., "A new PCR-ELISA for diagnosis of visceral leishmaniasis in blood of HIV-negative subjects," Transactions of the Royal Society of Tropical Medicine and Hygiene, vol. 99, no. 1, pp. 25–31, 2005.

75. S. Khosravi, S. H. Hejazi, M. Hashemzadeh, G. Eslami, and H. Y. Darani, "Molecular diagnosis of old world leishmaniasis: real-time PCR based on tryparedoxin peroxidase gene for the detection and identification of Leishmania spp," Journal of Vector Borne Diseases, vol. 49, no. 1, pp. 15–18, 2012.

76. E. E. Zijlstra, M. S. Ali, A. M. El-Hassan et al., "Kala-azar: a comparative study of parasitological methods and the direct agglutination test in diagnosis," Transactions of the Royal Society of Tropical Medicine and Hygiene, vol. 86, no. 5, pp. 505–507, 1992.

77. A. M. Allahverdiyev, M. Bagirova, S. Uzun et al., "The value of a new microculture method for diagnosis of visceral leishmaniasis by using bone marrow and peripheral blood," American Journal of Tropical Medicine and Hygiene, vol. 73, no. 2, pp. 276–280, 2005.

78. F. Chappuis, S. Rijal, A. Soto, J. Menten, and M. Boelaert, "A meta-analysis of the diagnostic performance of the direct agglutination test and rK39 dipstick for visceral leishmaniasis," British Medical Journal, vol. 333, no. 7571, pp. 723–726, 2006.

79. M. Gari-Toussaint, A. Lelièvre, P. Marty, and Y. Le Fichoux, "Contribution of serological tests to the diagnosis of visceral leishmaniasis in patients infected with the human immunodeficiency virus,"Transactions of the Royal Society of Tropical Medicine and Hygiene, vol. 88, no. 3, pp. 301–302, 1994.

80. H. D. F. H. Schallig, G. J. Schoone, C. C. M. Kroon, A. Hailu, F. Chappuis, and H. Veeken, "Development and application of 'simple' diagnostic tools for visceral leishmaniasis," Medical Microbiology and Immunology, vol. 190, no. 1-2, pp. 69–71, 2001.

81. S. Sundar, R. K. Singh, R. Maurya et al., "Serological diagnosis of Indian visceral leishmaniasis: direct agglutination test versus rK39 strip test," Transactions of the Royal Society of Tropical Medicine and Hygiene, vol. 100, no. 6, pp. 533–537, 2006.

82. C. B. Palatnik-de-Sousa, E. M. Gomes, E. Paraguai-de-Souza, M. Palatnik, K. Luz, and R. Borojevic,

"Leishmania donovani: titration of antibodies to the fucose-mannose ligand as an aid in diagnosis and prognosis of visceral leishmaniasis," Transactions of the Royal Society of Tropical Medicine and Hygiene, vol. 89, no. 4, pp. 390–393, 1995.

83. R. Kumar, K. Pai, K. Pathak, and S. Sundar, "Enzyme-linked immunosorbent assay for recombinant K39 antigen in diagnosis and prognosis of Indian visceral leishmaniasis," Clinical and Diagnostic Laboratory Immunology, vol. 8, no. 6, pp. 1220–1224, 2001.

84. R. L. Houghton, M. Petrescu, D. R. Benson et al., "A cloned antigen (recombinant K39) of Leishmania chagasi diagnostic for visceral leishmaniasis in human immunodeficiency virus type 1 patients and a prognostic indicator for monitoring patients undergoing drug therapy," Journal of Infectious Diseases, vol. 177, no. 5, pp. 1339–1344, 1998.

85. T. M. Mohapatra, D. P. Singh, M. R. Sen, K. Bharti, and S. Sundar, "Comparative evaluation of rK9, rK26 and rK39 antigens in the serodiagnosis of Indian visceral leishmaniasis," Journal of Infection in Developing Countries, vol. 4, no. 2, pp. 114–117, 2010.

86. F. Chappuis, Y. Mueller, A. Nguimfack et al., "Diagnostic accuracy of two rK39 antigen-based dipsticks and the formol gel test for rapid diagnosis of visceral leishmaniasis in northeastern Uganda," Journal of Clinical Microbiology, vol. 43, no. 12, pp. 5973–5977, 2005.

87. F. Chappuis, S. Sundar, A. Hailu et al., "Visceral leishmaniasis: what are the needs for diagnosis, treatment and control?" Nature Reviews Microbiology, vol. 5, no. 11, pp. 873–882, 2007. ·

88. M. J. Pérez-Alvarez, R. Larreta, C. Alonso, and J. M. Requena, "Characterisation of a monoclonal antibody recognising specifically the HSP70 from Leishmania," Parasitology Research, vol. 87, no. 11, pp. 907–910, 2001.

89. R. Piarroux, F. Gambarelli, H. Dumon et al., "Comparison of PCR with direct examination of bone marrow aspiration, myeloculture, and serology for diagnosis of visceral leishmaniasis in immunocompromised patients," Journal of Clinical Microbiology, vol. 32, no. 3, pp. 746–749, 1994.

90. S. De Doncker, V. Hutse, S. Abdellati et al., "A new PCR-ELISA for diagnosis of visceral leishmaniasis in blood of HIV-negative subjects," Transactions of the Royal Society of Tropical Medicine and Hygiene, vol. 99, no. 1, pp. 25–31, 2005.

91. R. K. Singh, H. P. Pandey, and S. Sundar, "Visceral leishmaniasis (kala-azar): challenges ahead," Indian Journal of Medical Research, vol. 123, no. 3, pp. 331–344, 2006.

92. T. K. Jha, "Evaluation of diamidine compound (pentamidine isethionate) in the treatment of resistant cases of kala-azar occurring in North Bihar, India," Transactions of the Royal Society of Tropical Medicine and Hygiene, vol. 77, no. 2, pp. 167–170, 1983.

93. S. N. Jha, N. K. Singh, and T. K. Jha, "Changing response to diamidine compounds in cases of kala-azar unresponsive to antimonial," The Journal of the Association of Physicians of India, vol. 39, no. 4, pp. 314–316, 1991.

94. S. Sundar, "Treatment of visceral leishmaniasis," Medical Microbiology and Immunology, vol. 190, no. 1-2, pp. 89–92, 2001.

95. S. L. Croft and V. Yardley, "Chemotherapy of leishmaniasis," Current Pharmaceutical Design, vol. 8, no. 4, pp. 319–342, 2002.

96. A. Jhingran, B. Chawla, S. Saxena, M. P. Barrett, and R. Madhubala, "Paromomycin: uptake and resistance in Leishmania donovani," Molecular and Biochemical Parasitology, vol. 164, no. 2, pp. 111–117, 2009.

97. N. Singh, M. Kumar, and R. K. Singh, "Leishmaniasis: current status of available drugs and new potential drug targets," Asian Pacific Journal of Tropical Medicine, vol. 5, no. 6, pp. 485–497, 2012.

98. A. Rochette, F. Raymond, J. M. Ubeda et al., "Genome-wide gene expression profiling analysis ofLeishmania major and Leishmania infantum developmental stages reveals substantial differences between the two species," BMC Genomics, vol. 9, pp. 255–281, 2008.

99. S. Krieger, W. Schwarz, M. R. Arlyanayagam, A. H. Fairlamb, R. L. Krauth-Siegel, and C. Clayton, "Trypanosomes lacking trypanothione reductase are avirulent and show increased sensitivity to oxidative stress," Molecular Microbiology, vol. 35, no. 3, pp. 542–552, 2000.

100. D. B. Castro-Pinto, M. Genestra, G. B. Menezes et al., "Cloning and expression of trypanothione reductase from a New World Leishmania species," Archives of Microbiology, vol. 189, no. 4, pp. 375–384, 2008.

101. R. F. Rodrigues, D. Castro-Pinto, A. Echevarria et al., "Investigation of trypanothione reductase inhibitory activity by 1, 3, 4- thiadiazolium-2-aminide derivatives and molecular docking studies,"Bioorganic & Medicinal Chemistry, vol. 20, no. 5, pp. 1760–1766, 2012.

102. P. Ascenzi, A. Bocedi, P. Visca, G. Antonini, and L. Gradoni, "Catalytic properties of cysteine proteinases from Trypanosoma cruzi and Leishmania infantum: a pre-steady-state and steady-state study,"Biochemical and Biophysical Research Communications, vol. 309, no. 3, pp. 659–665, 2003.

103. S. O. Lorente, R. Gómez, C. Jiménez et al., "Biphenylquinuclidines as inhibitors of squalene synthase and growth of parasitic protozoa," Bioorganic and Medicinal Chemistry, vol. 13, no. 10, pp. 3519–3529, 2005. ·

104. P. Bhargava, K. Kumar, S. S. Chaudhaery, A. K. Saxena, and U. Roy, "Cloning, overexpression and characterization of Leishmania donovani squalene synthase," FEMS Microbiology Letters, vol. 311, no. 1, pp. 82–92, 2010.

105. J. A. Urbina, J. L. Concepcion, S. Rangel, G. Visbal, and R. Lira, "Squalene synthase as a chemotherapeutic target in Trypanosoma cruzi and Leishmania mexicana," Molecular and Biochemical Parasitology, vol. 125, no. 1-2, pp. 35–45, 2002.

106. C. Jiménez-Jiménez, J. Carrero-Lérida, M. Sealey-Cardona, L. M. Ruiz-Pérez, J. A. Urbina, and D. González-Pacanowska, "Δ24 (25)-sterol methenyltransferase: intracellular localization and azasterol sensitivity in Leishmania major promastigotes overexpressing the enzyme," Molecular and Biochemical Parasitology, vol. 160, no. 1, pp. 52–59, 2008.

107. C. W. Roberts, R. McLeod, D. W. Rice, M. Ginger, M. L. Chance, and L. J. Goad, "Fatty acid and sterol metabolism: potential antimicrobial targets in apicomplexan and trypanosomatid parasitic protozoa,"Molecular and Biochemical Parasitology, vol. 126, no. 2, pp. 129–142, 2003.

108. O. Heby, L. Persson, and R. Madhubala, "Targeting the polyamine biosynthetic enzymes: a promising approach to therapy of African sleeping sickness, Chagas' disease, and leishmaniasis," Amino Acids, vol. 33, no. 2, pp. 359–366, 2007.

109. V. Iniesta, L. C. Gómez-Nieto, and I. Corraliza, "The inhibition of arginase by Nω-hydroxy-L-arginine controls the growth of Leishmania inside macrophages," Journal of Experimental Medicine, vol. 193, no. 6, pp. 777–783, 2001.

110. R. Balana-Fouce, E. Calvo-Álvarez, R. Álvarez-Velilla, C. F. Prada, Y. Pérez-Pertejo, and R. M. Reguera, "Role of trypanosomatid's arginase in polyamine biosynthesis and pathogenesis," Molecular and Biochemical Parasitology, vol. 181, no. 2, pp. 85–93, 2012.

111. B. M. Bakker, F. I. C. Mensonides, B. Teusink, P. Van Hoek, P. A. M. Michels, and H. V. Westerhoff, "Compartmentation protects trypanosomes from the dangerous design of glycolysis," Proceedings of the National Academy of Sciences of the United States of America, vol. 97, no. 5, pp. 2087–2092, 2000.

112. P. A. M. Michels, V. Hannaert, and F. Bringaud, "Metabolic aspects of glycosomes in Trypanosomatidae—new data and views," Parasitology Today, vol. 16, no. 11, pp. 482–489, 2000.

113. P. Hassan, D. Fergusson, K. M. Grant, and J. C. Mottram, "The CRK3 protein kinase is essential for cell cycle progression of Leishmania mexicana," Molecular and Biochemical Parasitology, vol. 113, no. 2, pp. 189–198, 2001.

114. K. M. Grant, M. H. Dunion, V. Yardley et al., "Inhibitors of Leishmania mexicana CRK3 cyclin-dependent kinase: chemical library screen and antileishmanial activity," Antimicrobial Agents and Chemotherapy, vol. 48, no. 8, pp. 3033–3042, 2004.

115. E. Xingi, D. Smirlis, V. Myrianthopoulos et al., "6-Br-5methylindirubin-3′oxime (5-Me-6-BIO) targeting the leishmanial glycogen synthase kinase-3 (GSK-3) short form affects cell-cycle progression and induces apoptosis-like death: exploitation of GSK-3 for treating leishmaniasis," International Journal for Parasitology, vol. 39, no. 12, pp. 1289–1303, 2009.

116. P. H. Liang and K. S. Anderson, "Substrate channeling and domain-domain interactions in bifunctional thymidylate synthase-dihydrofolate reductase," Biochemistry, vol. 37, no. 35, pp. 12195–12205, 1998. ·

117. O. Senkovich, N. Schormann, and D. Chattopadhyay, "Structures of dihydrofolate reductase-thymidylate synthase of trypanosoma cruzi in the folate-free state and in complex with two antifolate drugs, trimetrexate and methotrexate," Acta Crystallographica Section D, vol. 65, no. 7, pp. 704–716, 2009.

118. F. Zuccotto, A. C. R. Martin, R. A. Laskowski, J. M. Thornton, and I. H. Gilbert, "Dihydrofolate reductase: a potential drug target in trypanosomes and leishmania," Journal of Computer-Aided Molecular Design, vol. 12, no. 3, pp. 241–257, 1998.

119. I. D. Kuntz, "Structure-based strategies for drug design and discovery," Science, vol. 257, no. 5073, pp. 1078–1082, 1992.

120. P. S. T. Veras, C. I. Brodskyn, F. M. P. Balestieri et al., "A dhfr-ts- Leishmania major Knockout Mutant Cross-protects against Leishmania amazonensis," Memorias do Instituto Oswaldo Cruz, vol. 94, no. 4, pp. 491–496, 1999.

121. F. Fonseca-Silva, J. D. F. Inacio, M. M. Canto-Cavalheiro, and E. E. Almeida-Amaral, "Reactive oxygen species production and mitochondrial dysfunction contribute to quercetin induced death in Leishmania amazonensis," PLoS ONE, vol. 6, no. 2, article e14666, 2011.

CHAPTER 35

FIVE-MONTH COMPARATIVE EFFICACY EVALUATION OF THREE ECTOPARASITICIDES AGAINST ADULT CAT FLEAS (CTENOCEPHALIDES FELIS), FLEA EGG HATCH AND EMERGENCE, AND ADULT BROWN DOG TICKS (RHIPICEPHALUS SANGUINEUS SENSU LATO) ON DOGS HOUSED OUTDOORS

Marie Varloud, Elizabeth Hodgkins

Keywords: Cat flea, Ctenocephalides felis, Brown dog tick, Rhipicephalus sanguineus sensu lato, Acaricidal efficacy, Insecticidal efficacy

INTRODUCTION

Fleas and ticks are common and widespread blood-feeding ectoparasites which afflict dogs and cats. The cat flea *Ctenocephalides felis* is a prolific insect, and its population is mostly constituted by immature stages that infest the animal's environment. Regular and challenging infestations can easily be established from visiting and infested animals. On the animal, the adult cat flea can impair welfare of the host by gradual irritation and pruritus which can turn into flea bite hypersensitivity. It is also a competent vector for numerous diseases, including potentially zoonotic organisms such as *Dipylidium caninum* (Pugh 2001), *Rickettsia felis*(Wedincamp and Foil, 2000) or *Bartonella* spp. (Bouhsira et al. 2012a). The brown dog tick*Riphicephalus sanguineus* sensu lato is a monotropic three-host tick able to perform each stage on dogs, even indoors (Dantas-Torres 2010). It is widely distributed worldwide and within North America. In addition to causing blood loss and irritation, this tick is identified as a vector for different pathogens such as filaroids (*Cercopithifilaria* (Otranto et al. 2012)), protozoa (*Babesia* (Liebisch and Gillani 1979)) and bacteria (*Ehrlichia canis* (Aguiar et al. 2007; Wikswo et al. 2007)). *R sanguineus* is also suspected of being involved in the transmission of*Hepatozoon canis* (Nordgren and Craig 1984), *Anaplasma platys* (Ramcs et al. 2014),*Rickettsia* (Trotta et al. 2012), *Bartonella* (Wikswo et al. 2007) and *Coxiella burnetii*(Bernasconi et al. 2002). These pathogens can also be transmitted to humans. To protect companion animals from infestations by these parasites and to reduce the risk of zoonotic transmission, several ectoparasiticide products are available. Most of them are spot-on combinations of insecticide (dinotefuran, fipronil, imidacloprid) and acaricide (fipronil) or acaricide and repellent (permethrin) actives. Some of them also include an insect growth regulator (IGR, such as pyriproxyfen and (S)-methoprene) which provides control of the immature stages of fleas. Despite similar functions or actives, the products differ widely from each other through their formulation. This is based on chemistry, excipients and quality of ingredients and confers upon the products a large part of their efficacy properties (Endris et al.2003). In active

---

Citation: Varloud, M. & Hodgkins, E. Five-month Comparative Efficacy Evaluation of three Ectoparasiticides Against Adult cat Fleas (Ctenocephalides felis), Flea Egg Hatch and Emergence, and Adult Brown Dog Ticks (Rhipicephalus sanguineus sensu lato) on Dogs Housed Outdoors. doi:10.1007/s00436-014-4262-5.

dogs, these properties can make important differences in the final protection provided. Indeed, even companion dogs spend a large part of their time outdoors (Slater et al.2008) where they may encounter higher numbers of parasites. Because of climatic conditions (rain and UV light), time spent outdoors also increases the risk of removal or inactivation of the topical treatment and potentially reduces the level and duration of efficacy on these animals (Raveton et al. 2006; Schmahl et al. 2009). In order to assess the efficacy of three different spot-on ectoparasiticides for active dogs, their efficacy against fleas and ticks was compared on dogs for 5 months in outdoor conditions.

MATERIALS AND METHODS

The products were not administered to test animals by any individual involved in performing the post-treatment assessments and observations. Study groups were coded to blind the assessors.

Animals

Forty-two healthy adult Beagle dogs with short hair started the 15-day acclimation period. To be enrolled, the dogs should not have been treated with any ectoparasiticide for at least 3 months before the start of the study. The dogs were individually identified by a uniquely numbered tattoo and were fed commercial dog food once daily with water available ad libitum. During the acclimation period, the dogs were bathed with a non-insecticidal shampoo and infested with fleas. Counts were conducted to establish their flea retention level (Fig. 1). Seven dogs with the lowest flea counts and three dogs randomly selected were eliminated from the study and returned to the laboratory colony to reach the objective number of 32 dogs. The selected dogs, 17 males and 15 females, weighed from 10.6 to 16.1 kg and were from 1 to 9 years of age. They were housed individually in indoor pens during the pre-infestation and count period and for 5 days each month during the study for flea ova collection as well as for tick and flea infestation and counting. During the rest of the study period, the dogs were housed in compatible same sex pairs with dogs from the same treatment group in outdoor runs. The runs were designed to expose dogs to the outdoor environment but also enabled them to seek refuge from sunlight and rain, thus providing shelter at their pleasure. The last two allocated dogs were an intact male and a female that were separated in the pen with individual shelters. The general health of all dogs was observed once daily during the study. On each treatment day, clinical observations of all dogs were conducted at approximately 1, 2, 3 and 4 h post-treatment. This study plan was approved by the ethics committee of Nu-Era Farms.

Months	Jul		Aug							Sep						
Study days	-12	-11	-5	-3	0	14	15	18	19	28	30	44	46	50	51	55
Treatment					x						x					
Flea infestation	x					x										x
Flea count		x					x									
Flea reinfestation		x					x									
Flea eggs collection								x								
Flea eggs collection*									x							
Adult flea emergence count														x		
Adult flea emergence count**															x	
Tick infestation			x							x		x				
Tick count				x							x		x			

Months	Oct							Nov										Dec		Jan					Feb	
Study days	56	59	60	74	75	78	79	88	90	91	92	104	106	110	111	115	116	119	120	150	151	152	153	154	185	186
Treatment			x						x																	
Flea infestation				x												x				x						
Flea count	x				x												x							x		
Flea reinfestation	x				x												x									
Flea eggs collection		x				x												x					x			
Flea eggs collection*			x				x												x					x		
Adult flea emergence count										x				x							x				x	
Adult flea emergence count**											x				x							x				x
Tick infestation								x				x														
Tick count									x				x													

* if 50 ova not collected the previous day

** if second flea egg collection

Figure 1: Experimental design.

Allocation

Allocation to treatment groups was carried out on day 2. The 32 selected dogs were ranked, in descending order of day 2 body weights, into eight replicates of four animals each. Each dog within each replicate was randomly assigned, without regard to sex, to one of the four treatment groups (1, 2, 3 and 4). Each group consisted of eight dogs. Each dog was also randomly assigned to an indoor/outdoor run. Both male and female dogs were represented in each treatment group.

Treatment Application

Each dog was treated with the allocated treatment on days 0, 30, 60 and 90 of the study (Table 1, Fig. 1). Dogs in group 1 received the placebo control solution (CS) containing the vehicle of the commercial formulation Vectra 3D® (Ceva Animal Health LLC Lenexa, KS, USA). Dogs in group 2 were treated with the commercial formulation Vectra 3D® (DPP) containing dinotefuran (4.95 % *w/w*), pyriproxifen (0.44 %) and permethrin (36.08 %). Group 3 was treated with the commercial formulation Frontline Plus® (Merial Ltd., Duluth, GA) containing fipronil (9.8 %) and (S)-methoprene (8.8 %) (FM), and group 4 was treated with the commercial formulation K9 Advantix® 55 (Bayer HealthCare, Shawnee Mission, KS, USA) containing imidacloprid (8.8 %) and permethrin (44.0 %) (IP). The commercial formulations were administered topically, as spot-on, in accordance with the manufacturers' label directions. CS and DPP were administered at a rate of 3.6 mL per dog applied equally (1.2 mL per site) in three spots at the shoulder blades, mid-back and base of tail. FM was administered at a rate of 1.34 mL per dog, in one spot applied at the shoulder blades. IP was administered at a rate of 2.5 mL per dog, in three equal spots between the shoulder blades, mid-back and base of the tail.

Table 1: Study design

Study steps	**Study days**					
Treatment administration	0	30	60	90		
Flea infestation	−12	14	55	74	115	150
Flea count	−11	15	56	75	116	154
Flea reinfestation		15	56	75	116	
Flea eggs collection	18	59	78	119	153	
Flea eggs collection[a]	19	60	79	120	154	
Adult flea emergence count	50	91	110	151	185	
Adult flea emergence count[b]	51	92	111	152	186	
Tick infestation	−5	28	44	88	104	
Tick count	−3	30	46	90	106	

[a]If 50 ova not collected the previous day

[b]If second flea egg collection performed

Flea and Tick Challenge

The laboratory colonies of fleas and ticks used in the study were not known to be resistant to any pesticide, and both the fleas and ticks had been in culture for less than 3 years. All dogs were infested with 100 unfed *C. felis* adult fleas on days 12 (during acclimation), 14, 55, 74, 115 and 150 of the study. Flea counts were conducted 24 h after infestation except for the final infestation when flea counts were conducted 96 h post-infestation (on day 154). For counts, the hair coat on all parts of the dog including the tail was examined in a methodical manner so that fleas were combed off the dogs and live fleas were counted. Following the 24-h flea counts, all dogs were reinfested with new fleas (~100) on days −11, 15, 56, 75 and 116 for flea egg collection. Flea eggs were collected over a period of 48 h beginning 3 days after infestation, on egg collection liners placed under the indoor run resting areas. The liners were removed after overnight egg collection and carefully swept to collect the debris and eggs that had fallen from the animal. Following egg collection, the fleas were combed off the dogs but no counts were conducted. For each dog, available eggs (up to 50, if available) were counted and placed in dishes holding groups of 25 eggs per dish. The eggs were incubated with culture media for 4 days and examined to determine larval hatch. The dishes were held under the same conditions for an additional 28 days to determine the number of emerged adults.

All dogs were infested with 50 unfed *R. sanguineus* adult ticks (male:female ratio of 1:1) on days 5 (during acclimation), 28, 44, 88 and 104 of the study. Tick counts were conducted approximately 48 h after infestation (days 30, 46, 90 and 106) by systematically examining all areas of the animal. When performing the counts, the animal's hair was pushed against its nape so that the skin and the ticks were exposed. Ticks were removed with blunt pointed forceps and placed in a dish of alcohol for counting.

Statistical Analysis

Adult flea and Tick Effectiveness

To determine efficacy against adult fleas and ticks, the counts were transformed to the natural logarithm of (count+1) to calculate geometric means (GM). Percent efficacy for each treatment group on each flea or tick count day was calculated using the following equation:

$$\%\ \text{Efficacy} = \left(\frac{\text{Geometric Mean Count Control Group} - \text{Geometric Mean Count Treated Group}}{\text{Geometric Mean Count Control Group}}\right)*100$$

The treatments were compared using a *t* test for means with poolable variances or for means with unequal variances, as appropriate. Variances were compared using an F test, and Satterthwaite's approximation was used to determine the degree of freedom for the unequal variance tests; when one variance was 0, the variance was unequal by definition, and when both variances were 0, no comparisons were possible. Each treated group was compared to the CS group, and the group treated with DPP was compared to groups treated with FM and IP. Statistical significance was declared at a two-sided *p* value of 0.05.

Ovicidal and Adult Flea Emergence

Percentage hatch and adult emergence from flea eggs were transformed to the arcsine (radians) of the square root of the proportion to calculate means. Mean angle was then back transformed. This procedure maintained non-missing values for dogs participating in the study. Percent efficacy for each treatment group on each day was calculated using the following equation:

$$\%\ \text{Efficacy} = \left(\frac{\text{Retransformed Mean of Control Group} - \text{Retransformed Mean of Treated Group}}{\text{Retransformed Mean of Control Group}}\right)*100$$

The data were analyzed as described above for adult fleas and ticks. All analyses and calculations were performed using SAS Version 9.2 (SAS Institute, Cary, NC).

Guidelines

This study was carried out at Nu-Era Farms (Stillwater, OK, USA) in compliance with Good Clinical Practice requirements (VICH GL9, May 2001). In addition, the study was conducted in compliance with US EPA Product Performance Test Guidelines OPPTS 810.3300: Treatments to Control Pests of Humans and Pets.

RESULTS

No adverse effects to any of the treatment applications were observed in any dogs during the study. The climatic conditions in the location for the study duration were highly variable (Fig. 2).

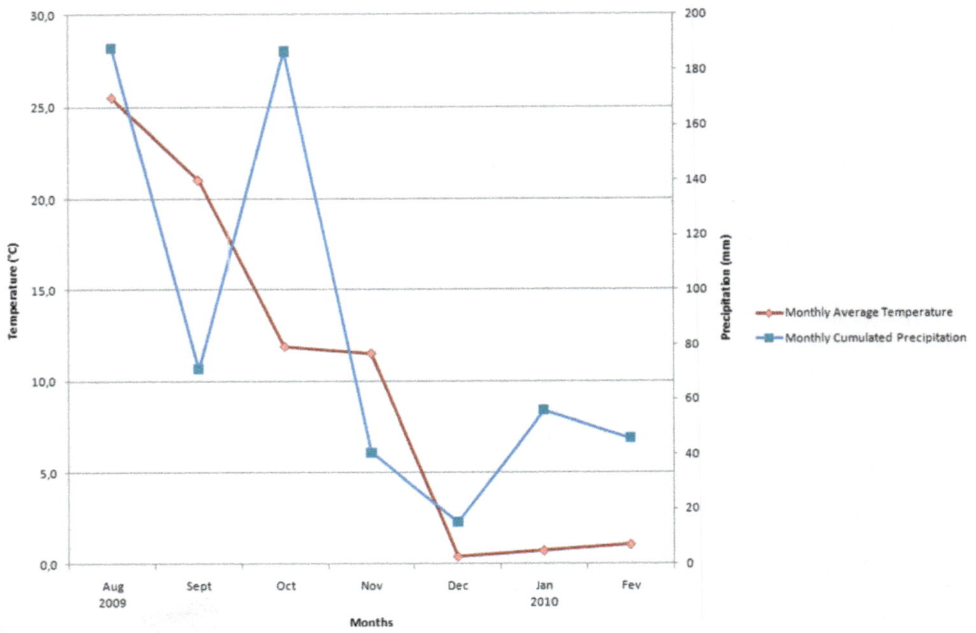

Figure 2: Climatological data of Stillwater, Oklahoma (US) between August 2009 and February 2010 (National Climatic Data Center).

Efficacy Against Adult Fleas (*Ctenocephalides felis*)

Pre-treatment GM flea counts ranged from 67.4 to 69.0 for all study groups. During the study, GM flea counts ranged from 67.4 to 81.6 for the CS group (Table 2).

Table 2: Geometric mean number of fleas (*Ctenocephalides felis*) per dog and the percent efficacy based on geometric mean flea counts for groups treated with either CS, DPP, FM or IP days 0, 30, 60 and 90 of the study.

		Geometric mean number of fleas/dog[a]				% Efficacy		
Study day	Days since last treatment[b]	CS	DPP	FM	IP	DPP	FM	IP
−11	NA	67.4	67.5	68.4	69.0	NA	NA	NA
15	15	76.3	1.1*	0.3*	1.1*	98.6	99.7	98.6
56	26	74.5	1.3*	0.7*	1.6*	98.3	99.1	97.9
75	15	81.6	0.1*	0.0*	0'0*	99.9	100	100
116	26	76.2	0.2*	0.5*	0.9*	99.8	99.4	98.9
154	64	76.4	6.3*	1.2*	8.4*	91.7	98.4	89.1

CS control solution, *DPP* dinotefuran, pyriproxifen and permethrin, *FM* fipronil and (S)-methoprene, *IP* imidacloprid and permethrin, *NA* not applicable

*Geometric mean flea counts significantly different from the CS group ($p<0.01$)

[a]Eight dogs in each group, flea counts conducted 24 h post-infestation

[b]Last or the most recent treatment

For dogs treated with DPP, FM or IP, efficacies ranged from 98.3 to 99.9 %, 99.1 to 100 % and 97.9 to 100 %, respectively, when counts were conducted 15 or 26 days after treatments and were 91.7, 98.4 and 89.1 %, respectively, when counts were conducted 64 days after the last treatment. Compared to the CS group, the three treated groups had lower ($p<0.005$) flea counts. When the DPP-treated group was compared to the FM- or IP-treated groups, it was not possible to detect any difference in efficacy at any of the assessment time points.

Efficacy against flea (*Ctenocephalides felis*) egg hatch and emerging adults

After the additional flea challenges on days 15, 56, 75 and 116 of the study, no eggs were available for collection on days 18–19, 59–60, 78–79 and 119–120 from all three treated groups. After the last challenge on day 150, eggs were collected from all groups on days 153–154 of the study (Table 3).

Table 3: Percent egg hatch and adult flea emergence with percent efficacies against*Ctenocephalides felis* for groups treated with CS DPP, FM or IP on days 0, 30, 60 and 90 of the study

		Egg hatch						
Egg collection		% hatch				% efficacy		
Study days	Days since last treatment	CS	DPP	FM	IP	DPP	FM	IP
18–19	18–19	78.1	na*	na*	na*	na	na	na
59–60	29–30	74.6	na*	na *	na*	na	na	na
78–79	18–19	75.1	na*	na*	na	na	na	na
119–120	29–30	80.7	na*	na*	na*	na	na	na
153–154	63–64	79.6	1.0*	0.2*	33.7*+	98.7	99.7	57.7
		Adult flea emergence						
Egg collection		% emergence				% efficacy		
Study days	Days since last treatment	CS	DPP	FM	IP	DPP	FM	IP
18–19	18–19	74.3	na*	na*	na*	na	na	na
59–60	29–30	73.9	na*	na*	na*	na	na	na
78–79	18–19	74.8	na*	na*	na*	na	na	na
119–120	29–30	80.4	na*	na*	na*	na	na	na
153–154	63–64	78.3	1.0*	0.1*	26.5*+	98.7	99.9	66.2

CS control solution, *DPP* dinotefuran, pyriproxifen and permethrin, *FM* fipronil and (S)-methoprene, *IP* imidacloprid and permethrin, *na* not applicable because no egg could be collected for incubation

*Significantly different from the CS group ($p<0.01$)

+Significantly different from the DPP group ($p<0.01$)

Except for two animals in the FM-treated group, flea eggs were collected from every animal in all four study groups on days 153–154 of the study (63–64 days after the last treatment). This measurement was added to measure the residual activity of all formulations. At this time point, for dogs treated with DPP, FM and IP, efficacy against egg hatch was 98.7, 99.7 and 57.7 %, respectively, and the efficacy against adult flea emergence was 98.7, 99.9 and 62.2 %, respectively. When compared, the CS group had a much higher ($p<0.0001$) percentage of egg hatch and adult flea emergence than the DPP- and FM-treated groups. The CS group had a higher percentage of egg hatch ($p=0.0019$) and of adult emergence ($p=0.0005$) than the IP-treated group. The DPP-treated group had a lower percentage of egg hatch ($p=0.0012$) and adult flea emergence ($p=0.0024$) than the IP-treated group, but no difference was detected between the DPP-treated group and the FM-treated group.

Efficacy against adult ticks (*R. Sanguineus*)

Pre-treatment GM tick counts for all study groups ranged from 19.5 to 21.9. For the CS group, GM tick counts ranged from 20.1 to 23.2 during the study (Table 4).

Table 4: Mean number of ticks (*Riphicephalus sanguineus*) per dog and the percent efficacy based on geometric mean tick counts for groups treated with CS, DPP, FM or IP on days 0, 30, 60 and 90 of the study

		Geometric mean number of tick/dog[a]				**% efficacy**		
Study day	**Days since last treatment[b]**	**CS**	**DPP**	**FM**	**IP**	**DPP**	**FM**	**IP**
3	NA	20.1	21.9	19.5	21.9	NA	NA	NA
30	30	21.8	1.5*	13.5*+	4.1*	93.2	38.0	81.4
46	16	22.5	0.4*	0.1*	0.3*	98.4	99.6	98.9
90	30	20.1	0.9*	10.5*+	0.3*	95.3	47.7	98.6
106	16	23.2	1.7*	3.3*	0.6*	92.6	85.8	97.4

[a]Eight dogs in each group, tick counts conducted 48 h post-infestation

[b]Last or the most recent treatment

CS control solution, *DPP* dinotefuran, pyriproxifen and permethrin, *FM* fipronil and (S)-methoprene, *IP* imidacloprid and permethrin, *NA* not applicable

*Geometric mean tick count significantly different from the CS (p<0.01)

+Significantly different from the DPP group (p<0.01)

For dogs treated with the DPP formulation, efficacies ranged from 92.6 to 98.4 % when tick counts were conducted 16 or 30 days after the most recent treatments. For FM-treated dogs, the tick efficacies ranged from 85.8 to 99.6 % for counts conducted 16 days after treatment and from 38.0 to 47.7 % for counts conducted 30 days after treatment. For the IP-treated dogs, the efficacies were between 97.4 to 98.9 % and 81.8 to 98.9 % when counts were conducted 16 or 30 days after the initial or the most recent treatments, respectively.

Whatever the time point, the CS group had higher (p<0.01) tick counts compared to any treated group. The DPP-treated group had lower tick counts than the FM group when counts were conducted 30 days after treatment (p=0.0034 at day 30 and p=0.0015 at day 90). It was not possible to detect any difference in tick counts between the DPP- and IP-treated groups at any of the assessment time points.

DISCUSSION

Methodological Considerations

The dogs spent 113 of the 171 days (66 %) of study duration after first treatment application, in outdoor housing. Their housing conditions can be considered as representative of a free-outdoor access. The study was run between 22 July 2009 and 8 February 2010 in Oklahoma (USA). One treatment was performed on the 6 August 2009, during one of the rainiest (188 mm of precipitation) and hottest (25.5 °C) months of the study (Fig. 2).

As demonstrated in the CS group, flea and tick challenges were successful during the whole duration of the study. Moreover, at the beginning of the experiment and before administration of the treatments, the four groups exhibited very similar levels of GM flea (from 67.4 to 69.0) and tick (from 19.5 to 21.9) counts.

In this study, infestations by the two parasites were artificial: the fleas and ticks were directly deposited on the haircoat of dogs, whereas in natural conditions, fleas jump on their targeted host and questing ticks crawl from down to upside positions. When they infest a permethrin-treated host, these parasites are repelled and leave the host. While the present experiment was designed to assess insecticidal and acaricidal efficacy, it was not designed to assess the repellency properties of IP and DPP permethrin-based combinations.

Efficacy against Adult Fleas

When efficacy was assessed 15 or 26 days after treatment, the three products exhibited very high adulticidal efficacy levels (>97.9–100 %). Because of these asymptotic levels, it was not possible to detect any difference between the products since all of them demonstrated a much lower (p<0.0001) adult flea count than the control. We can therefore consider them all suitable for flea adulticidal activity in outdoor dogs. In a previous field study, FM and DPP formulations already provided very similar levels of protection against fleas (Dryden et al. 2011).

Interestingly, adulticidal efficacy was assessed at the end of the study, 64 days after the last treatment, mimicking a lack of compliance. At this time point, again, all the groups treated with actives had lower adult flea counts than the CS group. The different treatments provided a 2-month protection against artificial infestations with adult fleas on dogs, without any negative interaction of outdoor housing conditions.

It is generally considered that permethrin (at 50 mg/Kg BW), one of the adulticidal actives of DPP, is deposited in the upper layers of the *stratum corneum* and on the surface of hairs (Lüssenhop et al. 2012). Fipronil, however, spreads across the body within the skin's sebum and accumulates in pilo-sebaceous glands and in superficial layers of the epidermis. This was demonstrated, in Beagle dogs, with a volume and dose of product (FM, 1.34 mL, 10 mg/Kg) similar to the one used in our study (Cochet et al. 1997). However, 2 months after treatment, in outdoor conditions, this property of FM did not confer any detectable advantage to this formulation as compared to DPP regarding flea adulticidal activity.

Efficacy Against Immature Stages of Fleas

For all DPP, FM and IP treatment groups and collection points, no eggs were collected up to day 120 of the study. This is probably the consequence of the high adulticidal efficacy of the products which killed the fleas before they laid their eggs as the animals were treated either 18–19 or 29–30 days before collection of eggs. Because no adult flea count was performed after egg collection, this hypothesis cannot be fully verified but the flea count conducted following day 115 infestation highly suggests this. Indeed, we counted only zero to one flea (six dogs without fleas) in the DPP-treated group, zero to three fleas (four dogs without fleas) in the FM-treated group and zero to nine fleas (five dogs without fleas) in the IP-treated group. Because of this high adulticidal activity, the adult flea population and the subsequent egg production may therefore have been highly reduced, falling under our detection limit.

In order to reduce the interaction between adulticidal and IGR actives, egg collection and subsequent evaluation of egg hatch and adult emergence were assessed 64 days after the last treatment. Despite the high adulticidal efficacy (>97.9 %), the number of flea-free dogs dropped to two, three and zero for DPP, FM and IP, respectively, and eggs were collected in every group. DPP and FM formulations contain a true IGR active: pyriproxyfen and (S)-methoprene, respectively, whereas IP has none. This resulted in a higher viability of the eggs, with larvae hatching more successfully in the IP-treated group than in the DPP- and FM-treated groups. The larvae were also more successful in their pupation and emergence process up to adults in the IP-treated group than in the DPP- and FM-treated groups. Both FM and DPP provided very satisfactory levels of protection against immature stages of fleas. These results confirmed previous observations with DPP performed on transplanted and ready to hatch fleas (Bouhsira et al. 2012b).

An increasing number of products without IGR actives is available to pet owners. These results demonstrate that such products cannot provide the same duration of protection against the immature population of fleas. Moreover, this experimental design was favourable to IGR-like activity. Indeed, it only mimicked the control of offspring production from fleas infesting the treated pets at specific time points. These fleas were directly exposed to the treated pets. Unlike in real situations, neither environmental infestation (wild animals, etc.) nor egg infestation of the dog surroundings occurred. In more realistic circumstances, more benefits of true IGR substances, which also prevent fleas from developing in the environment of the treated pets, would be expected.

Efficacy against ticks (*R. sanguineus*)

Despite the free outdoor access housing of the dogs, the tick counts were lower in all treated groups compared to the CS group. However, the different formulations provided different levels of protection. DPP, containing the acaricide permethrin, had higher efficacy than FM, containing the acaricide fipronil, as measured 30 days after the first (93.2 vs. 38.0 %) and third (95.3 vs. 47.7 %) monthly treatments. At these two time points, all the dogs treated with FM had at least 6 ticks attached and, more precisely, 7 to 16 ticks after the first treatment and 6 to 20 ticks after the third treatment. Moreover, a strong reduction in acaricidal efficacy was detected between the 16th (99.6–85.8 %) and the 30th (38.0–47.7 %) day after treatment in the FM-treated group. This phenomenon is compatible with a reduced residual concentration of the acaricide-active fipronil in the coat of the animals at the end of the expected treatment duration (1 month). In the outdoor conditions of our experiment, the spreading properties of the fipronil-based formulation did not provide any advantage as compared to the permethrin-based formulations. This difference in acaricidal activity between these fipronil-based and permethrin-based products has been documented in several studies: a laboratory experiment in dogs infested with *R. sanguineus* (Dryden et al. 2006), a multi-centre field study against adult*Ixodes* and *Rhipicephalus* ticks (Hellmann et al. 2003) and under natural conditions against both immature and adult stages of *R. sanguineus* (Otranto et al. 2005). These experiments all demonstrated that, at the end of the treatment duration, permethrin-based products such as IP and DPP are more effective against *R. sanguineus* than the fipronil-based combination FM. However, the residual acaricidal efficacy of the IP group was only 81.4 % 30 days after the first treatment.

DPP was already shown to be highly effective against *Amblyomma americanum* and *A. maculatum* (Coyne 2009). Our study confirms that DPP provides a satisfactory level of protection to dogs against *R. sanguineus*, without any adverse effect and despite the fact that dogs spent 5 months in challenging a free access outdoor housing. It can therefore be concluded that DPP is appropriate to protect active dogs with outdoor access against *R. sanguineus* ticks.

CONCLUSIONS

This experiment demonstrated that, under free outdoor-access housing, dogs treated with FM or DPP were protected against all stages of fleas for 2 months following four monthly applications. However, IP efficacy did not remain above 90 % 30 days after administration. The study also confirmed that fipronil-based formulations such as FM are not optimal for the control of artificial infestation by *R. sanguineus* ticks in dogs, especially with free outdoor access. Natural infestations can be even more challenging, with average tick loads already reported to reach 150 ticks per dog (Brianti et al. 2010). In the circumstances of this study, only permethrin-based formulations provided a satisfactory range of efficacy. However, with only 81.4 % efficacy, the IP formulation did not provide the expected minimum 90 % efficacy against ticks 30 days after the first treatment. DPP was therefore the only formulation providing both satisfactory efficacy levels against all stages of fleas (*C. felis*) and against ticks (*R. sanguineus*) on dogs housed with free outdoor access.

ACKNOWLEDGMENTS

The authors acknowledge Dr Sheila Gross for the statistical analysis. Dr Cathy Ball, Dr Sivaja Ranjan, Erick Hiott and the Nu-Era team are also acknowledged for their respective contributions in this experiment.

Conflict of Interests

Dr Elizabeth Hodgkins is the director of the Veterinary Services in CEVA USA and Dr Marie Varloud is the global technical manager for parasitology in companion animals in the medical services of CEVA.

Author contributions

The authors read and approved the final manuscript.

REFERENCES

1. Aguiar DM, Cavalcante GT, Pinter A, Gennari SM, Camargo LM, Labruna MB (2007) Prevalence of Ehrlichia canis (Rickettsiales: Anaplasmataceae) in dogs and *Rhipicephalus sanguineus* (Acari: Ixodidae) ticks from Brazil. J Med Entomol 44:126–132.
2. Bernasconi MV, Casati S, Péter O, Piffaretti JC (2002) *Rhipicephalus* ticks infected with*Rickettsia* and *Coxiella* in Southern Switzerland (Canton Ticino). Infec Genetic Evol 2:111–120.
3. Bouhsira E, Ferrandez Y, Liu MF, Franc M, Boulouis HJ, Biville F (2012a) *Ctenocephalides felis*an in vitro potential vector for five *Bartonella* species. Comp Immunol Microbiol Infect Dis 36:105–111.
4. Bouhsira E, Lienard E, Jacquiet P, Warin S, Kaltsatos V, Baduel L, Franc M (2012b) Efficacy of permethrin, dinotefuran and pyriproxyfen on adult fleas, flea eggs collection, and flea egg development following transplantation of mature female fleas (Ctenocephalides felis felis) from cats to dogs. Vet Parasitol 190:541–546.
5. Brianti E, Pennisi MG, Brucato G, Risitano AL, Gaglio G, Lombardo G, Malara D, Fogliazza A, Giannetto S (2010) Efficacy of the fipronil 10 %+(S)-methoprene 9 % combination against*Rhipicephalus sanguineus* in naturally infested dogs: speed of kill, persistent efficacy on immature and adult stages and effect of water. Vet Parasitol 170:96–103.

6. Cochet P, Birckel P, Bromet-Petit M, Bromet N, Weil A (1997) Skin distribution of fipronil by microautoradiography following topical administration to the beagle dog. Eur J Drug Metab Pharmacokinet 22:211–216.
7. Coyne MJ (2009) Efficacy of a topical ectoparasiticide containing dinotefuran, pyriproxyfen, and permethrin against *Amblyomma americanum* (Lone Star tick) and *Amblyomma maculatum* (Gulf Coast tick) on dogs. Vet Ther 10:17–23
8. Dantas-Torres F (2010) Biology and ecology of the brown dog tick, *Rhipicephalus sanguineus*. Parasit Vectors 3:26.
9. Dryden MW, Payne PA, Smith V, Hostetler J (2006) Evaluation of an imidacloprid (8.8 % w/w)–permethrin (44.0 % w/w) topical spot-on and a fipronil (9.8 % w/w)–(S)-methoprene (8.8 % w/w) topical spot-on to repel, prevent attachment, and kill adult Rhipicephalus sanguineus and Dermacentor variabilis ticks on dogs. Vet Ther 7:187–198
10. Dryden MW, Payne PA, Smith V, Riggs B, Davenport J, Kobuszewski D (2011) Efficacy of dinotefuran-pyriproxyfen, dinotefuran-pyriproxyfen-permethrin and fipronil-(S)-methoprene topical spot-on formulations to control flea populations in naturally infested pets and private residences in Tampa, FL. Vet Parasitol 182:281–286.
11. Endris RG, Hair JA, Anderson G, Rose WB, Disch D, Meyer JA (2003) Efficacy of two 65 % permethrin spot-on formulations against induced infestations of *Ctenocephalides felis* (Insecta: Siphonaptera) and *Amblyomma americanum* (Acari: Ixodidae) on beagles. Vet Ther 4:47–55
12. Hellmann K, Knoppe T, Krieger K, Stanneck D (2003) European multicenter field trial on the efficacy and safety of a topical formulation of imidacloprid and permethrin (Advantix) in dogs naturally infested with ticks and/or fleas. Parasitol Res 90:S125–S126.
13. Liebisch A, Gillani S (1979) Experimental transmission of canine babesiosis (*Babesia canis*) by native German ticks: 1. The brown dog tick (*Rhipicephalus sanguineus*). Dtsch Tierarztl Wochenschr 86:149–152
14. Lüssenhop J, Stahl J, Wolken S, Schnieder T, Kietzmann M, Bäumer W (2012) Distribution of permethrin in hair and stratum corneum after topical administration of four different formulations in dogs. J Vet Pharmacol Ther 35:206–208.
15. Nordgren RM, Craig TM (1984) Experimental transmission of the Texas strain of *Hepatozoon canis*. Vet Parasitol 16:207–214
16. Otranto D, Lia RP, Cantacessi C, Galli G, Paradies P, Mallia E, Capelli G (2005) Efficacy of a combination of imidacloprid 10 %/permethrin 50 % versus fipronil 10 %/(S)-methoprene 12 %, against ticks in naturally infected dogs. Vet Parasitol 130:293–304.
17. Otranto D, Brianti E, Latrofa MS, Annoscia G, Weigl S, Lia RP, Gaglio G, Napoli E, Giannetto S, Papadopoulos E, Mirò G, Dantas-Torres F, Bain O (2012) On a *Cercopithifilaria* sp. transmitted by *Rhipicephalus sanguineus*: a neglected, but widespread filarioid of dogs. Parasit Vectors 5:1–9.
18. Pugh RE (2001) Effects on the development of *Dipylidium caninum* and on the host reaction to this parasite in the adult flea (*Ctenocephalides felis felis*). Parasitol Res 73:171–177.
19. Ramos RA, Latrofa MS, Giannelli A, Lacasella V, Campbell BE, Dantas-Torres F, Otranto D (2014) Detection of *Anaplasma platys* in dogs and *Rhipicephalus sanguineus* group ticks by a quantitative real-time PCR. Vet Parasitol 205:285–288.
20. Raveton M, Aajoud A, Willison JC, Aouadi H, Tissut M, Ravanel P (2006) Phototransformation of the insecticide fipronil: identification of novel photoproducts and evidence for an alternative pathway of photodegradation. Environ Sci Technol 1:4151–4157.12
21. Schmahl G, Mehlhorn H, Abdel-Ghaffar F, Al-Rasheid K, Schumacher B, Jatzlau A, Pohle H (2009) Does rain reduce the efficacy of Butox 7.5 pour on (deltamethrin) against biting midges (*Culicoides* specimens)? Parasitol Res 105:1763–1765.
22. Slater MR, Di Nardo A, Pediconi O, Villa PD, Candeloro L, Alessandrini B, Del Papa S (2008) Cat and dog ownership and management patterns in central Italy. Preventive Veterinary Medicine 85:267–294.
23. Trotta M, Nicetto M, Fogliazza A, Montarsi F, Caldin M, Furlanello T, Solano-Gallego L (2012) Detection of *Leishmania infantum*, *Babesia canis*, and rickettsiae in ticks removed from dogs living in Italy. Ticks Tick Borne Dis 3:294–297.
24. Wedincamp J Jr, Foil LD (2000) Infection and seroconversion of cats exposed to cat fleas (*Ctenocephalides felis* Bouche) infected with *Rickettsia felis*. J Vector Ecol 25:123–126
25. Wikswo ME, Hu R, Metzger ME, Eremeeva ME (2007) Detection of *Rickettsia rickettsii* and*Bartonella henselae* in *Rhipicephalus sanguineus* ticks from California. J Med Entomol 44:158–162.

CHAPTER 36

FIPRONIL AND PERMETHRIN COMBINATION: A NOVEL ECTOPARASITICIDE FOR DOGS

Luís Cardoso

Arthropods may be ectoparasites of dogs, representing a nuisance and causing direct damage such as blood loss, irritation, skin lesions, hypersensitivity reactions, toxicosis and even paralysis. Many of those invertebrates are also a potential indirect threat to their vertebrate hosts due to the transmission, mainly while feeding on blood, of a range of vector-borne pathogens, including bacteria, protozoa, helminths and viruses, many of which are of zoonotic concern. Ticks, together with fleas, mosquitoes, sand flies and other insects, are among the haematophagous ectoparasites that have a major impact on the well-being and health not only of dogs but also of humans, thus providing factual examples of the "One Health" concept. The vector-borne diseases of dogs include anaplasmosis, babesiosis, bartonellosis, borreliosis, dipylidiosis, dirofilariosis, ehrlichiosis, leishmaniosis and rickettsiosis, most of which represent emergent veterinary medical and public health problems in many geographical regions worldwide.

Prevention of canine vector-borne diseases largely relies on ectoparasite control, aiming at protecting dogs and simultaneously limiting the risk of zoonotic infections. Due to changes in the distribution of arthropods, along with those in the lifestyle of pets, it is advisable to maintain protection against ectoparasites year-round. Regular application of effective anti-vector products on dogs remains the best approach to control infestations and associated diseases. The range of ectoparasiticides has expanded in recent years with the development of new active ingredients and formulations. Many active ingredients are available on the market as insecticides/acaricides, supplying veterinarians and dog owners with a wide variety of products to choose from, such as sprays, spot-on pipettes, impregnated collars and orally administered preparations. One current approach in the development of tools for parasite control is the use of existing molecules in combinations.

This *Parasites & Vectors* article collection represents a series of seven papers describing studies conducted on the efficacy of a novel combination of fipronil and permethrin in a spot-on formulation for dogs (Frontline Tri-Act®/Frontect®, Merial). Fipronil is a phenylpyrazole with both insecticidal and acaricidal properties; permethrin is a pyrethroid which combines insecticidal, acaricidal and repellent activities; both diffuse across the skin and accumulate in sebaceous glands and cutaneous lipids, remaining active for weeks. Although there is substantial available scientific literature on the efficacy of fipronil and permethrin as separate molecules, no previous study has been published on the performance of their combination. The efficacy of the current formulation has been demonstrated in controlled studies in dogs.

In five different studies with adult *Ctenocephalides felis*, a single application of fipronil and permethrin provided excellent levels of efficacy against fleas on dogs at 24 and 48 hours post-treatment or post-infestation, during one month. In two of those studies, efficacy was maintained at 100% during a full month after treatment in dogs that underwent either three water immersions or one shampooing, simulating an outdoor lifestyle. One of the articles presents interesting results on the repellency of the product against *Ctenocephalides canis* fleas at one hour post-infestation, which is a less investigated parameter of insecticide preparations. A successful flea control program aims at eliminating fleas quickly after infestation and preventing re-infestation from the environment. For fleas, insecticides should have rapid killing or repellent

Citation: Luís Cardoso, Fipronil and permethrin combination: a novel ectoparasiticide for dogs, DOI: 10.1186/s13071-015-0672-1.

activity. Adult fleas infesting the host must be eliminated, and further infestations by latent environmental stages should be prevented.

The new ectoparasiticide had the ability of killing ticks when administered to infested dogs (immediate or curative efficacy) and to prevent tick re-infestations for at least four weeks after treatment (persistent or protective efficacy). A single topical treatment with the fipronil and permethrin combination provided excellent acaricidal efficacy against both *Ixodes ricinus* and *Rhipicephalus sanguineus*. Regarding *Dermacentor reticulatus*, the new product demonstrated high repellency and prevention of attachment, at 12 and 24 hours after re-infestation, and excellent acaricidal efficacy, within 48 hours, with the effects persisting up to four weeks after treatment. Transmission of most pathogens from tick species to dogs usually requires an initial pre-activation period of about 24 to 48 hours after attachment. Taking these times into account, the results suggest that the application to dogs of the new combination can significantly reduce the potential for transmission of *Babesia canis* as well as other agents of tick-borne diseases.

The new fipronil and permethrin combination demonstrated a high repellency (*i.e.*, an anti-feeding effect) against the bites of *Phlebotomus perniciosus* sand flies, which lasted for three to four weeks. A single topical administration of the product also provided high repellency against mosquitoes (*Aedes aegypti*, *Aedes albopictus* and *Culex pipiens*) on dogs for at least four weeks. High protection (repellency and insecticidal efficacy) of the combination of fipronil and permethrin was also found against the biting stable fly *Stomoxys calcitrans* on dogs for at least five weeks after a single treatment. This overall repellent efficacy by inhibition of blood-feeding may contribute to the protection of dogs from sequelae of bites by mosquitoes and biting flies, as well as from major pathogens transmitted by mosquitoes and sand flies, *i.e.*, *Dirofilaria* spp. and*Leishmania infantum*, respectively.

In conclusion, a long lasting repellent effect against mosquitoes, sand flies and stable flies has been demonstrated, along with a long lasting efficacy against fleas and the main tick species infesting dogs in Europe. For one month following a single topical application, the new fipronil and permethrin ectoparasiticide combination offers a broad spectrum protection against the major canine ectoparasites, protecting the dogs themselves and also minimizing the risk of zoonotic pathogen transmission.

SECTION X: HOST RESISTANCE TO PARASITIC DISEASES

CHAPTER 37

SELECTION METHODS FOR RESISTANCE TO AND TOLERANCE OF HELMINTHS IN LIVESTOCK

Concepta McManus, Tiago do Prado Paim, Cristiano Barros de Melo,Bruno S. A. F. Brasil and Samuel R. Paiva

Keywords: Genome-wide selection, Selection indices, Heritability, Quantitative trait loci, Major histocompatibility complex, Animal genetic resources

INTRODUCTION

According to Perry et al. 96, helminthiases (i.e. diseases including those caused by nematode parasites) are the most important livestock diseases worldwide. Livestock selection to date has largely been based on production traits such as milk production or growth rate, with unfavourable correlated effects in fertility and health 93. The Resource Allocation Theory 13, 54 states that animals have limited resources for carrying out adaptation processes. As production (milk or meat) is increased through one biological process, this will affect other functions such as reproduction, maintenance, movement or disease resistance. Management factors, such as increasing access to quality feed and nutrients, could increase the overall health/robustness of the animal until resources became limited again. Any further increase would imply a reallocation of resources and thus change the response in other traits such as disease resistance or behaviour 13. Rauw et al. 101 reviewed the negative side effects of selection for high production and concluded that high productivity in livestock could mean that there are insufficient resources for adequate coping with stress factors, and hence poor welfare whenever resources are limiting.

Helminth control strategies worldwide are based almost entirely on the frequent use of dewormers (anthelmintic drugs), which are increasingly regarded as unsustainable given the emergence of multiple drug-resistant parasites 64, 129. The need for alternative methods of control is highlighted by the fact that few new classes of anthelmintic drugs have been launched in the last 25 years (e.g. amino-acetonitrile derivatives (ADDs) and spiroindoles). Many feel that anthelmintic resistance is inevitable. Each time an anthelmintic is administered, the animal eliminates susceptible parasites and selects for resistant parasites, who then pass their resistant genes onto the next generation of worms. Interest is, therefore, growing in integrated parasite management (IPM) programmes, of which breeding for genetic resistance is a component 109.

Parasitic diseases (such as those caused by *Haemonchus contortus*, *Nematodirus*, *Fasciola hepatica*, *Dicrocoelium dendriticum*, *Eimeria* and *Amblyomma* spp. among others) are important for the sheep industry and are considered some of the biggest bottlenecks to its development 81. Vieira et al. 127 recognised that economic losses are caused by these diseases. These include retarded growth, weight loss, reduced food consumption, decreased milk production, low fertility and, in cases of large infections, high mortality rates. The treatment of these diseases in ruminants has been affected by the emergence of nematode strains that are resistant to anthelmintics.

The acquisition and expression of immunity against gastrointestinal nematodes is genetically controlled and varies between breeds and between individuals of the same breed 81, 119. The proportion of animals found to be resistant or susceptible to nematodes is influenced by age and breed, as shown by Amarante et al. 4 comparing Santa Inês (hair breed) with Suffolk sheep. Santa Inês has been shown to be more resistant to GI nematodes than Suffolk, Ile de France and Poll Dorset in some studies 4, 28, 30, 87 but not in others 81. Studies show a negative correlation between the FEC and weight gain or weight of sheep of different breeds, where more resistant animals are more productive 4, although Eady et al. 46 found a positive correlation between FEC and wool production.

Genetic variation in resistance to internal parasites has been demonstrated in numerous species, including humans

Citation: McManus C, Paim TP, de Melo CB, Brasil BSAF & Paiva SR: Selection methods for resistance to and tolerance of helminths in livestock. Parasite, 2014, 21, 56.

and several livestock species 17, 71, 99. However, the genetic architecture underlying such traits is poorly understood 67. The genetic aspects related to helminth control are breed, genotype-environment interactions, heritability and correlations with other traits of interest, as well as genetic markers including quantitative trait loci (QTLs) and genomic selection. Therefore, the implementation of breeding programmes becomes one of the most important factors to take into consideration as the host-parasite interaction occurs on several levels. The selection schemes can confer resistance to or tolerance of infection. "Resistance" refers to the ability of the host to resist infection, while with "tolerance" the host is infected by the pathogen, but suffers little adverse effect. For example, where the objective is to prevent the spread of the disease to other populations (as in the case of zoonotic diseases), disease resistance rather than tolerance is required.

Infection transmission is usually impacted when genetic improvement is made in host resistance to infection. While genetic improvement of tolerance may reduce clinical signs of disease, it may not reduce transmission of infection to other animals 51. This review looks to investigate the use of genetic selection methods to improve animal response to challenges from helminths.

DEFINING WHAT TRAIT TO MEASURE

Direct Markers

An issue that is often debated by the scientific community is whether it is more appropriate to select for resistance or tolerance (resilience). If these are separated, then improvement of the two traits could have markedly different impacts. For example, improving resistance should also reduce the transmission of infection between animals, whereas improving tolerance will reduce clinical signs of disease but may not necessarily reduce the transmission of infection. In the former case, unselected animals introduced into the population would benefit from the improvement of the herd-level resistance, whereas in the latter case unselected animals in the same environment would be at risk from disease 73.

Although resilience is usually thought of as the ability of an animal to maintain performance in the face of parasitic challenge 20, it has also been defined in terms of anthelmintic treatment requirements and anaemia following *H. contortus* infection 9. Long-term selection for decreased treatment requirements has been shown to be successful and was accompanied by an increase in growth rate and a decrease in breech soiling 89; however, it was complex to implement under practical conditions and did not improve resistance. Conversely, selection for a combination of resistance and performance should encompass the concept of resilience, as well as include epidemiological benefits of selection. The choice of the optimal trait to select on will often depend on the feasibility of trait recording under practical conditions 20.

Genes controlling resistance *per se* and those influencing performance are generally not associated. Consequently, genetic relationships between resistance and performance may be thought of as the outcome of a balance between two opposing factors 13, 54: the resources used by the host to fight or protect against infection vs. the damage caused by infection. If the resources used to protect the host outweigh the benefits of being more resistant, then the relationship will be unfavourable. If the benefits of being resistant, that is, the damage that is avoided, outweigh the costs of achieving resistance, then the relationship will be favourable 20.

This framework also predicts genotype-by-environment interactions; for example, the ranking of animals on their performance may differ in environments with different challenge levels. This last prediction has been demonstrated in the comparison of Red Maasai (resistant to and tolerant of nematode infections) vs. Dorper sheep (susceptible) 8. In this comparison, breed differences in performance that were present in the face of strong nematode challenge (favouring the resistant Red Maasai) disappeared in an environment with a low-level challenge.

Several traits are used to determine resistance or resilience to helminths. Most within-breed studies of genetic resistance use the FEC as the indicator trait for resistance, and significant heritabilities are invariably found, coupled with extensive between-animal variation in FEC 17. The heritability of the FEC as a measure of resistance varies considerably depending on both the nematode species and breed surveyed. Estimates are generally moderate, ranging between 0.2 and 0.3 17; Safari et al. 106 estimated, from 16 published studies, a weighted mean heritability of 0.27 ± 0.02, with a coefficient for phenotypic variation of $31 \pm 7\%$. Importantly, resistance to different strongyle parasites is seen to be strongly genetically correlated, and even between *Strongyle* and *Nematodirus* FEC, genetic correlations are at least 0.5 18.

According to Bishop 21, FEC should not be the only trait considered when selecting for resistance. There are several alternative or additional indicator traits, such as: (i) measures of resistance: FEC, worm burden, worm size and fecundity; (ii) immune response: eosinophilia, and antibodies such as IgA, IgG and IgM; (iii) measures of impact of infection: anaemia, gastrin, pepsinogen or fructosamine concentrations; and (iv) resilience: growth rate and required treatment frequency.

For clinical diagnosis, the visual signs combined with the history of the animals are usually sufficient and a laboratory confirmation is not required 48. Faecal egg counts are not suitable for confirmation of the clinical diagnosis, as correlation between the FEC and adult infection levels is usually low, but are frequently used for the diagnosis of haemonchosis in small ruminants and the detection of anthelmintic resistance (Table 1). According to the authors, the value of DNA-based tests of faecal material is therefore limited and tests of nematode species-specific DNA will have little value for diagnosis and monitoring. While pasture larval and worm counts may be useful parameters for basic epidemiological studies, they are labour-intensive, which limits their use for routine diagnosis and monitoring, as well as selection criteria. Blood parameters (gastrin, pepsinogen and serology) may be considered valuable tools for diagnosis, while pepsinogen and ELISAs based on recombinant proteins show promise as parameters for herd health monitoring 48.

Table 1. Summary of quantitative trait loci for gastrointestinal nematode resistance in sheep.

Reference	QTL found or nearest marker	Chromosome number	Loci studied	Trait used
[12]	OARJMP29, McM130, McM357, TGLA67, OarVH130, McMA22, McM214,	1, 3, 6, 11, 12. 20	Genome-wide	FEC
[15]	BMS360, CSSM3, BM6465, CSAP39E, MCM158, RM96, CSSM37, MCM140, CMCA52, CSAP36E, CSSME76, MAF45, BM2818, FCB128	X, 1, 6, 12	251 markers – genome-wide	strongyle faecal egg count (FEC), the coccidia faecal oocyst count (FOC) and a count of keds (Melophagus ovinus)
[23]	None	20	MHC	FEC
[25]	None	20	MHC	faecal scouring
[33]	OMHC1, OLADRB1, OLADRB2	20	OMHC1, OLADRB1, OLADRB2	faecal egg count (FEC), blood packed cell volume (PCV), antibody (AB) levels, serum proteins (SP) and blood eosinophil count (EOS)
[37]	o(IFN)-γ	3	o(IFN)-γ	FEC, IgA
[38]	BM81124, BM3215, BM3215, BM9202, ILSTS65, ILSTS42	8, 11, 23	Genome-wide	FEC, total serum IgE, serum IgGspecific for the *T. colubriformis* L3 larvae
[40]	IFNG, MHC	2, 3, 14, 20	139 Microsatellite markers on Chr 1, 2, 3, 5, 14, 18, 20, 21	IgA, FEC
[43]	EPCDV010, ILSTS044	1	18 microsatellite markers	FEC, Nr adult larvae
[57]	OMCH1	20	MHC Class I	-
[58]	OLADRB1	20	MHC Class II	-
[62]	None	20	MHC Class II	FEC
[63]	OarCP73, DYMS1, BM1815	20	MHC	haemotocrit level, FEC, igL
[65]	Ovar-DQA1	20	MHC Class II	Transcription profiles
[77]	Between AC113228 & ILSTS62 *and* CP26 & BMS648; *between markers* URB060 & MCMA13; *between markers* ILSTS28 & ILSTS45; *between markers* DU363924 & BMS2572 *and* MCM37 & MCM137	1, 3, 4	223 markers in Genome scan	FEC
[85]	16 genomic regions including *CD53, CHI3L2, CHIA, DENND2D, RELN, NSUN2, HRH1*	1, 4, 16, 19	*Genome-wide*	Selection signatures
[88]	Not specified	5, 12, 13, 21	50 K SNP chip	FEC
[94]	OLADRB	3	MHC	FEC
[95]	IFNG region BL4; BMS1617	3	fine mapping	FEC
[97]	INRA132 CP101	20	BM1818, OarCP73, OarHH56, DYA, OLADRB, CP101, OMHC1, DQA2, DQA1, TFAP2A, DQBA27, Bf94_1, and INRA132	FEC
[102]	IRF3, TGF-B1 among others	4, 12, 14, 19, 20, as well as OAR1, 3, 4, 5, 7, 12, 19, 20 and 24 at suggestive level	Meta-analysis – Illumina OvineSNP50 BeadChip	FEC
[107]	s39968, OAR12_62301297, OAR12_62347621, OAR12_62371899	7, 9, 14, 15, 21, 4, 5, 6, 8, 12, 17, 18, 19, 23, 21, 13	160 microsatellite markers were used as well as the Illumina OvineSNP50 BeadChip	FEC, PCV, worm burden, length of females, IgG, and pepsinogen concentration
[111]	*MHC-DRB1*	20	*MHC-DRB1*	*FEC*
[119]	*MHC-DRB1*	20	*MHC-DRB1*	FEC, lymphocyte antigen

Indirect Markers

Despite its advantages, the FEC requires time to measure, and may fail to represent all of the pathways involved in internal nematode resistance due to physiological complexity 45. Increased levels of IgG1, IgE and IgM have been negatively correlated with FEC in Romney selection line sheep 22, 45, 112, although IgE was also negatively correlated with breech soiling. Immunoglobulin IgA, the isotype closely associated with intestinal mucosal immune responses, has also been positively associated with resistance 78, 114.

IgA, acting as an antibody to a *T. colubriformis* L3 carbohydrate surface antigen (CarLA), can prevent larvae from establishing in the gut, resulting in rapid expulsion 113. A commercial test (http://www.carlasalivatest.com) was subsequently developed to measure saliva IgA antibody response to CarLa from animals under parasite challenge; high CARLA™ animals have a lower FEC, and improved growth under challenge.

An important concept is that other disease-control measures also have an antagonistic effect on genetic resistance to disease as they allow the use of otherwise unfit animals in the breeding population by preventing natural selection to disease. Animal diseases significantly decrease profitability, and identification of the phenotype for disease resistance is difficult. In a population containing both healthy and sick animals, all healthy animals may not be disease-resistant. Animals that appear healthy may have sub-clinical infections. These could then be considered pathogen reservoirs. The level of exposure of susceptible animals may also not have been sufficient to cause illness. The clinical expression of a disease can also be confounded with a similar disease; for example, pneumonia can be confused with several other diseases; bronchitis, emphysema, pleuritis, pulmonary adenomatosis, upper respiratory infection and pleural fibrosis 116. Accurate disease diagnosis is therefore both costly and time-consuming.

The FAMACHA© method was introduced to support parasite control using target selective treatment 125, based on the principle of the correlation between eye mucous colour and the haematocrit values (level of anaemia). Riley and Van Wyk 103 proposed evaluations of a practical, relatively easily obtained phenotype such as the FAMACHA© score combined with simple penalties may permit rapid within-flock genetic evaluations. These could offer producers the ability to select from candidate sires and dams using ranked predicted breeding values for FAMACHA© scores to improve internal parasite resistance and/or resilience, with the ultimate objective of having sheep that are able to live and produce better under conditions of relatively severe internal parasite challenge. The fact that an animal survives and reproduces without deworming can be used as a selection criterion.

DIFFERENCES BETWEEN BREEDS

Genetic differences between and within breeds for the FEC have been seen 81. Most studies look at differences comparing locally adapted and commercial breeds, with results showing that the relatively unselected locally adapted breeds are more resistant to/tolerant of worm infections. This may be due to poor productivity of the locally adapted breeds, as their growth rate is frequently lower than commercial breeds. This lower genetic potential for growth affects resilience, as less demand is put on nutritional partition of factors which affect both growth and resilience such as protein level in the feed 76. In a study in the Federal District, Brazil, McManus et al. 84, in a study with several breeds and crosses, found that locally adapted Morada Nova and Bergamasca showed the lowest FEC for Strongylida, while the locally adapted Santa Inês and its cross with Ile de France (Ile X SI) had the lowest values for *Strongyloides*. On the other hand, the lowest faecal oocyst count (FOC –*Eimeria* spp.) was found in Ile de France sheep. Genetic correlations between the FEC or FOC and parasite species in these sheep were low, and heritabilities varied from 0.09 to 0.31. Nieto et al. 91 estimated heritability for the FEC using a threshold model as 0.08, but in this study animals found to have higher FECs were dewormed, which may have affected this result. Lôbo et al. 75 found FEC heritability to be highly variable throughout the life of the animal, ranging from 0.04 to 0.27 in the first challenge and 0.01 to 0.52 during the second.

The maintenance of diversity in terms of the genes underlying resistance provides an important resource for combating the effects of possible future pathogen evolution. There is much anecdotal evidence pointing to the greater disease resistance of indigenous livestock breeds to environments where they face a heavy disease challenge. A study conducted under field conditions in subhumid coastal areas of Kenya found that lambs of the Red Maasai breed showed lower FECs for *Haemonchus contortus* and lower mortality than Dorper lambs (another breed widely kept in Kenya). The Red Maasai flocks were estimated to be two to three times as productive as the Dorper animals under these subhumid conditions favourable to the parasites 10. Likewise, Indonesian Thin-Tailed sheep have been found to show greater resistance than sheep of the St. Croix and Merino breeds 104.

Selection and crossbreeding may affect breed resistance. In Brazil, although the locally adapted Santa Inês are frequently cited as being resistant to endoparasites, usually in comparisons with commercial breeds 4, 30, 105, this was not confirmed in other studies 81. Bricarello et al. 28 also found no significant differences between Ile de France and Santa Inês lambs in terms of their haematological and biochemical profiles under mild *H. contortus* infection. Genetic studies 82 have shown a division in this breed where crossbred animals are registered as purebred, and this may account for the lack of resistance in this "new" Santa Inês.

When resistant and susceptible breeds are crossed, studies have shown that the degree of resistance of the crossbred offspring varies depending on the breeds evaluated, the age of the animals and whether the evaluations were from natural or artificial infections 5. Within-breed selection for the FEC has been shown to be an effective means of reducing the need for treatment with anthelmintics and reducing the contamination of pastures with the eggs of nematode parasites 18, 90, 130,131. Managing genetic resources in order to enhance the resistance or resilience found in livestock populations offers an additional tool for disease control.

SELECTION

Few studies calculate economic values for resistance to gastrointestinal parasites 52, 74, 83. The FAO 49 stated a number of advantages of incorporating genetic elements in disease management strategies, including: (i) permanence of genetic change once it is established; (ii) consistency of the effect; (iii) absence of the need for purchased inputs once the effect is established; (iv) effectiveness of other methods is prolonged as there is less pressure for the emergence of resistance; (v) possibility of broad-spectrum effects (increasing resistance to more than one disease); (vi) possibility of having less impact on the evolution of macroparasites such as helminths, compared with other strategies such as chemotherapy or vaccination; and (vii) adding to the diversity of disease management strategies.

Depending on the nature of the problem and the resources available, genetic management of the disease may be undertaken in a number of ways. These include appropriate breed selection for the production environment; cross-breeding to introduce desirable genes into breeds that are otherwise well adapted; and the selection of individuals that have been seen to be disease-resistant/tolerant. Genetic diversity is a fundamental requirement in all cases and populations that are diverse in terms of the number of distinct genotypes conferring disease resistance are less susceptible to catastrophic disease epidemics 117.

Selective breeding to take advantage of within-breed variation in disease resistance is an important strategy in the control of a number of diseases. Selection for resistance alone can result in negative traits such as lower live weight gains, increased breech soiling and decreased fleece weight 116. Appropriate selection policies are therefore necessary, but the main indirect benefit of resistance is reduced pasture contamination. According to these authors, selecting for resilient animals is difficult in a commercial farming situation, although it results in animals with higher productivity, fewer dags and lower drench requirements. The major issue with resilience is pasture contamination; as there is no reduction in FEC, non-resilient animals in the flock receive a higher parasite challenge from the resilient animals, who are essentially asymptomatic carriers.

There has been considerable debate on the merits of the two approaches. Genetic correlations between resistance and resilience as high as 0.56 have been seen 3 and a heritability of resistance (0.3) significantly higher than resilience (not detectable). Bisset and Morris 22 also found low/moderate heritability (0.14 ± 0.03 to 0.34 ± 0.07), and no correlation with the FEC. Genotype × Environment interactions are thought to be low compared with the genetic factors. Kemper et al. 67 found that when *H. contortus* and *T. colubriformis* were exposed to genetically resistant or susceptible sheep over a long period of time (30 nematode generations) they did not adapt, supporting the hypothesis that resistance is determined by many genes, each with relatively small effect. This result also supports the use of selection flocks, as selection for parasite resistance based on the FEC is sustainable in the medium to long term.

It is thought that host genetic resistance may break down over time, as nematodes evolve to adapt to the resistant hosts. According to Bishop 21, the polygenic nature of parasite resistance suggests that worm evolution should be slower than that of anthelmintic resistance, as worms would have to evolve against many more targets. This author also affirms that there is no published evidence for apparently resistant breeds losing their relative advantage compared with those that are more susceptible.

Kemper et al. 68 explored three postulated mechanisms for the sheep genotype to influence the FEC in sheep: (i) reduce worm establishment, (ii) increase adult worm mortality and (iii) reduce adult egg production. These authors found that when the sheep resistance acts by reducing the adult egg production, it puts less selective pressure on the worm population, as the genes affect only the female worms and not the male. Thus, the magnitude of increase for resistant worms is only half of that when the resistance genes act on both sexes. These same authors concluded that adaptation of worms to sheep that are selected for low worm egg count (WEC) is unlikely to be detected in the short term. The authors state that the proper worm may have mutations with properties that are suitable for adaptation, i.e. mutations that are favourable for survival in low WEC sheep but unfavourable in unselected sheep. Many generations may be needed for these mutations to increase in frequency or they may be neutral (or near neutral) with respect to overall worm survival in the current population. Despite the issues, studies based on artificial conditions can be tested against natural populations, potentially providing independent validation of the results obtained. Therefore, multiple evolutionary solutions to the same problem can be tested.

According to Gibson and Bishop 51, when making decisions on the priorities for genetic improvement, the following should be taken into account: genetic improvement is an effective, low-risk method of control for the target disease; sufficient genetic variation exists for disease resistance between or within breeds to allow effective genetic improvement; there are clear economic and social benefits due to the genetic improvement of resistance, allowing for the use of other methods of disease control (used as an alternative to, or in conjunction with, host resistance).

Direct selection where heritabilities are generally medium to low which brings about slow results to selection for these traits and economic values tend to be low 74, 80, 83, but are highly affected by the price of detection and treatment.

GENOTYPE × ENVIRONMENT INTERACTION

Animals tend to adapt to the environment they are selected in, so it is unlikely that selection for increased production levels leads to environmental sensitivity. Castillo-Juarez et al. 34 and Kearney et al. 66 showed that unfavourable genetic correlations of milk yield with somatic cell score and conception rate were significantly higher in a poor environment relative to a good environment. McManus et al. 84 showed that breeds respond differently on different pasture types, related to feed quality and availability, with differing results for FECs. Vaminisetti et al. 126 also found that breed differences were more apparent when infection levels were higher.

According to Scholtz et al. 110, due to expected changes in environments with global warming and climate change, the matching of the genotype to the environment will be important to ensure a sustainable increase in production. According to these authors, this will also be important in defining breeding objectives and to develop selection criteria that ensure that breeding is effective and aimed at sustainable production in changing environments. Definition of breeding objectives and criteria is commonly lacking in breeding programmes, especially in developing countries where the impact of environmental change is expected to be higher. In these countries, the aim of achieving maximum production may not be feasible or recommended, which is in contrast to livestock production systems in developed countries located in the northern hemisphere temperate zone. Optimal production systems are those that are in harmony with the environment and utilise appropriate genotypes, and these should be developed where they are not already in place. During the development of these systems, factors such as definition of breeding objectives should be considered and linked to factors of sustainability of production systems in changing environments 110.

GENETIC MARKERS

The maintenance of local adapted breeds depends directly on their insertion into existing production systems. Important characteristics need to be identified in these breeds that may play an important role for specific market niches. With the development of molecular techniques, a great variety of tools are being used to improve the identification of desirable traits 117.

According to Kemper et al. 67, a further issue is that most association studies using molecular markers have relied on within-family linkage to detect polymorphisms. Thus, replicating results in a second family where the polymorphism is not segregating is almost impossible. Polymorphisms may not be segregating in families due to low allele frequencies in the breed, or because the polymorphism is fixed in a particular breed. Reproducing linkage results by identification of multiple linked QTLs is also difficult because of changes to the linkage phase between families. Many authors have studied the major histocompatibility complex (MHC) and the region containing the interferon gamma (IFNG) gene for resistance to worms 37,40.

The MHC involves a series of highly polymorphic genes which are responsible for the initiation of the immune response when an animal is challenged by pathogens or parasites 14, 42, 50, 57, 108. Its structure is relatively well conserved between different ruminant species, making it a candidate for comparative studies 11. The MHC is divided into three regions: class 1 (telomeric), class 2 (centromeric) and class 3 (central). In ruminants there is a division of the class 2 region into two sub-regions: class 2a and class 2b 6. Several studies have shown the existence of polymorphisms in each of these regions 57,58, 72, 94. The MHC is located on chromosome 20 in sheep 41 and its polymorphic portion is known as OLA (Ovine Leukocyte Antigen). The MHC is associated with a wide range of production traits in livestock, including sheep 25.

Several studies have been published linking nematode resistance to QTLs (Table 1) found on chromosomes 1 12, 43, 2 40, 3 12, 37, 40, 95, 6 12, 111, 14 40 and 20 40, 63, 111. The QTLs on chromosome 20 found by these authors include DRB1, OARCP73, DYMS1 and BM1815. The indicator trait used by Janen et al. 63 was haematocrit level and not faecal egg count as in the majority of studies. Davies et al. 40 found two QTLs on chromosome 20 close to the MHC regions. In this case, they did not specify specific microsatellites but these QTLs were close to DRB1, OLARB, PMHC1 and CP73.

Schwaiger et al. 111 looked at the association between MHC II-DRB1 alleles and FEC following natural infection by *T.(Ostertagia) circumcincta* in Scottish Blackface sheep. Least-squares regression analysis indicated that substitution of the most common allele (I) by G2 would result in a 58-fold reduction in FEC in 6-month-old lambs, suggesting that the MHC plays an important role in the development of resistance. Since this initial study, other studies, using differing breeds and nematode species, have found the same association 36, 118, 128. Variation in the microsatellite loci associated with functional MHC genes was also found to be correlated with juvenile FEC and survival in Soay sheep 94. The unmanaged population of Soay sheep on the remote island of Hirta, St. Kilda, are a good model for nematode resistance. This population is persistently unstable, with numbers fluctuating between 600 and 1600 individuals 120. Population crashes occur approximately every 3 years, primarily due to winter food shortages, although parasitism by nematodes is a contributing factor 121. A further three markers within the MHC region had significant association with the haematocrit level (CP73), IgL (immunoglobulin lambda) level (DYMS1) and FEC (BM1815) following an artificial challenge of a Roehnschaf flock with *H. contortus* 63. In Scottish Blackface sheep, microsatellite markers on chromosome 20 have been associated with non-*Nematodirus Strongyle* FEC 40.

Other studies using genetic marker approaches on various flocks have found no evidence for an effect of genes in the MHC on either *H. contortus* 23 or *T. colubriformis* resistance in sheep 62. This may be explained by the alleles themselves not causing resistance or susceptibility *per se*, but being in linkage disequilibrium (LD) with additional polymorphisms in the region 65; a combination of these polymorphisms may then contribute to resistance or susceptibility in some populations. As the extent of LD between those populations is likely to vary between breeds and populations, the MHC alleles previously implicated may not show up as being significant.

Quantitative trait loci (QTL) mapping has been widely used to try to understand the complexity of parasite resistance. This is carried out by identifying regions of the genome involved in variation in the phenotype. Diverse experimental approaches have been used, mainly based on comparing sheep breeds and nematode species at different ages and under different climatic/management conditions. Because of this, different chromosomal regions of interest have been suggested as being involved in this resistance/resilience. The results suggest that several different pathways are involved in nematode resistance. The region near the MHC on chromosome 20, and the region containing the IFNG gene on chromosome 3 are two regions that are frequently targeted during these studies.

The IFNG gene codes for a cytokine secreted by Th1 lymphocytes that plays a critical role in regulating the type 1 vs. type 2 immune responses in vertebrates. It activates macrophages, which can kill intracellular pathogens, and display increased ability to present antigens 129. INFG is used as a candidate for nematode resistance as it is associated with host response following an immune challenge. It also helps to determine whether a humoral or cell-mediated response predominates.

A QTL for parasite resistance in Romney divergent selection lines after multi-species challenge was fine-mapped to a region near the IFNG gene 95. Subsequently, polymorphism in the region near the IFNG gene was linked to reduced FEC and increased parasite-specific IgA in a wild population of Soay sheep on the island of Hirta in the St Kilda archipelago in the Outer Hebrides 37. This region has been implicated in a number of host resistance traits, including specific IgA activity,*Nematodirus* FEC, non-*Nematodirus* and strongyle FEC. These have all been identified to be associated with a QTL on chromosome 3 in Scottish Blackface sheep 40, using a partial genome scan of 139 microsatellite markers. Likewise, using 133 markers, a QTL in the IFNG region was also observed in Merino divergent selection lines after challenge with *T. colubriformis* 12. Finally, a whole genome scan using 247 markers was performed on the Soay sheep of St. Kilda, using the coccidian FOC as a measurement of resistance to parasites. Several other regions on chromosome 3 have also been found to have linkage to parasite resistance, although they are not found near the IFNG 15, 77.

A region at the distal end of chromosome one was also found in Merino selection lines to be significantly associated with a mean FEC of three counts after secondary artificial challenge with *T. colubriformis* 12, using an incomplete genome scan of 133 markers. A genome scan using 203 microsatellites and divergent Romney FEC selection line outcrosses naturally infected by *Trichostrongylus* species detected a significant QTL on the telomeric end of chromosome 8 38. A further partial association screen using 139 microsatellite markers has been used to also identify QTLs associated with *Nematodirus* FEC in Scottish Blackface sheep on chromosomes 2 and 14 40. These QTLs are known to affect egg production by *Nematodirus*species, although potential candidate genes have not yet been identified.

Over three successive population crashes in the Soay sheep of St. Kilda, Gulland 105 showed that mortality was significantly different among individuals of the three different genotypes at the diallelic adenosine deaminase (ADA) locus on chromosome 13 16. Three independent lines of evidence suggested that nematode burdens differ among the three genotypes, consistent with the idea that allele frequencies at the ADA locus are maintained by parasite-induced selection. Microsatellite work on the same breed, with 251 markers covering the whole genome, later failed to find any linkage between FOC and the ADA locus, INFG or MHC, all regions previously proposed to be candidate loci 15. The failure to detect linkage could be due to insufficient power, or low marker coverage, although good marker coverage was achieved in the putative regions 16. More recent studies with this population 29 have concluded that there is little evidence that the candidate gene approach will lead to the identification of loci explaining variation in parasitological and immunological traits.

The same genome scan produced a high LOD score for chromosome X, in the vicinity of one of the telomeres 15. This was the only study to analyse the X chromosome for linkage until recently, when Marshall et al. 77 discovered a QTL in the X-chromosome pseudoautosomal region, using resistance to *H. contortus* infestation in Merino sheep. This study used 223 microsatellite markers on all autosomes, plus the X-chromosome pseudoautosomal region. The QTL on the X chromosome was discovered alongside many other QTLs, of which only three (located on chromosomes 1, 3 and 4) were fine-mapped. While the locations for the significant markers were given, it did not appear that any of these QTLs were located in known genes.

Breeding plans should be constructed to implement strategies designed to maintain genetic variability and prevent the increase of inbreeding. This can be accomplished by: (i) including health, fertility and other fitness traits in breeding objectives along with production traits; (ii) taking genotype-by-environment interactions into account; (iii) implementing selection strategies to reduce inbreeding; and (iv) taking advantage of the molecular genetics tools.

DIFFERENCES AMONG STUDIES

The search for QTLs for nematode resistance in sheep is a difficult area of research. This is primarily due to the physiological and phenotypic complexity of the trait, and most studies derive from initial low-resolution genome screens, often resulting in very wide confidence intervals. More consistency in experimental protocols, materials and analysis approaches would allow a more accurate comparison of results; the studies have differed in the breed of sheep and their immune status, nematode species used in the experiments, measurement of internal nematode resistance and the challenge regimes. Comparisons between breeds of sheep, such as locally adapted and commercial breeds, are also problematic for many reasons including differences in environment, age structure, treatment history and parasitological methods. Considering the complexity of nematode resistance, it is unsurprising that previous studies have not necessarily yielded the same results.

Differences in experimental design aside, due to the moderate size of the effect of each QTL, it is likely that a panel of QTLs would be required for significant genetic gains to be achieved within the industry via marker-assisted selection. The information gained from such QTL studies can be used alongside new technology to gain a greater understanding of nematode resistance in sheep; as noted by Crawford et al. 38, the large number of suggestive QTLs discovered suggests that most of the genes controlling parasite resistance are of relatively small effect.

GENOME-WIDE SELECTION

Single nucleotide polymorphisms (SNPs) are DNA sequence variations that occur when a single nucleotide differs between different homologous chromosomes. Studies of variation at a single base pair level can provide information of two kinds; firstly, it can be used to study polymorphisms within protein coding regions, and secondly, variation can also be studied in non-protein coding regions, including regulatory regions. It has been suggested that much of the evolution of morphology, physiology and behaviour rests on changes in regulatory sequences, and thus they can have a profound effect 32. Recent studies have also shown the role of non-coding RNAs, including microRNAs and nsRNAs, in regulating various levels of gene function 79.

Due to their abundance, ease of scoring and low unit cost, SNPs are now the most widely used markers in genetics, allowing the development of dense catalogues of variation within a species 123. In the field of ovine genomics, technology such as the Illumina® OvineSNP50 or OvineSNP700 K BeadChips (www.sheephapmap.org) now enables researchers to characterise the genetic variation at more than 50,000 SNPs in the ovine genome simultaneously. This first genome-wide set of SNPs for sheep has opened the gateway for further research 69, 70.

Progress in genomics, along with technology, statistical techniques and bioinformatics advances, has led to the implementation of genome-wide association studies (GWAS) which aim to understand the genetic basis of common diseases. Infectious diseases are important on a global scale and there is strong epidemiological evidence that host genetic factors are important determinants of the interactions between host and pathogen. However, the application of GWAS to infectious diseases has been limited when compared with non-communicable diseases. Gilleard 53 has reviewed the literature on using this approach with *H. contortus* as a model.

Association studies with candidate genes, which look for a statistical correlation between specific genetic markers and a disease, have been widely used for the study of complex diseases 31, yet this approach had been criticised due to inability to replicate results and limits on its ability to include all possible causative genes and polymorphisms 122. These limitations have been overcome by population genomics 1, where the genome, or at least a large number of loci (often well into the 10,000 s) that are likely to be representative of the whole genome, is surveyed without any prior assumptions regarding which genes are under selection, resulting in less bias.

Kemper et al. 67 used a mixed-breed population of sheep to show that the detectable polymorphisms affecting resistance to worm infections have relatively small effects. Considering that the additive genetic effects for the WEC accounted for between 10 and 24% of the phenotypic variance in this population, this means that there are likely to be hundreds or thousands of underlying mutations influencing these phenotypes. These mutations are probably spread across the genome. This is in line with Al Kalaldeh et al. 2, who concluded that disease resistance is a largely polygenic trait. This implies that there are a large number of genes involved in the mechanisms of resistance but there are some chromosomal regions that explain a larger proportion of the variation. When all markers were used, a moderate proportion of the genetic variance in the trait was explained. However, improvements are still necessary and previous research in dairy cattle shows clearly how the accuracies of genomic predictions can be increased.

The first step is to increase the size of the reference population. Deterministic predictions indicate a steady, almost linear, increase in GEBV accuracy if up to 20,000 extra records were added to the reference dataset 55. The rate of increase is conditional on the heritability of the trait, and thus artificial challenges for the reference population may still be required to maximise exposure to infection and the potential heritability for WEC 19. The next step is to increase the potential LD between markers and polymorphisms by increasing the density of SNP markers. Low LD between markers in breeds such as Merinos suggests that the value of increasing the size of the reference population will be limited unless the density of markers is increased.

PROBLEMS WITH GWAS

While GWAS have identified hundreds of common genetic variants associated with complex disease so far, most confer relatively small increments in risk, in contrast with the initial "common disease, common variant" hypothesis 125. The question was then raised how the remaining, so called "missing", heritability can be explained. While it has been postulated that rare variants, epistasis, epigenetics and genotype-environment interactions might explain the missing genetic influence 47, the more likely reason is that complex traits are affected by thousands of variants that each have a small effect. The genetic variants now used in most studies were identified in a small number of presumably healthy humans/animals, whereas it may be the rare and low-frequency variants (MAF $< 5\%$) that are in fact contributing to the "missing" heritability.

This hypothesis has been validated by Yang 131, who concluded that much of the heritability for height can be captured by common variants undetected by GWAS, due to individual effects being too small to pass the stringent significance tests. The authors also provided evidence that the remaining heritability is due to incomplete linkage disequilibrium between the SNPs genotyped and the causal variants, which would be exacerbated by the causal variants having a low minor allele frequency 128.

Greater than 70% power to detect QTLs explaining 0.1–0.48% of the phenotypic variance requires a higher level of LD between markers and polymorphism, and a greater number of observations 67. Increased marker density or using a single breed with low effective population size, such as Poll Dorset, would increase the likely LD between markers and polymorphism. Reliable detection of polymorphism explaining about 0.5% of the phenotypic variance (e.g. 70% power), could be achieved when the LD between markers and QTLs is 0.4 and with about 10,000 records 67. Detection of smaller polymorphisms, such as those estimated for the WEC found by this author, would require greater marker density and many more phenotypes.

SELECTIVE SWEEPS

When an advantageous allele fixes in a population, it does so on a particular haplotype background. The advantageous mutations sweep through the population, along with linked variation, in a process referred to as a "selective sweep" 111. When this occurs, it leaves a characteristic signal in patterns of variation in genomic regions linked to the selected site. In the absence of recombination, all neutral SNPs on the chromosome also become fixed, thus losing all variability in the region. New haplotypes emerge through recombination, with the effect of the selective sweep (linkage disequilibrium) diminishing with distance from the advantageous allele. Incomplete selective sweeps denote any stage prior to the fixation of the advantageous allele.

Predictions of genetic merit from all markers are being implemented in livestock breeding programmes, typically within a single breed or strain of animals 56, 60, 61, 124. Kemper et al. 67 found that there are many polymorphisms of small effect underlying variation in FEC. These authors found the largest effects were estimated to explain between 0.12 and 0.48% of the phenotypic variance for the WEC following challenge with *T. colubriformis*, and between 0.02 and 0.08% of the phenotypic variance following *H. contortus* challenge. The additive genetic effects for the WEC accounted for between 10 and 24% of the phenotypic variance in this population; this means that there are likely to be hundreds or thousands of underlying mutations influencing these phenotypes. These mutations are probably spread across the genome.

LOOKING AT THE WORMS

The relationship between the parasite and its host leads to the establishment of a co-evolutionary process where the selective pressures imposed by both players shape each other's genome through time. Thereby, changes in gene frequencies leading to the fixation/loss of favourable/unfavourable alleles from both host and parasite populations become constant and counterbalanced, giving rise to a process that can be compared with an endless arms race 59. Thus, the modification of genetic features of host populations during breeding programmes is expected to have an impact on the parasites' genetic pool.

In this context, although resistance and resilience may have a similar impact on individual health and productivity, they can have contrasting effects on disease prevalence at a population level 44. For example, breeding for resistance has the potential to decrease the parasite load in the pasture, therefore providing clear epidemiological benefits. On the other hand, breeding for resilience is not expected to enhance the pathogen-host arms race at a rate as fast as the selective pressure imposed by resistance would do. This is a theoretical prediction that is important to highlight, since nematode infections are highly prevalent and several nematode species have a broad host spectrum 21. Together, these characteristics hinder pathogen eradication, the ultimate consequence of resistance, unlikely.

It is possible to speculate that the selective pressure imposed by anthelmintic treatment has similar effects to those the resistant host background would have upon the parasite population. Thus, it might be useful to take a look at the extensive amount of data gathered in the last decades regarding anthelmintic resistance rise and spread (reviewed by Prichard 98 and Molento et al. 86). After years of widespread use of drugs for the control of parasitic infections, the increasing prevalence of resistant nematodes now threatens the production of livestock in several parts of the world. The continued use of anthelmintic drugs did not eradicate the parasites, mainly because the majority of the nematode populations were in*refugia* (e.g. eggs and larvae in the pasture, inside asymptomatic animals or inside animals of other host species), and therefore not submitted to drug selection. Moreover, the genetic pool present in the populations in *refugia* started to continuously supply drug resistance-conferring mutations, which eventually became fixed. The situation is further complicated by the usually low genetic structure of parasite populations and their high mutation rates 7, 24, 26, 27, 39, 92, 114. Indeed, there are many reports describing that resistance can originate through different ways such as animal movement among farms 24, 26, 35 and novel/recurrent mutations 27, 114, 115.

When looking at the possibility of gastrointestinal worms adapting to sheep bred for a low faecal egg count, Kemper et al. 68 concluded that this requires an allele segregating in worms that is favourable in animals with improved resistance but less favourable in other animals. They state that the chance of obtaining alleles with this specific property seems unlikely and conclude that selection for a low faecal egg count should be stable over a short time frame (e.g. 20 years).

Another important feature of the anthelmintic resistance rise is that it took decades to become a major production problem. It seems that the same populations in *refugia* also functioned as buffers to the drug's selective pressure and slowed the process of resistance rise. This hypothesis is supported by the expectation that a low-prevalence, host-restricted pathogen would have become either quickly eradicated or resistant 44.

Therefore, given the different outcomes that breeding for resistance or resilience might have on the parasite populations it would be useful and more sustainable to combine both features. Indeed, breeding for resistance might be more effective in the short term, especially given its higher heritability compared with resilience traits 21. Furthermore, the selection of more virulent parasite populations might progress slowly, similarly to what happened to anthelmintic resistance. Nonetheless, resilience will be an important trait since it is unlikely that resistance will eventually lead to the eradication of these highly prevalent and broad-spectrum nematodes. In addition, there is no reason to believe that these traits are mutually exclusive 100, so greater performance gains should be achieved by the coupling of resistance and resilience.

CONCLUSIONS

The co-evolution of hosts and parasites is one of the most interesting examples of the evolutionary history of organisms, yet the complexity of both parasitic infections and host immunity makes it a challenging field to study. Studies aimed at understanding the underlying genetic factors in mammals can help with our understanding of the ongoing struggle between the parasite and host for evolutionary dominance. Whereas studies in humans traditionally lack statistical power, with sheep, the ability to manipulate breeding lines, replicate studies, and have accurate recorded pedigrees offers significant advantages, including increased statistical power. It also allows us the potential to test whether there are multiple evolutionary solutions to the same problem, through having independent selection lines.

Integrated disease control strategies are indicated in the control of these parasites. These include improved management, nutrition and careful use of anthelmintics. More recently, there has been increased interest in the selection of small ruminants for improved nematode resistance to complement other control measures 20. The existence of genetic variation in resistance, both within and between breeds, means that this may be successful. This involves the choice of appropriate breeds that are adapted to local environmental conditions, followed by phenotypic selection for resistance. Selection objective traits include performance (e.g. growth rate) under conditions of parasite challenge, FEC and measures of anaemia (Table 1).

There may be genotype-by-environment interactions, especially when animals are reared in environments that differ in the level of parasite challenge or the quality of available nutrition 74, 82. Nevertheless, antagonistic genetic relationships between performance and resistance are not expected, and selection indices should be constructed that improve both traits. If the FEC is decreased, then pasture contamination should also decrease 20, leading to additional benefits for all sheep grazing the same pasture. These authors state that breeding for nematode resistance should lead to lasting and sustained improvements in resistance or resilience. It is thought that nematodes will not evolve rapidly in response to resistant hosts, and research suggests that resistance should be sustainable.

REFERENCES

1. Akey JM. 2009. Constructing genome maps of positive selection in humans: where do we go from here? Genome Research, 19, 711–722.

2. Al Kalaldeh M, Gibson JP, Van der Werf JHJ, Gondro C. 2013. Partitioning the genetic variance into genomic and pedigree components for parasite resistance in sheep. Proceeding of Association of Advances in Animal Breeding and Genetics, 20, 412–415.

3. Albers GA, Gray GD, Piper LR, Barker JS, Le Jambre LF, Barger IA. 1987. The genetics of resistance and resilience to*Haemonchus contortus* infection in young Merino sheep. International Journal for Parasitology, 17(7), 1355–1363.

4. Amarante AFT, Bricarello PA, Rocha RA, Gennari RM. 2004. Resistance of Santa Inês, Suffolk and Ile de France sheep to naturally acquired gastrointestinal nematode infections. Veterinary Parasitology, 120(2), 91–106.

5. Amarante AFT, Susin I, Rocha RA, Silva MB, Mendes CQ, Pires AV. 2009. Resistance of Santa Inês and

crossbred ewes to naturally acquired gastrointestinal nematode infections. Veterinary Parasitology, 165(120), 273–280.

6. Andersson L. 1996. Major histocompatibility complex evolution, in The major histocompatibility complex region of domestic animal species. Schook LB, Lamont SJ, Editors. CRC Press: Boca Raton, Florida. p. 1–15.

7. Archie EA, Ezenwa VO. 2011. Population genetic structure and history of a generalist parasite infecting multiple sympatric host species. International Journal for Parasitology, 41, 89–98.

8. Baker RL, Mugambi JM, Audho JO, Carles AB, Thorpe W. 2004. Genotype by environment interactions for productivity and resistance to gastro-intestinal nematode parasites in Red Maasai and Dorper sheep. Animal Science, 79, 343–353.

9. Baker RL, Nagda S, Rodriguez-Zas SL, Southey BR, Audho JO, Aduda EO, Thorpe W. 2003. Resistance and resilience to gastro-intestinal nematode parasites and relationships with productivity of Red Maasai, Dorper and Red Maasai × Dorper crossbred lambs in the sub-humid tropics. Animal Science, 76, 119–136.

10. Baker RL. 1998. Genetic resistance to endoparasites in sheep and goats: a review of genetic resistance to gastrointestinal nematode parasites in sheep and goats in the tropics and evidence for resistance in some sheep and goat breeds in sub-humid coastal Kenya. Animal Genetic Resources Information, 24, 13–30.

11. Ballingall KT, Mckeever DJ. 2005. Conservation of promoter, coding and intronic regions of the non-classical MHC class II DYA genes suggests evolution under functional constraints. Animal Genetics, 36(3), 237–239.

12. Beh KJ, Hulme DJ, Callaghan MJ. 2002. A genome scan for quantitative trait loci affecting resistance to*Trichostrongylus colubriformis* in sheep. Animal Genetics, 33, 97–106.

13. Beilharz RG, Luxford BG, Wilkinson JL. 1993. Quantitative genetics and evolution: is our understanding of genetics sufficient to explain evolution? Journal of Animal Breeding and Genetics, 110, 161–170.

14. Benevides MV, Sacco AMS, Weimer TA. 2002. Marcadores genéticos como indicadores de resistência a parasitos gastrintestinais em ovinos. Embrapa Pecuária Sul (Documentos 31): Bagé.

15. Beraldi D, McRae AF, Gratten J, Pilkington JG, Slate J, Visscher PM, Pemberton JM. 2007. Quantitative trait loci (QTL) mapping of resistance to strongyles and coccidia in the free-living Soay sheep (*Ovis aries*). International Journal for Parasitology, 37, 121–129.

16. Beraldi D, McRae AF, Gratten J, Slate J, Visscher PM, Pemberton JM. 2006. Development of a linkage map and mapping of phenotypic polymorphisms in a free-living population of Soay sheep (*Ovis aries*). Genetics, 173, 1521–1537.

17. Bishop SC, Morris CA. 2007. Genetics of disease resistance in sheep and goats. Small Ruminant Research, 70, 48–59.

18. Bishop SC, Woolliams JA. 2004. Genetic approaches and technologies for improving the sustainability of livestock production. Journal of the Science of Food and Agriculture, 84(9), 911–919.

19. Bishop SC, Woolliams JA. 2010. On the genetic interpretation of disease data. PLoS One, 5, e8940.

20. Bishop SC. 2012. A consideration of resistance and tolerance for ruminant nematode infections. Frontiers in Genetics, 3, 1–7.

21. Bishop SC. 2012. Possibilities to breed for resistance to nematode parasite infections in small ruminants in tropical production systems. Animal, 6(5), 741–747.

22. Bisset SA, Morris CA. 1996. Feasibility and Implications of breeding sheep for resilience to nematode challenge. International Journal for Parasitology, 26(8/9), 857–868.

23. Blattman AN, Hulme DJ, Kinghorn BP. 1993. A search for associations between major histocompatibility complex restriction fragment length polymorphism bands and resistance to *Haemonchus contortus* infection in sheep. Animal Genetics, 24, 277–282.

24. Blouin MS, Yowell CA, Courtney CH, Dame JB. 1995. Host movement and the genetic structure of populations of parasitic nematodes. Genetics, 141, 1007–1014.

25. Bot J, Kaelsson LJE, Greef J. 2004. Association of the MHC with production traits in Merino ewes. Livestock Production Science, 86, 85–91.

26. Braisher TL, Gemmell NJ, Grenfell BT, Amos W. 2004. Host isolation and patterns of genetic variability in three populations of *Teladorsagia* from sheep. International Journal for Parasitology, 34, 1197–1204.

27. Brasil BSAF, Nunes RL, Bastianetto E, Drummond MG, Carvalho DC, Leite RC, Molento MB, Oliveira DAA. 2012. Genetic diversity patterns of *Haemonchus placei* and *Haemonchus contortus* populations isolated from domestic ruminants in Brazil. International Journal for Parasitology, 42(5), 469–479.

28. Bricarello PA, Amarante AFT, Rocha RA. 2005. Influence of dietary protein supply on resistance to experimental infections with *Haemonchus contortus* in Ile de France an Santa Inês lambs. Veterinary Parasitology, 134(11), 99–109.

29. Brown EA, Pilkington JG, Nussey DH, Watt KA, Hayward AD, Tucker R, Graham AL, Paterson S, Beraldi D, Pemberton JM, Slate J. 2013. Detecting genes for variation in parasite burden and immunological traits in a wild population: testing the candidate gene approach. Molecular Ecology, 22(3), 757–773.

30. Bueno MS, Cunha EA, Veríssimo CJ, Santos LE, Lara MAC, Oliveira SM, Spósito Filha E, Rebouças MM. 2002. Infección por nematódeos em razas de ovejas carnicas criadas intensivamente en la región del sudeste del Brasil. Archivos de Zootecnia, 51, 273–280.

31. Cardon LR, Bell JI. 2001. Association study designs for complex diseases. Nature Review Genetics, 2, 91–99.

32. Carroll S. 2000. Endless forms: the evolution of gene regulation and morphological diversity. Cell, 101, 577–580.

33. Castillo JAF, Medna RDM, Villalobos JMB, Gayosso-

Vázquez A. 2010. Association between major histocompatibility complex microsatellites, fecal egg count, blood packed cell volume and blood eosinophilia in Pelibuey sheep infected with *Haemonchus contortus*. Veterinary Parasitology, 177(3–4), 339–344.

34. Castillo-Juarez H, Oltenacu PA, Blake RW, McCulloch CE, Cienfuegos-Rivas EG. 2000. Effect of herd environment on the genetic and phenotypic relationships among milk yield, conception rate, and somatic cell score in Holstein cattle. Journal of Dairy Science, 83, 807–814.
35. Cerutti MC, Citterio CV, Bazzocchi C, Epis S, D'Amelio S, Ferrari N, Lanfranchi P. 2010. Genetic variability of*Haemonchus contortus* (Nematoda: Trichostrongyloidea) in alpine ruminant host species. Journal of Helminthology, 84, 276–283.
36. Charon K, Moskwa B, Kuryl J, Gruzcynska J, Rutkowski R. 2001. Relationship between polymorphism in locus OMHC1(MHC class I) and resistance to nematodes in Polish Heatherhead sheep. Animal Science Papers and Reports, 19(4), 285–292.
37. Coltman DW, Wilson K, Pilkington JG, Stear MJ, Pemberton JM. 2001. A microsatellite polymorphism in the gamma interferon gene is associated with resistance to gastrointestinal nematodes in a naturally parasitized population of Soay sheep. Parasitology, 122, 571–582.
38. Crawford AM, Paterson KA, Dodds KG, Tascon CD, Williamson PA, Thomson MR, Bisset SA, Beattie AE, Greer GJ, Green RS, Wheeler R, Shaw RJ, Knowler K, McEwan J. 2006. Discovery of quantitative trait loci for resistance to parasitic nematode infection in sheep: I. Analysis of outcross pedigrees. BMC Genomics, 7, 178.
39. Dame JB, Blouin MS, Courtney CH. 1993. Genetic structure of populations of *Ostertagia ostertagi*. Veterinary Parasitology, 46, 55–62.
40. Davies G, Stear MJ, Benothman M, Abuagob O, Kerr A, Mitchell S, Bishop SC. 2006. Quantitative trait loci associated with parasitic infection in Scottish Blackface sheep. Heredity, 96, 252–258.
41. De Gotari MJ, Freking BA, Cuthbertson RP. 1998. A second-generation linkage map of the sheep genome. Mammalian Genome, 9, 204–209.
42. Díaz S, Ripoli MV, Peral-García P. 2005. Marcadores genéticos para resistência y susceptibilidad a enfermedades infecciosas en animales domésticos. Los loci del complejo principal de histocompatibilidade (mhc) como genes candidatos. Analecta. Veterinaria, 25(1), 40–52.
43. Diez-Tascón C, Mcdonald PA, Doods KG. 2002. A screen of chromosome 1 for QTL affecting nematode resistance in an ovine outcross population, in Proceedings of the 7th World Congress on Genetics Applied to Livestock Production, Montpellier, France, August, 2002. Communication 13-37. p. 1–4.
44. Doeschl-Wilson AB, Kyriazakis I. 2012. Should we aim for genetic improvement in host resistance or tolerance to infectious pathogens? Frontiers in Genetics, 3, 1–2.
45. Douch PGC, Green RS, Morris CA, McEwan JC, Windon RG. 1996. Phenotypic markers for selection of nematode-resistant sheep. International Journal for Parasitology, 26(8–9), 899–911.
46. Eady SJ, Woolaston RR, Lewer RP. 1998. Resistance to nematode parasites in Merino sheep: correlation with production traits. Australian Journal of Agricultural Research, 49, 1201–1211.
47. Eichler EE, Flint J, Gibson G, Kong A, Leal SM, Moore JH, Nadeau JH. 2010. Missing heritability and strategies for finding the underlying causes of complex disease. Nature Reviews Genetics, 11, 446–450.
48. Eysker M, Ploeger HW. 2000. Value of present diagnostic methods for gastrointestinal nematode infections in ruminants. Parasitology, 120, 109–119.
49. FAO. 1999. Opportunities for incorporating genetic elements into the management of farm animal diseases: policy issues, in Background Study Paper Number 18. Commission on Genetic Resources for Food and Agriculture. Bishop S, de Jong M, Gray D, Editors. FAOSTAT: Rome (available at http://faostat.fao.org).
50. Geldermann H, Mir MR, Kuss AW. 2006. OLA-DRB1microssatellite variants are associated with ovine growth and reproduction traits. Genetic Selection and Evolution, 38, 431–444.
51. Gibson JP, Bishop SC. 2005. Use of molecular markers to enhance resistance of livestock to disease: a global approach. Revue Scientifique et Technique (International Office of Epizootics), 24(1), 343–353.
52. Gicheha MG, Kosgey IS, Bebe BO, Kahi AK. 2005. Economic values for resistance to gastrointestinal helminths in meat sheep in Kenya. Journal of Animal Breeding and Genetics, 122(3), 165–171.
53. Gilleard JS. 2013. *Haemonchus contortus* as a paradigm and model to study anthelmintic drug resistance. Parasitology, 140, 1506–1522.
54. Goddard ME, Beilharz RG. 1997. Natural selection and animal breeding. Proceedings of the 3rd International Congress SABRAO, Canberra, Australia. p. 4.19–4.21.
55. Goddard ME, Hayes BJ. 2009. Mapping genes for complex traits in domestic animals and their use in breeding programmes. Nature Reviews Genetics, 10, 381–391.
56. Gonzalez-Recio O, Gianola D, Rosa G, Weigel K, Kranis A. 2009. Genome-assisted prediction of a quantitative trait measured in parents and progeny: application to food conversion rate in chickens. Genetics Selection Evolution, 41, 3.
57. Gruszczynska J, Charon KM, Swiderek W. 2002. Microsatellite polymorphism in locus OMHC1 (MHC Class I) in Polish Heath sheep and Polish Lowland sheep (Zelazna variety). Journal of Applied Genetics, 43(2), 217–222.
58. Gruszczynska J. 1999. Polymorphism of the OLADRB1 (MHC Class II) gene in German Merino sheep. Annals of Warsaw Agricultural University – SGSW, Animal Science, 35, 125–132.
59. Guy SZY, Thomson PC, Hermesch S. 2012. Selection of pigs for improved coping with health and environmental challenges: breeding for resistance or tolerance?

Frontiers in Genetics, 3, 1–9.

60. Harris BL, Johnson DL. 2010. Genomic predictions for New Zealand dairy bulls and integration with national genetic evaluation. Journal of Dairy Science, 93, 1243–1252.

61. Hayes BJ, Bowman PJ, Chamberlain AJ, Goddard ME. 2009. Invited review: genomic selection in dairy cattle: progress and challenges. Journal of Dairy Science, 92, 433–443.

62. Hulme DJ, Nicholas FW, Windon RG. 1993. The MHC class II region and resistance to an intestinal parasite in sheep. Journal of Animal Breeding and Genetics, 110, 459–472.

63. Janem M, Weimann C, Gauly M. 2002. Association between infections with *Haemonchus contortus* and genetic markers on ovine chromosome 20, in Proceedings of the 7th World Congress on Genetics Applied to Livestock Production, Montpellier, France, August, 2002. Communication 13–37. p. 1–4.

64. Kaplan RM. 2004. Drug resistance in nematodes of veterinary importance: a status report. Trends in Parasitology, 20(10), 477–481.

65. Keane OM, Dodds KG, Crawford AM, McEwan JC. 2007. Transcriptional profiling of *Ovis aries* identifies *Ovar-DQA1* allele frequency differences between nematode-resistant and susceptible selection lines. Physiological Genomics, 30(3), 253–261.

66. Kearney JF, Schutz MM, Boettcher PJ. 2004. Genotype × environment interaction for grazing vs. confinement II. Health and reproduction traits. Journal of Dairy Science, 87, 510–516.

67. Kemper KE, Emery DL, Bishop SC, Oddy H, Hayes BJ, Dominik S, Henshall JM, Goddard ME. 2011. The distribution of SNP marker effects for faecal worm egg count in sheep, and the feasibility of using these markers to predict genetic merit for resistance to worm infections. Genetic Research, 93, 203–219.

68. Kemper KE, Goddard ME, Bishop SC. 2013. Adaptation of gastrointestinal nematode parasites to host genotype: single locus simulation models. Genetics Selection Evolution, 45(14), 1–14.

69. Kijas JW, Lenstra JA, Hayes B, Boitard S, Porto Neto LR. 2012. Genome-wide analysis of the world's sheep breeds reveals high levels of historic mixture and strong recent selection. PLoS Biology, 10(2), e1001258.

70. Kijas JW, Townley D, Dairymple BP, Heaton MP, Maddox JF, McGrath A, Wilson P, Ingersoll RG, McCulloch R, McWilliam S, Tang D, McEwan J, Cockett N, Oddy VH, Nicholas FW, Raadsma H. 2009. A genome wide survey of SNP variation reveals the genetic structure of sheep breeds. PLoS One, 4(3), e4668.

71. Kloosterman A, Parmentier HK, Ploeger HW. 1992. Breeding cattle and sheep for resistance to gastrointestinal nematodes. Parasitology Today, 8, 330–335.

72. Kulski JK, Shiina T, Anzai T. 2002. Comparative genome analysis of the MHC: the evolution of class I duplication blocks, diversity and complexity from shark to man. Immunology Review, 190, 95–122.

73. Lewis CRG, Ait-Ali T, Clapperton M, Archibald AL, Bishop S. 2007. Genetic perspectives on host responses to porcine reproductive and respiratory syndrome (PRRS). Viral Immunology, 20(3), 343–357.

74. Lôbo RNB, Pereira IDC, Facó O. 2011. Economic values for production traits of Morada Nova meat sheep in a pasture based production system in semi-arid Brazil. Small Ruminant Research, 96, 93–100.

75. Lôbo RNB, Vieira LS, Oliveira AA. 2009. Genetic parameters for fecal egg count, packed cell volume and body weight of Santa Inês lambs. Genetics and Molecular Biology, 32(2), 288–294.

76. Louvandini H, Veloso CFM, Paludo GR. 2006. Influence of protein supplementation on the resistance and resilience on young hair sheep naturally infected with gastrointestinal nematodes during rainy and dry seasons. Veterinary Parasitology, 137(4), 103–111.

77. Marshall K, Maddox JF, Lee SH, Zhang Y, Kahn L, Graser HU, Gondro C, Walkden-Brown SW, Van der Werf JHJ. 2009. Genetic mapping of quantitative trait loci for resistance to *Haemonchus contortus* in sheep. Animal Genetics, 40(3), 262–272.

78. Martínez-Valladares M, Varadel rio MP, Cruz-rojo MA, Rojovázquez FA. 2005. Genetic resistance to *Teladorsagia circumcincta*: IgA and parameters at slaughter in Churra sheep. Parasite Immunology, 27(6), 213–218.

79. Mattick JS, Makunin IV. 2006. Non-coding RNA. Human Molecular Genetics, 15(1), R17–R29.

80. McManus C, Louvandini H, Gugel R. 2011. Skin and coat traits in sheep in Brazil and their relation with heat tolerance. Tropical Animal Health and Production, 43, 121–126.

81. McManus C, Louvandini H, Paiva SR, Oliveira AA, Azevedo HC, Melo CB. 2009. Genetic factors of sheep affecting gastrointestinal parasite infections in the Distrito Federal, Brazil. Veterinary Parasitology, 166, 308–313.

82. McManus C, Paiva SR, Araújo RO. 2010. Genetics and breeding of sheep in Brazil. Revista Brasileira de Zootecnia, 39(Suppl. Esp.), 236–246.

83. McManus C, Pinto BF, Martins RFS, Louvandini H, Paiva SR, Braccini Neto J, Paim TP. 2011. Selection objectives and criteria for sheep in Central Brazil. Revista Brasileira de Zootecnia, 40(12), 2713–2720.

84. McManus CM, Dallago BSL, Louvandini H, Melo CB, Seixas LS, Oliveira FJG. 2013. Gastrointestinal parasitism in sheep kept on *Andropogon* and *Panicum* pastures in the Federal District, Brazil. Journal of Animal Science Advances, 3(5), 214–218.

85. McRae KM, McEwan JC, Dodds KG, Gemmell NJ. 2014. Signatures of selection in sheep bred for resistance or susceptibility to gastrointestinal nematodes. BMC Genomics, 15, 637.

86. Molento MB, Fortes FS, Pondelek DAS, Borges FA, Chagas ACS, Torres-Acosta JF, Geldhof P. 2011. Challenges of nematode control in ruminants: focus on Latin America. Veterinary Parasitology, 180, 126–132.

87. Moraes FR, Thomas-Soccol V, Rossi Junior P. 2000. Susceptibilidade de ovinos das raças Suffolk e Santa Inês à infecção natural por tricostrigilídeos. Archives of Veterinary Science, 6, 63–69.

88. Moreno CR, Jacquiet P, Bouvier F, Cortet J, Blanchard-Letort A, Guégnard F, Francois D, Bourdillon Y, Grisez C, Prevot F, Averadère A, Demars J, Sarry J, Stella A, Woloszyn F, Canale-Tabet K, Cabaret J, Tosser-Klopp G, Salle G. 2014. Validation of QTL affecting resistance to nematodes in sheep identified in a back-cross design in a pure breed population. Proceedings of the 10th World Congress on Genetics Applied to Animal Production, Vancouver, Canada, August 2014, Communication 516.

89. Morris CA, Bisset SA, Vlassoff A, Wheeler M, West CJ, Devantier BP, Mackay AD. 2010. Selecting for resilience in Romney sheep under nematode parasite challenge. New Zealand Journal of Agricultural Research, 53, 245–261.

90. Morris CA, Vlassoff A, Bisset SA, Baker RL, Watson TG, West CJ, Wheeler M. 2000. Continued selection of Romney sheep for resistance or susceptibility to nematode infection: estimates of direct and correlated responses. Animal Science, 70(1), 17–27.

91. Nieto LM, Martins EN, Macedo FAF. 2003. Utilização de um modelo de limiar na estimação da herdabilidade de resistência dos ovinos aos endoparasitos. Acta Scientiarum, 25(1), 151–155.

92. Nunes RL, Dos Santos LL, Bastianetto E, De Oliveira DAA, Brasil BSAF. 2013. Frequency of benzimidazole resistance in*Haemonchus contortus* populations isolated from buffalo, goat and sheep herds. Revista Brasileira de Parasitologia Veterinária, 22, 548–553.

93. Oltenacu PA, Broom DM. 2010. The impact of genetic selection for increased milk yield on the welfare of dairy cows. Animal Welfare, 19(S), 39–49.

94. Paterson S, Wilson K, Pemberton JM. 1998. Major histocompatibility complex variation associated with juvenile survival and parasite resistance in a large unmanaged ungulate population (*Ovis aries L.*). Proceedings of the National Academy of Science of the United States of America, 98, 3714–3719.

95. Patterson KA, McEwan JC, Dodds KG. 2001. Fine mapping a locus affecting host resistance to internal parasites in sheep, in Association for Advancement in Animal Breeding and Genetics Proceedings, Vol. 13. Queenstown, New Zealand. p. 91–94.

96. Perry BD, McDermott JJ, Randolph TF, Sones KR, Thornton PK. 2002. Investing in animal health research to alleviate poverty. Nairobi International Livestock Research Institute: Nairobi.

97. Petroli CD, Paiva SR, Paim TP, McManus CM. 2014. Association of microsatellite markers with production traits in Santa Inês and crossbred sheep. Archives of Veterinary Science, 19, 7–16.

98. Prichard R. 2001. Genetic variability following selection of *Haemonchus contortus* with anthelmintics. Trends in Parasitology, 17, 445–453.

99. Quinnell RJ. 2003. Genetics of susceptibility to human helminth infection. International Journal for Parasitology, 33, 1219–1231.

100. Raberg L, Graham AL, Read AF. 2009. Decomposing health: tolerance and resistance to parasites in animals. Philosophical Transactions of the Royal Society B: Biological Sciences, 364, 37–49.

101. Rauw WM, Kanis E, Noordhuizen-Stassen EN, Grommers FJ. 1998. Undesirable side effects of selection for high production efficiency in farm animals: a review. Livestock Production Science, 56, 15–33.

102. Riggio V, Pong-Wong R, Sallé G, Usai MG, Casu S, Moreno CR, Matika O, Bishop SC. 2014. A joint analysis to identify loci underlying variation in nematode resistance in three European sheep populations. Journal of Animal Breeding and Genetics, 8. Ahead of print (http://onlinelibrary.wiley.com/doi/10.1111/jbg.12071/full).

103. Riley DG, Van Wyk JA. 2011. The effects of penalization of FAMACHA scores of lambs treated for internal parasites on the estimation of genetic parameters and prediction of breeding values. Small Ruminant Research, 99, 122–129.

104. Roberts JA, Estuningsih E, Widjayanti S, Wiedosari E, Partoutomo S, Spithill TW. 1997. Resistance of Indonesian thin tail sheep against *Fasciola gigantica* and *F. hepatica*. Veterinary Parasitology, 68(1–2), 69–78.

105. Rocha RA, Amarante AFT, Bricarello PA. 2004. Comparison of the susceptibility of Santa Inês and Ile de France ewes to nematode parasitism around parturition and during lactation. Small Ruminant Research, 55(1), 65–75.

106. Safari E, Fogarty NM, Gilmour AR. 2005. A review of genetic parameter estimates for wool, growth, meat and reproduction traits in sheep. Livestock Production Science, 92(3), 271–289.

107. Sallé G, Jacquiet P, Gruner L, Cortet J, Sauvé C, Prévot F, Grisez C, Bergeaud JP, Schibler L, Tircazes A, François D, Pery C, Bouvier F, Thouly JC, Brunel JC, Legarra A, Elsen JM, Bouix J, Rupp R, Moreno CR. 2012. A genome scan for QTL affecting resistance to *Haemonchus contortus* in sheep. Journal of Animal Science, 45, 4690–4705.

108. Santucci F, Ibrahim KM, Hewit GM. 2007. Selection on MHC-linked microsatellite loci in sheep populations. Heredity, 99, 340–348.

109. Sayers G, Sweeney T. 2005. Gastrointestinal nematode infection in sheep – a review of the alternatives to antihelmintics in parasite control. Animal Health Research Reviews, 6(2), 159–171.

110. Scholtz MM, Maiwashe A, Neser FWC, Theunissen A, Olivier WJ, Mokolobate MC, Hendriks J. 2013. Livestock breeding for sustainability to mitigate global warmimg, with the emphasis on developing countries. South African Journal of Animal Science, 43(3), 269–281.

111. Schwaiger FW, Gostomski D, Stear MJ. 1995. An ovine major histocompatibilty complex DRB1 allele is associated with low faecal egg counts following natural, predominantly *Ostertagia circumcincta* infection.

International Journal of Parasitology, 25, 815–822.

112. Shaw RJ, McNeill MM, Gatehouse TK, Douch PG. 1997. Quantification of total sheep IgE concentration using anti-ovine IgE monoclonal antibodies in an enzyme immunoassay. Veterinary Immunology and Immunopathology, 57(3–4), 253–265.

113. Shaw RJ, Morris CA, Wheeler M. 2013. Genetic and phenotypic relationships between carbohydrate larval antigen (CarLA) IgA, parasite resistance and productivity in serial samples taken from lambs after weaning. International Journal for Parasitology, 43(8), 661–667.

114. Silvestre A, Sauve C, Cortet J, Cabaret J. 2009. Contrasting genetic structures of two parasitic nematodes, determined on the basis of neutral microsatellite markers and selected anthelmintic resistance markers. Molecular Ecology, 18, 5086–5100.

115. Skuce P, Stenhouse L, Jackson F, Hypša V, Gilleard J. 2010. Benzimidazole resistance allele haplotype diversity in United Kingdom isolates of *Teladorsagia circumcincta* supports a hypothesis of multiple origins of resistance by recurrent mutation. International Journal for Parasitology, 40, 1247–1255.

116. Snowder G. 2006. Genetic selection for disease resistance: challenges and opportunities. Beef Improvement Federation Conference Proceedings, 38, 52–60.

117. Springbett AJ, MacKenzie K, Woolliams JA, Bishop SC. 2003. The contribution of genetic diversity to the spread of infectious diseases in livestock populations. Genetics, 165(3), 1465–1474.

118. Stear MJ, Innocent GT, Buitkamp J. 2005. The evolution and maintenance of polymorphism in the major histocompatibility complex. Veterinary Immunology and Immunopathology, 108(1–2), 53–57.

119. Stear MJ, Murray M. 1994. Genetic resistance to parasitic disease: particularly of resistance in ruminants to gastrointestinal nematodes. Veterinary Parasitology, 54, 161–176.

120. Strain SAJ, Bishop SC, Henderson NG, Kerr A, Mickellar QA, Mitchell S, Stear MJ. 2002. The genetic control of IgA activity against *Teladorsagia circumcincta* and its association with parasite resistance in naturally infected sheep. Parasitology, 124(5), 545–552.

121. Sutherland I, Scott I. 2010. Gastrointestinal nematodes of sheep and cattle. Wiley-Blackweell: Ames, Iowa, USA. ISBN 978-4051-8582-0.

122. Tabor HK, Risch NJ, Myers RM. 2002. Candidate-gene approaches for studying complex genetic traits: practical considerations. Nature Reviews Genetics, 3, 391–397.

123. Thorisson GA, Smith AV, Krishnan L, Stein LD. 2005. The international HapMap project web site. Genome Research, 15, 1592–1593.

124. Van Raden PM, Van Tassell CP, Wiggans GR, Sonstegaard TS, Schnabel RD, Taylor JF, Schenkel F. 2009. Invited review: reliability of genomic predictions for North American Holstein bulls. Journal of Dairy Science, 92, 16–24.

125. Van Wyk JA, Bath GF. 2002. The FAMACHA© system for managing haemonchosis in sheep and goats by clinically identifying individual animals for treatment. Veterinary Research, 33, 509–529.

126. Vanimisetti HB, Greiner SP, Zajac AM, Notter DR. 2004. Performance of hair sheep composite breeds: resistance of lambs to *Haemonchus contortus*. Journal of Animal Science, 82, 595–604.

127. Vieira LS, Cavalcante ACR, Ximenes LJF. 1997. Epidemiologia e controle das principais parasitoses de caprinos nas regiões semi-áridas do Nordeste. Embrapa Caprinos, Circular Técnica, Embrapa Caprinos: Sobral, CE. 49p.

128. Visscher PM, McEvoy B, Yang J. 2010. From Galton to GWAS: quantitative genetics of human height. Genetics Research, 92(5–6), 371–379.

129. Wakelin D. 1996. Immunity to parasites: how parasitic infections are controlled. Press Syndicate of the University of Cambridge: New York, USA. ISBN 0521562457.

130. Woolaston RR, Windon RG. 2001. Selection of sheep for response to *Trichostrongylus colubriformis* larvae: genetic parameters. Animal Science, 73(1), 41–48.

131. Woolaston RR. 1992. Selection of Merino sheep for increased and decreased resistance to *Haemonchus contortus*: peri-parturient effects on faecal egg counts. International Journal for Parasitology, 22(7), 947–953.

CHAPTER 38

REDEFINING THE LIMITS OF BIOCHEMISTRY IN MULTIDRUG RESISTANT NEMATODES: IMPLICATIONS FOR FUTURE DRUG DEVELOPMENT

Hany Elsheikha and Cyril Rauch

MDR AND NEMATODE PARASITES

Chemotherapy remains the foremost available tool for the control of nematode parasites. However, the substantial use of anthelmintics, combined with a scarcity of new anthelmintic classes, has led to a gradual increase in the resistance of nematode parasites to these compounds. Multi-Drug Resistance (MDR) in economically important livestock nematodes, such as Haemonchus contortus enables the parasite to effectively 'escape' the effects of existing anthelmintics and represents a major obstacle to sustainable livestock farming and food production [1]. The growth in anthelmintic resistance has led to an increasing need for novel chemotherapeutic compounds.

Despite this unmet need, there has been a decline in anthelmintic research and development due to contraction of the industry, economic factors and regulatory requirements, among others [2]. Recently, two new anthelmintics have been released; however, resistant parasites are anticipated to appear in about a decade after the lunching of products, regardless their chemical structure or their mode of action. Hence, understanding the mechanisms of Drug Resistance (DR) in parasites is crucial for medical, veterinary, economic and eco-toxicological reasons and for maintaining the effectiveness of current anthelmintic drugs.

Among the different tactics by which nematode parasites tolerate the action of anthelmintic, those affecting influx and efflux are of special significance, as they limit the interaction of the chemical compound with its intracellular targets and hence, its lethal effects on the parasite. Mechanisms of drug evasion based on the intracellular extrusion of the drug and/or modification of target molecules have been described [3,4]. Cellular mechanisms related to metabolic activity have also been seen in eukaryotic systems, e.g. cancer cells. Recent observations suggest that such mechanism may occur in nematodes [5].

Drug Transporter Mediating MDR: Beyond the Obvious

Albeit an important body of works, fundamental questions remain unsolved that may, once understood allow us to design new therapeutic strategies. A structural study has enabled the molecular basis of P-gp (the archetypal drug transporter in cancer cells) to be defined with remarkable precision [6].

Citation: Elsheikha H, Rauch C (2012) Redefining the Limits of Biochemistry in Multidrug Resistant Nematodes: Implications for Future Drug Development. J Vet Sci Technol 3:e110 doi:10.4172/2157-7579.1000e110.

This study confirms that when ATP molecules bind to Pgp, conformational changes promote a "power stroke", leading to the passage of drugs from the membrane inner leaflet into the outer milieu [6,7]. Although the molecular model of Pgp has permitted a relatively simple representation of MDR in agreement with the usual concepts from the field of biochemistry, how a single protein can expel structurally different drugs, is still poorly understood. How P-gp recognizes hundreds of different hydrophobic drugs and pump them out of the cell is still debatable [8]. Nonetheless, there is something far more important at stake: the Pgp-like-mediated MDR model does not conform to the fundamental notion of specificity and seems to challenge the roots of biochemistry. This conceptual issue was noted very early in this field, and raised clearly by Paul Roepe [9]: "...MDR cells are resistant to, and/or exhibit decreased retention of literally hundreds of different hydrophobic compounds that are structurally divergent. Membrane transporters, like soluble enzymes, are exquisitely substrate-specific. If transporters were not specific, the cell would eventually become a high entropy chaotic mess, as there are no structural molecular motifs common to all the many different agents to which MDR cells are resistant. MDR protein is a very unusual enzyme with extraordinarily broad substrate recognition capabilities; that is, it violates the law of enzyme specificity".

Given the central importance of the notion of "specificity" in classical biochemistry, various models were put forward to explain MDR without absolutely requiring a drug-handling activity; by characterizing the interactions between the physico-chemical properties of drugs and biophysical changes recurrent in MDR cells, i.e. involving membrane potential [10], cytosolic pH [10,11] and membrane recycling [12,13]. Although conceptually satisfying and in accordance with the notion of specificity and hence, basic laws of biochemistry, it is worth noting that these models have their own limits and that they cannot rule out completely, the involvement of drug-handling by transporters. Are we back in a conceptual dead-lock?

Not necessarily, as recent works have demonstrated that membrane changes, reflected by alteration of parameters stated above (electric potential, pH and membrane recycling), may be central to maintain drugs in the membrane for a sufficient long time and hence allow drug pumping. Indeed, if we assume that, the specificity is not central to drug pumping, the only possibility for efficient drug extrusion relies on repeated collisions between a drug and the set of membrane transporters. For example, all chemists know that increasing the temperature accelerates the reaction rate. Albeit temperature is unlikely to be directly involved as such in drug pumping, it is worth mentioning that physicists have demonstrated a similar role to diffusion in two dimensions [14,15]. This would mean that extrusion is warranted by the diffusion properties and membrane changes. Looking at the MDR problem from this angle, opens new possibilities for the development of novel therapeutic strategies.

If the membrane diffusion is so important why not targeting the membrane itself to change the ability of transporters to interact with drugs. Doing so, we would impair the drug/transporter interaction allowing more drug uptake by cells. These membrane changes that seem so important in MDR have to be related to how parasites "handle" their membrane, i.e. what happen to parasites' membrane when they reach the drug resistant state. Thus, if one wants to eradicate MDR, it is the membrane of parasites that needs to be focused upon and targeted by specific drugs.

REFERENCES

1. Kaplan RM (2004) Drug resistance in nematodes of veterinary importance: a status report. Trends Parasitol 20: 477-481.
2. Woods DJ, Knauer CS (2010) Discovery of veterinary antiparasitic agents in the 21st century: a view from industry. Int J Parasitol 40: 1177-1181
3. McCavera S, Walsh TK, Wolstenholme AJ (2007) Nematode ligand-gated chloride channels: an appraisal of their involvement in macrocyclic lactone resistance and prospects for developing molecular markers. Parasitology 134: 1111-1121.
4. Riou M, Guégnard F, Sizaret PY, Le Vern Y, Kerboeuf D (2010) Drug resistance is affected by colocalization of P-glycoproteins in raft-like structures unexpected in eggshells of the nematode Haemonchus contortus. Biochem Cell Biol 88: 459-467.
5. Kerboeuf D, Riou M, Neveu C, Issouf M (2010) Membrane drug transport in helminths. Anti-Infective Agents in Med Chem 9: 113-129.
6. Aller SG, Yu J, Ward A, Weng Y, Chittaboina S, et al. (2009) Structure of P-glycoprotein reveals a molecular basis for poly-specific drug binding. Science 323: 1718-1722.
7. Sauna ZE, Ambudkar SV (2007) About a switch: how P-glycoprotein (ABCB1) harnesses the energy of ATP binding and hydrolysis to do mechanical work. Mol Cancer Ther 6: 13-23.
8. Gottesman MM, Ambudkar SV, Xia D (2009) Structure of a multidrug transporter. Nat Biotechnol 27: 546-547.
9. Roepe PD (2000) What is the precise role of human MDR 1 protein in chemotherapeutic drug resistance? Curr Pharm Des 6: 241-260.
10. Wadkins RM, Roepe PD (1997) Biophysical aspects of P-glycoprotein-mediated multidrug resistance. Int Rev Cytol 171: 121-165.
11. Simon SM, Schindler M (1994) Cell biological mechanisms of multidrug resistance in tumors. Proc Natl Acad Sci U S A 91: 3497-3504.
12. Rauch C (2009) On the relationship between drug's size, cell membrane mechanical properties and high levels of multi drug resistance: a comparison to published data. Eur Biophys J 38: 537-546.
13. Rauch C (2009) Toward a mechanical control of drug delivery. On the relationship between Lipinski's 2nd rule and cytosolic pH changes in doxorubicin resistance levels in cancer cells: a comparison to published data. Eur Biophys J 38: 829-846.

14. Panagiotopoulou V, Richardson G, Jensen OE, Rauch C (2010) On a biophysical and mathematical model of Pgp-mediated multidrug resistance: understanding the "space-time" dimension of MDR. Eur Biophys J 39: 201-211.

15. Rauch C (2011) The "multi" of drug resistance explained by oscillating drug transporters, drug-membrane physical interactions and spatial dimensionality. Cell Biochem Biophys 61: 103-113.

SECTION XI: IMMUNITY TO PARASITIC INFECTIONS

CHAPTER 39

THE EFFECT OF ANTHELMINTIC TREATMENT ON COCCIDIA OOCYST SHEDDING IN A WILD MAMMAL HOST WITH INTERMITTENT CESTODE INFECTION

Radovan Václav and Jana Blažeková

INTRODUCTION

Under natural conditions, hosts are routinely exploited by a community of parasite species [1–3]. It is not surprising, therefore, that organisms evolved elaborate responses towards parasites under the selective pressure of multiple infection [1, 2, 4, 5]. As the complexity of host-parasite and parasite-parasite interactions in natural multiparasite disease systems is not sufficiently described, the principles governing these interactions and host responses towards parasites are far from clear [6, 7].

From an applied perspective, identifying the health outcomes of coinfections involving helminth macroparasites and microparasites such as protozoa, bacteria, or viruses is of utmost importance to public and domestic animal health officials [4, 8]. This is, on one hand, because macroparasite control has become widely available and efficient for human populations and domestic animals. On the other hand, before any such macroparasite control programme is incorporated in the fight against microparasites, its potential effects on the focal microparasites should be carefully taken into account. For example, despite intensive research, it is still controversial whether deworming in humans leads to decrease or increase in malaria incidence or severity [8].

Citation: Radovan Václav and Jana Blažeková, "The Effect of Anthelmintic Treatment on Coccidia Oocyst Shedding in a Wild Mammal Host with Intermittent Cestode Infection," The Scientific World Journal, vol. 2014, Article ID 302903, 6 pages, 2014. doi:10.1155/2014/302903.

Current theoretical and empiric work suggests that the outcome of coinfection can be different even for the same parasite system (e.g., [9]), depending on the level of resource competition between macro- and microparasites [4] or macroparasite burden and pathogenicity [2]. The optimal host immune response towards microparasites evolved not only under a bias of the immune response towards chronically infective macroparasites [10, 11], but also under fluctuating physiological states and parasite burdens [6]. Although host-parasite interactions have been intensively studied using domestic and laboratory animals [5, 12], it is questionable how relevant these studies are for understanding how free-living mammals respond to concurrent macro- and microparasite infection [6, 7, 13, 14].

Here, we study the effect of anthelmintic treatment on coccidia infection intensity in the free-living Alpine marmot, M. marmota latirostris. Alpine marmots are commonly coinfected with a tapeworm Ctenotaenia marmotae and coccidia Eimeria spp. [15–18]. While Eimeria spp. persist in marmots during hibernation, C. marmotae is expulsed by marmots before hibernation and reinfects them in the subsequent spring [16]. Our study has two goals. First, we determine the seasonal pattern in the infection intensity for the two commonest endoparasites of the Alpine marmot. Second, we test the hypotheses on the effect of helminth infection on microparasite infection intensity. If helminths affect microparasites via a reduction in the host's immune response [4], we predict that the coccidia oocyst shedding rate for marmots exposed to anthelmintic treatment should be lower than that for marmots from the control group. Alternatively, if helminths affect microparasites via a reduction in the host's resource levels [4], we predict that the coccidia oocyst shedding rate for marmots exposed to anthelmintic treatment should be higher than that for marmots from the control group.

MATERIALS AND METHODS

Study System

We investigated the endoparasites of the Alpine marmot, M. marmota latirostris, in an alpine grassland of the Great Cold Valley in the High Tatra Mountains (49°10′N, 20°09′E), Slovakia, in 2011. The study site (ca. 200 ha) consists of about 16 territories (the number fluctuates between years) of a marmot subpopulation that is under investigation since 2010. The basic habitat features of the subpopulation studied are presented in [19]. The Alpine marmot is a true hibernating, territorial rodent (Rodentia: Sciuridae), living in social units of 2–20 individuals [20]. The active season of the Alpine marmots in the study population in the High Tatras spans from approximately mid-April to the beginning of October (Radovan Václav, unpublished data).

An anoplocephalid cestode Ctenotaenia (Cittotaenia) marmotae (Platyhelminthes: Cestoda) is the most prevalent and abundant helminth endoparasite of the Alpine marmot across its whole range, including Slovakia [15, 16, 18, 21–23]. Tapeworms are composed of successive reproductively viable segments, proglottids. After maturation, proglottids containing embryonated eggs detach from the tapeworm and are shed with host faeces. The weight of the cestode can reach more than 3% of a marmot's total body mass [17]. C. marmotae is expulsed from the marmot gastrointestinal tract before hibernation in autumn and the parasite recolonizes its definite host in the subsequent spring [15, 16]. A variety of oribatid mite species act as intermediate hosts for the tapeworm [24] with marmots acquiring infection by accidentally ingesting infected mites [18].

Coccidia from the genus Eimeria are the most common microparasites of the Alpine marmot [15, 16]. In contrast to C. marmotae, they do not require intermediate hosts for transmission and persist in marmots even during hibernation [17]. Moreover, in contrast to C. marmotae for which the peak in the proglottid shedding rate takes place in late summer, the peak in the coccidia oocyst shedding rate occurs in early spring [17]. It is assumed that the number of oocysts discharged and the length of time they are shed depend on the number of sporulated oocysts in the initial infective dose (e.g., [25]). If the host becomes exposed again to the same coccidia, the host's protective immunity is responsible for a reduced oocysts shedding rate [25].

Experimental Design and Data Collection

In spring 2011 (late April-mid-May), we captured Alpine marmots in two-door, live-capture traps, following a procedure by Cohas et al. [26]. After capture, marmots were tranquillized with Zolétil 100 (0.10 mL/kg) and marked with a numbered ear tag and a transponder. In order to address the effect of helminth macroparasite infection on coccidia microparasites, each marmot was administered a broad-spectrum anthelmintic drug combination consisting of Ivermectinum and Praziquantelum. A broad-spectrum anthelmintic treatment was used to eliminate the potential effects of infection on coccidia not only by the most prevalent tapeworms but also by any helminth taxa known to infect Alpine marmots [18]. We administered 0.025 mL/kg of Ivermectinum (Biomectin, 10 mg/mL) and 0.1 mL/kg of Praziquantelum (Bancid, 56.8 mg/mL) intramuscularly to each marmot from the experimental group and 0.125 mL/kg of physiological solution intramuscularly to each marmot from the control group. The treatment was only applied once for each marmot. The effect of the treatment was examined considering all sampling units (individual faecal samples) at the level of marmot territories with four and three territories being assigned to the experimental (11 marmots) and control (13 marmots) groups, respectively.

From mid-May, we conducted intensive behavioural observations to confirm the structure of marmot social units within territories and started to collect fresh marmot faeces at seven territories where all (24) marmots were captured and either anthelmintic or physiological solution had been administered to them. Forty-five faecal samples were collected during field visits in May, July, and September at the specific defecation sites, latrines, which were used exclusively by territory members. For this study, we did not include faeces collected from marmot pastures because it was not possible to assign them unambiguously, due to territory overlaps, to individual territories. Also, juvenile marmots, which normally emerge during July, do not use latrines and defecate freely within territories (personal observations). Therefore, the faeces of untreated juveniles, which also can be classified visually based on their size, were not included in our analysis.

Fresh faecal samples were weighed to the nearest 0.1 g and stored in vials containing 2.5% (w/v) aqueous $K_2Cr_2O_7$. The vials were stored at ambient temperature for five days to allow oocyst sporulation while the content of each vial was mixed thoroughly twice every day. After five days, the aqueous content of vials was extracted into clean vials and stored in a cool place and then in the fridge until examination (within 3 months). Oocysts and tapeworm eggs and proglottids were isolated by flotation in saturated sucrose solution and identified using oil immersion lenses on a compound microscope and Nomarski differential interference contrast microscopy. The oocyst numbers were quantified using the FLOTAC technique. Because most tapeworm proglottids containing eggs were crushed and did not allow exact quantification, the rate of tapeworm proglottid shedding was assigned to four levels at the scale from 0 to 3 based on the number of unambiguously identified C. marmotae proglottids. All coprological samples were analysed at the University of Veterinary and Pharmaceutical Sciences in Brno, the Czech Republic.

Data Analysis

The effect of anthelmintic treatment on C. marmotae and Eimeria spp. shedding rates was examined with general linear mixed models (GLMM). Both response variables, C. marmotae proglottid shedding rate and log-transformed Eimeria spp. oocyst numbers per gram (OPG) and faecal sample, were analysed assuming normally distributed errors. A visual inspection of model validation graphs (residuals versus fitted values and Q-Q plot) did not suggest a clear violation of the assumptions of homogeneity and normality for neither model [27]. Both models contained treatment, month, and the interaction between treatment and month as fixed factors. The tapeworm proglottid shedding rate was used as a covariate in the model on Eimeria spp. oocyst shedding. Because samples collected from the same territories are not statistically independent, territory identity was entered as a random factor. All tests were conducted with R software [28], using the lme4 package and the lmer function [29]. The Type III tests with denominator degrees of freedom were calculated based on a Satterthwaite's approximation and the least-square means were calculated using the lmerTest package [30]. The slice tests, examining the equality of simple effects of one factor for a given level of the other factor, were calculated using the lsmeans package and the glht function [31] with the P values reported being adjusted for multiple comparisons using the Bonferroni single-step procedure.

RESULTS

Faecal Parasite Community Structure

Examining 45 marmot faecal samples collected from mid-May to the end of September at seven marmot territories, the presence of eggs or proglottids of a tapeworm Ctenotaenia marmotae (Platyhelminthes: Anoplocephalidae), the eggs of a nematode Strongyloides sp. (Nematoda: Strongyloididae), and the oocysts of coccidia Eimeria spp. (Apicomplexa: Eimeriidae) was detected in 58% (26/45: 2/12, 14/23, and 10/10 for May, July, and September), 9% (4/45: 1/12, 3/23, and 0/10 for May, July, and September), and 80% (36/45: 9/12, 20/23, and 7/10 for May, July, and September) samples, respectively.

Effect of Anthelmintic Treatment on Tapeworm Faecal Shedding

Considering the whole active season of marmots, anthelmintic treatment conducted shortly after hibernation did not significantly lower the total shedding rate of Ctenotaenia marmotae (effect of treatment: $F_{1,4.64}$=0.24, P=0.644, effect of time of season:$F_{2,38.78}$=8.83, P<0.001, and interaction between treatment and time of season: $F_{2,33.78}$=1.12, P<0.333). Yet, examination of the interaction between experimental treatment and time of season revealed that anthelmintic treatment affected the dynamics of tapeworm faecal shedding during specific periods. Namely, the shedding rate increased from July to September but only for marmots in the control group (effect of time of season sliced by experimental treatment: difference between July and September for control group,P=0.012; difference between July and September for experimental group, P=0.637; Figure 1). Also, the proglottid shedding rate tended to increase from May to July but only for marmots in the experimental group (effect of time of season sliced by experimental treatment: difference between May and July for control group,P=0.631; difference between May and July for experimental group,P=0.078; Figure 1). That is to say, while the tapeworm shedding rate for the control group increased exponentially from May to September, the tapeworm shedding rate for the experimental group was sigmoidal, increasing abruptly from May to July and remaining high thereafter.

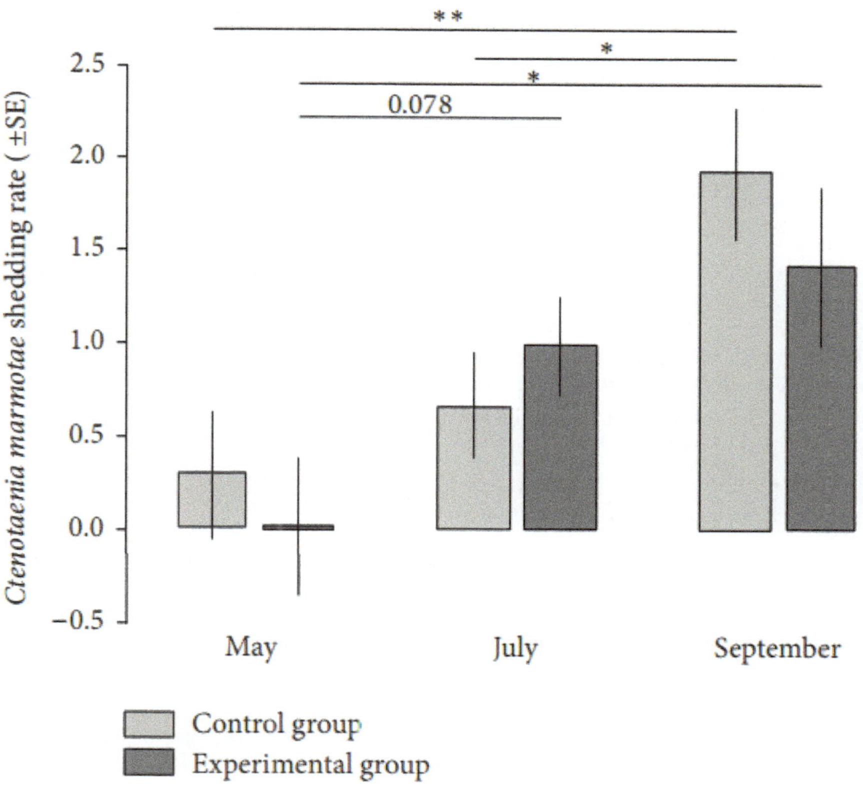

Figure 1: Effect of anthelmintic treatment on the faecal shedding rate of Ctenotaenia marmotae proglottids in the Alpine marmot, M. marmota latirostris. The C. marmotaeshedding rate represents proglottid numbers on the scale from 0 to 3 per gram of a faecal sample, as more precise proglottid/egg quantification was not possible due to the physical damage of most proglottids. The symbols above lines **, *, and 0.078 refer to P<0.001, P<0.05 and P=0.078, respectively. The P values reported are adjusted for multiple comparisons using the Bonferroni single-step procedure.

Effect of Anthelmintic Treatment on Coccidia Faecal Shedding

While the shedding rate of tapeworm proglottids and Eimeria spp. oocysts was negatively associated (estimate ± SE = −1.02 ± 0.49, $t_{37,12}$=--2.07, P=0.045), we did not find a significant difference in the shedding rate of oocysts between anthelmintic and control groups (effect of treatment:$F_{1,5.62}$=0.452, P=0.528, effect of time of season:$F_{2,36.46}$=3.48, P=0.041, and interaction between treatment and time of season: $F_{2,37.51}$=1.417, P=0.255). Nevertheless, similarly, as for the dynamics of tapeworm shedding, we found that the shedding rate of Eimeria spp. oocysts increased from May to July but only for marmots in the experimental group (effect of time of season sliced by experimental treatment: difference between May and July for control group, P=0.858; difference between May and July for experimental group, P=0.036; Figure 2).

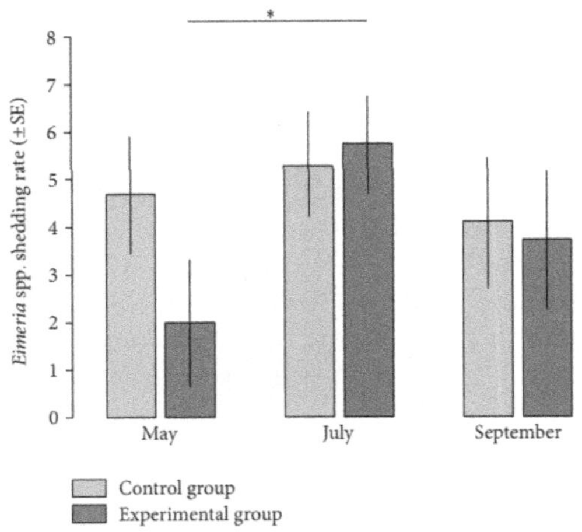

Figure 2: Effect of anthelmintic treatment on the faecal shedding rate of Eimeria spp. oocysts in the Alpine marmot, M. marmota latirostris. The Eimeria spp. shedding rate represents log-transformed oocyst numbers per gram of a faecal sample. The symbol above line * refers to P<0.05. The P value reported is adjusted for multiple comparisons using the Bonferroni single-step procedure.

DISCUSSION

Our experimental results suggest that helminth infection has a protective effect on the reproductive rates of coccidia microparasites in free-living Alpine marmots (hereafter referred to as marmots). Specifically, we found that when helminth infection was postponed in the beginning of the marmot active season via anthelmintic treatment, an increase in the shedding rate of Eimeria spp. oocysts also was postponed. Interestingly, a correlative result revealed a negative association between the infection intensity of a tapeworm macroparasiteC. marmotae and the coccidia microparasites of the genus Eimeria, indicating that, under increased host exploitation, tapeworms negatively affect coccidia reproductive rates.

We stress that our deworming treatment affected only existing helminth infections because the shedding rates of tapeworm proglottids were comparable between experimental and control marmot groups from the mid active season (cf. [32]). Thus, our treatment can be considered as a postponement rather than prevention of helminth infection, and larger sample size would unlikely lead to revealing a significant effect of deworming treatment on tapeworm infection during the whole season. Importantly, this study shows that marmots of the study population in the High Tatras started to shed the proglottids of C. marmotae already in the second half of May. Assuming the prepatent period of C. marmotae to be 39–50 days [17], this study indicates that marmots can acquire infections with C. marmotae already during early April, that is, after hibernation but before emergence. This finding, suggesting that the first tapeworm infections take place in the underground burrow system, is important because the mechanism of host infections with Anoplocephalid tapeworms is still unclear [19].

Similar to previous studies conducted elsewhere [15–17], we found that Eimeria spp. prevalence is high in marmots in the High Tatras. However, compared to a previous study by Callait et al. [17], which revealed the peak in coccidia oocyst shedding during early spring, we found that the Eimeria spp. oocyst shedding rates in control marmots remained high through summer. It is possible that this difference is due to higher coccidia diversity in the High Tatras and a correspondingly longer time taking marmots to acquire resistance against this complex parasite group. In addition, this pattern can be due to a longer time taking marmots in the High Tatras to accumulate or sustain growing helminths, thereby allowing coccidia to reproduce for a longer time without elevated competition for host resources. The importance of coccidia diversity and seasonal changes in tapeworm burdens warrants further studies.

Our work lends support to the hypothesis [4] that helminth infection has a protective effect on concurrent microparasite infections via modulated host immunity. Nevertheless, our work also points to the fact that within-host interactions between helminths and microparasites can be context-dependent [2], and they can change to negative ones once helminth parasites mature and start to reproduce. This is feasible in our study system because both tapeworms C. marmotae and coccidia Eimeria spp. share the same body sections of their marmot hosts.

Based on our results, we suggest that coccidia benefit from intermittent helminth infection in marmots due to the protective effects of helminth infection during the first phase of the host active season. In turn, from the host perspective, this study indicates that marmot immune response towards continuous coccidia infection would be optimal only under no helminth infection when the host immune response is not compromised by a downregulated Th1-like response (e.g., [4, 5]). Even if this situation is hardly possible under natural conditions, we propose that intestinal worm expulsion by marmots, regularly taking place just before hibernation, might represent not only intestinal self-cure of worm infections [15, 17] but also an optimal strategy to control microparasite infection intensity during an important part of the host life cycle shortly after hibernation.

Coinfection with multiple parasites or parasite strains has an important bearing on parasite virulence because under competition parasites are thought to increase host resource exploitation [7]. Our study suggests that coccidia virulence might not be heightened in marmot populations if tapeworm infections are low or occur later in the season because competition between the two parasites groups is likely to be low (cf. [33]). In contrast, Eimeria virulence can be higher in seasons or marmot populations exhibiting higher worm burden or earlier worm infections when interspecific competition among parasites is likely to be elevated. Finally, interstrain competition also can affect parasite virulence in marmots because we detected a complex of distinct morphotypes of Eimeria spp. in faecal samples. A future work needs to establish whether specific Eimeriamorphotypes prevail under different tapeworm burdens.

CONCLUSION

This experimental work demonstrates that correlational studies as well as those studies limiting their scope to macroparasite prevalence are not sufficient to depict the complexity of macroparasite-microparasite interactions. Our results suggest that the synergic effects of tapeworm infection on Eimeria spp. microparasites change into antagonistic ones under increased host exploitation by grown and reproducing macroparasites. We suggest that studying host-parasite and parasite-parasite interactions in free-ranging host species such as marmots, showing intermittent helminth infections, would be rewarding because this system mimics the one involving human populations receiving intermittent anthelmintic treatment while concurrently fighting microparasite diseases such as malaria.

Conflict of Interests

The authors declare that there is no conflict of interests regarding the publication of this paper.

ACKNOWLEDGMENTS

The authors are indebted to Dr. David Modrý and his team for help with coccidia analysis. Dr. Martina Miterpáková helped with helminth identification. Four anonymous reviewers helped to improve this paper. Ľudovít Záhor and the staff of the Zbojnícka chata cabin provided invaluable logistic support during the field season. Dr. Ľubomír Vidlička helped with sample logistics. This study was funded by a VEGA grant of the Ministry of Education, Science, Research and Sport of the Slovak Republic (no. 2/0176/10). The study was conducted under approval from the Ministry of Environment of the Slovak Republic (no. 4983/2010-2.1.1).

REFERENCES

1. F. E. G. Cox, "Concomitant infections, parasites and immune responses," Parasitology, vol. 122, supplement, pp. S23–S38, 2001.
2. A. Fenton, "Dances with worms: the ecological and evolutionary impacts of deworming on coinfecting pathogens," Parasitology, vol. 140, no. 9, pp. 1119–1132, 2013.
3. T. N. Petney and R. H. Andrews, "Multiparasite communities in animals and humans: frequency, structure and pathogenic significance," International Journal for Parasitology, vol. 28, no. 3, pp. 377–393, 1998.
4. A. L. Graham, "Ecological rules governing helminth-microparasite coinfection," Proceedings of the National Academy of Sciences of the United States of America, vol. 105, no. 2, pp. 566–570, 2008.
5. E. Moreau and A. Chauvin, "Immunity against helminths: interactions with the host and the intercurrent infections," Journal of Biomedicine and Biotechnology, vol. 2010, Article ID 428593, 9 pages, 2010.
6. Z. M. Weil, L. B. Martin II, and R. J. Nelson, "Interactions among immune, endocrine, and behavioural response to infection," in Micrommals and Microparasites: From Evolutionary Ecology to Management, S. Morand, B. R. Krasnov, and R. Poulin, Eds., pp. 443–474, Springer, Tokyo, Japan, 2006.
7. S. Bordes and S. Morand, "The impact of multiple infections on wild animal hosts: a review," Infection Ecology & Epidemiology, vol. 1, Article ID 7346, 2011.
8. M. Nacher, "Interactions between worms and malaria: good worms or bad worms?" Malaria Journal, vol. 10, article 259, 2011.
9. G. Karadjian, D. Berrebi, N. Dogna et al., "Co-infection restrains Litomosoides sigmodontis filarial load and plasmodial P. yoelii but not P. chabaudi parasitaemia in mice," Parasite, vol. 21, article 16, 2014.
10. O. O. Barriga, "Evidence and mechanisms of immunosuppression in tick infestations," Genetic Analysis: Biomolecular Engineering, vol. 15, no. 3–5, pp. 139–142, 1999.
11. J. A. Jackson, I. M. Friberg, S. Little, and J. E. Bradley, "Review series on helminths, immune modulation and the hygiene hypothesis: immunity against helminths and immunological phenomena in modern human populations: coevolutionary legacies?" Immunology, vol. 126, pp. 18–27, 2009.
12. W. C. Gause, J. F. Urban Jr., and M. J. Stadecker, "The immune response to parasitic helminths: insights from murine models," Trends in Immunology, vol. 24, no. 5, pp. 269–277, 2003.
13. S. C. L. Knowles, A. Fenton, O. L. Petchey, T. R. Jones, R. Barber, and A. B. Pedersen, "Stability of within-host-parasite communities in a wild mammal system," Proceedings of the Royal Society B, vol. 280, no. 1762, Article ID 20130598, 2013.
14. A. B. Pedersen and J. Antonovics, "Anthelmintic treatment alters the parasite community in a wild mouse host," Biology Letters, vol. 9, no. 4, Article ID 20130205, 2013.
15. B. Bassano, B. Sabatier, L. Rossi, and E. Macchi, "Parasitic fauna of the intestinal tracts of Marmota marmota in the western Alps," in Proceedings of 1st International Symposium on Alpine Marmot and on Genus Marmota, B. Bassano, P. Durio, U. Gallo-Orsi, and E. Macchi, Eds., pp. 13–24, Torino, Italy, 1992.
16. M. P. Callait and D. Gauthier, "Parasite adaptations to hibernation in Alpine marmots (Marmota marmota)," in Proceedings of the 11th International Hibernation Symposium: Life in the Cold, G. Heldmaier and M. Klingenspor, Eds., pp. 139–146, Springer, Jungholz, Austria, 2000.
17. M. P. Callait, D. Gauthier, and C. Prud'homme, "Alpine marmots and their digestive parasites: infection kinetic and parasitic strategy," in Holarctic Marmots As a Factor of Biodiversity, Abstracts of the 3rd International Conference on Marmots, K. B. Armitage and V. Y.

Rumiantsev, Eds., pp. 113–122, ABF, Moscow, Russia, 1997.

18. M. Preleuthner, "Parasiten des Alpenmurmeltieres (Marmota marmota): Systematik, Entwicklung, Verbreitung," Stapfia, vol. 146, pp. 77–92, 1999.

19. R. Václav and S. Kalúz, "The effect of herbivore faeces on the edaphic mite community: implications for tapeworm transmission," Experimental and Applied Acarology, vol. 62, no. 3, pp. 377–390, 2014.

20. C. Perrin, D. Allainé, and M. Le Berre, "Socio-spatial organization and activity distribution of the alpine marmot Marmota marmota: preliminary results," Ethology, vol. 93, pp. 21–30, 1993.

21. C. Gortázar, J. Herrero, A. García-Serrano, J. Lucientes, and D. F. Luco, "Preliminary data on the parasitic fauna of the digestive system of Marmota marmota in the Western Pyrenees," in Biodiversity in Marmots, M. Le Berre, R. Ramousse, and L. Le Guelte, Eds., pp. 105–108, International Marmot Network, Moscow, Russia, 1996.

22. M. T. Manfredi, E. Zanin, and A. P. Rizzoli, "Helminth community on alpine marmots," in Proceedings of the 1st International Symposium on Alpine Marmot and Genus Marmota, B. Bassano, P. Durio, U. Gallo-Orsi, and E. Macchi, Eds., pp. 203–207, Torino, Italy, 1992.

23. F. Tenora, "Discovery of a tapeworm Ctenotaenia marmotae/Frölich, 1802/Railliet 1893 in ČSSR," Foolia Zoologica, vol. 10, p. 396, 1961.

24. E. Ebermann, "Oribatiden (Oribatei, Acari) als Zwischenwirte des Murmeltier-Bandwurmes Ctenotaenia marmotae (Frölich , 1802)," Parasitology Research, vol. 50, pp. 303–312, 1976.

25. D. W. Duszynski and S. J. Upton, "Cyclospora, Eimeria, Isospora, and Cryptosporidium spp," in Parasitic Diseases of Wild Animals, W. M. Samuel, M. J. Pybus, and A. A. Kocan, Eds., pp. 416–459, Iowa State University Press, Ames, Iowa, USA, 2001.

26. A. Cohas, N. G. Yoccoz, C. Bonenfant et al., "The genetic similarity between pair members influences the frequency of extrapair paternity in alpine marmots," Animal Behaviour, vol. 76, no. 1, pp. 87–95, 2008. ·

27. A. F. Zuur, E. N. Ieno, N. J. Walker, A. A. Saveliev, and G. M. Smith, Mixed Effects Models and Extensions in Ecology with R, Springer, New York, NY, USA, 2009.

28. R Core Team, R: A Language and Environment for Statistical Computing, R Foundation for Statistical Computing, Vienna, Austria, 2014, http://www.R-project.org/.

29. D. Bates, M. Maechler, B. Bolker, and S. Walker, "lme4: Linear mixed-effects models using Eigen and S4. R package version 1.1-6," 2014, http://CRAN.R-project.org/package=lme4.

30. A. Kuznetsova, P. B. Brockhoff, and R. H. B. Christensen, "lmerTest: Tests for random and fixed effects for linear mixed effect models (lmer objects of lme4 package). R package version 2.0-6," 2014, http://CRAN.R-project.org/package=lmerTest.

31. R. V. Lenth, "lsmeans: Least-Squares Means. R package version 2.00-5," 2014, http://CRAN.R-project.org/package.

32. M. P. Callait, "Marmotte alpine et endoparasites: biologie des parasites et comparaison del'infestation sur différents sites," in Proceedings of the 4ème Journée d'Étude sur la Marmotte Alpine, R. Ramousse and M. Le Berre, Eds., pp. 53–58, International Marmot Network, Lyon, France, 1997.

33. S. Schjørring and J. C. Koella, "Sub-lethal effects of pathogens can lead to the evolution of lower virulence in multiple infections," Proceedings of the Royal Society B: Biological Sciences, vol. 270, pp. 189–193, 2003.

CHAPTER 40 IMMUNE REGULATION DURING HELMINTH INFECTIONS

Natasha M. Girgis, Uma Mahesh Gundra, P'ng Loke

THE CO-EVOLUTION OF HELMINTHS AND THE MAMMALIAN IMMUNE SYSTEM

Helminth is a nonphylogenetic term that refers to multicellular animals (or metazoans) that have adopted a parasitic lifestyle in mammalian hosts. They are more commonly referred to as parasitic worms. These worms generally (with the exception of *Strongyloides stercoralis*) cannot replicate within the host, and they have evolved distinct methods to co-exist with their host through the activation of an immune regulatory network. Until quite recently in human history, the majority of *Homo sapiens* were likely colonized by one type of worm or another, just like many mammals are in the wild. This close relationship has led to the evolution of "disease tolerance" by the host [1], [2], in the presence of these parasites [3]. In other words, the mammalian host has evolved mechanisms to minimize the virulence of helminths, even without necessarily reducing worm burden. While helminths cause disease in hundreds of millions of people [4], nonetheless a large proportion of infected individuals are relatively tolerant to colonization with helminths.

Heterogeneity in Susceptibility to Infection and Pathology

Maintaining variation in immunity to any parasite is critical toward the survival of a host population. In an endemic population, a large proportion of helminth-infected individuals are relatively asymptomatic. Pathology often occurs in individuals that have a reduced immunity and are therefore highly susceptible to infection with very high worm burdens. Seventy percent of the worm burden in a population may occur in only 15% of the infected individuals [4]. Pathology can also occur in individuals that are very immunologically reactive, despite having low worm burdens [5], [6]. In this case, a breakdown of the immune-regulatory environment established by the host and the parasite may have occurred. Maintaining a disease-tolerant or asymptomatic state requires an appropriate immune regulatory relationship between each host and helminth, which is unlikely to occur for every individual host. Hence, there is a strong need to understand the natural variation in immune responses against helminths [7]. There is evidence that resistance to helminth infection could improve survivability during harsh conditions, but brings with it the cost of autoimmune susceptibility and reduced reproduction [8]. As clinical trials reintroducing helminths as treatment for autoimmunity are ongoing [9], [10], there is an urgency to understand heterogeneity in immune responses against helminths in order to personalize treatment regiments to maximize clinical benefit.

Type 2 Responses Minimize the Virulence of Helminth Infections

A key component of the immune system that has evolved to minimize the virulence of helminths is the type 2 (or T_H2) response [11]. Instead of giving us allergies and asthma, the type 2 response likely evolved both to provide resistance by limiting the number helminths that can live in our intestinal tract [12] and to repair the tissue damage that is caused by the helminths that have colonized our tissues [3]. This response is characterized by the production of cytokines such as interleukin-4 (IL-4), IL-5, IL-9, and IL-13. While it is still unclear how this response is initiated during helminth infection, a broad range of effector mechanisms are activated by these cytokines [11], [13].

Signaling through IL-4Ra and STAT6 in intestinal epithelial cells (IECs) promotes goblet cell differentiation and

Citation: Girgis NM, Gundra UM, Loke P (2013) Immune Regulation during Helminth Infections. PLoS Pathog 9(4): e1003250. doi:10.1371/journal.ppat.1003250.

increases mucus production, as well as increases proliferation and turnover of the IECs [12]. This may help maintain the mucosal barrier and limit aberrant responses triggered by the gut bacteria [10]. Increased contraction of intestinal muscles and the activation and release of mast cell proteases that can increase fluid flow into the lumen may also help flush the worms out of the gut [12]. Macrophages are alternatively activated by IL-4Ra/STAT6 signaling to adopt an anti-inflammatory tissue repair function [3]. The type 2 response will also increase secretion of Immunoglobulin E (IgE) by B cells that can in turn activate cells that express Fc receptors (FcRs), such as basophils, eosinophils, and mast cells to amplify the type 2 response by producing more IL-4. The absence of this type 2 response during helminth infections in mice is often associated with lethal sepsis from compromised gut integrity and leakage of gut bacteria [3].

Host Mechanisms of Immune Regulation during Helminth Infection

During chronic helminth infection, peripheral T cells from infected patients are unresponsive to stimulation with parasite antigens, and responses to other antigens are also reduced [6]. This observation led to studies to define the immune regulatory mechanisms at play during helminth infection. In addition to the T_H2 response described above, regulatory T cells [14], regulatory B cells [15], and alternatively activated (or M2) macrophages [16] were identified as key components of the immune regulatory network functioning during helminth infections[13].

Foxp3+ Treg cells expand during helminth infections and may promote the survival of helminths as well as limit immune-driven pathology [14]. Depletion of these Treg cells can increase resistance to the parasites and reduce worm burden, but can also lead to increased immune-driven pathology [14]. IL-10 producing regulatory B cells was first identified to play an important role in limiting disease severity during autoimmune diseases and then later found to be induced by helminths [15]. In several mouse studies whereby helminths could suppress allergic inflammation, suppression could be reversed by depleting these B cells or transferred to a recipient animal by transferring B cells [15]. Alternatively activated macrophages that are expanded during helminth infections have been shown to promote Foxp3+ Treg differentiation [17] and, by up-regulating arginase 1, play an important immune regulation and tissue repair role, respectively, by competing for L-arginine and generating proline [13], [16]. The expansion and increased functionality of these regulatory cells during helminth infection may be responsible for the bystander suppression of autoimmune diseases, which has been noted in several study cohorts [5],[18]. Additionally, activation of this immune regulatory network likely contributes toward the deficiency in generating protective immunity when exposed to natural helminth infection [6].

Helminth Products That Enhance Immune Regulation

In order to promote the host immune regulatory network described above, helminths have evolved the production of immuno-modulating molecules that are just being elucidated [19],[20]. A few examples include a TGF-β-like ligand identified from the secreted products of the intestinal nematode parasite *Heligmosomoides polygyrus bakeri* can induce the differentiation of regulatory T cells [20]. A glycoprotein secreted *by Schistosoma mansoni*eggs called omega-1 has been shown to condition dendritic cells to promote T_H2 differentiation [19]. The phosphorylcholines covalently attached to the N-type glycans of ES-62, a protein secreted by filarial nematodes, have been shown to suppress inflammatory responses [19]. While the mechanisms of action are still unclear, some of these molecules have been shown to act through Toll-like receptors (TLRs) and can in turn suppress pro-inflammatory responses triggered by other TLR ligands such as lipopolysaccharide (LPS)[19]. Since many helminths share the intestinal tract with commensal bacteria and can cause tissue damage to the intestines, there could be an evolutionary advantage toward suppressing the host responses against bacterial TLR ligands and preventing sepsis from a leaky gut.

Suppression of Autoimmunity by Helminth Infection

In the last 50 years there has been an exponential increase in various diseases of immune dysregulation in the developed world. Regions of the world where helminth parasites are still endemic because of poor sanitation have a lower prevalence of allergies and autoimmune diseases [5], [21]. Studies on individuals from endemic regions treated with anti-helminthic medications have generally shown an increase in allergen reactivity posttreatment [5]. Through mouse models, various helminths have been shown in many studies to suppress the symptoms of many different types of experimental autoimmune diseases (e.g., experimental autoimmune encephalomyelitis, type 1 diabetes, arthritis, and colitis) as well as allergic conditions of the skin, intestines, and the airways [21]. Based on these studies, investigators began to conduct clinical trials introducing live helminths to patients with autoimmune diseases [9], [10], [21]. *Trichuris suis* (the pig whipworm) and *Necator americanus* (human hookworm) are the two worms that have been investigated as therapeutic agents for diseases as wide ranging as autism, multiple sclerosis, asthma, allergic rhinitis, celiac disease, Crohns disease, and ulcerative colitis. FDA-regulated clinical trials are ongoing for the treatment of Crohns disease with *Trichuris suis* ova (TSO). While these large trials will establish if treatment is efficacious, a small pilot mechanistic trial on ulcerative colitis patients is also ongoing to investigate the mechanism of action for TSO in the intestinal tract [10]. Recently, it has become clear that the gut microbiota plays an important role in establishing a balanced immune response and is often dysregulated in autoimmune diseases [22]. In addition to the mechanisms already discussed above, helminth exposure may also restore the gut microbiota to a healthy state [23], which will enhance the immune regulatory network of the mammalian host [24].

REFERENCES

1. Medzhitov R, Schneider DS, Soares MP (2012) Disease tolerance as a defense strategy. Science 335: 936–941. doi: 10.1126/science.1214935
2. Little TJ, Shuker DM, Colegrave N, Day T, Graham AL (2010) The coevolution of virulence: tolerance in

perspective. PLoS Pathog 6: e1001006 doi:10.1371/journal.ppat.1001006.

3. Allen JE, Wynn TA (2011) Evolution of Th2 immunity: a rapid repair response to tissue destructive pathogens. PLoS Pathog 7: e1002003 doi:10.1371/journal.ppat.1002003.

4. Hotez PJ, Brindley PJ, Bethony JM, King CH, Pearce EJ, et al. (2008) Helminth infections: the great neglected tropical diseases. J Clin Invest 118: 1311–1321. doi: 10.1172/jci34261

5. Wiria AE, Djuardi Y, Supali T, Sartono E, Yazdanbakhsh M (2012) Helminth infection in populations undergoing epidemiological transition: a friend or foe? Semin Immunopathol 34: 889–901. doi: 10.1007/s00281-012-0358-0

6. McSorley HJ, Maizels RM (2012) Helminth infections and host immune regulation. Clin Microbiol Rev 25: 585–608. doi: 10.1128/cmr.05040-11

7. Babayan SA, Allen JE, Bradley JE, Geuking MB, Graham AL, et al. (2011) Wild immunology: converging on the real world. Ann N Y Acad Sci 1236: 17–29. doi: 10.1111/j.1749-6632.2011.06251.x

8. Graham AL, Hayward AD, Watt KA, Pilkington JG, Pemberton JM, et al. (2010) Fitness correlates of heritable variation in antibody responsiveness in a wild mammal. Science 330: 662–665. doi: 10.1126/science.1194878

9. Jouvin MH, Kinet JP (2012) Trichuris suis ova: Testing a helminth-based therapy as an extension of the hygiene hypothesis. J Allergy Clin Immunol 130: 3–10. doi: 10.1016/j.jaci.2012.05.028

10. Wolff MJ, Broadhurst MJ, Loke P (2012) Helminthic therapy: improving mucosal barrier function. Trends Parasitol 28: 187–194. doi: 10.1016/j.pt.2012.02.008

11. Pulendran B, Artis D (2012) New paradigms in type 2 immunity. Science 337: 431–435. doi: 10.1126/science.1221064

12. Artis D, Grencis RK (2008) The intestinal epithelium: sensors to effectors in nematode infection. Mucosal Immunol 1: 252–264. doi: 10.1038/mi.2008.21

13. Allen JE, Maizels RM (2011) Diversity and dialogue in immunity to helminths. Nat Rev Immunol 11: 375–388. doi: 10.1038/nri2992

14. Taylor MD, van der Werf N, Maizels RM (2012) T cells in helminth infection: the regulators and the regulated. Trends Immunol 33: 181–189. doi: 10.1016/j.it.2012.01.001

15. Hussaarts L, van der Vlugt LE, Yazdanbakhsh M, Smits HH (2011) Regulatory B-cell induction by helminths: implications for allergic disease. J Allergy Clin Immunol 128: 733–739. doi: 10.1016/j.jaci.2011.05.012

16. Gordon S, Martinez FO (2010) Alternative activation of macrophages: mechanism and functions. Immunity 32: 593–604. doi: 10.1016/j.immuni.2010.05.007

17. Broadhurst MJ, Leung JM, Lim KC, Girgis NM, Gundra UM, et al. (2012) Upregulation of retinal dehydrogenase 2 in alternatively activated macrophages during retinoid-dependent Type-2 immunity to helminth infection in mice. PLoS Pathog 8: e1002883 doi:10.1371/journal.ppat.1002883.

18. Correale J, Farez MF (2011) The impact of environmental infections (parasites) on MS activity. Mult Scler 17: 1162–1169. doi: 10.1177/1352458511418027

19. Harnett W, Harnett MM (2010) Helminth-derived immunomodulators: can understanding the worm produce the pill? Nat Rev Immunol 10: 278–284. doi: 10.1038/nri2730

20. Hewitson JP, Grainger JR, Maizels RM (2009) Helminth immunoregulation: the role of parasite secreted proteins in modulating host immunity. Mol Biochem Parasitol 167: 1–11. doi: 10.1016/j.molbiopara.2009.04.008

21. Elliott DE, Weinstock JV (2011) Helminth-host immunological interactions: prevention and control of immune-mediated diseases. Ann N Y Acad Sci 1247: 83–96. doi: 10.1111/j.1749-6632.2011.06292.x

22. Cho I, Blaser MJ (2012) The human microbiome: at the interface of health and disease. Nat Rev Genet 13: 260–270. doi: 10.1038/nrg3182

23. Broadhurst MJ, Ardeshir A, Kanwar B, Mirpuri J, Gundra UM, et al. (2012) Therapeutic helminth infection of macaques with idiopathic chronic diarrhea alters the inflammatory signature and mucosal microbiota of the colon. PLoS Pathog 8: e1003000 doi:10.1371/journal.ppat.1003000.

24. Hooper LV, Littman DR, Macpherson AJ (2012) Interactions between the microbiota and the immune system. Science 336: 1268–1273. doi: 10.1126/science.1223490

CHAPTER 41

IMMUNITY AGAINST HELMINTHS: INTERACTIONS WITH THE HOST AND THE INTERCURRENT INFECTIONS

Emmanuelle Moreau and Alain Chauvin

INTRODUCTION

Many species of helminths are parasitic multicellular organisms of medical and economic importance as they infect humans and animals and sometimes provoke fatal diseases such as schistosomiasis. They can also be responsible for economic losses due to decreased milk or meat production and the cost of anthelminthic treatments of parasitized individuals. Helminths are extremely diverse. They can be classified into 3 taxonomic groups, that is, nematodes, trematodes, and cestodes, often with very different parasitic cycles. For example, (i) they may be transmitted orally (Strongyles, Fasciola sp., etc.) by transcutaneous route (Ankylostoma sp.,Strongyloïdes sp., Schistosoma sp., etc.) by an arthropod vector (Onchocerca volvulus, Dirofilaria immitis, etc.); (ii) their definitive and intermediate hosts range from mammals, birds, reptiles to fish, molluscs and arthropods, and so forth; (iii) they may be localized in organ lumen or in tissues such as gut, liver (parenchyma and bile ducts), lung, lymphatic vessels, and so forth; (iv) the successive developmental stages of parasitic species may infect different tissues and cells of different organs.

Despite this great complexity, helminths usually cause asymptomatic or subclinical chronic infection, although some parasitized individuals can suffer from severe disease which may be fatal. Indeed, worms tend to be aggregated in their distribution, with a large number of hosts harboring few parasites and few heavily infected hosts [1, 2]. This remarkable equilibrium between most hosts and parasites is the product of long-term coevolution of the two partners and particularly of the immune defence of the host and the immune evasion of the parasite. The immune responses of the hosts to helminth infection are generally characterized by a skewed Th2-like response. Helminths have developed several means of escaping these immune responses. Recently, Maizels et al. [3] called them "masters of immunomodulation". These immunomodulatory abilities enable the worm to persist in the host and can lead to interactions with inflammatory and immune mechanisms involved in other infections or to vaccines or in allergic and autoimmune diseases. The focus in this review is on pathogenic helminths of veterinary importance, especially in Ruminants medicine, and includes Fasciola spp. and gastrointestinal nematodes.

Citation: Emmanuelle Moreau and Alain Chauvin, "Immunity against Helminths: Interactions with the Host and the Intercurrent Infections," Journal of Biomedicine and Biotechnology, vol. 2010, Article ID 428593, 9 pages, 2010. doi:10.1155/2010/428593.

EFFECTOR IMMUNE MECHANISMS AGAINST HELMINTHS AND THEIR REGULATION

Helminth infections are typically associated with hypereosinophilia, considerable IgE production, mucous mastocytosis, and goblet cells hyperplasia [4]. These immune parameters are involved in different effector mechanisms highly depending on where the helminth is localized.

Effector Mechanisms against Tissue-Dwelling Parasites and Escape Mechanisms Developed by the Parasite

Several mechanisms against tissue-dwelling parasites have been described. These parasites are mainly larval stages, for example, of trematodes (Schistosoma spp., Fasciola spp.) or nematodes, which migrate through tissue.

Antibody Dependent Cellular Cytotoxicity (ADCC) is dependent on eosinophils, neutrophils, macrophages, or platelets as effector cells and IgE, IgG, or IgA as antibodies. The parasitic structures covered by antibodies are destroyed by cells carrying receptors to the Fc fragment (RFc) (Figure 1). When these cells are activated by fixation of the antibodies to the RFc, they release products that are toxic to the worm (major basic protein, eosinophil cationic protein, eosinophil-derived neurotoxin, reactive nitrogen intermediates, ...). ADCCs are also able to immobilize nematode larval stages as they migrate through the gut mucosa [5–8].

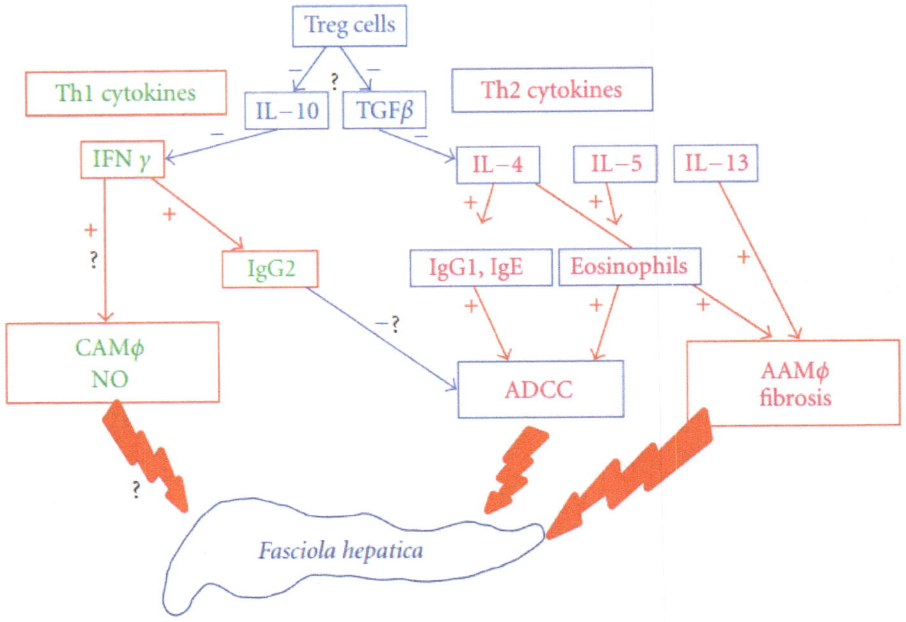

Figure 1: Immune mechanisms and regulation induced against Fasciola hepatica. Two main immune mechanisms are directed against F. hepatica in the liver parenchyma: (i) during the early phase of infection, classically activated macrophages may induce nitric oxide production which is toxic for the fluke. This mechanism needs to be confirmed and may be upregulated by Th1-type cytokines and downregulated by IL-10 produced by T regulatory cells. (ii) During the chronic phase of infection, antibody-dependent cellular cytotoxicity (ADCC) allows the release of toxic mediators such as major basic protein, eosinophil cationic protein, and reactive nitrogen intermediates. This mechanism is upregulated by Th2-type cytokines. T regulatory cells (Treg cells) produce IL-10 TGF β which inhibit the production and function of Th1 cytokines. They downregulate any excessive Th2 response in the immunopathogenesis of fasciolosis. Finally, alternative activated macrophage (AAM ϕ) produces molecules that are toxic to the fluke and participates in fibrosis and tissue repair.

A granuloma can occur around the parasite in the tissue which stops the worm migration and development. This phenomenon has been well investigated for Schistosoma mansoni. The granuloma is composed of eosinophils, macrophages, and lymphocytes with an increasingly fibrotic extracellular matrix [4], which surrounds and segregates the eggs from the hepatic tissue [9]. In the long term, fibrosis may develop as the eggs die and the granuloma is resolved [9].

Finally, nitric oxide (NO), toxic to the worm, is released by the macrophages classically activated by IFNγ and TNF (Figure 1). This mechanism has been described mainly against trematodes (Schistosoma sp., Fasciola sp.) during acute infection, before egg production in Schistosoma mansoni [10–12].

Tissue-dwelling parasites have developed several mechanisms to escape to the effector response of the host (Figure 2). For example, Fasciola sp. escapes from the immune responses by different means as follows:

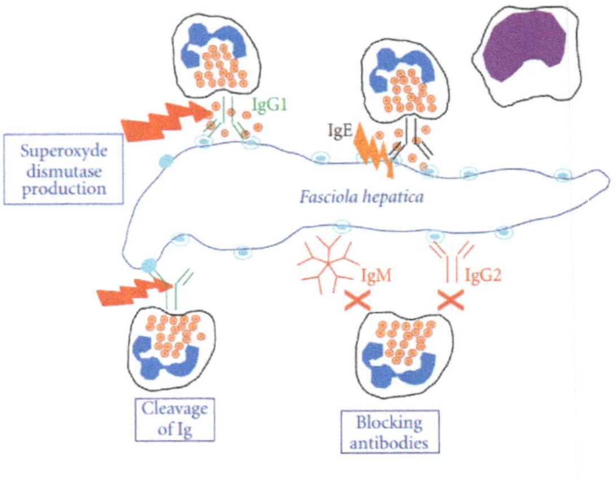

Figure 2: Main evasion mechanisms developed by Fasciola spp. against ADCC. Three main evasion mechanisms have been described: (i) production of superoxide dismutase and Glutathione S-transferase which neutralize superoxide radicals, (ii) cleavage of IgE and IgG involved in the ADCC, and (iii) production of blocking antibodies IgM and IgG2 which could inhibit eosinophil adhesion to flukes.

- Fasciola gigantica produces superoxide dismutase which neutralizes superoxide radicals toxic for juveniles [13, 14].
- F. hepatica releases cathepsin L-protease which cleaves IgE and IgG involved in the ADCC [15].
- Juvenile flukes were found to be covered by IgM [16]. While eosinophils do not express Fc μ receptor, IgM deposition on fluke tegument could inhibit eosinophil adhesion. IgG2 produced during fasciolosis in susceptible sheep [17] has been also suspected to be a blocking immunoglobulin of the ADCC.

Furthermore, F. hepatica secretes several molecules able to modulate the immune response. Excretory-secretory products of F. hepatica (ESPFh) can depress the sheep and rat lymphocytes stimulation [18, 19] and induce eosinophil apoptosis [20]. Milbourne and Howell (1990, 1993) [21, 22] have shown that there is an "IL5-like" substance in the excretory-secretory products (ESPs) probably responsible in part of the local and systemic eosinophilia observed during fasciolosis. Cathepsin L-proteases induce a decrease of lymphoproliferation in sheep and of the CD4 expression on human and ovine T cells [23]. GST from F. hepatica induces a significant inhibition of nitrite production by rat peritoneal macrophages [18].

Effector Mechanisms against Parasites Localized in the Lumen of Ducts and Escape Mechanisms Developed by the Parasite

Intestinal anaphylaxis, with IgE-induced mast cells degranulation, is responsible for changes in the intestine physiology as well as architecture and chemistry of the gut epithelium, including stimulation of fluid, electrolyte and mucus secretion, smooth muscle contractility, increased vascular and epithelial permeability, and recruitment of immune cells such as eosinophil or mast cells [24] (Figure 3). This can lead to rapid elimination of the gastrointestinal larvae, before they reach their tissue niche, and to expulsion of the adult [25]. Furthermore, IgA on the surface of the gut mucosa helps to neutralize the metabolic enzymes released by digestive strongyles and interfere with the worm's ability to feed [26, 27].

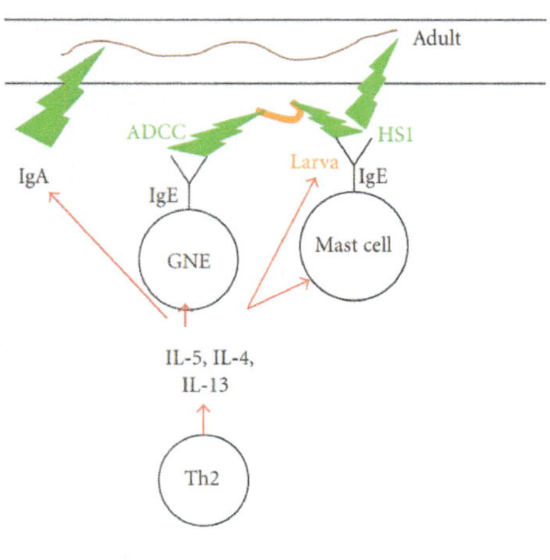

Figure 3: Immune response against gastrointestinal nematodes (GNE: eosinophil granulocyte, HS1: type 1 hypersensitivity). Against larva, ADCC and type 1 hypersensitivity are involved to block their migration in gut mucosa and to eliminate the parasite. Against adult in the lumen of gut, intestinal anaphylaxis responsible for muscle contractility, mucus secretion, and so forth, leads to the expulsion of the parasite. IgA neutralizes the metabolic enzymes and interferes with the worm's ability to feed.

As for tissue-dwelling parasites, parasites localized in the lumen of ducts are able to produce immunomodulatory substances to escape to the host immune responses. For example, Necator americanussecretes a metalloprotease which cleaves eotaxin, a chemotactic factor for eosinophils [28]. Gastrointestinal nematodes produce also superoxide dismutase and glutathione S-transferase which neutralize toxic oxide radicals [29]. A cystatin produced by H. contortus and N. brasiliensis modulates the antigen presentation to T cells by inhibiting cysteine proteases of antigen presenting cells, involved in the processing of the antigen [30,31].

Regulation of Immune Responses against Helminths

All these mechanisms, except the classically activated macrophages, are regulated by Th2-like cytokines and immunomodulatory cell types (Figure 1). Interleukin-4 is involved in the IgE isotype-switched B-cell responses, IL-5 is involved in the production of eosinophils, and IL-13 has similar functions to IL-4 and is involved mainly in the effector phase of inflammation and the development of fibrosis [9]. T regulatory cells produce the suppressive cytokines IL-10 and TGF-β which have antiinflammatory effects and could be involved in the skewed Th2-like responses. Immune deviation may also be promoted by the development of a Th2-driving dendritic cell population induced by excretory-secretory antigens from N. brasiliensis [32] or soluble egg antigen from schistosome [33]. Finally, IL-4 and IL-13 are able to alternatively activate macrophages (AAMps) which have strong antiinflammatory properties, enhance Th2 cell differentiation, contribute to fibrosis, and repair at the site of injury [34]. Thus, an environment, with downregulated proinflammatory responsiveness, activated damage repair mechanisms, and a controlled development of Th2-like anti-parasite effector responses is created during infection with helminths [35].

Several proteins produced by helminths were involved in the regulation of cytokine production [36, 37]. Schistosome soluble egg antigen contains molecules as alpha-1 or omega-1 that initiate a Th2-like response [38–40]. ES-62, a leucine aminopeptidase secreted by Acanthocheilonema vitae, reduces CD4+ cell IL-4 and IFN γ production but promotes IL-10 production by peritoneal B1 cells [41, 42]. It also inhibits the antigen-presenting cells ability to produce IL12p70 and drives Th2-like differentiation in vitro [43, 44]. Helminths could also secrete cytokine homologues as macrophage migration inhibitory factor (MIF) which induces, with IL-4, the development of alternatively activated macrophage [45].

PROTECTIVE AND IMMUNOPATHOLOGICAL EFFECTS OF THE IMMUNE RESPONSE AGAINST HELMINTHS

Despite the Th2-like response induced against helminths, these parasites are often able to persist in the host for a long time, resulting in chronic infection. However 2 types of immunity evaluated from the partial elimination of settled parasites and from host resistance to reinfection have been described, namely, premune immunity and partial immunity.

Premune immunity against helminths is very common and particularly observed against gastrointestinal strongyles. Premunition or concomitant immunity has been defined by MacDonald et al. [9] as a state wherein the host is protected from further infection with a given species by ongoing persistent infection with the same organism. Thus immune mechanisms existing concomitantly with parasites (adults and encysted larval stages) in animals infected by gastrointestinal nematodes prevent the establishment of new larvae. In contrast, the elimination of adult worms by the phenomenon of "self-cure" (spontaneous expulsion of adults by massive larval invasion during a short period of exposure) or by anthelminthic treatment results in the installation of new larvae until an equilibrium state is obtained. Premune immunity can also be expressed as a reduction in adult worm size and in female worm fertility. In contrast, the primary immune response against Fasciola hepatica in bovine limits the number of metacercariae which develops in adults and reduces the fertility of the females [46]. However it is unable to prevent the establishment of new parasites, which is a great difference with the premune immunity [46]. It also permits partial expulsion of adults in the bile ducts of infected cattle. So, immune responses against Fasciola hepatica partially protect the host against the infection.

Effector mechanisms regulated by Th2-like responses play a major role in immune protection to strongyles. Comparison of the immune responses of different breeds of sheep to Haemonchus contortus revealed a greater production of Th2-like cytokines (IL-4, IL-5, IL-13) in resistant breeds [47]. Similarly, Balb/c mice, which develop a Th2-like response against Trichuris muris, were soon able to eliminate the parasite, in contrast to AKR mice which express Th1-like responses and chronic infection with the same parasite [48]. The protective role of Th1- and Th2-like responses during fluke infection is less clear: Th1-like responses might act on larvae migrating through the liver parenchyma whereas the chronic phase with F. hepatica might be due to Th2-like responses against which the fluke has developed several escape mechanisms [46]. As described during infection with Schistosoma mansoni, Th2-like responses are predominant during infection by F. hepatica but early Th1-like responses seem to be involved in protection against this parasite. Indeed, sheep susceptible to F. hepaticadevelop a mixed Th1- and Th2-like response with IFNγ and IL-10 production during the first 6 weeks of infection, whereas the immune response of sheep resistant to F. gigantica is Th1 like, with production of IFNγ only. This suggests that protection against Fasciola sp. is linked with Th1-cytokine production [49]. Similarly, vaccinal trials with cathepsin L-protease from F. hepatica proved that protection induced by this antigen is mediated by a Th1-like response [50].

Although the host immune reaction against helminths may control the infection, it can also be responsible for tissue lesions and symptoms which are often the primary cause of disease during worm infection. Immunopathologic phenomena have been thoroughly investigated in infections with Schistosoma spp. As described above for F. hepatica infection, acute schistosomosis is associated with Th1-like responses against adult parasites. The Th2-like responses, induced as a result of egg antigens secretion, downregulate the production and effector functions of Th1-like mediators [51, 52]. When Th2-like responses against the eggs were blocked experimentally, an exacerbated granuloma driven by Th1 and Th17 cells resulted in hepatic damage and death [53]. Granulomatous responses evolve from an early Th1- to a sustained and dominant Th2-like response [54]. Whereas tissue fibrosis stimulated by Th2-like cytokine (IL-13) promotes tissue healing, excessive fibrosis may become pathogenic with loss of hepatic functions and portal hypertension [54, 55]. It seems that during trematode infections Th1-like responses are more protective than Th2-like responses against which these parasites have developed many escape mechanisms. Although Th1-like responses are closely associated with immunopathogenesis, Th2-like responses may also contribute to inflammatory damage. Treg cells seem to regulate this detrimental immune response by suppressing the Th1-like response and by downregulating any excessive Th2-like response during granuloma formation [56].

Granuloma formation dependent on the Th2-like response is also observed during gastrointestinal nematode infection. A recent study has shown that experimental downregulation of the Th2-like response to Nippostrongylus brasiliensis suppresses resistance to gastrointestinal nematode infection, pulmonary granulomatous inflammation, and fibrosis [57]. Similarly bovine ostertagiosis is associated with diarrhoea, inappetence, and weight loss. These clinical signs could result from smooth muscle contractility, increased mucus production, loss of specialized cells in the abomasal epitheliums induced by IgE-mediated immediate hypersensitivity reactions, and degranulation of mast and goblet cells and of proinflammatory mediators [24,58].

Hence, protection against gastrointestinal nematodes and against tissue-dwelling trematodes is controlled by Th2- and Th1-like responses, respectively [59]. The migration step in tissue is considered an immunoevasive strategy due to the predominant Th2-like response during helminth infection whereas protection in tissue is mediated by the Th1-like response [59]. However, the immune mechanisms, particularly those regulated by Th1-like cytokines, are responsible for considerable immunopathological damage and for the clinical signs observed during a helminthic disease. Even if the immune responses against most of helminths are orchestrated by Th2-like cytokines, the worms are still able to persist in the host for a long time. Indeed, the immune response during the chronic phase of infection was recently reported to be a modified Th2-like response, that is, a Th2-like response associated with Treg activity and the production of antiinflammatory cytokines such as IL-10 and TGFβ [60]. The induction of immunomodulatory Th2/Treg responses would allow the survival of both partners, by downregulating the host's inflammatory response and the immunopathological lesions observed during helminth infection, and also the protective immune mechanisms directed against the parasite [61, 62].

HELMINTHS AND COINFECTION

Some helminths are able to downregulate the Th1-like response because their high immunomodulator activity allows the induction of Th2/Treg-type responses. Indeed F.

hepatica inhibits the Th1-like response induced byBordetella pertussis in mice [63]. Similarly F. hepatica is also able to change the predictive value of the tuberculosis diagnosis test by modifying the immune response against Mycobacterium bovis [64]. Helminths can affect the evolution of coinfection by making animals more resistant to pathogens in which protection is mediated by the Th2-like response and more susceptible to pathogens in which protection is mediated by the Th1-like response [9]. For example, the expulsion of T. muris by mice is dependent on the Th2-like response. Curry et al. [65] demonstrated that mice susceptible to T. muris and coinfected with S. mansoni which induced the Th2-like response were able to eliminate T. muris by producing Th2-like cytokines. In contrast, mice infected with S. mansoni were more susceptible to Toxoplama gondii (protected by the Th1-like response) by inducing high mortality and weak production of IFNγ and NO, compared to mice solely infected with T. gondii[66]. Helminths were also able to inhibit the development of protective immunity regulated by Th1-like cytokines against Plasmodium sp. [62]. Many analyses of helminth - Plasmodium coinfections have provided controversial results as the parasite burden of Plasmodium sp. is dependent on the helminth species used, the intensity and duration of worm infection, and the age of the individual under study [67].

Helminths influence not only host resistance to another pathogen but also the gravity of the resulting disease. Cerebral malaria is associated with an overproduction of proinflammatory cytokines. Helminth infections are able to decrease the production of these cytokines by secreting IL-10 and TGF β and thereby diminish the risk of severe disease [62]. The nematode Heligmosomoides polygyrus promotes an immune response regulated by Th2-like cytokines, alternative activated macrophages, and regulatory T cells, and hence, prevents the inflammatory reaction controlled by Th1 cytokines and severe immunopathological lesions observed during schistosomosis [68]. Trichinella spiralis infection limits pulmonary damage induced by influenza virus in mice [69]. In contrast, H. polygyrus promotes intestinal lesions due to bacteria such as Citrobacter rodentium by alternative activation of macrophages [70].

However, other pathogens can also influence the immune response against helminths. For example, Miller et al. [71] recently showed that the production of Th1-like cytokines and classic activation of macrophages were little altered when F. hepatica infection preceded or succeeded T. gondii infections, whereas the production of F. hepatica-specific Th2-like cytokines and recruitment of AAMp were suppressed by T. gondii infection. Similarly, neutrophil-activating protein from Helicobacter pylori downmodulated the Th2-like response to Trichinella spiralis infection [72].

The effects of helminths on infections with other pathogens are complex and dependent on many factors such as the helminth species, coinfecting pathogen, protective and pathological immune mechanisms, and also the host and the individual.

HELMINTHS AND VACCINATION

Several studies have shown that helminths can influence vaccine efficacy by modulating host immune response, in particular when Th1-like and cellular-dependent responses are required. Schistosoma sp. and Onchocerca volvulus infections decrease the efficacy of vaccine against tuberculosis or tetanus [62], and Ascaris suum alters the efficacy of vaccine against Mycoplasma hyopneumoniae [73]. In mice, H. polygyrus was able to downregulate the strong immunity against Plasmodium chabaudi induced by blood stage antigens [74]. Effects of helminth infections on vaccine efficacy must be taken into account when using vaccines and also when developing new vaccines, in particular by choosing adapted adjuvants which are able to counterbalance the immunomodulatory activities of the helminth.

HELMINTHS AND ALLERGIC AND AUTOIMMUNE DISEASES

For several years, epidemiologic observations have shown that the prevalence ofhelminth infection is decreasing in westernized countries whereas the prevalence of diseases due to immune or inflammatory disorders such as allergic or autoimmune diseases is increasing. Epidemiologic and experimental data prove that chronic infection with helminths is protective against allergy. Humans infected with worms rarely develop allergic reactions [9] and an allergic reaction against ovalbumin was inhibited in mice infected with H. polygyrus or Schistosoma sp. [62, 75]. Similarly, immunization with Toxascaris leonina-derived proteins was able to inhibit allergy-specific Th2-like responses to ovalbumin [76]. Treatment against gastrointestinal nematodes increases cutaneous reactivity against house-dust mites [77]. These results are paradoxical because allergy is linked to mastocyte degranulation by IgE; the production of which is stimulated by helminths. In fact, worms induce the production of large quantities of antiinflammatory cytokines (IL-10, TGF β) by the regulatory T cells which then inhibit allergic inflammation.

In the same way, helminths can protect the host against autoimmune disease or at least decrease the gravity of symptoms induced by autoimmune inflammation. For example, S. mansoni infection inhibits the development of type 1 diabetes in NOD mice [78] or of experimental autoimmune encephalomyelitis in mice [79]. Helminth-specific Treg cells and their antiinflammatory cytokines (IL-10, TGF β) seem to be largely implicated in the inflammatory disorders associated with allergic diseases. Several studies are currently underway to investigate the possibility of treating allergic inflammatory diseases with immunomodulatory molecules from helminths, with special focus on the molecules involved and the ways in which helminths manipulate the host response, particularly how they activate and induce the expansion of Treg cells.

IMMUNOMODULATORY MOLECULES OF HELMINTHS AS NEW ANTIINFLAMMATORY DRUGS

Immunomodulatory function of helminths and their products could be used as antiinflammatory drugs.Trichuris suis has been tested recently to treat patients with inflammatory bowel disease and Crohn's disease with success [80, 81]. An excretory-secretory protein of Acanthocheilonema vitae, ES62, has been well studied for its antiinflammatory property. ES62 significantly decreases the severity of collagen-induced arthritis in mice [80] and of cutaneous hypersensitivity dependant on mast cells [81]. However, these immunomodulatory molecules could have side effects by increasing the risk of infections. Furthermore, they could be responsible for allergic reactions because they could be allergens or they could cross-react with allergens derived from pollen or another source [82].

In conclusion, helminth species have coevolved with their host for a long time. This has led to a strict adaptation which enables them to settle and persist in the host. Helminths are strong immunomodulators able to interfere with immune and inflammatory mechanisms induced by themselves and by coinfecting pathogens, inflammatory disorders, or vaccine. Immunomodulatory products from helminths are probably the antiinflammatory molecules of the future. Effects of helminths on the host immune system are not properly known because data are partial or can not be generalized between species. Nevertheless these effects need to be taken in account when controlling helminths and the diseases induced by worms. However, an individual could be infected by several pathogens and it will be necessary to evaluate the overall immune equilibrium resulting from the immune interaction between host and pathogens in different tissues and organs, which is still difficult, for instance.

REFERENCES

1. S. Gaba, V. Ginot, and J. Cabaret, "Modelling macroparasite aggregation using a nematode-sheep system: the Weibull distribution as an alternative to the negative binomial distribution?" Parasitology, vol. 131, no. 3, pp. 393–401, 2005.
2. A. Hall, S. Horton, and N. de Silva, "The costs and cost-effectiveness of mass treatment for intestinal nematode worm infections using different treatment thresholds," PLoS Neglected Tropical Diseases, vol. 3, no. 3, article e402, 2009.
3. R. M. Maizels, A. Balic, N. Gomez-Escobar, M. Nair, M. D. Taylor, and J. E. Allen, "Helminth parasites—masters of regulation," Immunological Reviews, vol. 201, pp. 89–116, 2004.
4. R. M. Anthony, L. I. Rutitzky, J. F. Urban Jr., M. J. Stadecker, and W. C. Gause, "Protective immune mechanisms in helminth infection," Nature Reviews Immunology, vol. 7, no. 12, pp. 975–987, 2007.
5. M. Capron and A. Capron, "Effector functions of eosinophils in schistosomiasis," Memorias do Instituto Oswaldo Cruz, vol. 87, no. 4, pp. 167–170, 1992.
6. E. N. T. Meeusen, A. Balic, and V. Bowles, "Cells, cytokines and other molecules associated with rejection of gastrointestinal nematode parasites," Veterinary Immunology and Immunopathology, vol. 108, no. 1-2, pp. 121–125, 2005.
7. D. Piedrafita, J. C. Parsons, R. M. Sandeman, et al., "Antibody-dependent cell-mediated cytotoxicity to newly excysted juvenile Fasciola hepatica in vitro is mediated by reactive nitrogen intermediates,"Parasite Immunology, vol. 23, no. 9, pp. 473–482, 2001.
8. P. F. Weller, "Eosinophils: structure and functions," Current Opinion in Immunology, vol. 6, no. 1, pp. 85–90, 1994.
9. A. S. MacDonald, M. I. Araujo, and E. J. Pearce, "Immunology of parasitic helminth infections," Infection and Immunity, vol. 70, no. 2, pp. 427–433, 2002.
10. L. Cervi, G. Rossi, H. Cejas, and D. T. Masih, "Fasciola hepatica-induced immune suppression of spleen mononuclear cell proliferation: role of nitric oxide," Clinical Immunology and Immunopathology, vol. 87, no. 2, pp. 145–154, 1998.
11. R. T. Gazzinelli, I. P. Oswald, S. L. James, and A. Sher, "IL-10 inhibits parasite killing and nitrogen oxide production by IFN-γ- activated macrophages," Journal of Immunology, vol. 148, no. 6, pp. 1792–1796, 1992.
12. P. Sibille, O. Tliba, and C. Boulard, "Early and transient cytotoxic response of peritoneal cells fromFasciola hepatica-infected rats," Veterinary Research, vol. 35, no. 5, pp. 573–584, 2004. ·
13. G. Ganga, J. P. Varshney, and R. C. Patra, "Activity of antioxidant enzymes in excretory-secretory fluid and somatic extracts of Fasciola gigantica," Journal of Veterinary Parasitology, vol. 21, no. 1, pp. 51–52, 2007.
14. D. Piedrafita, E. Estuningsih, J. Pleasance, et al., "Peritoneal lavage cells of Indonesian thin-tail sheep mediate antibody-dependent superoxide radical cytotoxicity in vitro against newly excysted juvenileFasciola gigantica but not juvenile Fasciola hepatica," Infection and Immunity, vol. 75, no. 4, pp. 1954–1963, 2007.
15. A. M. Smith, A. J. Dowd, M. Heffernan, C. D. Robertson, and J. P. Dalton, "Fasciola hepatica: a secreted cathepsin L-like proteinase cleaves host immunoglobulin," International Journal for Parasitology, vol. 23, no. 8, pp. 977–983, 1993.
16. A. Chauvin and C. Boulard, "Local immune response to experimental Fasciola hepatica infection in sheep," Parasite, vol. 3, no. 3, pp. 209–215, 1996.
17. D. S. Hansen, D. G. Clery, S. E. Estuningsih, S. Widjajanti, S. Partoutomo, and T. W. Spithill, "Immune responses in Indonesian thin tail and Merino sheep during a primary infection with Fasciola gigantica: lack of a specific IgG2 antibody response is associated with increased resistance to infection in Indonesian sheep," International Journal for Parasitology, vol. 29, no. 7, pp. 1027–1035, 1999.
18. L. Cervi, G. Rossi, and D. T. Masih, "Potential role for excretory-secretory forms of glutathione-S-transferase (GST) in Fasciola hepatica," Parasitology, vol. 119, no. 6, pp. 627–633, 1999.
19. E. Moreau, S. Hervé, Z. W. Yu, and C. Alain, "Modulation of sheep lymphocyte responses by Fasciola hepatica excretory-secretory products," Veterinary Parasitology, vol. 108, no. 3, pp. 207–215, 2002.
20. M. C. Serradell, L. Guasconi, L. Cervi, L. S. Chiapello, and D. T. Masih, "Excretory-secretory products from Fasciola hepatica induce eosinophil apoptosis by a caspase-dependent mechanism," Veterinary Immunology and Immunopathology, vol. 117, no. 3-4, pp. 197–208, 2007.
21. E. A. Milbourne and M. J. Howell, "Eosinophil responses to Fasciola hepatica in rodents," International Journal for Parasitology, vol. 20, no. 5, pp. 705–708, 1990.

22. E. A. Milbourne and M. J. Howell, "Eosinophil differentiation in response to Fasciola hepatica and its excretory/secretory antigens," International Journal for Parasitology, vol. 23, no. 8, pp. 1005–1009, 1993.

23. R. K. Prowse, P. Chaplin, H. C. Robinson, and T. W. Spithill, "Fasciola hepatica cathepsin L suppresses sheep lymphocyte proliferationin vitro and modulates surface CD4 expression on human and ovine T cells," Parasite Immunology, vol. 24, no. 2, pp. 57–66, 2002.

24. M. J. G. Farthing, "Immune response-mediated pathology in human intestinal parasitic infection,"Parasite Immunology, vol. 25, no. 5, pp. 247–257, 2003.

25. A. Balic, V. M. Bowles, and E. N. T. Meeusen, "Mechanisms of immunity to Haemonchus contortusinfection in sheep," Parasite Immunology, vol. 24, no. 1, pp. 39–46, 2002.

26. H. S. Gill, G. D. Gray, D. L. Watson, and A. J. Husband, "Isotype-specific antibody responses toHaemonchus contortus in genetically resistant sheep," Parasite Immunology, vol. 15, no. 2, pp. 61–67, 1993.

27. G. Smith, "The population biology of the parasitic stages of Haemonchus contortus," Parasitology, vol. 96, no. 1, pp. 185–195, 1988.

28. F. J. Culley, A. Brown, D. M. Conroy, I. Sabroe, D. I. Pritchard, and T. J. Williams, "Eotaxin is specifically cleaved by hookworm metalloproteases preventing its action in vitro and in vivo," Journal of Immunology, vol. 165, no. 11, pp. 6447–6453, 2000.

29. S. Liddell and D. P. Knox, "Extracellular and cytoplasmic Cu/Zn superoxide dismutases fromHaemonchus contortus," Parasitology, vol. 116, no. 4, pp. 383–394, 1998.

30. G. F. J. Newlands, P. J. Skuce, D. P. Knox, and W. D. Smith, "Cloning and expression of cystatin, a potent cysteine protease inhibitor from the gut of Haemonchus contortus," Parasitology, vol. 122, no. 3, pp. 371–378, 2001.

31. T. Dainichi, Y. Maekawa, K. Ishii, et al., "Nippocystatin, a cysteine protease inhibitor fromNippostrongylus brasiliensis, inhibits antigen processing and modulates antigen-specific immune response," Infection and Immunity, vol. 69, no. 12, pp. 7380–7386, 2001.

32. K. J. Else, "Have gastrointestinal nematodes outwitted the immune system?" Parasite Immunology, vol. 27, no. 10-11, pp. 407–415, 2005.

33. P. G. Thomas, M. R. Carter, O. Atochina, et al., "Maturation of dendritic cell 2 phenotype by a helminth glycan uses a Toll-like receptor 4-dependent mechanism," Journal of Immunology, vol. 171, no. 11, pp. 5837–5841, 2003.

34. T. Kreider, R. M. Anthony, J. F. Urban Jr., and W. C. Gause, "Alternatively activated macrophages in helminth infections," Current Opinion in Immunology, vol. 19, no. 4, pp. 448–453, 2007.

35. J. A. Jackson, I. M. Friberg, S. Little, and J. E. Bradley, "Review series on helminths, immune modulation and the hygiene hypothesis: immunity against helminths and immunological phenomena in modern human populations: coevolutionary legacies?" Immunology, vol. 126, no. 1, pp. 18–27, 2009.

36. D. A. Harn, J. McDonald, O. Atochina, and A. A. Da'dara, "Modulation of host immune responses by helminth glycans," Immunological Reviews, vol. 230, no. 1, pp. 247–257, 2009.

37. J. P. Hewitson, J. R. Grainger, and R. M. Maizels, "Helminth immunoregulation: the role of parasite secreted proteins in modulating host immunity," Molecular and Biochemical Parasitology, vol. 167, no. 1, pp. 1–11, 2009.

38. J.-M. Grzych, E. Pearce, A. Cheever, et al., "Egg deposition is the major stimulus for the production of Th2 cytokines in murine Schistomiasis mansoni," Journal of Immunology, vol. 146, no. 4, pp. 1322–1327, 1991.

39. G. Schramm, F. H. Falcone, A. Gronow, et al., "Molecular characterization of an interleukin-4-inducing factor from Schistosoma mansoni eggs," Journal of Biological Chemistry, vol. 278, no. 20, pp. 18384–18392, 2003.

40. B. Everts, G. Perona-Wright, H. H. Smits, et al., "Omega-1, a glycoprotein secreted by Schistosoma mansoni eggs, drives Th2 responses," Journal of Experimental Medicine, vol. 206, no. 8, pp. 1673–1680, 2009.

41. E. H. Wilson, E. Katz, H. S. Goodridge, M. M. Harnett, and W. Harnett, "In vivo activation of murine peritoneal B1 cells by the filarial nematode phosphorylcholine-containing glycoprotein ES-62," Parasite Immunology, vol. 25, no. 8-9, pp. 463–466, 2003.

42. F. A. Marshall, A. M. Grierson, P. Garside, W. Harnett, and M. M. Harnett, "ES-62, an immunomodulator secreted by filarial nematodes, suppresses clonal expansion and modifies effector function of heterologous antigen-specific T cells in vivo," Journal of Immunology, vol. 175, no. 9, pp. 5817–5826, 2005.

43. H. S. Goodridge, W. Harnett, F. Y. Liew, and M. M. Harnett, "Differential regulation of interleukin-12 p40 and p35 induction via Erk mitogen-activated protein kinase-dependent and -independent mechanisms and the implications for bioactive IL-12 and IL-23 responses," Immunology, vol. 109, no. 3, pp. 415–425, 2003.

44. M. Whelan, M. M. Harnett, K. M. Houston, V. Patel, W. Harnett, and K. P. Rigley, "A filarial nematode-secreted product signals dendritic cells to acquire a phenotype that drives development of Th2 cells,"Journal of Immunology, vol. 164, no. 12, pp. 6453–6460, 2000.

45. L. Prieto-Lafuente, W. F. Gregory, J. E. Allen, and R. M. Maizels, "MIF homologues from a filarial nematode parasite synergize with IL-4 to induce alternative activation of host macrophages," Journal of Leukocyte Biology, vol. 85, no. 5, pp. 844–854, 2009.

46. A. Chauvin, W. Zhang, and E. Moreau, "Fasciolosis of ruminants: immunity, immunomodulation and control strategies," Bulletin de l'Academie Veterinaire de France, vol. 160, pp. 85–92, 2007.

47. G. Terefe, C. Lacroux, O. Andreoletti, et al., "Immune response to Haemonchus contortus infection in susceptible (INRA 401) and resistant (Barbados Black

Belly) breeds of lambs," Parasite Immunology, vol. 29, no. 8, pp. 415–424, 2007.

48. W. C. Gause, J. F. Urban Jr., and M. J. Stadecker, "The immune response to parasitic helminths: insights from murine models," Trends in Immunology, vol. 24, no. 5, pp. 269–277, 2003.

49. W. Y. Zhang, E. Moreau, J. C. Hope, C. J. Howard, W. Y. Huang, and A. Chauvin, "Fasciola hepatica andFasciola gigantica: comparison ofcellularresponsetoexperimental infection in sheep," Experimental Parasitology, vol. 111, no. 3, pp. 154–159, 2005.

50. G. Mulcahy and J. P. Dalton, "Cathepsin L proteinases as vaccines against infection with Fasciola hepatica(liver fluke) in ruminants," Research in Veterinary Science, vol. 70, no. 1, pp. 83–86, 2001.

51. M. H. Kaplan, J. R. Whitfield, D. L. Boros, and M. J. Grusby, "Th2 cells are required for the Schistosoma mansoni egg-induced granulomatous response," Journal of Immunology, vol. 160, no. 4, pp. 1850–1856, 1998.

52. E. J. Pearce, C. M. Kane, J. Sun, J. J. Taylor, A. S. McKee, and L. Cervi, "Th2 response polarization during infection with die helminth parasite Schistosoma mansoni," Immunological Reviews, vol. 201, pp. 117–126, 2004.

53. M. J. Stadecker, H. Asahi, E. Finger, H. J. Hernandez, L. I. Rutitzky, and J. Sun, "The immunobiology of Th1 polarization in high-pathology schistosomiasis," Immunological Reviews, vol. 201, pp. 168–179, 2004. ·

54. T. A. Wynn, R. W. Thompson, A. W. Cheever, and M. M. Mentink-Kane, "Immunopathogenesis of schistosomiasis," Immunological Reviews, vol. 201, pp. 156–167, 2004.

55. E. J. Pearce and A. S. MacDonald, "The immunobiology of schistosomiasis," Nature Reviews Immunology, vol. 2, no. 7, pp. 499–511, 2002.

56. M. L. Burke, M. K. Jones, G. N. Gobert, Y. S. Li, M. K. Ellis, and D. P. McManus, "Immunopathogenesis of human schistosomiasis," Parasite Immunology, vol. 31, no. 4, pp. 163–176, 2009. ·

57. J. T. Pesce, T. R. Ramalingam, M. S. Wilson, et al., "Retnla (Relmα/Fizz1) suppresses helminth-induced Th2- type immunity," PLoS Pathogens, vol. 5, no. 4, Article ID e1000393, 2009.

58. G. Mulcahy, S. O'Neill, S. Donnelly, and J. P. Dalton, "Helminths at mucosal barriers—interaction with the immune system," Advanced Drug Delivery Reviews, vol. 56, no. 6, pp. 853–868, 2004.

59. G. Mulcahy, S. O'Neill, J. Fanning, E. McCarthy, and M. Sekiya, "Tissue migration by parasitic helminths—an immunoevasive strategy?" Trends in Parasitology, vol. 21, no. 6, pp. 273–277, 2005.

60. R. M. Maizels, "Infections and allergy—helminths, hygiene and host immune regulation," Current Opinion in Immunology, vol. 17, no. 6, pp. 656–661, 2005.

61. R. M. Maizels and M. Yazdanbakhsh, "Immune regulation by helminth parasites: cellular and molecular mechanisms," Nature Reviews Immunology, vol. 3, no. 9, pp. 733–744, 2003.

62. E. Van Riet, F. C. Hartgers, and M. Yazdanbakhsh, "Chronic helminth infections induce immunomodulation: consequences and mechanisms," Immunobiology, vol. 212, no. 6, pp. 475–490, 2007. ·

63. S. M. O'Neill, K. H. G. Mills, and J. P. Dalton, "Fasciola hepatica cathepsin L cysteine proteinase suppresses Bordetella pertussis-specific interferon-γ production in vivo," Parasite Immunology, vol. 23, no. 10, pp. 541–547, 2001.

64. R. J. Flynn, C. Mannion, O. Golden, O. Hacariz, and G. Mulcahy, "Experimental Fasciola hepaticainfection alters responses to tests used for diagnosis of bovine tuberculosis," Infection and Immunity, vol. 75, no. 3, pp. 1373–1381, 2007.

65. A. J. Curry, K. J. Else, F. Jones, A. Bancroft, R. K. Grencis, and D. W. Dunne, "Evidence that cytokine-mediated immune interactions induced by Schistosoma mansoni alter disease outcome in mice concurrently infected with Trichuris muris," Journal of Experimental Medicine, vol. 181, no. 2, pp. 769–774, 1995.

66. A. J. Marshall, L. R. Brunet, Y. van Gessel, et al., "Toxoplasma gondii and Schistosoma mansoni synergize to promote hepatocyte dysfunction associated with high levels of plasma TNF-α and early death in C57BL/6 mice," Journal of Immunology, vol. 163, no. 4, pp. 2089–2097, 1999.

67. S. Specht and A. Hoerauf, "Does helminth elimination promote or prevent malaria?" The Lancet, vol. 369, no. 9560, pp. 446–447, 2007.

68. L.E.Bazzone,P.M.Smith,L.I.Rutitzky,etal.,"Coinfection with the intestinal nematodeHeligmosomoides polygyrus markedly reduces hepatic egg-induced immunopathology and proinflammatory cytokines in mouse models of severe schistosomiasis," Infection and Immunity, vol. 76, no. 11, pp. 5164–5172, 2008.

69. R. C. Furze, T. Hussell, and M. E. Selkirk, "Amelioration of influenza-induced pathology in mice by coinfection with Trichinella spiralis," Infection and Immunity, vol. 74, no. 3, pp. 1924–1932, 2006.

70. M. Weng, D. Huntley, I.-F. Huang, et al., "Alternatively activated macrophages in intestinal helminth infection: effects on concurrent bacterial colitis," Journal of Immunology, vol. 179, no. 7, pp. 4721–4731, 2007.

71. C. M. D. Miller, N. C. Smith, R. J. Ikin, N. R. Boulter, J. P. Dalton, and S. Donnelly, "Immunological interactions between 2 common pathogens, Th1-inducing protozoan Toxoplasma gondii and the Th2-inducing helminth Fasciola hepatica," PLoS ONE, vol. 4, no. 5, article e5692, 2009. ·

72. G. Del Prete, L. Chiumiento, A. Amedei, et al., "Immunosuppression of TH2 responses in Trichinella spiralis infection by Helicobacter pylori neutrophil-activating protein," Journal of Allergy and Clinical Immunology, vol. 122, no. 5, pp. 908–913, 2008.

73. J. F. Urban Jr., N. R. Steenhard, G. I. Solano-Aguilar, et al., "Infection with parasitic nematodes confounds vaccination efficacy," Veterinary Parasitology, vol. 148, no. 1, pp. 14–20, 2007.

74. Z. Su, M. Segura, and M. M. Stevenson, "Reduced protective efficacy of a blood-stage malaria vaccine by concurrent nematode infection," Infection and Immunity, vol. 74, no. 4, pp. 2138–2144, 2006.

75. M. S. Wilson, M. D. Taylor, A. Balic, C. A. M. Finney, J. R. Lamb, and R. M. Maizels, "Suppression of allergic airway inflammation by helminth-induced regulatory T cells," Journal of Experimental Medicine, vol. 202, no. 9, pp. 1199–1212, 2005.

76. K. H. Lee, H. K. Park, H. J. Jeong, et al., "Immunization of proteins from Toxascaris leonina adult worm inhibits allergic specific Th2 response," Veterinary Parasitology, vol. 156, no. 3-4, pp. 216–225, 2008.

77. A. H. J. van den Biggelaar, L. C. Rodrigues, R. Van Ree, et al., "Long-term treatment of intestinal helminths increases mite skin-test reactivity in Gabonese schoolchildren," Journal of Infectious Diseases, vol. 189, no. 5, pp. 892–900, 2004.

78. A. Cooke, P. Tonks, F. M. Jones, et al., "Infection with Schistosoma mansoni prevents insulin dependent diabetes mellitus in non-obese diabetic mice," Parasite Immunology, vol. 21, no. 4, pp. 169–176, 1999.

79. D. Sewell, Z. Qing, E. Reinke, et al., "Immunomodulation of experimental autoimmune encephalomyelitis by helminth ova immunization," International Immunology, vol. 15, no. 1, pp. 59–69, 2003.

80. R. W. Summers, D. E. Elliott, K. Qadir, J. F. Urban Jr., R. Thompson, and J. V. Weinstock, "Trichuris suisseems to be safe and possibly effective in the treatment of inflammatory bowel disease," American Journal of Gastroenterology, vol. 98, no. 9, pp. 2034–2041, 2003.

81. R. W. Summers, D. E. Elliot, J. F. Urban Jr., R. Thompson, and J. V. Weinstock, "Trichuris suis therapy in Crohn's disease," Gut, vol. 54, no. 1, pp. 87–90, 2005.

82. W. Harnett, I. B. McInnes, and M. M. Harnett, "ES-62, a filarial nematode-derived immunomodulator with anti-inflammatory potential," Immunology Letters, vol. 94, no. 1-2, pp. 27–33, 2004.

SECTION XII: PROTOZOAL INFECTIONS

CHAPTER 42

IMMUNOLOGY AND INFECTION BY PROTOZOAN PARASITES

Edecio Cunha-Neto, Christophe Chevillard, Mauricio Martins Rodrigues, and Marcelo T. Bozza

Protozoan infection is the cause of diseases of high morbidity and mortality. Most are non-self-limiting chronic infections and neglected diseases; emergent antimicrobial-resistant strains pose a substantial problem; for many of them treatment either is highly toxic or has limited effectiveness. Vaccine development is still a formidable task and there is no licensed vaccine for human protozoan infection. The key to the control of protozoan infection is the understanding of the host immune response to protozoan parasites, which will guide the development of effective vaccines and immunotherapeutic agents. In this special issue, there are important studies on the immunology of T. cruzi infection, tegumentary and visceral leishmaniasis, malaria, and toxoplasmosis, both in patients and in animal models, which promote the understanding of immunopathological/immunoprotective parameters in these diseases.

The reviews by J. M. Álvarez and colleagues and by E. Cunha-Neto and C. Chevillard cover fundamental findings, mechanisms, and questions concerning the immune response and pathology of mouse and human disease. In this line, L. G. Nogueira and colleagues characterize the myocardial expression of transcriptional factors involved in effector CD4+ T cell differentiation and the characteristic cytokines produced by the distinct lymphocyte subsets and demonstrate a profound predominance of local Th1 response. L. C. J. Abel and coworkers characterized the proinflammatory effects of glicophosphatidyl inositol-anchored T. cruzi mucin (GPI-mucins) on human immune cells. It was observed that IL-12 production by GPI-mucins was dependent on IFN-γ and CD40-CD40L interactions. F. C. Dias and colleagues investigated the HLA-G expression in tissues and HLA-G 147 3′ UTR polymorphic site typing in patients presenting Chagas disease and the role of the mouse functional homolog in T. cruzi infection. F. Vorraro and colleagues studied the susceptibility to T. cruzi of mouse strains previously selected based on inflammatory and antibody responses to complex antigens. Q. Miao and M. Ndao review the potential impact of T. cruzi infection on the status of host lipid metabolism. The role of lipid mediators in T. cruzi infection is explored in two research articles. A. M. C. Canavaci and colleagues revisit the pathological role of 5-lipoxygenase in the acute infection of mice and A. D. Malvezi and coworkers investigate the role of cyclooxygenase and lipoxins in macrophage invasion by T. cruzi. In mouse models of chronic myocardial disease by T. cruzi, I. R. Pereira and colleagues show that treatment with infliximab, an anti-human TNF monoclonal antibody, reduced the frequency of mice with arrhythmias and cardiac fibrosis, while M. B. de Cuba and coworkers show the beneficial effect of cholinergic stimulation in reducing inflammation and fibrosis in the heart. Importantly, A. F. Araújo and coworkers demonstrate the beneficial effects of prophylactic vaccination using T. cruzi genes against acute and chronic pathologies caused by myotropic strains of the parasite. W. H. K. Cabrera and colleagues have characterized mouse lines selected for maximal (AIRmax) or minimal (AIRmin) acute inflammatory reaction and for high (HIII) or low (LIII) antibody (Ab) responses to complex antigens. Resistance to T. cruzi infection was found in female and in high responder lines AIRmax and HIII. It was correlated with enhanced production of IFN-γ and nitric oxide production by peritoneal and lymph node cells, in HIII males and females. Moreover, an Ab production QTL marker mapping to mouse chromosome 1 significantly cosegregated with survival after acute T. cruzi infection.

In the Leishmania field, M. F. Lopes and colleagues here review the interface between Leishmania and phagocytes, cells that are both targets and effector of the anti-Leishmania immune

Citation: Edecio Cunha-Neto, Christophe Chevillard, Mauricio Martins Rodrigues, and Marcelo T. Bozza, "Immunology and Infection by Protozoan Parasites," Mediators of Inflammation, vol. 2015, Article ID 504951, 2 pages, 2015. doi:10.1155/2015/504951.

response. The study by E. Svensjö and colleagues suggests that a serine peptidase (ISP-2) from L. major regulates macrophage phagocytosis by inhibiting the pericellular release of proinflammatory kinins from surface bound kininogens. C. M. V. Vendrame and coworkers have shown that insulin-like growth factor- (IGF-) I decreased nitric oxide production but increased arginase expression and activity, which lead to increased Leishmania parasitism. However, IGF-I did not result in altered cytokine levels. Moreover, stimulation with IGF-I induced phosphatidylserine exposure on amastigotes led to increased arginase activity in macrophages, and this process was not blocked by anti-TGF-β antibodies. M. D. T. Carvalho and colleagues investigated risk markers of L. infantum visceral leishmaniasis and found that lipoprotein and triglyceride levels are risk factors for development of visceral leishmaniasis. They also found that genetic polymorphisms at the Lpl and Pparγ were associated with differential levels of lipoproteins and thus related to the disease outcome. I. Naouar and coworkers investigated granzyme-positive CD4+ T cells activated by L. major antigens, in Leishmania-healed subjects. They found that even CD4+CD25+CD127$^{dim/-}$ Tregs expressed granzyme after exposure to Leishmania antigens.

A number of manuscripts published in this issue provide important new knowledge in the important field of malaria. A review from H. Zheng and colleagues highlighted important aspects of preerythrocytic stages biology and the immune evasion strategies of malaria parasites. The unraveling of these escape mechanisms may aid the development of a vaccine against malaria. In this same direction, the manuscript by the group of J. Huang and colleagues generated a new mouse model to study the immunity to these preerythrocytic stages. This new model employed transgenic MHC-I Kd mice. The results of their studies indicate that protective antimalaria immunity induced by radiation-attenuated sporozoites of Plasmodium yoelii in MHC-I-Kd-Tg mice is mediated by CS protein-specific, Kd-restricted CD8+ T cells. E. S. Fernandes and colleagues studied the effect of TRPV1 antagonism by capsazepine during mouse infection with Plasmodium berghei ANKA. Their result indicated that there was a modulation of the innate immune response in mice infected but it did not affect parasitemia. Two other studies dealt with malaria pathogenesis. L. S. Ortolan and coworkers described new predictive criteria to study the pathogenesis of malaria-2 associated ali/ards in mice. This method for accurately identifying mice suffering from ALI/ARDS before death will allow the use of this model to study the pathogenesis of this disease. Finally, J. C. Sánchez-Arcila and colleagues evaluated whether intestinal parasites coinfection would alter plasma cytokines profile elicited in acute malaria in subjects from endemic area of Brazil. They concluded that the infection with intestinal parasites (mainly protozoan) does not significantly modify the pattern of cytokine production in individuals infected with P. falciparum and P. vivax.

Finally, A. S. Machado and colleagues investigated the immunopathogenesis of toxoplasmosis in parturients and nonpregnant women. They measured the synthesis of Th1 and Th2 cytokines by mononuclear cells after culture with live T. gondii and identified Th17 (CD4+) and Tc17 (CD8+) cells in toxoplasma-seronegative and toxoplasma-seropositive parturient and nonpregnant women. They observed a lower level of IL-17-expressing CD4+ and CD8+ T lymphocytes in cultures of cells from seronegative and seropositive parturient and nonpregnant women that were stimulated with tachyzoites. It has been shown that the cytokine pattern and IL-17-expressing CD4+ and CD8+ T lymphocytes may have important roles in the inflammatory response to T. gondii, thus contributing to the maintenance of pregnancy and control of parasite invasion and replication. A. S. Machado and coworkers studied immunological and hematological biomarkers of ocular congenital toxoplasmosis in infants, finding differential immune parameter networks in each clinical group (active and cicatricial ocular toxoplasmosis).

CHAPTER 43 IMMUNITY TO PROTOZOAN PARASITES

Marcela F. Lopes, Dario S. Zamboni, Hugo D. Lujan and Mauricio M. Rodrigues

Protozoan parasites cause several diseases, such as Malaria, Leishmaniasis, and Trypanosomiasis, hampering human development worldwide. Many protozoa cause infections that often follow chronic courses, owing to coevolution between parasites and host immune system. The survival and transmission of pathogenic protozoa depends on their ability to evade or subvert host's innate and adaptive immune responses. A great challenge to research in immunology and parasitology is the development of strategies that favor immunity against protozoan parasites and prevent their evasion, chronic, or recurrent infections and associated pathologies. This special issue includes original papers and reviews that summarize current advances in our understanding on the mechanisms of immunity to protozoan parasites in humans and experimental animal models.

The discovery of pattern recognition receptors (PRRs) devoted to detection of pathogen- or microbe-associated molecular patterns (PAMPs/MAMPs) fostered a vibrant research in the past decade, identifying new receptors, new ligands on pathogens, and key signaling pathways inducing innate immunity [1–3]. Therefore, it is not surprising that about 70% of the papers published here deal with early steps of immune responses to protozoan infections, including the role of parasite products, host receptors, molecular mechanisms, and effector cells of innate immune system.

Four papers of this special issue discuss molecules present at initial encounter between hosts and protozoan parasites plus the secretions of their insect vectors. Macrophage migration inhibitory factor (MIF, "Macrophage migration inhibitory factor in protozoan infections") is a host inflammatory cytokine with protective or pathogenic actions in distinct protozoan infections. Interestingly, parasites also express their own MIFs, a relevant finding that deserves further investigation. During transmission of Trypanosoma cruzi, lysophosphatidylcholine (LPC, "Lysophosphatidylcholine: a novel modulator of Trypanosoma cruzi transmission") is introduced with vector's secretions and recruits host cells, promoting infection. Apoptotic cells also express LPC among other "find me" and "eat me" signals that favor their clearance by professional phagocytes. As described elsewhere, interactions between apoptotic cells and T. cruzi-infected macrophages induce intracellular parasite replication [4]. Similarly, Leishmania amazonensis parasites express phosphatidylserine (PS, "Subversion of immunity by Leishmania amazonensis parasites: possible role of phosphatidylserine as a main regulator"), mimicking apoptotic cells to inhibit host cell activation and exacerbate infection. In "New insights on the inflammatory role of Lutzomyia longipalpis saliva in Leishmaniasis", the authors discuss how immunization against vector's saliva components might help development of a new approach to prevent Leishmaniasis. Further research will be required to define target antigens involved in distinct biological activities of vector's saliva for novel vaccines against Leishmania spp. infections.

Another four papers review the role of Toll-like receptors (TLRs) on immunity to parasitic infections, their ligands, and how this knowledge can be translated into PAMP-based adjuvants for novel vaccine strategies. Authors present what we have learnt from experiments performed in mice defective in one or multiple TLRs or key signaling molecules to gain insight into their role on immunity triggered by protozoan PAMPs, with emphasis on T. cruzi and Leishmania infections. Other PRRs, such as Nod-like receptors (NLR), only recently came into spotlight in immunity to protozoan parasites [5]. Lack of putative PRRs not only affects innate immunity, but also the development of certain adaptive immune responses, presumably due to their role on antigen-presenting dendritic

Citation: Marcela F. Lopes, Dario S. Zamboni, Hugo D. Lujan, and Mauricio M. Rodrigues, "Immunity to Protozoan Parasites," Journal of Parasitology Research, vol. 2012, Article ID 250793, 3 pages, 2012. doi:10.1155/2012/250793.

cells (DCs). This is particularly relevant for new vaccine approaches aiming at inducing memory T cells against intracellular protozoan infections (The immune response to Trypanosoma cruzi: role of toll-like receptors and perspectives for vaccine development). Whereas protozoan PAMPs activate innate immunity through TLR-induced signaling pathways, other molecules, such as lipophosphoglycan (LPG, "Innate immune activation and subversion of mammalian functions by Leishmania lipophosphoglycan"), subvert the immune responses, allowing parasite escape (Toll-like receptors in Leishmania infections: guardians or promoters). Furthermore, detection of protozoan PAMPs by immune and target tissue cells can induce protective, regulatory, or even pathogenic reactions upon infection (Nonimmune cells contribute to crosstalk between immune cells and inflammatory mediators in the innate response to Trypanosoma cruzi infection). How responses to stress occur in pathogenic protozoa and host tissues has been a topic of increasing interest for development of drugs to treat parasitic diseases [6].

There are also three papers that address the major effector cells in innate immunity to protozoan parasites: neutrophils, macrophages, dendritic cells, and their arsenal of effector molecules. Lately, monocytes were also imputed as major effector and regulatory players against protozoan parasites [7, 8]. ETosis was recently described in neutrophils as a death process leading to extrusion of antimicrobial DNA traps, which can also be triggered by and act on protozoan parasites (ETosis: a microbicidal mechanism beyond cell death). In "Reactive oxygen species and nitric oxide in cutaneous Leishmaniasis", the authors describe effector molecules expressed by phagocytes and subsets of macrophages, with protective or regulatory roles in protozoan infections. In "The role of vitamin D and vitamin D receptor in immunity to Leishmania major infection", the authors take advantage of deficiency in vitamin D receptor to show that vitamin D controls susceptibility to Leishmania major infection in resistant, but not susceptible mice. Vitamin D receptor signaling seems to inhibit the ability of DCs both as effector cells and as promoters of Th1-protective adaptive immunity.

In four papers of this issue, the authors approach the role of adaptive immunity in both protection and pathogenesis of protozoan infections. "Thymus atrophy and double positive escape are common features in infectious diseases" and "B cell response during protozoan parasite infections" discuss how protozoan parasites negatively affect development and modulate functions of T and B lymphocytes in cellular and humoral responses to infections. In "Evidence for T cell help in the IgG response against tandemly repetitive Trypanosoma cruzi B13 protein in chronic Chagas disease patients", authors investigated how the cooperation between T and B cells result in humoral responses to a parasite antigen in chronic chagasic patients. In "Comparison of protective immune responses to apicomplexan parasites", the researchers focus on the immune responses to apicomplexan protozoa, including Plasmodium, Toxoplasma, and Cryptosporidium. They also discuss issues such as antigenic variation that precludes development of conventional or transmission vaccines against these infections. Recently, disruption of the mechanism of antigenic variation in the protozoan Giardia lamblia, which is regulated posttranscriptionally by an RNA interference-like mechanism [9], allowed the formulation of an effective vaccine against this intestinal parasite [10].

In another paper, the researchers propose a mathematical model to predict Malaria transmission in endemic areas under drug pressure, taking into account induction of relapses by Plasmodium vivax infection, which confer the ability to boost adaptive immunity and prevent clinical Malaria.

Hopefully, the strong body of information available in this special issue will facilitate research on new mechanisms of immunity as well as the development of novel vaccine and immunotherapeutic tools against parasitic diseases, which are some of the most deadly human infections.

REFERENCES

1. B. Lemaitre, E. Nicolas, L. Michaut, J. M. Reichhart, and J. A. Hoffmann, "The dorsoventral regulatory gene cassette spatzle/Toll/Cactus controls the potent antifungal response in Drosophila adults," Cell, vol. 86, no. 6, pp. 973–983, 1996.
2. R. Medzhitov, P. Preston-Hurlburt, and C. A. Janeway Jr., "A human homologue of the Drosophila toll protein signals activation of adaptive immunity," Nature, vol. 388, no. 6640, pp. 394–397, 1997.
3. A. Poltorak, X. He, I. Smirnova et al., "Defective LPS signaling in C3H/HeJ and C57BL/10ScCr mice: mutations in Tlr4 gene," Science, vol. 282, no. 5396, pp. 2085–2088, 1998.
4. C. G. Freire-De-Lima, D. O. Nascimento, M. B. P. Soares et al., "Uptake of apoptotic cells drives the growth of a pathogenic trypanosome in macrophages," Nature, vol. 403, no. 6766, pp. 199–203, 2000.
5. G. K. Silva, F. R. S. Gutierrez, P. M. M. Guedes et al., "Cutting edge: nucleotide-binding oligomerization domain 1-dependent responses account for murine resistance against Trypanosoma cruzi infection,"Journal of Immunology, vol. 184, no. 3, pp. 1148–1152, 2010.
6. A. Ferreira, I. Marguti, I. Bechmann et al., "Sickle hemoglobin confers tolerance to Plasmodiuminfection," Cell, vol. 145, no. 3, pp. 398–409, 2011.
7. R. Goncalves, X. Zhang, H. Cohen, A. Debrabant, and D. M. Mosser, "Platelet activation attracts a subpopulation of effector monocytes to sites of Leishmania major infection," Journal of Experimental Medicine, vol. 208, no. 6, pp. 1253–1265, 2011.
8. W. F. Pereira, F. L. Ribeiro-Gomes, L. V. C. Guillermo et al., "Myeloid-derived suppressor cells help protective immunity to Leishmania major infection despite suppressed T cell responses," Journal of Leukocyte Biology, vol. 90, no. 6, pp. 1191–1197, 2011.
9. C. G. Prucca, I. Slavin, R. Quiroga et al., "Antigenic variation in Giardia lamblia is regulated by RNA interference," Nature, vol. 456, no. 7223, pp. 750–754, 2008.
10. F. D. Rivero, A. Saura, C. G. Prucca, P. G. Carranza, A. Torri, and H. D. Lujan, "Disruption of antigenic variation is crucial for effective parasite vaccine," Nature Medicine, vol. 16, no. 5, pp. 551–557, 2010.

CHAPTER 44

IMMUNOLOGY AND MOLECULAR BIOLOGY OF PROTOZOAN INFECTIONS

Ali Ouaissi

The protozoan parasites, which cause important diseases affecting million of people worldwide especially in the tropical and subtropical areas, are responsible for high mortality and morbidity. Most of these parasites are transmitted by insect vectors and invade a range of different tissues in their mammalian hosts. Prophylactic and therapeutic strategies are far from satisfactory. Indeed, although significant progress has been made in our understanding of the immune response to parasites, no definitive step has yet been successfully done in terms of operational vaccines against parasitic diseases. Moreover, some drugs are available, but there are concerns over their effectiveness, toxicity, and emergence of resistant strains.

An acquired immune response is the expected outcome of invasion by any living foreign organism, yet in many hosts the parasites are able to survive for long periods and most of the host-parasite systems explored demonstrated their own peculiarities to reach this equilibrium.

In this issue of the Journal of Biomedicine and Biotechnology, functional lessons learned from a number of parasitic models: (Malaria, leishmaniasis, Chagas'disease, and toxoplasmosis) have been gathered. Analysis of plasmodium falciparum parasitized red blood cells cytoadherence to host cell receptors, a key step in the progression of parasitic infection, revealed that in the case of pregnancy-associated malaria (PAM), *P. falciparum* isolates from infected pregnant women and children have distinct adhesive and antigenic properties from that of parasites causing cerebral malaria. This strengthened the possibility that antigens expressed by parasites causing PAM could be potential targets for vaccine development. Furthermore, recent advances in DNA vaccines against protozoan parasites especially Leishmania and Trypanosoma cruzi have been reviewed in this special issue. The parasite and their released products elicit a complex series of cellular interactions leading to the activation/inhibition of the host immune system. This relies on ligand (s)-receptor (s) association among which CD40/CD40L costimulatory signaling, induction of immune cells such as dendritic cells, macrophages and T and B lymphocytes producing themselves various cytokines: IL-10, IL-12, IL-23, IL-27, IL-17, among others which create a microenvironment that may promote the development of defined Th cells. The balance between cytokine producing Th cells will determine the outcome of parasitic infection. This up-to-date information has been discussed in terms of physiological processes and therapeutic implications. The contributors convey both the state of the art and the direction of future studies in this particular area of research.

ACKNOWLEDGMENTS

As an Editor, I express my gratitude to the contributing authors as well as to the Editor-in-Chief, Dr. Abdelali Haoudi, for the opportunity provided by the Journal of Biomedicine and Biotechnology to present to the scientific community various facets of protozoan parasites-host interplay.

Citation: Ali Ouaissi, "Immunology and Molecular Biology of Protozoan Infections," Journal of Biomedicine and Biotechnology, vol. 2007, Article ID 67210, 1 pages, 2007. doi:10.1155/2007/67210.

SECTION XIII: PARASITE VACCINES

CHAPTER 45

TOXOPLASMA RHOPTRIES: UNIQUE SECRETORY ORGANELLES AND SOURCE OF PROMISING VACCINE PROTEINS FOR IMMUNOPREVENTION OF TOXOPLASMOSIS

Henryka Dlugonska

INTRODUCTION

Toxoplasma gondii is arguably the most successful protozoan parasite on earth. It infects humans and many species of endothermic animals with a great infection rate, achieving nearly 100% in some local populations [1]. The course, symptoms, and consequences of T. gondii infection depend strongly on the virulence and inoculum size of the parasite and the genetic background and immune status of the infected host. In general, most postnatal cases of toxoplasmosis are mild and subclinical, with lifelong persistence of the parasite in the host. However, in immunosuppressed beings, both primary infection and reactivation of chronic infection could occur very serious, causing even death. Primary infection acquired during pregnancy can lead to an abortion and neonatal malformations. Unfortunately, despite many efforts there are no satisfactory immunoprevention methods against toxoplasmosis. The only accepted vaccine against toxoplasmosis (Toxovax, Ovilis Toxovac) contains live tachyzoites of incomplete nonpersistent S48 strain and is used to prevent congenital toxoplasmosis in sheep. The vaccine causes a decrease in abortion cases frequency but not complete eradication of the parasite [2].

Citation: Henryka Dlugonska, "Toxoplasma Rhoptries: Unique Secretory Organelles and Source of Promising Vaccine Proteins for Immunoprevention of Toxoplasmosis," Journal of Biomedicine and Biotechnology, vol. 2008, Article ID 632424, 7 pages, 2008. doi:10.1155/2008/632424.

TOXOPLASMA GONDII: OBLIGATE INTRACELLULAR APICOMPLEXAN PARASITE

Successful parasitism by T. gondii is based on its ability to form within the host cell a replication permissive niche—parasitophorous vacuole (PV). This growing niche is delimited from the host cell cytoplasm by PV membrane (PVM), a unique and dynamic "organelle" found only in infected cells which prevents T. gondiidegradation by the host cell endocytic machinery and enables parasite's intracellular propagation. Unique to the apicomplexan protozoa including Toxoplasma gondii are also three types of electrodense secretory organelles: micronemes, rhoptries, and dense granules, carrying their characteristic proteins: MICs, RONs, ROPs, and GRAs, respectively; see Table 1. Host cell invasion is mediated by the sequential secretion of the contents of all three organelles, which are exocytosed at the apical region when the parasite invades the host cell. The processes, critical in the establishment of a productive infection, are highly regulated at possibly two levels: physical separation of exocytosis sites in the parasite's plasma membrane and different trigger mechanisms [3,4]. Micronemes are involved in the attachment and penetration of T. gondii, while rhoptries are required for creating a transient enigmatic structure, moving junction and then the establishment of PV. Host cell entry of the parasite is completed in 15–20 seconds [5, 6]. Dense granules secrete proteins throughout most of the parasite stages. The secretion process coincides with the formation of intravacuolar network and continues during the intracellular residence of T. gondii [3, 4].

Table 1: The participation of secretory organelles proteins in the invasion of the host cell by protozoan Toxoplasma gondii; PV: parasitophorous vacuole, MICs: micronemes proteins, TgAMA1: T. gondii apical membrane antigen 1, RONs: rhoptry neck proteins, ROPs: rhoptry proteins, GRAs: dense granule proteins.

Invasion stage	Secretory organelles/*secretion process* secreted proteins
Adhesion	Micronemes/*transient* TgAMA1,TgMICs etc.
Biogenesis of moving junction, PV and its association with host mitochondria and endoplasmic reticulum	Rhoptries/*transient* RONs, ROPs
Formation of the specific architecture and function of PV	Dense granules/*continuous* GRAs

RHOPTRIES AND RHOPTRIES PROTEINS

Unlike most secretory and lysosomal granules in mammalian cells, which are of a semispheroidal shape, the mature rhoptries are club shaped with a bulbous base and an extended duct (neck), connected to the extreme apical pole of the parasite. The rhoptries in the number of 8–12 per cell occupy 10–30% of the total cell volume. They are the only known acidified organelles in T. gondii; pH of immature rhoptries is 3.5–5.5 and of mature rhoptries is 5.0–7.0 [7]. Most probably each mature rhoptry originates from a separate immature rhoptry [8].

Current findings suggest that rhoptries are most analogous to secretory lysosomal granules because they receive material from both biosynthetic and endocytic cell pathways. In the exit site of endoplasmic reticulum, the rhoptry proteins (in a form of proproteins) are loaded into coated vesicles and then travel to the Golgi apparatus where they are sorted to an immature rhoptry using the specific sorting signals [9]. Both tyrosine-based and dileucine sorting motifs were detected within cytoplasmic tails of the predominant ROP2 family proteins [10]. Proproteins undergo proteolytic cleavage of an N-terminal prodomain, which occurs in post-Golgi compartment, probably in immature rhoptries [11]. In contrast to all known prominent ROP2 family members, a new described ROP5 protein is not processed during trafficking but is synthesized in the mature form [12]. Some rhoptry cargo is delivered by endosomal pathway via multivesicular body and immature rhoptry [9]. Immature rhoptries evolve into mature rhoptries characterized by specific morphology and subcompartmentalization of their contents: ROP proteins are located in the bulb body whereas RONs in the neck of the rhoptry [13].

A proteomic analysis revealed over 30 rhoptry proteins, all localized in the contents of the rhoptries, although many of the identified proteins have putative transmembrane domains [13]. As shown for ROP2, a prototype protein of ROP2 protein family, apart from an N-terminal signal sequence, the molecule is characterized by the high abundance of charged amino acids and proline residues, N- terminal arginine-rich stretches and hydrophobic sequence in C-terminus considered as transmembrane domain [14, 15]. The ROP2 protein was shown to be inserted in PVM during the invasion of a host cell and its N-terminal domain is exposed to host cytosol [14] mediating the association of parasitophorous vacuole with host cell mitochondria [14, 16]. Targeted depletion of ROP2 resulted in multiple effects, such as: (i) impairments of rhoptry biogenesis and cytokinesis, (ii) reduction in the association of host cell mitochondria with PVM of the parasite, and a reduced sterol uptake from the host cell, and (iii) reduced capacity to invade and replicate in vitro in human fibroblasts and attenuation of virulence in mice [17]. Besides, anti-ROP2 antibodies caused a decrease in the invasion ability of T. gondii RH tachyzoites in vitro [18]. The observed effects of ROP2 depletion or inactivation and simultaneous synthesis of several related proteins (ROP2 family) suggest that they serve crucial biological functions. All members of the ROP2 family contain a protein kinase-like domain but only some of them are catalytically active [15]. The exocytosis of rhoptry contents coincides with the formation of PV but the biological trigger of rhoptry secretion has not been identified. Mobilization of intracellular Ca^{2+} by ionophores triggers the discharge of micronemes but not rhoptries and dense granules [19]. In contrast to other secretory organelles, rhoptry proteins and lipids are exocytosed through the duct, whereas delimiting membrane is retained in the cell and the rhoptry is transiently empty. Secreted rhoptry proteins are subsequently discharged into nascent parasitophorous vacuole and localized in its membrane [14, 20].

As mentioned earlier, certain rhoptry proteins are preferentially localized in the neck of the rhoptry. During invasion, RON4 relocalizes at the moving junction and participates in the formation of this short living and very enigmatic structure between the host cell and the parasite, sliding over the parasite as it invades [21]. RON4, RON2, and RON5 (Ts4705) form protein trio that associates with adhesion microneme protein TgAMA1 (T. gondii apical membrane protein 1) forming an unusual complex derived from two distinct secretory organelles: rhoptries and micronemes [22]. Moving junction functions as a molecular sieve for the quick selective sorting of parasite surface components (like RONs-TgAMA1 complex mentioned above) as well as surface proteins of the host cell. Because of the exclusion of most host cell membrane proteins, developing parasitophorous vacuole is not recognized by the host cell fusogenic machinery enabling the vigorous parasite proliferation in this safe intracellular compartment [5, 23].

VIRULENCE OF T. GONDII AND NEW DESCRIBED RHOPTRY ANTIGENS AS MAJOR VIRULENCE COMPONENTS

Despite the very high genetic homology achieving ~98%, T. gondii strains express dramatic differences in many phenotype aspects, including virulence. The majority of T. gondii isolates from Europe and North America belong to three clonal lines (types) significantly differing in their virulence, which has been well characterized in the mouse model. Type I isolates have an LD100 of a single organism and lead to rapid death of the infected mice (6–10 days), whereas types II and III (called nonvirulent or avirulent) typically have LD100 of $\geq 10^3$ organisms; mice which survive acute phase of toxoplasmosis remain chronically infected and highly seropositive [24].

Dramatic differences in acute virulence between three major types of T. gondii enabled the mapping of virulence genes by an analysis of F1 progeny from genetic crosses between three toxoplasma types, using an experimental mouse model to test virulence. The method applied to types I×III recombinants revealed first two closely adjacent virulence loci on parasite chromosome VIIa and then single gene encoding ROP18 protein as a major virulence component. Type III and type I alleles of ROP18 differed significantly in nucleotide sequence and expression level. The contribution of ROP18 to virulence was confirmed by the transfection of the virulent ROP18 allele into nonpathogenic type III parasite strain. The obtained transformants showed an increased growth rate in vitro and an enhanced mortality by 4 to 5 logs in CD1 mice, as compared to wild nontransformed strain [25]. Saeij et al. [26] mapped virulence in F1 progeny derived from crosses between type II and type III strains. Five virulence loci were identified, and two of them coded rhoptry proteins: ROP18 and ROP16, both hypervariable protein kinases that are responsible for the high virulence of certain strains of the parasite. Contrary to ROP2 and several other members of this family that lost detectable kinase activity [15] and retained "molecular fossils" [27], newly described rhoptry proteins ROP16 and ROP18 are true kinases, the substrates of which are unknown. Both kinases presumably disrupt some signaling processes and alter intracellular environment in a way that favors parasite growth. The work of El Hajj et al. [28] brought many interesting data on ROP18. The protein showed a very strong tropism to PVM and during the invasion it was translocated from rhoptry to PVM. The mature recombinant ROP18 was able to phosphorylate two as yet unknown parasite's (but not host's) proteins, a major one of 70 kDa and a minor one of 68 kDa. The overexpression of ROP18 protein promoted dramatically parasite's proliferation, whereas the mutation (D394A) in ROP18 molecule resulted in the loss of both the enzyme activity and accelerated growth. In contrast to ROP18, the second recently described rhoptry protein, ROP16 is translocated to the host cell nucleus like phosphatase 2C [29], subverts STAT3/6 signaling, and, in consequence, IL-12 production in infected host cells. Allele shared by types I and III of the parasite induce prolonged phosphorylation of STAT3 (STAT3-PO_4) which results in a much lower level of IL-12 secretion, as compared to type II allele [30]. The observed type-specific effects show the key role of ROP kinases in T. gondii virulence and could explain different disease outcomes seen with type I, II, and III strains. The role of ROPs in virulence suggests that they could be promising vaccine candidates against toxoplasmosis.

In contrast to ROP18 and ROP16, another novel rhoptry protein, bradyzoite rhoptry protein 1 (BRP1), is expressed in bradyzoites but absent from tachyzoites. Bradyzoites are a low-replicating, inactive developmental stage, sequestered in tissue cysts, which are a typical marker of chronic toxoplasmosis. The biological function of BRP1 is not defined yet. This protein does not play an essential role in the development of the bradyzoite stage, brain cyst formation, and oral infection of new hosts [31].

IMMUNOPROPHYLAXIS OF TOXOPLASMOSIS

As mentioned earlier, the only vaccine against toxoplasmosis has been licensed for use in sheep in Europe and New Zealand [2]. This conventional vaccine contains live attenuated tachyzoites of the nonpersistent T. gondiiS48 strain and it cannot be considered for an application in humans because of the risk of reverting to tissue cyst formation. From both humanitarian and economic points of views, an effective anti-T. gondii vaccine(s) for humans and animals is still strongly desired. Taking into account the main sources and transmission routes ofT. gondii, host groups of a particularly high infection risk and consequences of congenital infection, as well as postnatal infections in immunocompromised individuals, targets for vaccination strategy should include (i) preventing tissue cyst formation in consumption animals (to avoid parasite transmission to humans and animals) and in people (to protect against reactivation of infection in immunosuppression state of persistently infected individuals), (ii) reducing oocyst shedding in cats (to limit environmental contamination and infection risk for all intermediate hosts), and (iii) preventing development of parasitemia in pregnant women and farm livestock (to avoid transplacental transmission to the fetus and congenital toxoplasmosis) [32].

Vaccine candidates should induce protective cellular TH1 and humoral responses as well, both at the level of intestinal mucosa (local) and whole organism (systemic). Many studies have shown that protective immunity toT. gondii is characterized by the development of cell-mediated immunity dominated by the production of IFN-γby T lymphocytes (a TH1 type response). Whereas immune CD8+ lymphocytes are cytotoxic for T. gondii-infected host cells, CD4+ lymphocytes exert their protective activity primarily by the production of many proinflammatory cytokines (IFN-γ, TNF-α, IL-12) and providing growth factor, IL-2. Specific antibodies limit multiplication of T. gondii by killing of extracellular tachyzoites, either by activating complement, or opsonizing the parasites for phagocytosis and next killing by macrophages [33]. The major challenge in novel vaccine construction is a selection of relevant T. gondii antigens and then their presentation to host immune system in an appropriate manner to induce strong and long-lasting protective immunity. Because of the complex life cycle of the parasite, the expression of numerous common and stage-dependent antigenic epitopes and host-dependent immune responses, the vaccination with multiantigen preparation comprising antigens from different life cycle stages is likely to be more efficacious than with a single antigen. Previous and current vaccine approaches focus not only on classic formulations (live attenuated or mutant T. gondii strains) [2, 34, 35] but more often on the defined subcellular components of the parasite such as biosynthetic (recombinant) antigens [36] and naked T. gondii DNA [37] or RNA [38]. Nonpathogenic recombinant microorganisms with the expression of immunoprotective antigens of T. gondii (live vector vaccines) [39] and synthetic peptides have also been tested as interesting antitoxoplasmic vaccine alternatives [40]. These new generation subunit vaccines require an addition of potent adjuvants enhancing the intensity of the immune response and inducing the desired TH1 profile. Several new compounds, for instance unmetylated CpG nucleotides, present satisfactory adjuvant TH1 activity [41].

RHOPTRY ANTIGENS AS A POTENTIAL VACCINE AGAINST TOXOPLASMOSIS

Most of the current vaccine candidates for T. gondii and other apicomplexa are either surface or secreted antigens that appear to be essential for the invasion process, rhoptry proteins among them. Until now several rhoptry proteins of T. gondii have been tested as vaccines. Garcia et al. [42] used crude native rhoptry antigens incorporated in the immunostimulating complexes (ISCOMs) to protect pigs against an infection with oocysts of T. gondii VEG strain (of type III). Two-fold subcutaneous immunization procedure led to a partial protection against cysts formation in muscles and brain during chronic infection (as confirmed by bioassay in mice) but it was not protective against acute infection, probably because of the lack of intestinal immunity after subcutaneous immunization. Taking into account epidemiological role of cats as an important source of T. gondii dissemination by shedding millions of oocysts in feces, the authors tested the same antigen material in domestic cats [43]. The cats were immunized intranasally three times (0, 21, 42 day) with crude rhoptry proteins adjuvanted with Quil-A and then challenged with tissue cysts of the T. gondii VEG strain. This vaccination procedure resulted in a partial protection only—two from three immunized cats did not shed oocysts.

Till now vaccine trials with individual ROPs of T. gondii have mostly focused on the ROP2 antigen, prominent member of ROP2 protein family. In majority, the experiments were performed with DNA vaccines which are believed to elicit a predominant TH1 response. Vercammen [44] showed that the immunization with ROP2 gene protected mice against lethal challenge with a highly virulent RH strain, but the observed protection was mouse strain dependent—inbred C3H mice were protected, whereas C57BL/6 and BALB/c were not.

Similar results were obtained by Leyva et al. [45] in mice of three inbred strains (CBA/J, C57BL/6, and BALB/c), vaccinated with plasmid encoding antigen ROP2. The mice did not resist a challenge with RH strain but the protection was achieved by vaccination with live tachyzoites of the T. gondii nonpersistent thermosensitive ts-4 strain. In the mice immunized with ROP2-plasmid, a mixed TH1/TH2 immune profile instead of a desirable TH1 profile and a significant variability in the response between individual mice was observed. Using similar vaccine material, that is, ROP2-plasmid, Wei et al. [46] reported both a high immune response and significant immunoprotection against a lethal dose of T. gondii RH strain in BALB/c mice.

Recently, live nonpathogenic microbes (viruses or bacteria) were used as vectors of selected ROP genes. Recombinant vaccinia virus carrying ROP2 gene induced in mice a specific humoral response very similar, in intensity and profile, to the thermosensitive ts-4 strain of T. gondii. Because the ts-4 strain as vaccine was able to fully protect mice against the challenge with the highly virulent RH strain, the authors conclude by analogy that ROP2-vaccinia virus could be equally effective in toxoplasmosis immunoprotection [47]. Mishima et al. [18] obtained recombinant feline herpesvirus 1 (FHV1) encoding ROP2 and evaluated its ability to induce antitoxoplasmic activity and protective immune responses. Antisera of ROP2-FHV1-immunized cats reduced significantly the invasion capacity of T. gondii RH tachyzoites in vitro. The number of parasites in the brains of immunized cats lowered, however oocyst shedding intensity was not reduced. Recently, Wang et al. [48] tested the efficacy of recombinant Mycobacterium bovis BCG expressing ROP2 gene as a vaccine, using mouse experimental toxoplasmosis model. BCG, widely applied in immunoprophylaxis of tuberculosis, is a particularly attractive vector for delivering heterologous antigens because mycobacteria elicit TH1-mediated immune response without an additional adjuvant [49]. Vaccine ROP2-BCG induced strong specific humoral and cellular (IL-2 and IFN-γ in supernatants of splenocytes cell cultures) immunity. A significant delay in mortality after the infection with the highly virulent RH strain was also observed [48].

The use of recombinant ROP2 antigen, instead of ROP2-plasmid, revealed again in mouse experimental model that the protective activity of ROP2 protein is mouse strain-dependent; ROP2 vaccination resulted in the partial protection (decrease in tissue cyst burden) only in C3H mice but not C57BL/6 mice [50]. The efficacy of ROP2 protein vaccine significantly increased by including new immunostimulatory components, Leishmania infantum heat shock protein 83 (Hsp83) fused with the ROP2 [51]. Immunization with this fusion protein elicited a predominant TH1 response in all mouse strains used (BALB/c, C57Bl/6, and C3H), whereas ROP2 alone or in mixture with Hsp83 induced a mixed TH1/TH2 profile.

Multiple endogenous and exogenous parameters can influence the type and intensity of vaccine-induced immune response. The results obtained on inbred mouse strains proved that the protection induced by ROP2 and other vaccine antigens of T. gondii is strongly dependent on the host genetic background [43, 50, 52]. In relation to the vaccine itself, the composition seems a very important factor in the context of both selected ROP antigens and adjuvants used. In the light of our current knowledge on rhoptry antigens, ROP18 protein, described recently as a major component of pathogenicity of T. gondii, seems a very promising candidate for a vaccine, as a single antigen or, more possibly, accompanied by other T. gondii antigens because many previous studies showed greater effectiveness of combined than single-antigen vaccines. However, the usefulness of ROP18 as a vaccine antigen for toxoplasmosis needs to be experimentally confirmed, especially in relation to the polymorphism of this protein. Whether protection across T. gondii species could be achieved with that polymorphic antigen remains an open question.

The advantages of combined vaccines as compared to single-antigen vaccines were recently emphasized by Zhang et al. [53] who constructed a multiantigenic DNA vaccine consisting of plasmid encoding both ROP2 and surface antigen 1 (SAG1) antigens and inoculated it to BALB/c mice with or without plasmid encoding murine IL-12. Multiantigenic (cocktail) vaccine elicited stronger antibody and cellular responses than single-gene vaccines and, additionally, coimmunization with IL-12 gene significantly enhanced the intensity of immune responses. The most immunostimulating vaccine, pSAG1+ROP2+pIL-12, delayed about three times the survival time of mice after a lethal challenge with RH tachyzoites. As found by Guo et al. [54] another genetic adjuvant, plasmid carrying IFN-γ, revealed also a potent stimulatory activity, enhancing the cellular immune response induced in mice by ROP1-plasmid.

In summary, all the above presented experimental vaccination strategies with ROP antigens still remain suboptimal but the vaccination results appear promising and therefore future research on ROP vaccine seems rational.

CONCLUDING REMARKS

Toxoplasmosis, widely dispersed in the populations of humans and endothermic animals all over the world, is a serious problem of human and veterinary medicine in the case of immunocompromised individuals (fetuses, AIDS patients, etc.). The consequences of primary infection in pregnant females and the possibility of reactivation of latent infection in immunodepressed individuals cause that both immunoprophylactic and immunotherapeutic vaccines are needed. Natural infection with Toxoplasma leads to strong, lifelong nonsterile protective immunity. The persistence of the memory T lymphocytes, stimulated by the regular rupture of T. gondii tissue cysts or by recurrent contact with infected food, prevents a reinfection in most individuals [33]. The effective and safe vaccine should mimic the immune response observed in natural infections and protect the hosts against T. gondii infection, however without the potential risk of tissue cyst generation in intermediate hosts and development of oocysts in cats, associated with the vaccination using live attenuated or incomplete parasite strains. In this context, for T. gondii ROP antigens as key molecules in biogenesis of parasite intracellular niche in the host cells and their association with host organelles, major virulence factors showing satisfactory immunogenicity [55] seem particularly valuable vaccine candidates for toxoplasmosis prophylactic approaches but their vaccine potential needs experimental confirmation. It is worth mentioning that rhoptry proteins are also vaccine candidates in other apicomplexa, including rhoptry-associated protein 1 (RAP1) and RAP2 proteins of Plasmodium falciparum [56]. Several rhoptry proteins are polymorphic, with T and B epitopes that are conserved among strains but not across species and over species, as found for instance forPlasmodium [57] and Eimeria [58]. The question, if it would be possible to construct universal anti-T. gondiivaccine, independent of the host and vaccination target, remains open. The results of the studies on ROP-vaccine presented in this paper are promising and could be a good starting point to develop an effective vaccine not only for the prevention of toxoplasmosis but also other parasitoses caused by apicomplexan protozoa. Recent advances in bioinformatics and experimental tools will make the selection of vaccine candidates easier.

ACKNOWLEDGMENT

The article was supported by Grant N N302 3196 33 of the Ministry of Science and Higher Education in Poland.

REFERENCES

1. A. M. Tenter, A. R. Heckeroth, and L. M. Weiss, "Toxoplasma gondii: from animals to humans,"International Journal for Parasitology, vol. 30, no. 12-13, pp. 1217–1258, 2000.
2. D. Buxton, "Toxoplasmosis: the first commercial vaccine," Parasitology Today, vol. 9, no. 9, pp. 335–337, 1993.
3. J. F. Dubremetz, A. Achbarou, D. Bermudes, and K. A. Joiner, "Kinetics and pattern of organelle exocytosis during Toxoplasma gondii/host-cell interaction," Parasitology Research, vol. 79, no. 5, pp. 402–408, 1993.
4. V. B. Carruthers and L. D. Sibley, "Sequential protein secretion from three distinct organelles ofToxoplasma gondii accompanies invasion of human fibroblasts," European Journal of Cell Biology, vol. 73, no. 2, pp. 114–123, 1997.
5. L. D. Saffer, O. Mercereau-Puijalon, J. F. Dubremetz, and J. D. Schwartzman, "Localization of aToxoplasma gondii rhoptry protein by immunoelectron microscopy during and after host cell penetration," Journal of Protozoology, vol. 39, no. 4, pp. 526–530, 1992.
6. D. G. Mordue, N. Desai, M. Dustin, and L. D. Sibley, "Invasion by Toxoplasma gondii establishes a moving junction that selectively excludes host cell plasma membrane proteins on the basis of their membrane anchoring," Journal of Experimental Medicine, vol. 190, no. 12, pp. 1783–1792, 1999.
7. M. K. Shaw, D. S. Roos, and L. G. Tilney, "Cysteine and serine protease inhibitors block intracellular development and disrupt the secretory pathway of Toxoplasma gondii," Microbes and Infection, vol. 4, no. 2, pp. 119–132, 2002.
8. L. Pelletier, C. A. Stern, M. Pypaert, et al., "Golgi biogenesis in Toxoplasma gondii," Nature, vol. 418, no. 6897, pp. 548–552, 2002.
9. H. M. Ngô, M. Yang, and K. A. Joiner, "Are rhoptries in Apicomplexan parasites secretory granules or secretory lysosomal granules?" Molecular Microbiology, vol. 52, no. 6, pp. 1531–1541, 2004.
10. H. C. Hoppe, H. M. Ngô, M. Yang, and K. A. Joiner, "Targeting to rhoptry organelles of Toxoplasma gondii involves evolutionarily conserved mechanisms," Nature Cell Biology, vol. 2, no. 7, pp. 449–456, 2000.
11. D. Soldati, A. Lassen, J. F. Dubremetz, and J. C. Boothroyd, "Processing of Toxoplasma ROP1 protein in nascent rhoptries," Molecular and Biochemical Parasitology, vol. 96, no. 1-2, pp. 37–48, 1998.
12. H. El Hajj, M. Lebrun, M. N. Fourmaux, H. Vial, and J. F. Dubremetz, "Inverted topology of theToxoplasma gondii ROP5 rhoptry protein provides new insights into the association of the ROP2 protein family with the parasitophorous vacuole membrane," Cellular Microbiology, vol. 9, no. 1, pp. 54–64, 2007.
13. P. J. Bradley, C. Ward, S. J. Cheng, et al., "Proteomic analysis of rhoptry organelles reveals many novel constituents for host-parasite interactions in Toxoplasma gondii," Journal of Biological Chemistry, vol. 280, no. 40, pp. 34245–34258, 2005.

14. C. J. Beckers, J. F. Dubremetz, O. Mercereau-Puijalon, and K. A. Joiner, "The Toxoplasma gondii rhoptry protein ROP2 is inserted into the parasitophorous vacuole membrane, surrounding the intracellular parasite, and is exposed to the host cell cytoplasm," The Journal of Cell Biology, vol. 127, no. 4, pp. 947–961, 1994.

15. H. El Hajj, E. Demey, J. Poncet, et al., "The ROP2 family of Toxoplasma gondii rhoptry proteins: proteomic and genomic characterization and molecular modeling," Proteomics, vol. 6, no. 21, pp. 5773–5784, 2006.

16. A. P. Sinai and K. A. Joiner, "The Toxoplasma gondii protein ROP2 mediates host organelle association with the parasitophorous vacuole membrane," Journal of Cell Biology, vol. 154, no. 1, pp. 95–108, 2001. ·

17. V. Nakaar, H. M. Ngô, E. P. Aaronson, I. Coppens, T. T. Stedman, and K. A. Joiner, "Pleiotropic effect due to targeted depletion of secretory rhoptry protein ROP2 in Toxoplasma gondii," Journal of Cell Science, vol. 116, no. 11, pp. 2311–2320, 2003.

18. M. Mishima, X. Xuan, N. Yokoyama, et al., "Recombinant feline herpesvirus type 1 expressingToxoplasma gondii ROP2 antigen inducible protective immunity in cats," Parasitology Research, vol. 88, no. 2, pp. 144–149, 2002.

19. V. B. Carruthers and L. D. Sibley, "Mobilization of intracellular calcium stimulates microneme discharge in Toxoplasma gondii," Molecular Microbiology, vol. 31, no. 2, pp. 421–428, 1999.

20. K. L. Carey, A. M. Jongco, K. Kim, and G. E. Ward, "The Toxoplasma gondii rhoptry protein ROP4 is secreted into the parasitophorous vacuole and becomes phosphorylated in infected cells," Eukaryotic Cell, vol. 3, no. 5, pp. 1320–1330, 2004.

21. M. Lebrun, A. Michelin, H. El Hajj, et al., "The rhoptry neck protein RON4 relocalizes at the moving junction during Toxoplasma gondii invasion," Cellular Microbiology, vol. 7, no. 12, pp. 1823–1833, 2005. ·

22. D. L. Alexander, J. Mital, G. E. Ward, P. Bradley, and J. C. Boothroyd, "Identification of the moving junction complex of Toxoplasma gondii: a collaboration between distinct secretory organelles," PLoS Pathogens, vol. 1, no. 2, p. e17, 2005.

23. A. J. Charron and L. D. Sibley, "Molecular partitioning during host cell penetration by Toxoplasma gondii," Traffic, vol. 5, no. 11, pp. 855–867, 2004.

24. L. D. Sibley, D. G. Mordue, C. Su, P. M. Robben, and D. K. Howe, "Genetic approaches to studying virulence and pathogenesis in Toxoplasma gondii," Philosophical Transactions of the Royal Society B, vol. 357, no. 1417, pp. 81–88, 2002.

25. S. Taylor, A. Barragan, C. Su, et al., "A secreted serine-threonine kinase determines virulence in the eukaryotic pathogen Toxoplasma gondii," Science, vol. 314, no. 5806, pp. 1776–1780, 2006.

26. J. P. J. Saeij, J. P. Boyle, S. Coller, et al., "Polymorphic secreted kinases are key virulence factors in toxoplasmosis," Science, vol. 314, no. 5806, pp. 1780–1783, 2006.

27. A. P. Sinai, "The Toxoplasma kinase ROP18: an active member of a degenerate family," PLoS Pathogens, vol. 3, no. 2, p. e16, 2007.

28. H. El Hajj, M. Lebrun, S. T. Arold, H. Vial, G. Labesse, and J. F. Dubremetz, "ROP18 is a rhoptry kinase controlling the intracellular proliferation of Toxoplasma gondii," PLoS Pathogens, vol. 3, no. 2, p. e14, 2007.

29. L. A. Gilbert, S. Ravindran, J. M. Turetzky, J. C. Boothroyd, and P. J. Bradley, "Toxoplasma gondii targets a protein phosphatase 2C to the nuclei of infected host cells," Eukaryotic Cell, vol. 6, no. 1, pp. 73–83, 2007. ·

30. J. P. J. Saeij, S. Coller, J. P. Boyle, M. E. Jerome, M. W. White, and J. C. Boothroyd, "Toxoplasma co-opts host gene expression by injection of a polymorphic kinase homologue," Nature, vol. 445, no. 7125, pp. 324–327, 2007.

31. J. A. Schwarz, A. E. Fouts, C. A. Cummings, D. J. P. Ferguson, and J. C. Boothroyd, "A novel rhoptry protein in Toxoplasma gondii bradyzoites and merozoites," Molecular and Biochemical Parasitology, vol. 144, no. 2, pp. 159–166, 2005.

32. E. A. Innes and A. N. Vermeulen, "Vaccination as a control strategy against the coccidial parasitesEimeria, Toxoplasma and Neospora," Parasitology, vol. 133, supplement 2, pp. S145–S168, 2006.

33. C. A. Hunter and G. Reichmann, "Immunology of Toxoplasma infection," in Toxoplasmosis. A Comprehensive Clinical Guide, D. H. M. Joynson and T. G. Wreghitt, Eds., pp. 43–56, Cambridge University Press, Cambridge, UK, 2001.

34. J. K. Frenkel, E. R. Pfefferkorn, D. D. Smith, and J. L. Fishback, "Prospective vaccine prepared from a new mutant of Toxoplasma gondii for use in cats," American Journal of Veterinary Research, vol. 52, no. 5, pp. 759–763, 1991.

35. D. S. Lindsay, B. L. Blagburn, and J. P. Dubey, "Safety and results of challenge of weaned pigs given a temperature-sensitive mutant of Toxoplasma gondii," Journal of Parasitology, vol. 79, no. 1, pp. 71–76, 1993.

36. J. Gatkowska, A. Gasior, J. Kur, and H. Dlugonska, "Toxoplasmagondii: chimericDrfimbriaeasarecombinant vaccine against toxoplasmosis," Experimental Parasitology, vol. 118, no. 2, pp. 266–270, 2008.

37. K. N. Couper, H. V. Nielsen, E. Petersen, F. Roberts, C. W. Roberts, and J. Alexander, "DNA vaccination with the immunodominant tachyzoite surface antigen (SAG-1) protects against adult acquiredToxoplasma gondii infection but does not prevent maternofoetal transmission," Vaccine, vol. 21, no. 21-22, pp. 2813–2820, 2003.

38. I. Dimier-Poisson, F. Aline, D. Bout, and M.-N. Mévélec, "Induction of protective immunity against toxoplasmosis in mice by immunization with Toxoplasma gondii RNA," Vaccine, vol. 24, no. 10, pp. 1705–1709, 2006.

39. H. Cong, Q. M. Gu, Y. Jiang, et al., "Oral immunization with a live recombinant attenuated Salmonella typhimurium protects mice against Toxoplasma gondii," Parasite Immunology, vol. 27, no. 1-2, pp. 29–

35, 2005.

40. H. Siachoque, F. Guzman, J. Burgos, M. E. Patarroyo, and J. E. Gomez-Marin, "Toxoplasma gondii: immunogenicity and protection by P30 peptides in a murine model," Experimental Parasitology, vol. 114, no. 1, pp. 62–65, 2006.

41. J. A. Spencer, B. F. Smith, A. J. Guarino, B. L. Blagburn, and H. J. Baker, "The use of CpG as an adjuvant to Toxoplasma gondii vaccination," Parasitology Research, vol. 92, no. 4, pp. 313–316, 2004.

42. J. L. Garcia, S. M. Gennari, I. T. Navarro, et al., "Partial protection against tissue cysts formation in pigs vaccinated with crude rhoptry proteins of Toxoplasma gondii," Veterinary Parasitology, vol. 129, no. 3-4, pp. 209–217, 2005.

43. J. L. Garcia, I. T. Navarro, L. Biazzono, et al., "Protective activity against oocyst shedding in cats vaccinated with crude rhoptry proteins of the Toxoplasma gondii by the intranasal route," Veterinary Parasitology, vol. 145, no. 3-4, pp. 197–206, 2007.

44. M. Vercammen, T. Scorza, K. Huygen, et al., "DNA vaccination with genes encoding Toxoplasma gondiiantigens GRA1, GRA7, and ROP2 induces partially protective immunity against lethal challenge in mice," Infection and Immunity, vol. 68, no. 1, pp. 38–45, 2000.

45. R. Leyva, P. Hérion, and R. Saavedra, "Genetic immunization with plasmid DNA coding for the ROP2 protein of Toxoplasma gondii," Parasitology Research, vol. 87, no. 1, pp. 70–79, 2001.

46. Q. K. Wei, J. Li, T. X. Fu, et al., "Studies on the immunoprotection of ROP2 nuclei acid vaccine inToxoplasma gondii infection," Zhongguo Ji Sheng Chong Xue Yu Ji Sheng Chong Bing Za Zhi, vol. 24, no. 5, pp. 337–341, 2006.

47. J. L. Roque-ReséNdiz, R. Rosales, and P. Herion, "MVA ROP2 vaccinia virus recombinant as a vaccine candidate for toxoplasmosis," Parasitology, vol. 128, no. 4, pp. 397–405, 2004.

48. H. Wang, Q. Liu, K. Liu, et al., "Immune response induced by recombinant Mycobacterium bovis BCG expressing ROP2 gene of Toxoplasma gondii," Parasitology International, vol. 56, no. 4, pp. 263–268, 2007. ·

49. G. Dietrich, J.-F. Viret, and J. Hess, "Novel vaccination strategies based on recombinant Mycobacterium bovis BCG," International Journal of Medical Microbiology, vol. 292, no. 7-8, pp. 441–451, 2003.

50. V. Martin, A. Supanitsky, F. C. Echeverria, et al., "Recombinant GRA4 or ROP2 protein combined with alum or the gra4 gene provides partial protection in chronic murine models of toxoplasmosis," Clinical and Diagnostic Laboratory Immunology, vol. 11, no. 4, pp. 704–710, 2004.

51. P. C. Echeverria, N. de Miguel, M. Costas, and S. O. Angel, "Potent antigen-specific immunity toToxoplasma gondii in adjuvant-free vaccination system using Rop2-Leishmania infantum Hsp83 fusion protein," Vaccine, vol. 24, no. 19, pp. 4102–4110, 2006.

52. V. Letscher-Bru, A. W. Pfaff, A. Abou-Bacar, et al., "Vaccination with Toxoplasma gondii SAG-1 protein is protective against congenital toxoplasmosis in BALB/c mice but not in CBA/J mice," Infection and Immunity, vol. 71, no. 11, pp. 6615–6619, 2003.

53. J. Zhang, S. He, H. Jiang, et al., "Evaluation of the immune response induced by multiantigenic DNA vaccine encoding SAG1 and ROP2 of Toxoplasma gondii and the adjuvant properties of murine interleukin-12 plasmid in BALB/c mice," Parasitology Research, vol. 101, no. 2, pp. 331–338, 2007.

54. H. Guo, G. Chen, F. Lu, H. Chen, and H. Zheng, "Immunity induced by DNA vaccine of plasmid encoding the rhoptry protein 1 gene combined with the genetic adjuvant of pcIFN-γ against Toxoplasma gondii in mice," Chinese Medical Journal, vol. 114, no. 3, pp. 317–320, 2001 (English).

55. J. F. Dubremetz, "Rhoptries are major players in Toxoplasma gondii invasion and host cell interaction,"Cellular Microbiology, vol. 9, no. 4, pp. 841–848, 2007.

56. W. E. Collins, A. Walduck, J. S. Sullivan, et al., "Efficacy of vaccines containing rhoptry-associated proteins RAP1 and RAP2 of Plasmodium falciparum in Saimiri boliviensis monkeys," American Journal of Tropical Medicine and Hygiene, vol. 62, no. 4, pp. 466–479, 2000.

57. J.-C. Doury, S. Bonnefoy, N. Roger, J. F. Dubremetz, and O. Mercereau-Puijalon, "Analysis of the high molecular weight rhoptry complex of Plasmodium falciparum using monoclonal antibodies,"Parasitology, vol. 108, no. 3, pp. 269–280, 1994.

58. F. M. Tomley, "Characterization of rhoptry proteins of Eimeria tenella sporozoites: antigenic diversity of rhoptry epitopes within species of the genus Eimeria and among three asexual generations of a single species, E. tenella," Infection and Immunity, vol. 62, no. 10, pp. 4656–4658, 1994.

CHAPTER 46

DNA VACCINES AGAINST PROTOZOAN PARASITES: ADVANCES AND CHALLENGES

Eric Dumonteil

INTRODUCTION

In spite of the success of vaccines in public health, there are still numerous pathogens, and in particular protozoan parasites such as *Plasmodium falciparum, Trypanosoma* sp., or *Leishmania* sp. against which there are still no effective vaccine. However, the discovery that the direct injection of plasmid DNA encoding foreign proteins could lead to endogenous protein biosynthesis and a specific immune response against it opened new perspectives in vaccine development. Over 15 years later, DNA vaccines have gone from a scientific curiosity to one of the most dynamic fields of research and may offer new alternatives for the control of infectious diseases [1]. Indeed, the first two DNA vaccines have been licenced, in recent years, to protect horses from west nile virus and salmons from infectious hematopoietic necrosis virus, confirming the usefulness of this biotechnology. We review here some of the advances and challenges for the development of DNA vaccines against two well-studied protozoan parasites, *Leishmania* sp. and *Trypanosoma cruzi*. Both belong to the trypanosomatidae family and are ranked among the three major protozoan parasites affecting humans. Leishmaniasis is a complex disease caused by at least 18 species of parasites from the *Leishmania* genus and transmitted to humans by hematophagous sandflies. With an estimated 12 million cases, it has a major public health impact in several regions, and in particular in India, Sudan, and Brazil [2]. Clinical manifestations range from self-healing cutaneous lesion to fatal visceral form, and this variety can be attributed in part to the respective parasite species, and each presents specific relationships with the host and diverse mechanisms of pathogenesis [3, 4], which represents an additional difficulty for the development of treatments and vaccines. On the other hand, *T. cruzi* is the agent of Chagas disease, which is present from southern Argentina to the southern USA. An estimated 16–18 million persons are infected in the Americas and close to 100 million people are at risk of infection. After a short benign acute phase (a few weeks) and a very long (several years) asymtomatic phase, about 30–40% of infected patients develop chronic chagasic cardiomyopathy and eventualy die of heart failure. Current chemotherapy relies on nitrofurans (Nifurtimox), or nitroimidazoles (Benznidazole). However, the usefulness of these drugs is limited by their reduced efficacy (mostly during the early stages of the infection), serious side effects, and the emergence of drugresistant strains of parasites, and new treatments are slow to develop [5].

Citation: Eric Dumonteil, "DNA Vaccines against Protozoan Parasites: Advances and Challenges," Journal of Biomedicine and Biotechnology, vol. 2007, Article ID 90520, 11 pages, 2007. doi:10.1155/2007/90520.

WHY DNA VACCINES?

DNA vaccines induce a complete immune response against the encoded antigen. The exact mechanisms involved in this proccess are still poorly understood, and particularly the type of $CD4^+$ and $CD8^+$ effector and memory cells activated, and some of these aspects have been reviewed in detail elsewhere [1]. Apart from their immunogenicity and efficacy that will be discussed below, there are several features of DNA vaccines that make them very advantageous against tropical diseases. First, they are extremely safe as they do not contain any pathogenic organism that may revert in virulence. The major concern of genomic integration of the plasmid DNA has also extensively been studied in safety studies and found to be rather unlikely [6]. Additional safety issues such as anti-DNA antibodies or autoimmunity have also been addressed in a growing number of preclinical and clinical studies [7], which confirmed the high safety of these vaccines. With respect to manufacturing, storage, and distribution, they also present major benefits in that the production process is the same for any DNA vaccine, which is not the case for other types of biologicals and vaccines, for which a specific protocol has to be developed for each. This makes production easy and costs will likely go down as this type of vaccines become mainstream and future technological improvements are implemented. Also, plasmid DNA is a very stable molecule, specially compared to recombinant or live attenuated vaccines, which would greatly facilitate storage and distribution of DNA vaccine in tropical settings with limited health infrastructure as the huge costs associated with the cold chain may be offset. Administration is also easy as simple IM or ID injections can be sufficient, and multiple plasmids can be combined for the elaboration of multivalent vaccines [1]. Overall, DNA vaccines may thus represent an ideally affordable alternative for disease control, which explains in part the growing interest in their development for the control of tropical parasitic diseases such as malaria, Leishmaniasis, or Chagas disease.

DNA VACCINES AGAINST LEISHMANIA

Correlates for Protection

As mentioned above, leishmaniasis is caused by at least 18 species of parasites with diverse relationships with the host and mechanisms of pathogenesis [3, 4]. Early studies of cross-protection between *Leishmania*species clearly showed that it is a complex problem, with infection by one species protecting or not from subsequent infection by another species, depending on the species and the order of infections. Most vaccine studies have thus been focusing on homologous protection, although a single vaccine able to protect against all pathogenic species would be ideal.

The correlates for protection have been extensively studied in the case of *L. major*, and contributed considerably to the development of the Th1/Th2 paradigm [8]. Thus, there is a general agreement that a Th1-type immune response, characterized by a high IFNγ and low IL-4 and IL-10 production, leads to control of*L. major* infection, while a Th2-type immune response does not [8]. Antibodies may have an exacerbatory role [9], but may also contribute to T cell responses [10, 11]. Both IFNγ producing CD4$^+$ and CD8$^+$T cells seem to contribute to protective immunity, and induction of NO production by macrophages is central to parasite elimiation [12, 13]. While it was assumed for a long time that this Th1/Th2 paradigm was applied to all *Leishmania* species, it has become clear in recent years that each species has a distinct relationship with the host, different mechanisms of pathogenesis, and possibly different correlates for protection [3, 4]. Nonetheless, IFNγ production seems to be a general requirement, although not necessarily sufficient, for protection against most if not all *Leishmania* species.

Single antigen DNA vaccines

The earliest DNA vaccine experiments against *Leishmania* used *L. major* GP63 antigen, which has been extensively used as a recombinant or peptide vaccine. Immunization with a plasmid encoding GP63 was able to induce a Th1-type cytokine profile and a significant reduction of lesion size after challenge of the immunized mice with *L. major* [14–17]. Subsequent studies investigated DNA vaccines encoding a large variety of *Leishmania* proteins (Table 1) and showed that many different DNA vaccines were able to induce a Th1 immune response, and confer variable degrees of protection as assessed by reduction in skin lesion size and/or parasite burdens in mouse models. However, given the large variety in experimental models and designs, it is difficult to compare the effectiveness of the different vaccines to induce a protective immune response. Nonetheless, it is clear from studies comparing different DNA vaccines that the nature of the antigen encoded by the vaccine is a key parameter for efficacy.

Table 1: DNA vaccines tested against murine leishmaniasis

Antigen	Dose	Challenge	Immune response	Protection	Reference
GP63	2 × 100 μg IM	*L. major*	Th1	+++	[14–17]
LACK	2 × 100 μg IM	*L. major*	Th1, IFNγ	+++	[18–21]
LACK	2 × 30 μg IN	*L. amazonensis*		+++	[22]
LACK	2 × 100 μg IM	*L. mexicana*		–	[23]
LACK	2 × 100 μg IM or SC	*L. chagasi*	Th1, IFNγ	–	[24]
LACK	2 × 100 μg ID or SC	*L. chagasi*	Th1	–	[25]
LACK	Prime/boost	*L. major*	Th1	+++	[26]
LACK	Prime/boost	*L. major*	Th1	+++	[27]
LACK	Prime/boost	*L. major*	Th1, IFNγ	+++	[28]
LACK	Prime/boost	*L. infantum*	IFNγ	+++	[29]
TRYP	Prime/boost	*L. major*	IFNγ	+++	[30]
LiP0	2 × 100 μg im	*L. major*	Th1	++	[31]
SP1	2 × 100 μg SC or prime/boost	*L. major*	IFNγ	++	[32]
Histones mix: H2A, H2B, H3, H4	3 × 200 μg IM	*L. major*	Th1, IFNγ	+++	[22]
LmSTI1,TSA	3 × 100 μg IM	*L. major*	Th1	+++	[33]
LACK, LmSTI1, TSA	1 × 300 μg SC	*L. major*	Th1	+++	[13]
CPb/CPa	2 × 100 μg IM	*L. major*	Th1	+++	[34]
PSA-2	2 × 20–50 μg IM	*L. major*	Th1	+++	[35]
LACK, PSA2, Gp63, LeIF, p20 Ribosomal like protein	1 × 50 μg IM	*L. major*		– to +++	[36]
Meta 1	3 × 100 μg IM	*L. major*	Th2	–	[37]
P4	3 × 100 μg various sites	*L. amazonensis*	Th1	+++	[38]
CPb, GP63, GP46	2 × 100 μg IM	*L. mexicana*		+ to +++	[23, 39]
NH36	2 × 100 μg IM	*L. domovani*		+++	[40]
		L. mexicana		++	
NH36, GP63	2 × 20 μg IM	*L. mexicana*	IFNγ	+++	[41]
CPa/CPb	Prime/Boost	*L. infantum*	Th1, IFNγ	+++	[42]
ORFF	3 × 100 μg IM	*L. donovani*		+++	[43]

IM: intramuscular; IN: intranasal; SC: subcutaneous; –: no protection; +: little protection; ++: fair protection; +++: very good protection.

Also, a few studies provided interesting comparisons of the same antigens administered as recombinant protein or DNA vaccines and showed that the latter were overall more effective than their recombinant protein counterparts. Indeed, DNA vaccines were able to induce a stronger Th1 bias in the immune response, a longer-lasting immunity, and/or a better protection against disease progression [19, 31, 32, 35, 40, 44]. While most of these studies have used a rather artificial infectious challenge based on the injection via nonnatural routes of high parasite doses, an experimental system criticized by some authors, the superior efficacy of DNA vaccines was also observed using a low-dose intradermal challenge in the ear, which was proposed to more closely mimick natural infection [45]. In these studies, both DNA and protein vaccination were able to induce very similar level of short-term (2 weeks postvaccination) protection against infection with *L. major*, but only DNA vaccine was able to induce long-term (12 weeks postvaccination) protection [45].

These results thus confirmed the strong potential of DNA vaccines against *Leishmania*, but also indicated that in most cases only partial protection was achieved. Prime-boost immunization protocols have been tested with various antigens to increase vaccine potency (Table 1). They are based on priming the immune response with a DNA vaccine and boosting with the corresponding recombinant vaccine based on recombinant virus or protein (Table 1). In some studies, such immunization protocol resulted in increased immunogenicity of the vaccines and better protection levels [26, 27], but in others, DNA only remained the best formulation for optimum efficacy [32]. Nonetheless, a major drawback of such vaccine formulation remains its complexity, which may limit their practical use.

Multiple Antigen DNA Vaccines

An alternative way to broaden vaccine immunogenicity and increase its efficacy has been to use combination of plasmids encoding various antigens. For examples, cysteine proteinase (CP) a and b DNA vaccines are not protective when used individually, but immunization with a combination of both plasmids induces long-term protective immunity [34]. Alternatively, gene fusion has also been successively used to achieve expression of an antigenic fusion protein from a single plasmid construct [33]. Overall, expression of several antigens mostly resulted in increased efficacy, but this also depended on the antigen combination [13, 22, 23,41, 45]. Most authors thus argue that a successful *Leishmania* vaccine is likely to be based on multiple antigens.

Antigen Discovery

Immunization with large number of plasmids is also the basis for expression library immunization, a powerful but labor intensive strategy for vaccine discovery [46], which has been used with *Leishmania*. Immunization of mice with *L. major* genomic expression library fractions was able to induce significant protection, but these authors did not pursue library fractionation further [47]. In another study, the identification of protective library subsets from an *L. donovani* amastigote cDNA library and their successive fractionation into smaller protective libraries lead to the identification of novel protective antigens [48]. Interestingly, most of the antigens identified would not have been predicted to be good vaccine candidates. Indeed, they were not surface or secreted proteins, neither stage-specific, but were intracellular and some very conserved such as histones, or ribosomal proteins [48]. Vaccine discovery is also the next logical step following the recent completion of the *L. major* genome sequencing [49]. In one approach, the random screening of 100 genes upregulated in amastigotes tested as DNA vaccine allowed the identification of 14 novel protective and 7 exacerbating antigens [50, 51]. Again, function and cellular localization would have been poor predictors of the protective efficacy of these antigens, as most were not predicted to be localized on the surface, but shared similarity with ribosomal proteins, cytoskeleton, or metabolic enzymes [51]. It is thus becoming increasingly clear that there is little rationale to limit *Leishmania* vaccine discovery searches to surface or secreted antigens. Rather, new criteria need to be considered for the rational identification of vaccine candidates as strategies based on such random screening cannot be applied to large genomes such as that of *Leishmania*, with over 8000 annotated genes.

Therapeutic Vaccines

An additional advantage of DNA vaccines is their potential as therapeutic vaccines, aimed at reinforcing or redirecting the immune response of an infected host to control disease progression [58]. The major advantage of this strategy in addition to its efficacy is that it relies on short treatment regimens, and it is thus an attractive alternative to chemotherapy, particularly in the case of *Leishmania* with so few chemotherapeutic options. Thus, administration of as little as two doses of a DNA vaccine encoding PSA-2 can control an ongoing infection with *L. major* in mice [59]. The therapeutic effect is due to a shift of the immune response towards a Th1 immune response [59]. Similarly, a DNA vaccine encoding *L. donovani* nucleoside hydrolase NH36 has therapeutic activity against murine visceral leishmaniasis caused by *L. chagasi* [60]. The simplicity of such treatment makes them very advantageous compared to chemotherapy. In addition, the fact that the same DNA vaccine can be effective for both the prophylaxis [40] and the therapy of *Leishmania* infection is thus very promising as this would provide a versatile tool for the control of this parasite.

Cross-Protection Against Multiple Leishmania Species

As mentioned above, an added challenge to *Leishmania* vaccine development is the large number of species, as well as the variability within species. Indeed, studies on the polymorphism of leading antigens such as GP63 quickly revealed that it was a very polymorphic [61, 62]. Such polymorphism has important implication for vaccine development as it may limit their efficacy against variant strains of parasites or novel escape mutants, and thus restrict vaccine protection to a single species [63, 64]. Antigen polymorphism between multiple strains and species is thus becoming a major issue in many vaccine development studies [65, 66]. In the case of *Leishmania*, few DNA vaccines have been tested against multiple species. LACK antigen, initially identified in *L. major*, and found to be very conserved between *Leishmania* species, can protect mice against *L. major* [20] and *L. amazonensis* [67], but not against *L. mexicana* [23], *L. donovani*[25], or *L. chagasi* [24]. On the other hand, *L. amazonensis* nuclease protein P4 can protect against both *L. amazonensis* and *L. major*, but cross-protection requires a different formulation (IL-12 or HSP70 as adjuvant, resp.) [38]. In other studies, antigens from one species were used to induce protection against another species [31], but the extent of cross-protection against various species was not investigated. More recently, a single formulation of *L. donovani* NH36 DNA vaccine was found to induce a very good protection against both *L. chagasi* and *L. mexicana*, suggesting that this DNA vaccine may be able to provide broad protection against various *Leishmania* species [40]. Importantly, no DNA vaccine has yet been tested against *L. braziliensis*, in spite of this species being responsible of most cases of cutaneous leishmaniasis in South America.

Non-Leishmania Antigens as Vaccines

While all the above DNA vaccines were based on *Leishmania* antigens, an alternative approach has used antigens derived from sand-fly saliva. Indeed, it has been shown that sand-fly saliva can exacerbate*Leishmania* infection [68, 69], and preexposure of mice to saliva components may be sufficient to induce protection against infection [70]. Thus, a number of salivary antigens have been tested as vaccines against*Leishmania*. Maxadilan is a potent vasodilator from sand-fly saliva and was found to be responsible of most of the exacerbatory effects of whole saliva on *Leishmania* infection [71]. Immunization with this antigen (as a recombinant vaccine) protected mice against *L. major* infection [71]. Other salivary components, such as*Phlebotomus papatasi* SP15, have been tested as DNA vaccines and found to protect mice against *L. major*and while the vaccine induced both humoral and DTH responses, protection seemed to be mostly accounted for by the latter, as B-cell deficient mice remain protected [72]. Thus, characterization of sand-fly salivary proteins may lead to the identification of new vaccine candidates [73, 74]. However, as for *Leishmania*antigens, salivary protein polymorphism remains an important issue and may limit the usefulness of such antigens as vaccine candidates [75, 76].

DNA Vaccines against Nonmurine Leishmaniasis

Based on the success of many of these DNA vaccine studies in mice, a few vaccine candidates have been tested in additional animal models, possibly more relevants for the development of a veterinary or human vaccine (Table 2). PFR-2 and KMP11 antigens were tested as DNA vaccines in hamsters, a highly susceptible animal model. PFR-2 was tested as protein, DNA, or DNA-protein immunization, and protection levels against *L. mexicana* varied greatly depending on vaccine formulation, route of immunization, and sex of the animals [52]. Also, contrary to mouse studies, protein vaccination seemed more protective than DNA only vaccination. However, as in mouse studies, heterologous prime-boost vaccination with DNA and protein seemed better than DNA only [52]. Another DNA vaccine encoding PapLe22 was found to be immunogenic in hamsters and decreased parasitemia after infection with *L. infantum*, but further assessment of disease was not performed [54]. Immunization with KPM11 DNA induced a mixed Th1/Th2 response, but was able to protect hamsters against visceral leishmaniasis caused by *L. donovani* [53]. In dogs, while several protein vaccines have been tested and a purified protein vaccine has now been licenced for veterinary use [77], very few DNA vaccine studies have been performed. A heterologous prime-boost strategy using CPa and CPb DNA and protein was reported as immunogenic and protective [57], but the study was of limited power given the reduced number of animals. In another study, dogs were immunized with a mixture of DNA vaccines encoding 10 different antigens previously tested in mouse models, and this immunization induced a very good immune response, with a high production of IFNγ [56]. However, evaluation of protection was limited to an acute *in vitro* assay [56] and further studies will be required to assess the potential of this vaccine in dogs. In spite of their limitations, these studies clearly showed that several DNA vaccines can induce a potent immune response in nonmurine animal models, and it is likely that a good level of protection can be achieved in these as well, provided the correct antigens and vaccine formulation are used.

Table 2: Preclinical studies *Leishmania* DNA vaccines in nonmurine models.

Antigen	Dose	Challenge	Host	Immune response	Protection	Reference
PFR-2	Variable	*L. mexicana* *L. panamensis*	Hamster		− to +++	[52]
KMP11	2 × 100 μg IM	*L. donovani*	Hamster	Th1-Th2	+++	[53]
PapLe22	1 × 100 μg IM	*L. infantum*	Hamster		+++	[54]
LACK	2 × 100 μg IM or Prime/boost	*L. infantum*	Dog	Th1/Th2 Th1	+ to +++	[55]
10 antigens mix	2 × 500 μg IM	*L. donovani*	Dog	Th1		[56]
CPa/b	Prime/boost	*L. infantum*	Dog	IFNγ	+++	[57]

−: no protection; +: little protection; ++: fair protection; +++: very good protection.

DNA VACCINES AGAINST TRYPANOSOMA CRUZI

Correlates for Protection

Vaccine development against Chagas disease has been dramatically limited because of extensive debate on the mechanisms involved in this pathology [78, 79]. Indeed, some studies suggested that tissue damage was associated with the presence and replication of intracellular amastigotes, while others proposed that autoimmunity induced by parasite antigens mimicking host proteins was responsible for it. It was thus unclear if the immune response needed to be inhibited, to reduce autoimmunity, or stimulated, to eliminate the parasite. It is now accepted that the presence of parasites in cardiac tissue is necessary to initiate and maintain the inflammatory response, and that therapeutic treatments or vaccines aimed at eliminating *T. cruzi* would limit or prevent the progression towards chronic chagasic cardiomyopathy [80, 81]. There is a growing consensus that protection against *T. cruzi* relies on a Th1 immune response and the activation of cytotoxic CD8+T cells [82–85].

Single Antigen DNA Vaccines

The first DNA vaccines to be tested against *T. cruzi* encoded an antigen from the well characterized trans-sialidase family of proteins. There are over 1400 members in this family, making it one of the largest protein families of the parasite, and they are very abundant surface proteins. Several studies have used different members of this family, such as TS or TSA-1 (Table 3) [84, 86–88]. Immunization with TS was found to induce significant antibody titers able to inhibit trans-sialidase enzyme activity, a strong DTH, and lymphoproliferative response [86]. This immune response was protective as determined by an increase in survival and a decrease in parasitemia. Immunization with TSA-1 DNA was found to induce a specific CTL response which also lead to a lower parasitemia and increased survival in both BALB/c and C57BL/6 mice [88].

Table 3: DNA vaccines tested against *Trypanosoma cruzi.*

Antigen	Type of antigen	Dose	Mouse strain	Immune response	Protection	Reference
TS 154	TS family		BALB/c	Th1, CTL	+++	[84, 89, 90]
			A/Sn		–	
TSA-1	TS family	2 × 100 μg IM	C57BL/6 BALB/c	CTL	+++	[87, 91]
ASP-1	TS family	2 × 100 μg IM	C57BL/6	CTL	+++	[87]
ASP-2	TS family	2 × 100 μg IM	C57BL/6	CTL	+++	[87]
Tc13	TS family	5 × 50 μg IM	BALB/c		–	[92]
ASP-clone9	TS family	4 × 100 μg IM	BALB/c	IFNγ	+++	[93]
TSSA	TS family	2 to 4 × 100 μg IM	BALB/c, C57BL/6 C3H/Hej	CTL	– to +++	[94, 95]
TS (7 members mix)	TS family	2 × 25 μg IM	C57BL/6		+++	[96]
ASP-clone9, TS	TS family	4 × 200 μg IM	BALB/c	IFNγ	+++	[97]
CRP		2 × 100 μg IM	BALB/c		+++	[98]
cruzipain			BALB/c	CTL		[99]
DHOD		2 to 4 × 100 μg IM	BALB/c, C57BL/6 C3H/Hej		–	[94]
LYT1		2 × 25 μg	C57BL/6	IFNγ, CTL	+++	[96]
FCaBP/Tc24		2 × 25 μg	C57BL/6	IFNγ, CTL	–	[96]
Tcβ3		2 × 25 μg	C57BL/6	IFNγ, CTL	++	[96]
Mucin (6 members)		2 × 25 μg	C57BL/6		–	[96]
KMP11		4 doses IM	BALB/c	CTL	– to +–	[100]

IM: intramuscular; CTL: cytolytic activity; –: no protection; +: little protection; ++: fair protection; +++: very good protection.

As in *Leishmania* vaccine studies, a few authors addressed the question of comparing protein and DNA vaccines encoding the same antigen [90, 98]. In A/Sn mice, immunization with recombinant TS induced a higher antibody titer than TS DNA, but a comparable decrease in parasitemia. However, the DNA vaccine was unable to increase survival, which the author attributed to the strain of the mice used, since this DNA vaccine was protective in BALB/c mice [90]. On the other hand, immunization with recombinant CRP or CRP DNA induced a comparable Th1 immune response, but only the DNA vaccine was protective against infection [98].

A number of other studies showed that DNA vaccines encoding various antigens could induce significant protection against *T. cruzi* infection, as evidenced by decreased parasitemia and improved survival of vaccinated mice (Table 3). In addition, a few studies also presented evidence of a reduction in cardiac tissue damage and inflammation at the histopathologic level [87, 97]. Furthermore, T cell analysis confirmed that protection relied on CD8+T cells [84, 91] and recent studies showed that these cells were very rapidly activated following infection of mice immunized with DNA vaccines [101]. DNA vaccines based on defined T cell epitopes from TS antigen have also been tested and it was found that both CD4+ and CD8+T cell epitopes were necessary and sufficient to induce a protective immune response [102].

Taken together, these data clearly demonstrated that vaccination did not result in increased pathology, as initially feared, but allowed at least partial control of disease progression, thus confirming the central role of parasite persistence for Chagas disease pathogenesis and opening the way to further assessment of DNA vaccines against *T. cruzi*. However, it has to be noted that many of the antigens tested belonged to the trans-sialidase family of protein, so that there is still little diversity in terms of the antigens tested as vaccines against *T. cruzi* (Table 3).

Strategies for Potentiating T. cruzi DNA Vaccines

Because protection induced by single antigen DNA vaccine remained partial, a number of studies have evaluated strategies to increase vaccine efficacy. These include the use of cytokine/chemokine encoding plasmids to potentiate the immune response induced by the vaccine, and two of the most studied molecules have beens IL-12 and GM-CSF, which both were generally able to potentiate protection (Table 2). Alternatively, mixtures of plasmids encoding distinct antigens were used for immunization, and as mentioned above for *Leishmania* vaccines. For example, immunization of mice with plasmids encoding TS and ASP-2 proteins resulted in a specific immune response against both antigens and an increased protection against infection [97]. On the other hand, an immunization with a mixture of DNA vaccines encoding up to 6 proteins from the mucin family resulted poorly protective, while a mixture of up to 7 proteins from the TS family was protective, but not as much as a single antigen vaccine encoding the TS-like antigen ASP-2 [96]. Similarly, a mixture of DNA vaccines encoding ASP-1, ASP-2, and TSA-1 had a similar protective activity as TSA-1 alone [87]. The lack of efficacy of these multivalent vaccines may be attributed to the presence of shared or immunodominant epitopes since they have significant sequence similarity that may not have resulted in a broader immune reponse.

Heterologous prime-boost approach has also been evaluated and immunization with some combinations of DNA and recombinant TS was found to enhance Th1 immune response, but protection was not significantly different from that obtained with DNA alone [103]. Taken together, these studies suggest that additional strategies need to be investigated to potentiate DNA vaccine efficacy against *T. cruzi*.

Therapeutic DNA Vaccines

Therapeutic administration of DNA vaccines to control an ongoing infection with *T. cruzi* may represent an additional alternative for Chagas disease control. The concept was demonstrated in mice acutely or chronically infected, and in both cases the administration of only two doses of DNA vaccine encoding TSA-1 or Tc24 antigens was sufficient to limit disease progression, as treated mice presented increased survival and reduced cardiac tissue damage, as assessed by histopathologic analysis [104]. A comparative study of different DNA vaccines identified Tc52 antigen as another therapeutic vaccine candidate, while DNA vaccines encoding antigens from the TS family previously found to be protective had no signifiacnt therapeutic effect [105]. It was found that therapeutic vaccination rapidly induced spleen cell proliferation, including IFNγ-producing CD4$^+$ and CD8$^+$T cells, while the effects on cardiac tissue inflammation and parasite burden take longer to be detectable [106]. Importantly, in all these studies, therapeutic vaccination of*T. cruzi* infected mice did not result in an increased inflammatory reaction in the heart, confirming that it is safe to stimulate the immune response of *T. cruzi* infected mice and that attacking the parasite can lead to a reduction of pathology. These studies thus open very attractive perspectives for the control of *T. cruzi*infection, and further studies on the efficacy of DNA vaccines encoding other antigens and on the immune mechanisms underlying their therapeutic effect should provide clues for the optimization of this strategy.

Antigen Discovery

As for any vaccine, the nature of the antigen used remains a key factor for vaccine efficacy, and there is still little variety in terms of antigens evaluated as DNA vaccine candidates against *T. cruzi*. Thus, a number of studies have aimed at identifying novel antigens through various strategies. The most classical approach has been the screening of cDNA libraries using antibodies and screening an amastigote library allowed the identification of a novel antigen Tcβ3, and two previously characterized ones, LYT1 and FcaBP/Tc24 [96]. DNA vaccines encoding these antigens induced variable levels of protection, the best one being LYT [96]. Alternatively, expression-library immunization, described above for *Leishmania*, was also tested with *T. cruzi*, and found to be immunogenic, but there was no attempt at fractionating the library or identifying protective antigens [107]. A likely reason is that such strategy may be too labor-intensive for large genomes/libraries, and its usefulness may be limited to pathogens with small genomes. The availability of *T. cruzi* genome sequence also opens new possibilities for antigen discovery. In one of the first studies using such resource, a combination of bioinformatics analysis were used to identify GPI-anchored or secreted proteins, and most of the identified clones were immunogenic as DNA vaccines [108]. Further studies may confirm the usefulness of these new vaccines to protect against *T. cruzi* infection. Nonetheless, as discussed above for *Leishmania*, the rationale for limiting antigen searches to surface proteins may not be totally relevant, and additional strategies should also be used to include unbiaised genome-wide surveys for antigen discovery.

FUTURE DIRECTIONS

As detailed in this review, there have been considerable advances in DNA vaccines against *Leishmania* and*T. cruzi* in recent years. Taken together, these studies clearly validated the concept of using DNA vaccines for both protection and therapy against these protozoan parasites in a variety of mouse models. While sterile immunity seems to be an irrealistic goal for either *Leishmania* or *T. cruzi*, a reduction in disease severity and in the development of the pathology seems clearly within the reach of DNA vaccines. Nonetheless, the relevance of such mouse models for the development of veterinary or human vaccines against these parasites has been challenged by some authors. The few DNA vaccine studies in nonmurine models of Leishmaniasis suggest that some extrapolation may be feasible, but certainly not completely. Additional advanced preclinical studies of DNA vaccine candidates in nonmurine animal models such as rats, hamsters, dogs, or monkeys are thus warranted in the next few years, to further explore the immunology and efficacy of DNA vaccines against these parasites. As already observed in such studies for other pathogens, this will lead to the challenge of achieving in these species an immunogenicity of comparable level and protective efficacy as that obtained in murine models. However, advances in adjuvants, DNA vaccine formulation, and delivery systems are likely to contribute to such results [1, 109].

Another major issue is that of antigen discovery, and while a number of DNA vacines tested so far against *Leishmania* or *T. cruzi* have shown promise, we are still unsure if these are the best possible antigens, particularly since these parasites have relatively large genomes, and only a limited variety of antigens have been tested. The availability of the genome sequences of these parasites will without doubt be a key resource for genome-wide screenings for new protective antigens. A key lesson from the initial studies reviewed here [48, 51, 108], together with other similar antigen discovery studies, seems to be that cellular localization and protein function are poor predictors of the antigenicity and protective efficacy of a protein. Alternative criteria should thus be used so that potent vaccine candidates are not missed, and the important development of genome-mining and bioinformatic tools is providing new tools for a more rational search of vaccine candidates [110].

To conclude, those DNA vaccines represent a promising approach for the control of *Leishmania* sp. and *T. cruzi*, and such vaccines would have a major impact in developing endemic countries. Thus the question does not seem to be if DNA vaccines can control these parasites, since many studies have clearly showed that this is the case, but how to translate what has been achieved in mouse models into veterinary or human vaccines of comparable efficacy.

ACKNOWLEDGMENT

This work was funded by Grant SEP-2004-C01-47122 from the Consejo Nacional de Ciencia y Tecnología (CONACYT).

REFERENCES

1. Liu MA, Wahren B, Hedestam GBK. DNA vaccines: recent developments and future possibilities.*Human Gene Therapy*. 2006;17(11):1051–1061.
2. Murray HW, Berman JD, Davies CR, Saravia NG. Advances in leishmaniasis. *The Lancet*.2005;366(9496):1561–1577.
3. Alexander J, Bryson K. T helper (h)1/Th2 and *Leishmania*: paradox rather than paradigm. *Immunology Letters*. 2005;99(1):17–23.
4. McMahon-Pratt D, Alexander J. Does the *Leishmania major* paradigm of pathogenesis and protection hold for New World cutaneous leishmaniases or the visceral disease? *Immunological Reviews*.2004;201(1):206–224.
5. Castro JA, de Mecca MM, Bartel LC. Toxic side effects of drugs used to treat Chagas' disease (American trypanosomiasis) *Human and Experimental Toxicology*. 2006;25(8):471–479.
6. Sheets RL, Stein J, Manetz TS, et al. Biodistribution of DNA plasmid vaccines against HIV-1, Ebola, Severe Acute Respiratory Syndrome, or West Nile virus is similar, without integration, despite differing plasmid backbones or gene inserts. *Toxicological Sciences*. 2006;91(2):610–619.
7. Sheets RL, Stein J, Manetz TS, et al. Toxicological safety evaluation of DNA plasmid vaccines against HIV-1, Ebola, Severe Acute Respiratory Syndrome, or West Nile virus is similar despite differing plasmid backbones or gene-inserts. *Toxicological Sciences*. 2006;91(2):620–630.
8. Louis J, Himmelrich H, Parra-Lopez C, Tacchini-Cottier F, Launois P. Regulation of protective immunity against *Leishmania major* in mice. *Current Opinion in Immunology*. 1998;10(4):459–464.
9. Miles SA, Conrad SM, Alves RG, Jeronimo SMB, Mosser DM. A role for IgG immune complexes during infection with the intracellular pathogen *Leishmania* . *The Journal of Experimental Medicine*.2005;201(5):747–754.
10. Stäger S, Alexander J, Kirby AC, et al. Natural antibodies and complement are endogenous adjuvants for vaccine-induced CD8+ T-cell responses. *Nature Medicine*. 2003;9(10):1287–1292.
11. Woelbing F, Kostka SL, Moelle K, et al. Uptake of *Leishmania major* by dendritic cells is mediated by Fcγ receptors and facilitates acquisition of protective immunity. *The Journal of Experimental Medicine*.2006;203(1):177–188.
12. Bogdan C, Röllinghoff M. The immune response to *Leishmania*: mechanisms of parasite control and evasion. *International Journal for Parasitology*. 1998;28(1):121–134.
13. Méndez S, Belkaid Y, Seder RA, Sacks D. Optimization of DNA vaccination against cutaneous leishmaniasis. *Vaccine*. 2002;20(31-32):3702–3708.
14. Walker PS. American Academy of Dermatology 1997 Awards for Young Investigators in Dermatology. Direct targeting of skin with DNA vaccines for genetic immunization against *Leishmania* in a murine model.*Journal of the American Academy of Dermatology*. 1997;37(5, part 1):776–777.
15. Walker PS, Scharton-Kersten T, Rowton ED, et al. Genetic immunization with glycoprotein 63 cDNA results in a helper T cell type 1 immune response and protection in a murine model of leishmaniasis. *Human Gene Therapy*. 1998;9(13):1899–1907.
16. Xu D, Liew FY. Genetic vaccination against leishmaniasis. *Vaccine*. 1994;12(16):1534–1536.
17. Xu D, Liew FY. Protection against leishmaniasis by injection of DNA encoding a major surface glycoprotein, gp63, of *L. major* . *Immunology*. 1995;84(2):173–176.
18. Gurunathan S, Sacks DL, Brown DR, et al. Vaccination with DNA encoding the immunodominant LACK parasite antigen confers protective immunity to mice infected with *Leishmania major* . *The Journal of Experimental Medicine*. 1997;186(7):1137–1147.
19. Gurunathan S, Prussin C, Sacks DL, Seder RA. Vaccine requirements for sustained cellular immunity to an intracellular parasitic infection. *Nature Medicine*. 1998;4(12):1409–1415.
20. Gurunathan S, Stobie L, Prussin C, et al. Requirements for the maintenance of Th1 immunity in vivo following DNA vaccination: a potential immunoregulatory role for CD8+ T cells. *The Journal of Immunology*. 2000;165(2):915–924.
21. Stobie L, Gurunathan S, Prussin C, et al. The role of antigen and IL-12 in sustaining Th1 memory cells in vivo: IL-12 is required to maintain memory/effector Th1 cells sufficient to mediate protection to an infectious parasite challenge. *Proceedings of the National Academy of Sciences of the United States of America*. 2000;97(15):8427–8432.
22. Iborra S, Soto M, Carrión J, Alonso C, Requena JM. Vaccination with a plasmid DNA cocktail encoding the nucleosomal histones of *Leishmania* confers protection against murine cutaneous leishmaniosis. *Vaccine*.2004;22(29-30):3865–3876.
23. Dumonteil E, Ramirez-Sierra MJ, Escobedo-Ortegonr J,

García-Miss MR. DNA vaccines induce partial protection against *Leishmania mexicana* . *Vaccine.* 2003;21(17-18):2161–2168.

24. Marques-da-Silva EA, Coelho EAF, Gomes DCO, et al. Intramuscular immunization with p36(LACK) DNA vaccine induces IFN-γ production but does not protect BALB/c mice against *Leishmania chagasi*intravenous challenge. *Parasitology Research.* 2005;98(1):67–74.
25. Melby PC, Yang J, Zhao W, Perez LE, Cheng J. *Leishmania donovani* p36(LACK) DNA vaccine is highly immunogenic but not protective against experimental visceral leishmaniasis. *Infection and Immunity.*2001;69(8):4719–4725.
26. Gonzalo RM, del Real G, Rodriguez JR, et al. A heterologous prime-boost regime using DNA and recombinant vaccinia virus expressing the *Leishmania infantum* P36/LACK antigen protects BALB/c mice from cutaneous leishmaniasis. *Vaccine.* 2002;20(7-8):1226–1231.
27. Tapia E, Pérez-Jiménez E, López-Fuertes L, Gonzalo R, Gherardi MM, Esteban M. The combination of DNA vectors expressing IL-12 + IL-18 elicits high protective immune response against cutaneous leishmaniasis after priming with DNA-p36/LACK and the cytokines, followed by a booster with a vaccinia virus recombinant expressing p36/LACK. *Microbes and Infection.* 2003;5(2):73–84.
28. Pérez-Jiménez E, Kochan G, Gherardi MM, Esteban M. MVA-LACK as a safe and efficient vector for vaccination against leishmaniasis. *Microbes and Infection.* 2006;8(3):810–822.
29. Dondji B, Pérez-Jimenez E, Goldsmith-Pestana K, Esteban M, McMahon-Pratt D. Heterologous prime-boost vaccination with the LACK antigen protects against murine visceral leishmaniasis. *Infection and Immunity.* 2005;73(8):5286–5289.
30. Stober CB, Lange UG, Roberts MTM, Alcami A, Blackwell JM. Heterologous priming-boosting with DNA and modified vaccinia virus Ankara expressing tryparedoxin peroxidase promotes long-term memory against *Leishmania major* in susceptible BALB/c mice. *Infection and Immunity.* 2007;75(2):852–860.
31. Iborra S, Soto M, Carrión J, et al. The *Leishmania infantum* acidic ribosomal protein P0 administered as a DNA vaccine confers protective immunity to *Leishmania major* infection in BALB/c mice. *Infection and Immunity.* 2003;71(11):6562–6572.
32. Rafati S, Ghaemimanesh F, Zahedifard F. Comparison of potential protection induced by three vaccination strategies (DNA/DNA, Protein/Protein and DNA/Protein) against *Leishmania major* infection using Signal Peptidase type I in BALB/c mice. *Vaccine.* 2006;24(16):3290–3297.
33. Campos-Neto A, Webb JR, Greeson K, Coler RN, Skeiky YAW, Reed SG. Vaccination with plasmid DNA encoding TSA/LmSTI1 leishmanial fusion proteins confers protection against *Leishmania major*infection in susceptible BALB/c mice. *Infection and Immunity.* 2002;70(6):2828–2836.
34. Rafati S, Salmanian A-H, Taheri T, Vafa M, Fasel N. A protective cocktail vaccine against murine cutaneous leishmaniasis with DNA encoding cysteine proteinases of *Leishmania major* . *Vaccine.*2001;19(25-26):3369–3375.
35. Sjölander A, Baldwin TM, Curtis JM, Handman E. Induction of a Th1 immune response and simultaneous lack of activation of a Th2 response are required for generation of immunity to leishmaniasis.*The Journal of Immunology.* 1998;160(8):3949–3957.
36. Ahmed SBH, Bahloul C, Robbana C, Askri S, Dellagi K. A comparative evaluation of different DNA vaccine candidates against experimental murine leishmaniasis due to *L. major* . *Vaccine.* 2004;22(13-14):1631–1639.
37. Serezani CHC, Franco AR, Wajc M, et al. Evaluation of the murine immune response to *Leishmania*meta 1 antigen delivered as recombinant protein or DNA vaccine. *Vaccine.* 2002;20(31-32):3755–3763.
38. Campbell K, Diao H, Ji J, Soong L. DNA immunization with the gene encoding P4 nuclease of*Leishmania amazonensis* protects mice against cutaneous leishmaniasis. *Infection and Immunity.*2003;71(11):6270–6278.
39. Dumonteil E, Andrade-Narvarez F, Escobedo-Ortegon J, et al. Comparative study of DNA vaccines encoding various antigens against *Leishmania mexicana* . *Developments in Biologicals.* 2000;104:135–141.
40. Aguilar-Be I, da Silva Zardo R, Paraguai de Souza E, et al. Cross-protective efficacy of a prophylactic*Leishmania donovani* DNA vaccine against visceral and cutaneous murine leishmaniasis. *Infection and Immunity.* 2005;73(2):812–819.
41. Rosado-Vallado M, Mut-Martin M, García-Miss MR, Dumonteil E. Aluminium phosphate potentiates the efficacy of DNA vaccines against *Leishmania mexicana* . *Vaccine.* 2005;23(46-47):5372–5379.
42. Rafati S, Zahedifard F, Nazgouee F. Prime-boost vaccination using cysteine proteinases type I and II of*Leishmania infantum* confers protective immunity in murine visceral leishmaniasis. *Vaccine.*2006;24(12):2169–2175.
43. Sukumaran B, Tewary P, Saxena S, Madhubala R. Vaccination with DNA encoding ORFF antigen confers protective immunity in mice infected with *Leishmania donovani* . *Vaccine.* 2003;21(11-12):1292–1299.
44. Sjölander A, Baldwin TM, Curtis JM, Bengtsson KL, Handman E. Vaccination with recombinant Parasite Surface Antigen 2 from *Leishmania major* induces a Th1 type of immune response but does not protect against infection. *Vaccine.* 1998;16(20):2077–2084.
45. Méndez S, Gurunathan S, Kamhawi S, et al. The potency and durability of DNA- and protein-based vaccines against *Leishmania major* evaluated using low-dose, intradermal challenge. *The Journal of Immunology.* 2001;166(8):5122–5128.
46. Barry MA, Lai WC, Johnston SA. Protection against mycoplasma infection using expression-library immunization. *Nature.* 1995;377(6550):632–635.

47. Piedrafita D, Xu D, Hunter D, Harrison RA, Liew FY. Protective immune responses induced by vaccination with an expression genomic library of *Leishmania major* . *The Journal of Immunology*.1999;163(3):1467–1472.

48. Melby PC, Ogden GB, Flores HA, et al. Identification of vaccine candidates for experimental visceral leishmaniasis by immunization with sequential fractions of a cDNA expression library. *Infection and Immunity*. 2000;68(10):5595–5602.

49. Ivens AC, Peacock CS, Worthey EA, et al. The genome of the kinetoplastid parasite, *Leishmania major* . *Science*. 2005;309(5733):436–442.

50. Stober CB. From genomes to vaccines for leishmaniasis. *Methods in Molecular Biology*. 2004;270:423–438.

51. Stober CB, Lange UG, Roberts MTM, et al. From genome to vaccines for leishmaniasis: screening 100 novel vaccine candidates against murine *Leishmania major* infection. *Vaccine*. 2006;24(14):2602–2616.

52. Saravia NG, Hazbón MH, Osorio Y, et al. Protective immunogenicity of the paraflagellar rod protein 2 of*Leishmania mexicana* . *Vaccine*. 2005;23(8):984–995.

53. Basu R, Bhaumik S, Basu JM, Naskar K, De T, Roy S. Kinetoplastid membrane protein-11 DNA vaccination induces complete protection against both pentavalent antimonial-sensitive and -resistant strains of*Leishmania donovani* that correlates with inducible nitric oxide synthase activity and IL-4 generation: evidence for mixed Th1- and Th2-like responses in visceral leishmaniasis. *The Journal of Immunology*.2005;174(11):7160–7171.

54. Fragaki K, Suffia I, Ferrua B, Rousseau D, Le Fichoux Y, Kubar J. Immunisation with DNA encoding*Leishmania infantum* protein papLe22 decreases the frequency of parasitemic episodes in infected hamsters. *Vaccine*. 2001;19(13-14):1701–1709.

55. Ramiro MJ, Zárate JJ, Hanke T, et al. Protection in dogs against visceral leishmaniasis caused by*Leishmania infantum* is achieved by immunization with a heterologous prime-boost regime using DNA and vaccinia recombinant vectors expressing LACK. *Vaccine*. 2003;21(19-20):2474–2484.

56. Saldarriaga OA, Travi BL, Park W, Perez LE, Melby PC. Immunogenicity of a multicomponent DNA vaccine against visceral leishmaniasis in dogs. *Vaccine*. 2006;24(11):1928–1940.

57. Rafati S, Nakhaee A, Taheri T, et al. Protective vaccination against experimental canine visceral leishmaniasis using a combination of DNA and protein immunization with cysteine proteinases type I and II of *L. infantum* . *Vaccine*. 2005;23(28):3716–3725.

58. Autran B, Carcelain G, Combadiere B, Debre P. Therapeutic vaccines for chronic infections. *Science*.2004;305(5681):205–208.

59. Handman E, Noormohammadi AH, Curtis JM, Baldwin T, Sjölander A. Therapy of murine cutaneous leishmaniasis by DNA vaccination. *Vaccine*. 2000;18(26):3011–3017.

60. Gamboa-León R, Paraguai de Souza E, Borja-Cabrera GP, et al. Immunotherapy against visceral leishmaniasis with the nucleoside hydrolase-DNA vaccine of *Leishmania donovani* . *Vaccine*.2006;24(22):4863–4873.

61. Espinoza JR, Skinner AC, Davies CR, et al. Extensive polymorphism at the Gp63 locus in field isolates of *Leishmania peruviana* . *Molecular and Biochemical Parasitology*. 1995;72(1-2):203–213.

62. Guerbouj S, Victoir K, Guizani I, et al. Gp63 gene polymorphism and population structure of*Leishmania donovani* complex: influence of the host selection pressure? *Parasitology*. 2001;122(1):25–35.

63. Alvarez-Valin F, Tort JF, Bernardi G. Nonrandom spatial distribution of synonymous substitutions in the GP63 gene from *Leishmania* . *Genetics*. 2000;155(4):1683–1692.

64. Guerbouj S, Guizani I, Victoir K, Le Ray D, Dujardin J-C. Parasite candidate vaccines: a warning from polymorphic *Leishmania* populations. *Parasitology Today*. 2000;16(6):265–266.

65. Fitzpatrick DA, Creevey CJ, McInerney JO. Evidence of positive Darwinian selection in putative meningococcal vaccine antigens. *Journal of Molecular Evolution*. 2005;61(1):90–98.

66. Kumkhaek C, Phra-Ek K, Rénia L, et al. Are extensive T cell epitope polymorphisms in the *Plasmodium falciparum* circumsporozoite antigen, a leading sporozoite vaccine candidate, selected by immune pressure?*The Journal of Immunology*. 2005;175(6):3935–3939.

67. Pinto EF, Pinheiro RO, Rayol A, Larraga V, Rossi-Bergmann B. Intranasal vaccination against cutaneous leishmaniasis with a particulated leishmanial antigen or DNA encoding LACK. *Infection and Immunity*.2004;72(8):4521–4527.

68. Belkaid Y, Kamhawi S, Modi G, et al. Development of a natural model of cutaneous leishmaniasis: powerful effects of vector saliva and saliva preexposure on the long-term outcome of *Leishmania major*infection in the mouse ear dermis. *The Journal of Experimental Medicine*. 1998;188(10):1941–1953.

69. Mbow ML, Bleyenberg JA, Hall LR, Titus RG. Phlebotomus papatasi sand fly salivary gland lysate down-regulates a Th1, but up-regulates a Th2, response in mice infected with *Leishmania major* . *The Journal of Immunology*. 1998;161(10):5571–5577.

70. Kamhawi S, Belkaid Y, Modi G, Rowton E, Sacks D. Protection against cutaneous leishmaniasis resulting from bites of uninfected sand flies. *Science*. 2000;290(5495):1351–1354.

71. Morris RV, Shoemaker CB, David JR, Lanzaro GC, Titus RG. Sandfly maxadilan exacerbates infection with *Leishmania major* and vaccinating against it protects against *L. major* infection. *The Journal of Immunology*. 2001;167(9):5226–5230.

72. Valenzuela JG, Belkaid Y, Garfield MK, et al. Toward a defined anti-*Leishmania* vaccine targeting vector antigens: characterization of a protective salivary protein. *The Journal of Experimental Medicine*.2001;194(3):331–342.

73. Anderson JM, Oliveira F, Kamhawi S, et al. Comparative

salivary gland transcriptomics of sandfly vectors of visceral leishmaniasis. *BMC Genomics*. 2006;7:52.

74. Valenzuela JG, Garfield M, Rowton ED, Pham VM. Identification of the most abundant secreted proteins from the salivary glands of the sand fly *Lutzomyia longipalpis*, vector of *Leishmania chagasi* . *The Journal of Experimental Biology*. 2004;207(21):3717–3729.
75. Elnaiem D-EA, Meneses C, Slotman M, Lanzaro GC. Genetic variation in the sand fly salivary protein, SP-15, a potential vaccine candidate against *Leishmania major* . *Insect Molecular Biology*. 2005;14(2):145–150.
76. Milleron RS, Mutebi J-P, Valle S, et al. Antigenic diversity in maxadilan, a salivary protein from the sand fly vector of American visceral leishmaniasis. *American Journal of Tropical Medicine and Hygiene*.2004;70(3):286–293.
77. Saraiva EM, de Figueiredo Barbosa A, Santos FN, et al. The FML-vaccine (Leishmune®) against canine visceral leishmaniasis: a transmission blocking vaccine. *Vaccine*. 2006;24(13):2423–2431.
78. Gironés N, Cuervo H, Fresno M. *Trypanosoma cruzi*-induced molecular mimicry and Chagas' disease.*Current Topics in Microbiology and Immunology*. 2005;296:89–123.
79. Tarleton RL. Parasite persistence in the aetiology of Chagas disease. *International Journal for Parasitology*. 2001;31(5-6):549–553.
80. Bhatia V, Garg N. Current status and future prospects for a vaccine against American trypanosomiasis.*Expert Review of Vaccines*. 2005;4(6):867–880.
81. Kierszenbaum F. Where do we stand on the autoimmunity hypothesis of Chagas disease? *Trends in Parasitology*. 2005;21(11):513–516.
82. Hoft DF, Schnapp AR, Eickhoff CS, Roodman ST. Involvement of CD4+ Th1 cells in systemic immunity protective against primary and secondary challenges with *Trypanosoma cruzi* . *Infection and Immunity*. 2000;68(1):197–204.
83. Martin D, Tarleton R. Generation, specificity, and function of CD8+ T cells in *Trypanosoma cruzi*infection. *Immunological Reviews*. 2004;201(1):304–317.
84. Rodrigues MM, Ribeirão M, Pereira-Chioccola V, Renia L, Costa F. Predominance of CD4 Th1 and CD8 Tc1 cells revealed by characterization of the cellular immune response generated by immunization with a DNA vaccine containing a *Trypanosoma cruzi* gene. *Infection and Immunity*. 1999;67(8):3855–3863.
85. Rodrigues MM, Boscardin SB, Vasconcelos JR, Hiyane MI, Salay G, Soares IS. Importance of CD8 T cell-mediated immune response during intracellular parasitic infections and its implications for the development of effective vaccines. *Anais da Academia Brasileira de Ciências*. 2003;75(4):443–468.
86. Costa F, Franchin G, Pereira-Chioccola VL, Ribeirão M, Schenkman S, Rodrigues MM. Immunization with a plasmid DNA containing the gene of *trans*-sialidase reduces *Trypanosoma cruzi* infection in mice. *Vaccine*. 1998;16(8):768–774.
87. Garg N, Tarleton RL. Genetic immunization elicits antigen-specific protective immune responses and decreases disease severity in *Trypanosoma cruzi* infection. *Infection and Immunity*. 2002;70(10):5547–5555.
88. Wizel B, Nunes M, Tarleton RL. Identification of *Trypanosoma cruzi* trans-sialidase family members as targets of protective CD8+ TC1 responses. *The Journal of Immunology*. 1997;159(12):6120–6130.
89. Costa F, Pereira-Chioccola VL, Ribeirão M, Schenkman S, Rodrigues MM. *Trans*-sialidase delivered as a naked DNA vaccine elicits an immunological response similar to a *Trypanosoma cruzi* infection. *Brazilian Journal of Medical and Biological Research*. 1999;32(2):235–239.
90. Pereira-Chioccola VL, Costa F, Ribeirão M, et al. Comparison of antibody and protective immune responses against *Trypanosoma cruzi* infection elicited by immunization with a parasite antigen delivered as naked DNA or recombinant protein. *Parasite Immunology*. 1999;21(2):103–110.
91. Wizel B, Garg N, Tarleton RL. Vaccination with trypomastigote surface antigen 1-encoding plasmid DNA confers protection against lethal *Trypanosoma cruzi* infection. *Infection and Immunity*.1998;66(11):5073–5081.
92. García GA, Arnaiz MR, Laucella SA, et al. Immunological and pathological responses in BALB/c mice induced by genetic administration of *Tc*13 Tul antigen of *Trypanosoma cruzi* . *Parasitology*.2006;132(6):855–866.
93. Boscardin SB, Kinoshita SS, Fujimura AE, Rodrigues MM. Immunization with cDNA expressed by amastigotes of *Trypanosoma cruzi* elicits protective immune response against experimental infection.*Infection and Immunity*. 2003;71(5):2744–2757.
94. Katae M, Miyahira Y, Takeda K, et al. Coadministration of an interleukin-12 gene and a *Trypanosoma cruzi* gene improves vaccine efficacy. *Infection and Immunity*. 2002;70(9):4833–4840.
95. Miyahira Y, Katae M, Takeda K, et al. Activation of natural killer T cells by α-galactosylceramide impairs DNA vaccine-induced protective immunity against *Trypanosoma cruzi* . *Infection and Immunity*.2003;71(3):1234–1241.
96. Fralish BH, Tarleton RL. Genetic immunization with *LYT1* or a pool of *trans*-sialidase genes protects mice from lethal *Trypanosoma cruzi* infection. *Vaccine*. 2003;21(21-22):3070–3080.
97. Vasconcelos JR, Hiyane MI, Marinho CRF, et al. Protective immunity against *Trypanosoma cruzi*infection in a highly susceptible mouse strain after vaccination with genes encoding the amastigote surface protein-2 and trans-sialidase. *Human Gene Therapy*. 2004;15(9):878–886.
98. Sepulveda P, Hontebeyrie M, Liegeard P, Mascilli A, Norris KA. DNA-based immunization with*Trypanosoma cruzi* complement regulatory protein elicits complement lytic antibodies and confers protection against *Trypanosoma cruzi* infection. *Infection and Immunity*. 2000;68(9):4986–4991.

99. 99 . Schnapp AR, Eickhoff CS, Scharfstein J, Hoft DF. Induction of B- and T-cell responses to cruzipain in the murine model of *Trypanosoma cruzi* infection. *Microbes and Infection*. 2002;4(8):805–813.

100. Planelles L, Thomas MC, Alonso C, López MC. DNA immunization with *Trypanosoma cruzi* HSP70 fused to the KMP11 protein elicits a cytotoxic and humoral immune response against the antigen and leads to protection. *Infection and Immunity*. 2001;69(10):6558–6563.

101. Tzelepis F, de Alencar BCG, Penido MLO, Gazzinelli RT, Persechini PM, Rodrigues MM. Distinct kinetics of effector $CD8^+$ cytotoxic T cells after infection with *Trypanosoma cruzi* in naïve or vaccinated mice. *Infection and Immunity*. 2006;74(4):2477–2481.

102. Fujimura AE, Kinoshita SS, Pereira-Chioccola VL, Rodrigues MM. DNA sequences encoding $CD4^+$and $CD8^+$ T-cell epitopes are important for efficient protective immunity induced by DNA vaccination with a*Trypanosoma cruzi* gene. *Infection and Immunity*. 2001;69(9):5477–5486.

103. Vasconcelos JR, Boscardin SB, Hiyane MI, Kinoshita SS, Fujimura AE, Rodrigues MM. A DNA-priming protein-boosting regimen significantly improves type 1 immune response but not protective immunity to *Trypanosoma cruzi* infection in a highly susceptible mouse strain. *Immunology and Cell Biology*. 2003;81(2):121–129.

104. Dumonteil E, Escobedo-Ortegon J, Reyes-Rodriguez N, Arjona-Torres A, Ramirez-Sierra MJ. Immunotherapy of *Trypanosoma cruzi* infection with DNA vaccines in mice. *Infection and Immunity*.2004;72(1):46–53.

105. Sanchez-Burgos G, Mezquita-Vega G, Escobedo-Ortegon J, et al. Comparative efficacy of DNA vaccines encoding various *Trypanosoma cruzi* antigens. *FEMS Immunology and Medical Microbiology*,(Online Early Articles) Doi:10.1111/j.1574-695X.2007.00251.X, 2007.

106. Zapata-Estrella H, Hummel-Newell C, Sanchez-Burgos G, et al. Control of *Trypanosoma cruzi*infection and changes in T-cell populations induced by a therapeutic DNA vaccine in mice. *Immunology Letters*. 2006;103(2):186–191.

107. Alberti E, Acosta A, Sarmiento ME, et al. Specific cellular and humoral immune response in Balb/c mice immunised with an expression genomic library of *Trypanosoma cruzi* . *Vaccine*. 1998;16(6):608–612.

108. Bhatia V, Sinha M, Luxon B, Garg N. Utility of the *Trypanosoma cruzi* sequence database for identification of potential vaccine candidates by in silico and in vitro screening. *Infection and Immunity*.2004;72(11):6245–6254.

109. Manoj S, Babiuk LA, van Drunen Littel-van den Hurk S. Approaches to enhance the efficacy of DNA vaccines. *Critical Reviews in Clinical Laboratory Sciences*. 2004;41(1):1–39.

110. Moutaftsi M, Peters B, Pasquetto V, et al. A consensus epitope prediction approach identifies the breadth of murine T_{CD8+}-cell responses to vaccinia virus. *Nature Biotechnology*. 2006;24(7):817–819.

INDEX